D1162030

ABDOMINAL ULTRASOUND

Commissioning Editor: Claire Wilson
Development Editor: Catherine Jackson
Project Manager: Priya Dauntess
Designer: Kirsteen Wright

ABDOMINAL ULTRASOUND

How, Why and When

Third Edition

Jane Bates MPhil DMU DCR
Cons Practitioner, Ultrasound, Leeds, UK

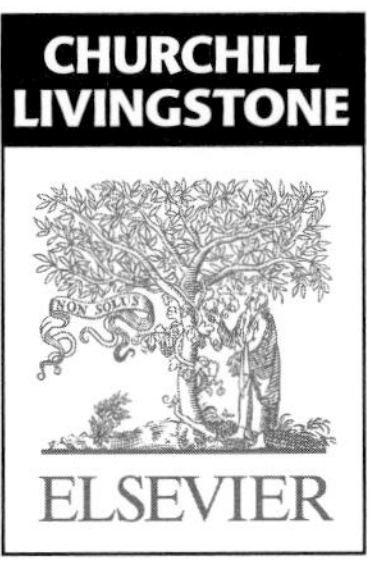

Edinburgh • London • New York • Oxford • Philadelphia • St Louis • S

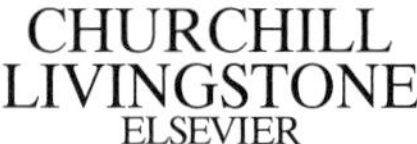

First edition 1999
Second edition 2004
Third edition 2011

ISBN 978 0 443 06919 2

British Library Cataloguing in Publication Data
A catalogue record for this book is available from the British Library

Library of Congress Cataloging in Publication Data
A catalog record for this book is available from the Library of Congress

Notices
Knowledge and best practice in this field are constantly changing. As new research and experience broaden our understanding, changes in research methods, professional practices, or medical treatment may become necessary.

Practitioners and researchers must always rely on their own experience and knowledge in evaluating and using any information, methods, compounds, or experiments described herein. In using such information or methods they should be mindful of their own safety and the safety of others, including parties for whom they have a professional responsibility.

With respect to any drug or pharmaceutical products identified, readers are advised to check the most current information provided (i) on procedures featured or (ii) by the manufacturer of each product to be administered, to verify the recommended dose or formula, the method and duration of administration, and contraindications. It is the responsibility of practitioners, relying on their own experience and knowledge of their patients, to make diagnoses, to determine dosages and the best treatment for each individual patient, and to take all appropriate safety precautions.

To the fullest extent of the law, neither the Publisher nor the authors, contributors, or editors, assume any liability for any injury and/or damage to persons or property as a matter of products liability, negligence or otherwise, or from any use or operation of any methods, products, instructions, or ideas contained in the material herein.

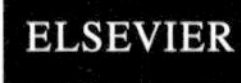

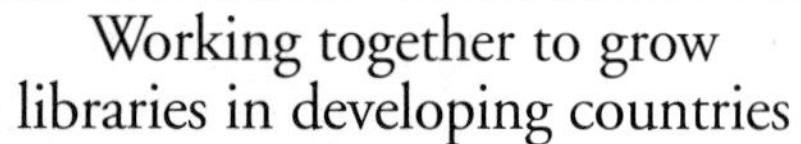

Printed in China

Contents

Contributors

Grant Baxter FRCR
Consultant Radiologist, Department of Radiology, Western Infirmary, Glasgow, UK

Terry M Humphrey MHSC DMU DCR
Sonographer Practitioner – Paediatric Specialist, Ultrasound Department, St James's University Hospital, Leeds, UK

Preface

Ultrasound is one of the most important and most frequently used diagnostic tools at our disposal. It is used by a range of health professionals from various clinical backgrounds, and its contribution covers a broad spectrum from first-line triage to focused definitive diagnostic tool, from basic exclusion tool to guided interventional therapy. Ultrasound is operator dependent to a degree unrivalled by most diagnostic instruments, and, in the hands of the unwary operator, has the potential for great harm as well as good.

This book is intended as a practical, easily accessible guide to sonographer practitioners and those wishing to learn and develop in the field of ultrasound. It seeks to enable the operator to maximize the diagnostic information available and, most importantly, to recognize the limitations of the scan and to avoid diagnostic pitfalls.

Where possible it presents a wider, more holistic approach to the patient, including presenting symptoms, complementary imaging procedures and further management options. It does not aim to be in any way comprehensive, but is intended as a springboard from which practical skills and clinical knowledge can further develop.

The book seeks to increase the student's awareness of the contribution of ultrasound in patient management, and to encourage the sonographer to explore the enormous potential of diagnostic ultrasound in a properly supervised environment.

The author gratefully acknowledges the help and support of staff working in diagnostic ultrasound in Leeds.

Jane Bates
2010

Abbreviations

ADPCDK	autosomal dominant polycystic disease of the kidney
AFP	alpha-fetoprotein
AI	acceleration index
AIDS	acquired immune deficiency syndrome
AIUM	American Institute for Ultrasound in Medicine
ALARA	as low as reasonably achieved
ALT	alanine aminotransferase
AML	angiomyolipomas
APKD	autosomal dominant (adult) polycystic kidney
ARPCDK	autosomal recessive polycystic disease of the kidney
AST	aspartate aminotransferase
AT	acceleration time
AV	arteriovenous
BCS	Budd–Chiari syndrome
CAPD	continuous ambulatory peritoneal dialysis
CBD	common bile duct
CD	common duct
CF	cystic fibrosis
CT	computed tomography
DIC	disseminated intravascular coagulation
DMSA	dimercaptosuccinic acid
DTPA	diethylene triaminepenta-acetic acid
EDF	end-diastolic flow
ERCP	endoscopic retrograde cholangiopancreatography
ESWL	extracorporeal shock wave lithotripsy
EUS	endoscopic ultrasound
FAST	focused assessment with sonography for trauma
FDA	Food and Drug Administration
FDG-PET	[18F]2-fluoro-2-deoxy-d-glucose positron emission tomography
FPS	frames per second
HA	hepatic artery
HCC	hepatocellular carcinoma
HELLP	haemolytic anaemia, elevated liver enzymes and low platelet count
HIDA	hepatic iminodiacetic acid
HOP	head of pancreas
HPS	hypertrophic pyloric stenosis
HV	hepatic vein
INR	international normalized ratio
IOUS	intraoperative ultrasound
IVC	inferior vein cava
IVU	intravenous urogram
LFT	liver function test
LPV	left portal vein
LRV	left renal vein
LS	longitudinal section
LUQ	left upper quadrant
MCKD	multicystic dysplastic kidney
MHA	middle hepatic artery
MHV	middle hepatic vein
MI	mechanical index
MPV	main portal vein
MRA	magnetic resonance angiography
MRCP	magnetic resonance cholangiopancreatography
MRI	magnetic resonance imaging
MRV	main renal vein

ODS	output display standard
PAC	photographic archiving and communications
PACS	photographic archiving and communications systems
PBC	primary biliary cirrhosis
PCKD	polycystic kidney disease
PCS	pelvicalyceal system
PD	pancreatic duct
PI	pulsatility index
PID	pelvic inflammatory disease
PRF	pulse repetition frequency
PSC	primary sclerosing cholangitis
PTLD	post-transplant lymphoproliferative disorder
PV	portal vein
RAS	renal artery stenosis
RCC	renal cell carcinoma
RF	radiofrequency
RHV	right hepatic vein
RI	resistance index
RIF	right iliac fossa
RK	right kidney
RPV	right portal vein
RRA	right renal vein
RUQ	right upper quadrant
RVT	renal vein thrombosis
SA	splenic artery
SLE	systemic lupus erythematosus
SMA	superior mesenteric artery
SV	splenic vein
TB	tuberculosis
TGC	time gain compensation
THI	tissue harmonic imaging
TI	thermal index
TIB	bone-at-focus index
TIC	cranial index
TIPSS	transjugular intrahepatic portosystemic shunt
TIS	soft-tissue thermal index
TOP	tail of pancreas
TORCH	toxoplasmosis, rubella, cytomegalovirus and HIV
TS	transverse section
UTI	urinary tract infection
VHL	von Hippel–Lindau disease
VUJ	vesicouretic junction
WRMSD	work-related musculoskeletal disorders
XGP	xanthogranulomatous pyelonephritis

Optimizing the diagnostic information

1

CHAPTER CONTENTS

INTRODUCTION

Ultrasound is operator dependent to a greater degree than any other diagnostic imaging modality. The potential for misdiagnosis is significant, and the only acceptable way to undertake diagnostic ultrasound is:

1. After appropriate training – practical as well as theoretical
2. Preferably following independent assessment by a qualified ultrasound practitioner (as not everyone can reach the desired standard)
3. By continuing to develop your knowledge and technique with regular relevant practice
4. By employing audit of your practice, preferably within a team setting, as prolonged isolated practice is more likely to result in poor standards of diagnosis.

Importantly, the introduction of smaller, cheaper machines (increasingly hand-held) while improving accessibility to a valuable diagnostic technique on the one hand, has opened it up to potential abuse by untrained users on the other hand. This has focused attention on more rigorous quality control measures, and on the need for comprehensive practical training and competency assessment to supplement theoretical 'courses'.

TECHNIQUE

Ultrasound is devolving rapidly from radiology departments to other clinical environments, such as surgeries and clinics. The potential for ultrasound to be carried out by untrained personnel is therefore increasing. A lack of understanding by some has led to theoretical courses being considered as 'training'. This is very far from the case, and possibly one of the most dangerous legacies of this rapidly developing type of service provision.

Whatever the limitations of your equipment, a comprehensive and properly executed technique is essential. This is not about taking pictures (unlike many other radiological imaging tests). It is about a comprehensive and confident evaluation of the organs (with representative images for audit and recording purposes). This can only be achieved with practical experience, closely supervised by qualified practitioners.

Knowing your own limitations, knowing when you have not been able to execute a satisfactory scan, and being able to request assistance from expert practitioners, is one of the most valuable lessons you will learn.

Although the dynamic nature of the scan is a huge advantage over other forms of imaging, the potential for misdiagnosis is significant. The skilled operator continuously adjusts his or her technique to obtain the maximum diagnostic information. In any abdominal ultrasound survey the operator assesses the limitations of the scan and the level of confidence with which pathology can be excluded or confirmed. The confidence limits help in determining the subsequent investigations and management of the patient.

It is important, too, to retain an open mind about the diagnosis when embarking on the scan; an operator who 'decides' the likely diagnosis on a clinical basis may sometimes be correct but, in trying to 'fit' the scan to match the symptoms, risks serious misdiagnosis.

IMAGE OPTIMIZATION

Misinterpretation of ultrasound images is a significant risk in ultrasound diagnosis. The skill of effective scanning lies in the operator's ability to maximize the diagnostic information available, and in being able to properly interpret the appearances. This is dependent on:

- Technical skill – knowing how to interrogate the organ(s) fully, and obtain the most useful and relevant images
- Knowledge of how the sound interacts with tissue – recognizing and being able to avoid artefacts and the pitfalls of scanning
- Clinical knowledge – knowing what to look for and why, knowing how to interpret the appearances on the image and an understanding of physiological and pathological processes
- Knowledge of the equipment being used, i.e. making the most of your machine Box 1.1).

There are numerous ways in which different manufacturers allow us to make compromises during the scanning process in order to maximize image quality and enhance diagnostic information.

BOX 1.1 Making the most of your equipment

1. Use the highest frequency possible – try increasing the frequency when examining the pancreas or anterior gallbladder
2. Use the lowest frame rate and highest line density possible. Restless or breathless patients will require a higher frame rate
3. Use the smallest field practicable – sections through the liver require a relatively wide sector angle and a large depth of view, but when examining the common duct, for example, the field can be greatly reduced, thereby improving the resolution with no loss of frame rate
4. Use the focal zone at relevant correct depth
5. Use tissue harmonic imaging to increase the signal to noise ratio and reduce artefact
6. Try different processing curves to highlight subtle abnormalities and increase contrast resolution

The diagnostic quality of the image can be improved by:

- Increasing the frequency – at the expense of poorer penetration (Fig. 1.1)
- Increasing the line density – this may be achieved by reducing the frame rate and/ or reducing the sector angle and/or depth of field (Fig. 1.2)
- Using the focal zones correctly – focus at the level under investigation, or use multiple focal zones at the expense of a decreased frame rate (Fig. 1.3)
- Using different pre- and post-processing options, which may highlight particular areas (Fig. 1.4)
- Using tissue harmonics to reduce artefact (Fig. 1.5). This technique uses the second harmonic frequency using pulse inversion.[1] This results in a higher signal to noise ratio, which demonstrates particular benefits in many difficult scanning situations, including obese or gassy abdomens.

The bottom line is, it is far better to have a scan performed properly on a low-tech piece of equipment by a knowledgeable and well-trained operator than to have a poorly performed scan on the latest high-tech machine (Fig. 1.6). A good operator will get the best out of even the lowliest scanning device and produce a result that will promote the correct patient management. A misleading result from a top-of-the-range scanner can be highly damaging and at best, delay the correct treatment or at worst promote incorrect management.

The operator should know the limitations of the scan in terms of equipment capabilities, operator skills, clinical problems and patient limitations, take those limitations into account and communicate them where necessary.

THE USE OF DOPPLER

Many pathological processes in the abdomen affect the haemodynamics of relevant organs and the judicial use of Doppler is an essential part of the diagnostic procedure. This is discussed in more detail in subsequent chapters.

Colour Doppler is used to assess the patency and direction of flow of vessels in the abdomen, to establish the vascularity of masses or lesions and to identify vascular disturbances such as stenoses. Flow information is colour coded (usually red towards and blue away from the transducer) and superimposed on the image. This gives the operator an immediate impression of a vascular 'map' of the area (Fig. 1.7). This Doppler information is obtained simultaneously, often from a relatively large area of the image, at the expense of the grey-scale image quality. The extra time taken to obtain the Doppler information for each line results in a reduction in frame rate and line density, which worsens as the colour Doppler area is enlarged. It is advisable, therefore, to use a compact colour 'box' to maintain image quality.

Power Doppler also superimposes Doppler information on the grey-scale image, but without any directional information. It displays only the amount of energy (Fig. 1.8). It has the advantage of a stronger signal, allowing identification of smaller vessels with lower velocity flow than colour Doppler. As it is less angle-dependent than colour Doppler it is particularly useful for vessels which run perpendicular to the beam – such as the inferior vena cava (IVC).

Pulsed Doppler uses pulses of Doppler from individual elements or small groups of elements within the array. This allows the operator to select

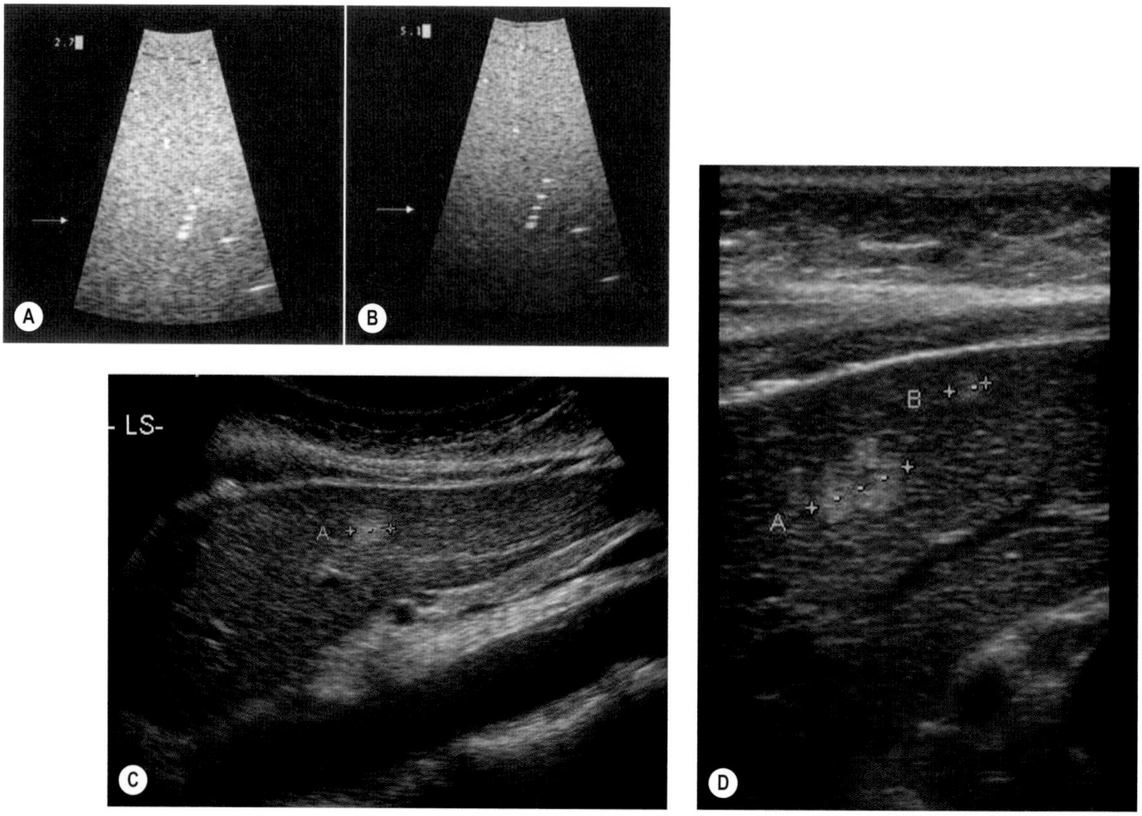

Fig. 1.1 • The effect of changing frequency. (A) At 2.7 MHz the wires are poorly resolved and the background 'texture' of the test object looks coarse. (B) The same transducer is switched to a resonant frequency of 5.1 MHz. Without changing any other settings, the six wires are now resolved and the background texture appears finer. (C) A small nodule in the anterior portion of the left lobe of liver demonstrated with a 5.0 MHz transducer. (D) Using 7.5 MHz, the nodule in (C) has improved detail, and a further small nodule (calipers B), not seen on the lower frequency, is detected near the anterior surface.

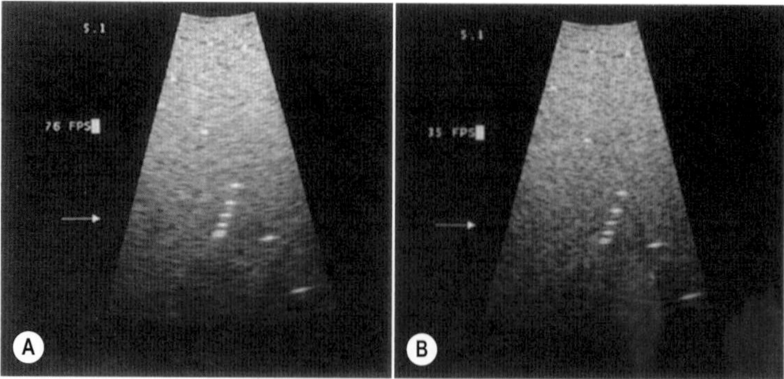

Fig. 1.2 • The effect of line density. (A) 76 frames per second (FPS). (B) 36 FPS – the resulting higher line density improves the image, making it sharper.

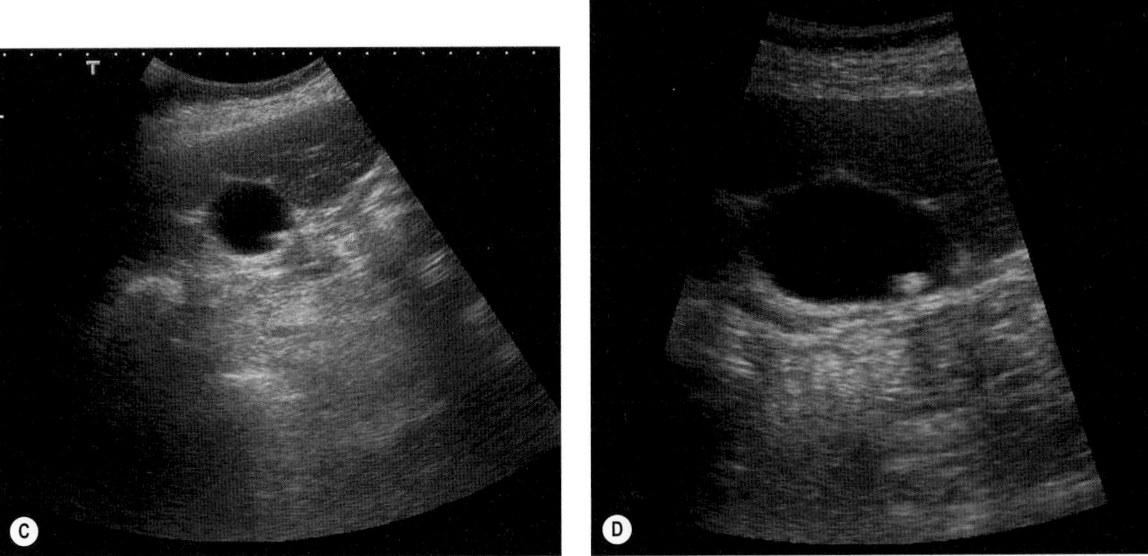

Fig. 1.2, cont'd • (C) The gallbladder is displayed with a low line density, as the scanning area is large. (D) By reducing the field of view, the line density is increased, clarifying the small stone in the gallbladder.

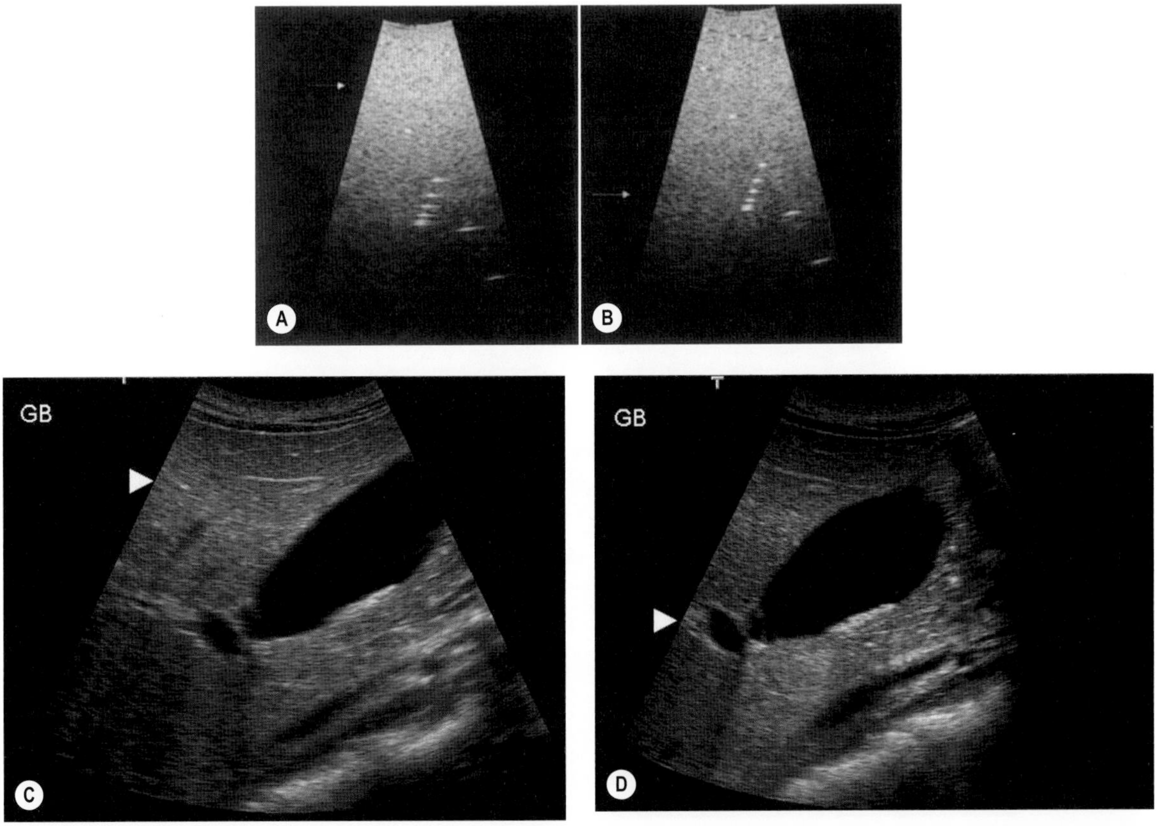

Fig. 1.3 • The effect of focal zone placement. (A) With the focal zone in the near field, structures in the far field are poorly resolved. (B) Correct focal zone placement improves both axial and lateral resolution of the wires. (C) The focal zone incorrectly set in the near field (arrowhead) makes it difficult to demonstrate small gallstones. (D) With the focal zone correctly set (arrowhead), the stones are resolved with a clear, diagnostic band of posterior shadowing.

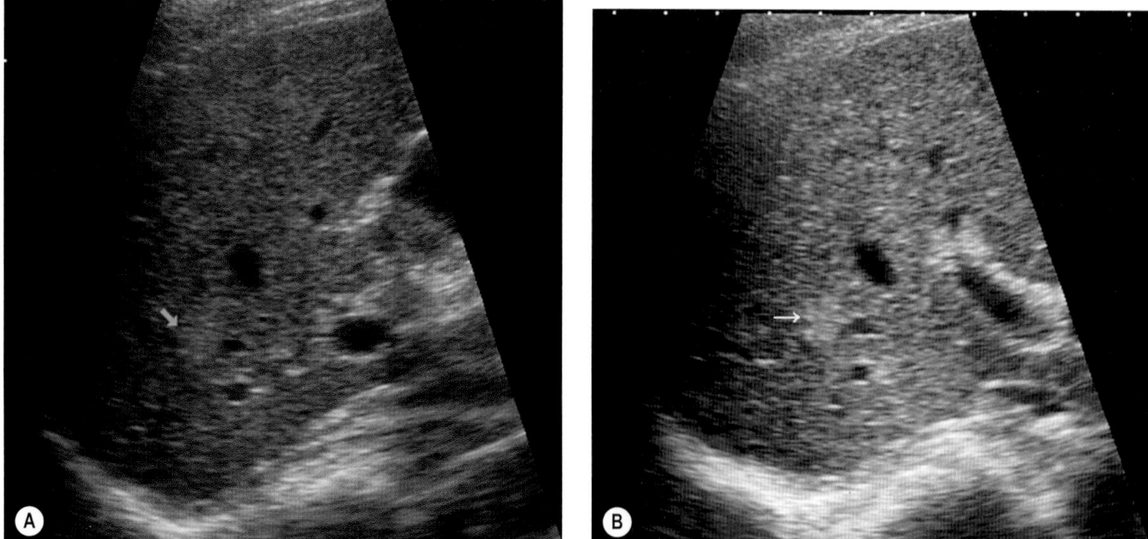

Fig. 1.4 • The effect of using post-processing options. (A) A small nodule in a cirrhotic liver merges into the background and is difficult to detect. (B) A post-processing option that allocates the range of grey shades in a non-linear manner enhances contrast resolution and improves the lesion's conspicuity.

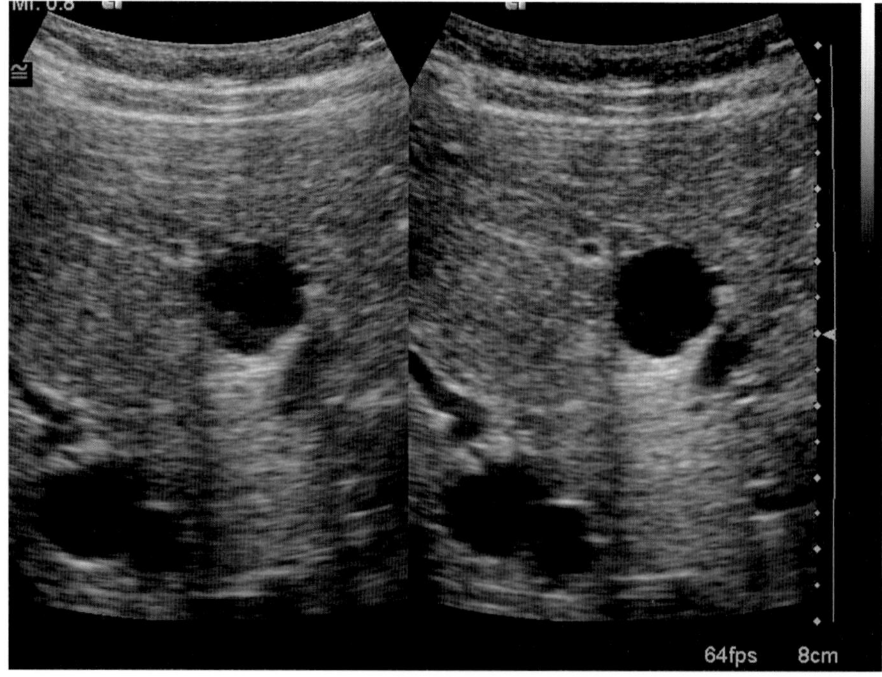

Fig. 1.5 • The effect of tissue harmonic imaging: the left image shows a liver containing cysts. The right image has tissue harmonic imaging applied, which reduces artefact and clarifies the structures.

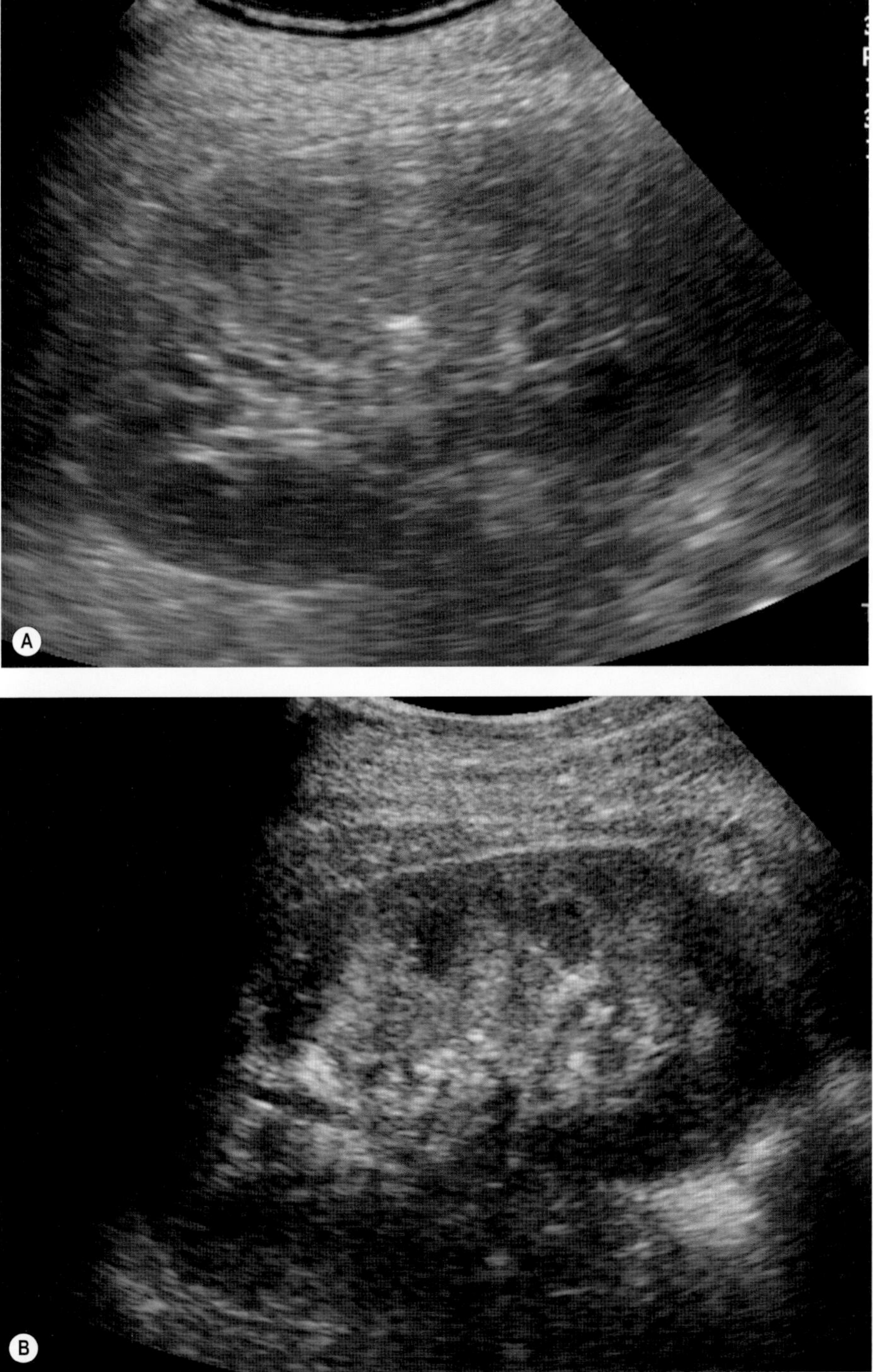

Fig. 1.6 • The importance of using correct equipment settings: (A) Incorrect use of equipment settings makes it difficult to appreciate the structures in the right kidney. (B) By increasing the resonant frequency, decreasing the frame rate (increasing line density) and adjusting the focal zone, structures in the kidney are clarified.

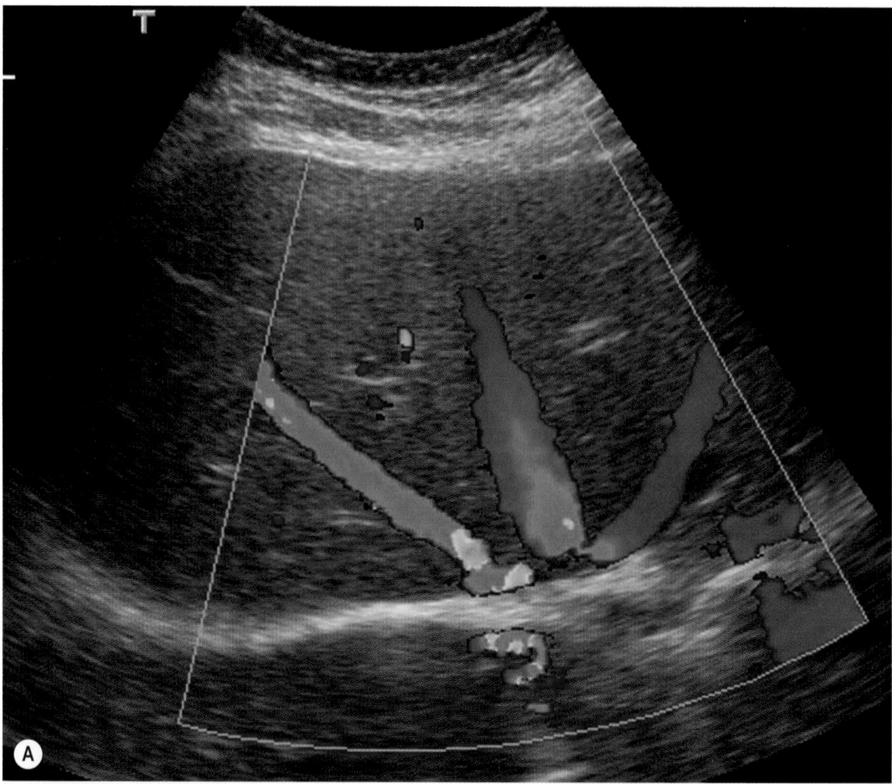

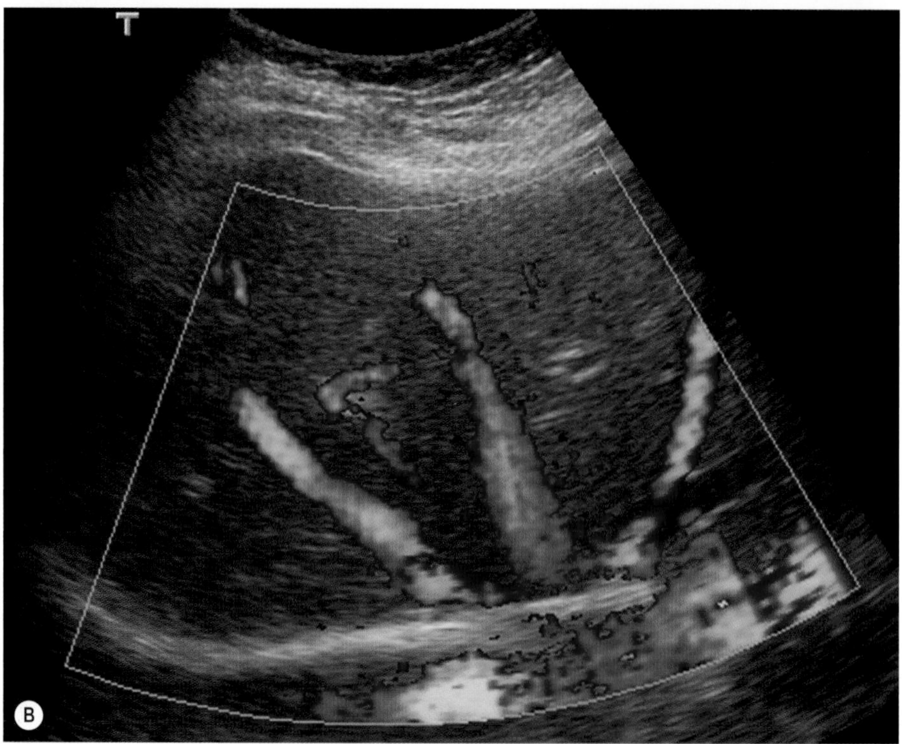

Fig. 1.7 • Colour Doppler of the hepatic vein confluence. Flow is coloured blue to indicate a direction away from the transducer.

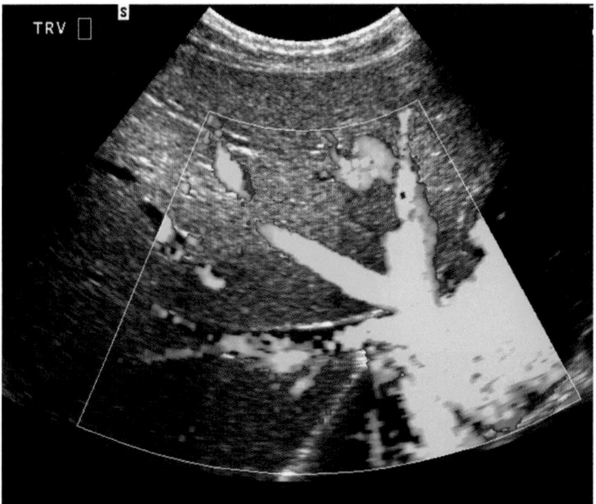

Fig. 1.8 • Power Doppler of the hepatic vein confluence. Directional information is lost, but power Doppler can be superior to colour in demonstrating low velocity flow.

a specific vessel, which has been identified on the grey-scale or colour Doppler image, from which to obtain a spectrum. This gives further information regarding the flow envelope, variance, velocity and downstream resistance of the blood flow (Fig. 1.9).

GETTING THE BEST OUT OF DOPPLER

Familiarity with Doppler controls is essential in order to avoid the pitfalls and increase confidence in the results. It is relatively straightforward to demonstrate flow in major vessels and to assess the relevant spectral waveform; most problems arise when trying to diagnose the *lack* of flow in a suspected thrombosed vessel, and in displaying low velocity flow in difficult-to-access vessels.

Doppler is known to produce false positive results for vessel occlusion (Fig. 1.10) and the operator must avoid the pitfalls. It is essential that the Doppler settings are sensitive enough to detect the velocity of flow in the vessel (Box 1.2). This means that the angle of insonation to the direction

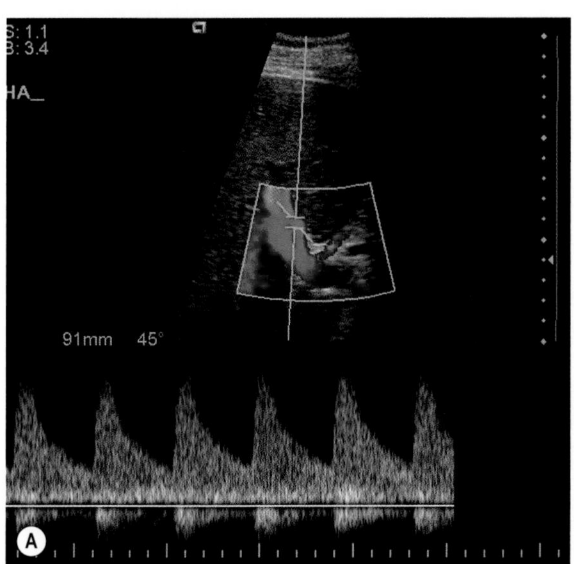

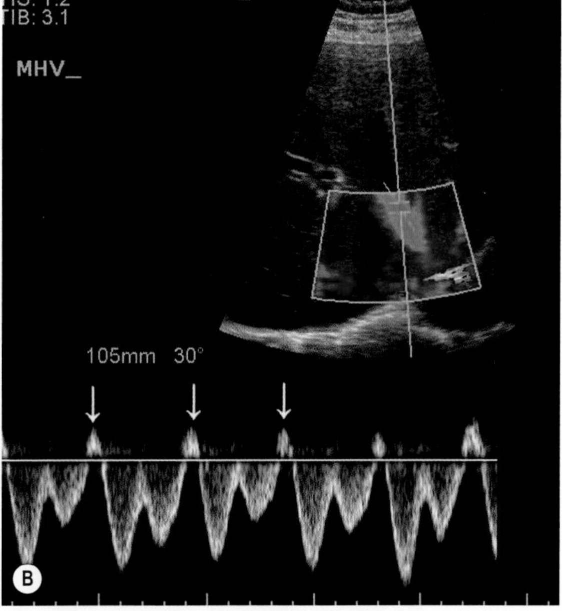

Fig. 1.9 • Flow velocity waveforms. (A) Low resistance flow towards the transducer from a normal hepatic artery. Good end diastolic flow throughout the cycle with a 'filled in' waveform indicating variance in flow. (B) In contrast, this hepatic vein trace with flow away from the transducer is triphasic, with a clear 'envelope' consistent with less variance. The pulsatile nature of the flow incorporates brief flow towards the transducer (arrows) at the end of each cycle.

of flow must be as close to 0° as possible (i.e. the vessel must be flowing towards or away from the beam, not perpendicular to it), the pulse repetition frequency (PRF) must be set to detect slow flow and the Doppler gain must be turned up sufficiently.

It is also possible to make mistakes if the settings are *too* sensitive, i.e. non-occlusive thrombus can be masked by too much colour flow, and a very low PRF can result in aliasing – giving a confusing picture if the operator is unaware (Fig. 1.10).

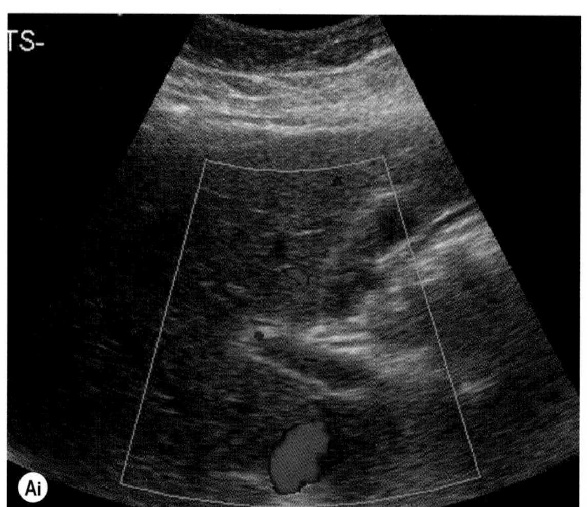

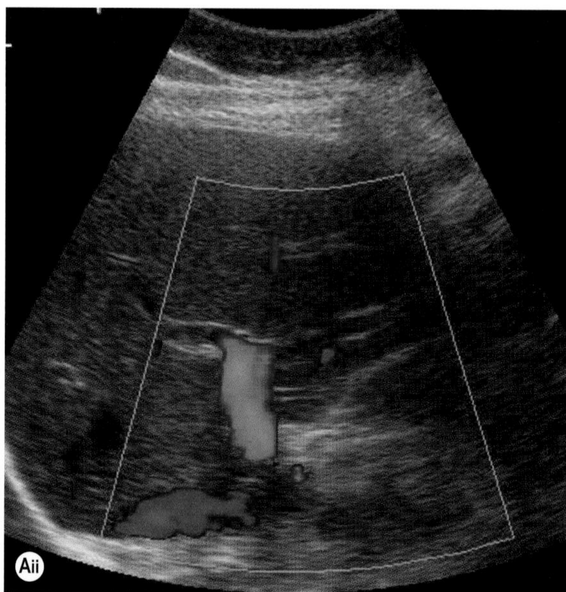

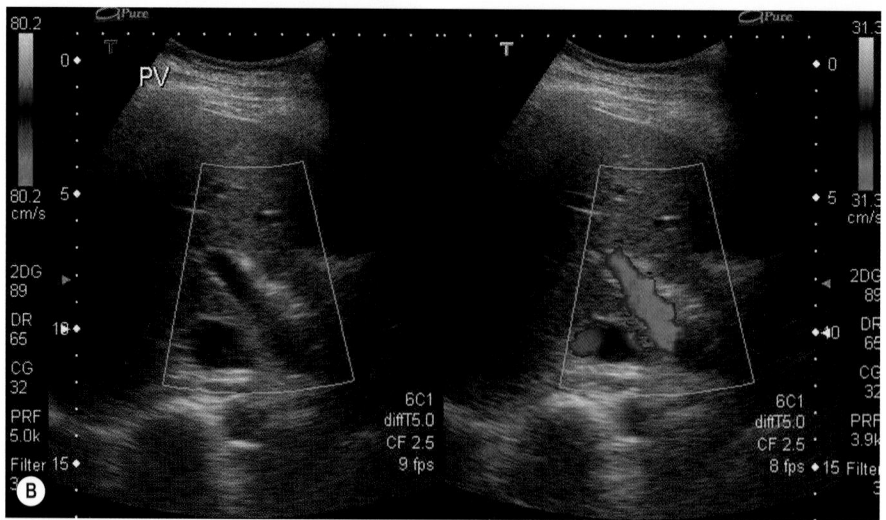

Fig. 1.10 • (Ai) The portal vein appears to have no flow when it lies at 90° to the beam – a possible misinterpretation for thrombosis. (Aii) When scanned intercostally, the vein is almost parallel to the beam and flow is easily demonstrated. (B) Too high a PRF results in the false appearances of no flow in the left image. Reducing the PRF demonstrates flow in the right portal vein (RPV) on the right image.

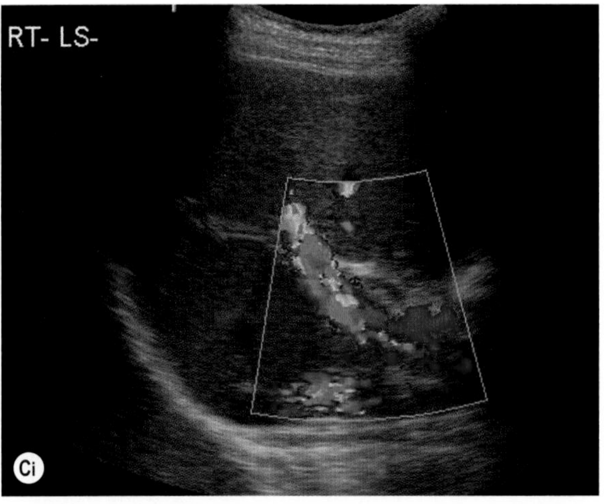

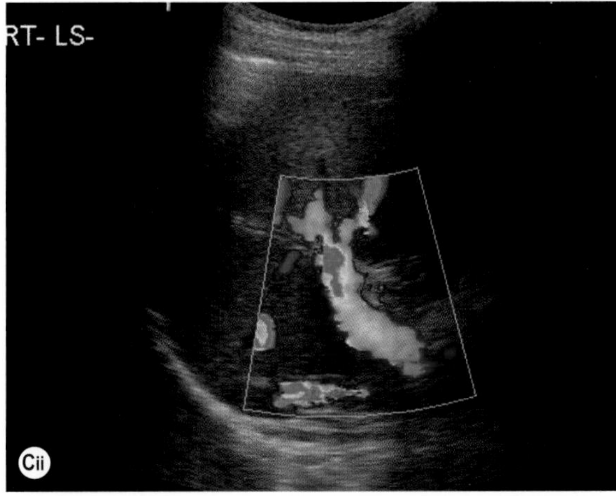

Fig. 1.10, cont'd • (Ci) This portal vein looks blue due to a low PRF and aliasing, which could be mistaken for reversed flow. (Cii) Reducing the PRF displays normal hepatopetal flow in red.

BOX 1.2 Steps to take if you can't detect flow with colour Doppler

1. Ensure the angle of insonation between the vessel and the transducer is <60°. Colour and pulsed Doppler are highly angle dependent.
2. Ensure the Doppler gain is set at the correct level (colour and pulsed Doppler gain settings should be just below background noise level)
3. Ensure the Doppler power/output setting is sufficient
4. Ensure the PRF is set correctly. A low PRF ('range' or 'scale' setting) is required to pick up low velocity flow
5. Ensure the wall thump filter setting is low (if the setting is too high, real low velocity flow is filtered out)
6. Use power Doppler, which is more sensitive and is not angle dependent
7. Reduce the field of view and enlarge or zoom the vessel in question to give yourself the best chance of seeing and sampling flow from small vessels
8. Know the limitations of your machine. Machines differ in their ability to detect low velocity flow
9. If in doubt, test it on a reference vessel you know should contain flow

ADDITIONAL IMAGING MODES

Tissue harmonic imaging

Tissue harmonic imaging processes the harmonic frequency (usually twice the fundamental, transmitted frequency) by using pulse inversion. The reflected beam consists of the fundamental (transmitted) frequency together with diminishing amounts of harmonic frequencies. Using the harmonic has the effect of reducing artefact, improving spatial resolution and consequently the conspicuity of structures.[1,2] Different manufacturers have different ways of employing this mode, and therefore the results can differ from machine to machine. In some cases the dynamic range may be reduced, or the penetration impaired, so it is useful to be familiar with both fundamental and harmonic modes on your machine to get the best from the examination.

Compound imaging

There are two types of ultrasound compound imaging. The first, spatial compound imaging, insonates the tissues from several different angles. Theoretically, this enables the beam to be perpendicular to the various reflective surfaces for a greater proportion of the image, thus improving the definition around lesions and reducing artefact due to edge attenuation. It has been shown to improve the conspicuity of liver lesions and sharpen their margins.[3]

The second type of compound imaging uses several different transmission frequencies to achieve an optimum display of the tissues. With spatial compounding, the different angles of insonation may achieve better definition and improvement in clarity, but also has the disadvantage of reducing or eliminating useful artefacts, which may assist the interpretation and diagnosis.[4]

Volume ultrasound

This features the use of either a multi-element transducer being moved mechanically over a region, producing a large number of slices which may be displayed as a three-dimensional image, or the use of a matrix of elements within a two-dimensional transducer. The acquisition of these volume data sets may help to eliminate measurement errors, movement artefacts (in the case of the matrix) and speed up the process of acquiring ultrasound information. A further advantage is that such datasets may be examined and manipulated when the patient has left the department.[5] However, its use requires further validation and examination before it is adopted in the clinical department.

Elastography

This is a method of estimating the stiffness of the tissue by sending in a pulse of sound and analysing the velocity of the returning pulse. Various methods are available, including a 'blind' transient elastography using a thin pencil probe, and also methods that are linked to real time ultrasound images. The latter have the advantage of allowing the operator to know exactly where the pulse is transmitted, so avoiding potential miscalculations from cysts or vessels. Elastography has been shown to be a reliable method of estimating liver fibrosis, and may therefore avoid the need for some biopsy procedures.[6]

CHOOSING A MACHINE

The practitioner is confronted with a confusing range of equipment, from hand-held kit the size of a large mobile phone (usually relatively low cost) to high-end complex and expensive machines. Choosing the right machine for the job can be a daunting task.

The best advice here is: you get what you pay for. Cheaper machines frequently have an inferior image quality (do not be taken in by a tiny monitor that makes the image look crisper than it really is). As far as abdominal scanning is concerned you need to go for the *best grey-scale image* you can possibly afford. Do not be tempted by lavish (expensive) functionality on a machine, which increases the price of equipment with an indifferent or inferior basic grey-scale image.

Many machines, purchased in the first enthusiastic flush of setting up a new service, turn out to be unsuitable a couple of years down the line. Mistakes are made by insufficient forward planning. Take careful stock of the range of examinations you expect your machine to perform. Future developments that may affect the type of machine you buy include:

- Increase in numbers of patients calculated from trends in previous years
- Increase in range of possible applications – an impending peripheral vascular service, for example, or regional screening initiative
- Clinical developments and changes in patient management which may require more, or different, ultrasound techniques – for example, medical therapies which require ultrasound monitoring, applications involving the use of contrast agents, surgical techniques which may require intraoperative scanning, increases or decreases in hospital beds, introduction of new services and enlargement of existing ones
- Impending political developments by government or hospital management, resulting in changes in the services provided, the funding or the catchment area
- Other impending ultrasound developments – such as the use of contrast media or ultrasound-guided therapies which may be required in future.

The following points are useful to bear in mind when purchasing new equipment:

- Involve someone who knows about ultrasound kit – the local radiology department, for example.
- Probe number and design (Fig. 1.11).

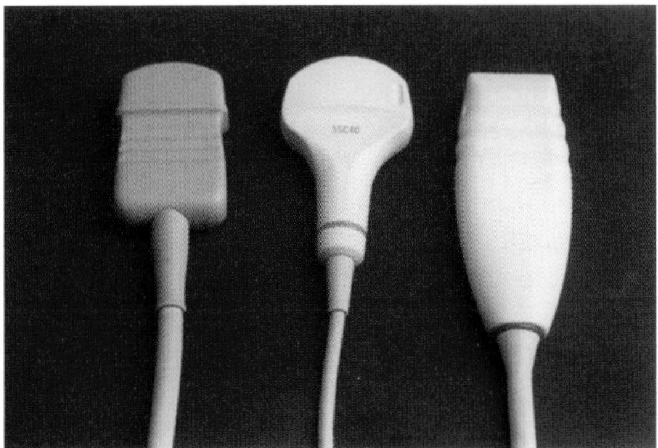

Fig. 1.11 • Curved arrays (left and centre) suitable for abdominal scanning. A 5 or 7.5 MHz linear array (right) is useful for superficial structures, e.g. gallbladder and anterior abdominal wall.

Consider the footprint, shape and frequencies required: most modern transducers are broadband in design, enabling the operator to use a wide range of frequencies in one probe. This is a potential advantage as it limits the number of probes required for a general service. A curved array probe is suitable for most general abdominal applications, operating in the 3.5–6 MHz region. Additional higher frequency probes are useful for paediatrics and for superficial structures. A small footprint is essential if neonatal and paediatric work is undertaken and a 7–10 MHz frequency will probably be required.

A biopsy attachment may be needed for invasive procedures, and, depending on the range of work to be undertaken, linear probes, endoprobes, intraoperative probes and other designs can be considered.

Image quality

There are very few applications where this is not of paramount importance, and abdominal scanning requires the very best you can afford. A machine capable of producing a high-quality image is likely to remain operational for much longer than one capable of only poor quality, which will need replacement much sooner.

A poor-quality image is a false economy in abdominal scanning (you are better compromising on functionality if funding is tight).

Machine capabilities and functions

The availability and ease of use of various functions differ from machine to machine. Some of the important issues to consider when buying a machine are:

- Probe selection and switching process, simultaneous connection of several probes
- Dynamic frequency capability
- Dynamic focusing control, number and pattern of focal zones
- Functions such as beam steering, sector angle adjustment, zoom, frame rate adjustment, trackerball controls
- Time gain compensation (TGC) and power output controls
- Cine facility – operation and size of memory
- Programmable presets
- Tissue harmonic and/or contrast harmonic imaging
- Body marker and labelling functions
- Measurement packages – operation and display
- Colour/power and spectral Doppler through all probes
- Doppler sensitivity
- Doppler controls – ease of use, programmable presets
- Output displays
- Report package option.

Ergonomics

Good ergonomics contribute considerably to the success of the service provided. The machine must be usable by various operators in all the required situations. There is a significant risk of work-related musculoskeletal disorders (WRMSDs)[7] if careful consideration is not given to the scanning environment (see below). When choosing and setting up a scanning service, forethought should be given not only to the design of the ultrasound machine, but also to the seating arrangements and examination couch. These should all be adjustable in order to facilitate the best scanning position for the operator.

Other considerations are:

- System dimensions and steering. The requirement for the system to be portable –

for example for ward or theatre work – or mobile for transportation to remote clinics. Machines used regularly for mobile work should be robust and easy to move
- Moveable (swivel and tilt) monitor and control panel, including height adjustment for different operators and situations
- Keyboard design – to facilitate easy use of the required functions, without stretching or twisting.

Hand-held portable machines are an option that may be considered.

Maintenance issues

It is useful to consider the reliability record of the chosen equipment, particularly if it is to operate in outreach clinics, or without available backup in the case of breakdown. Contacting other users may prove useful.

Various maintenance contract options and costs are available, including options on the replacement of probes, which should be taken into account when purchasing new equipment.

Upgradeability

A machine which is potentially upgradeable has a longer, more cost-effective life and will be supported by the manufacturer over a longer period of time. Consider:
- Future software upgrades – possible effects and costs
- Other available options for the future, such as additional transducers or add-on Doppler facilities.

RECORDING OF IMAGES

There are no hard and fast rules about the recording of ultrasound scans and departmental practices vary. It is good practice for departments to have guidelines for taking and retaining images within individual schemes of work, outlining the minimum expected.[8]

The advantages of recording images are:
- They provide a record of the quality of the scan and how it has been conducted, the organs examined, the extent of the scan, the type and standard of equipment, the settings used and other scanning factors that can be an invaluable tool in providing a medicolegal defence
- They provide a valuable teaching aid
- They help to ensure quality control within departments: promoting the use of good technique, they can be used to ensure protocols are followed and provide an excellent audit tool
- They can be used to obtain a second opinion on difficult or equivocal cases and provide a basis for discussion with clinical colleagues.

The disadvantages are:
- The cost of buying, running and maintaining the recording device or system
- The quality of images in some cases may not accurately reflect that of the image on the ultrasound monitor
- The scanning time must be slightly increased to accommodate the taking of images
- Storage and retrieval of images may be time- and space-consuming
- Hard-copy may be mislaid or lost
- If the examination has been *badly* performed, the image may demonstrate that too!

Generally speaking the recording of images is encouraged. It reduces the operator's vulnerability to litigation and supports the ultrasound diagnosis.[9] The operator must take the responsibility for ensuring the scan has been performed to the required standard; any images produced for subsequent discussion are only *representative* of the examination and have been chosen by the operator as an appropriate selection. If you have missed a small metastasis in the liver while scanning, or a gallstone in the gallbladder, you are unlikely to have included it on an image.

Digital imaging networks (picture archiving and communications systems, or PACS) are convenient, quick and relatively easy to use. The image quality is excellent, suffering little or no degradation in capture and subsequent retrieval, and the system can potentially be linked to a conventional imager should hard copy be required.

The number of workstations in the system, while theoretically unlimited, may be limited by financial considerations, and this may be inconvenient in busy departments. The operator has the flexibility to transmit images immediately to remote locations – for example clinical meetings, outpatient clinics etc., making this ideal for outreach clinics. Digital storage and retrieval avoids loss of films and affords considerable savings in time, labour and space.

Many systems now incorporate patient registration and reporting, further streamlining the ultrasound examination. Beware – some systems do not accommodate video clips or even colour images and there are considerable differences between the facilities available on different systems. The potential purchaser is advised to plan carefully for the needs of the ultrasound service.

SAFETY OF DIAGNOSTIC ULTRASOUND

Within the field of clinical diagnostic ultrasound, it is currently accepted that there is insufficient evidence for any deleterious effects at diagnostic levels, and that the benefits to patients outweigh the risks. As new techniques and technological developments come onto the market, new biophysical conditions may be introduced, which require evaluation with regard to safety,[10] and we cannot afford to become complacent about the possible effects. The situation remains under constant review.

Several international bodies continue to consider the safety of ultrasound in clinical use. The European Federation for Ultrasound in Medicine and Biology (EFSUMB) has confirmed the safety of diagnostic ultrasound and endorsed its 'informed' use.[11] While the use of pulsed Doppler is considered inadvisable for the developing embryo during the first trimester, no such exceptions are highlighted for abdominal ultrasound. The European Committee for Ultrasound Radiation Safety (ECURS) confirms that no deleterious effects have yet been proven in clinical medicine. It recommends, however, that equipment is used only when designed to national or international safety standards and that it is used only by competent and trained personnel. The World Federation for Ultrasound in Medicine and Biology (WFUMB) confirms that the use of B-mode imaging is not contraindicated,[12] concluding that exposure levels and duration should be reduced to the minimum necessary to obtain the required diagnostic information.

The increase in use of contrast agents in abdominal ultrasound has given rise to concern for safety, and while this is generally considered low risk, provided the appropriate contraindications are observed,[13,14] there is a theoretical risk of cavitation (see below). Once again, the requirement for proper training is emphasized.

Ultrasound intensities used in diagnostic ultrasound vary according to the mode of operation – pulsed Doppler usually has a higher level than B-mode scanning, which operates at lower intensities, although there may be overlap with colour or power Doppler. The American Institute for Ultrasound in Medicine (AIUM) has suggested that ultrasound is safe below 100 Wcm^{-2}.[15] This figure refers to the spatial peak temporal average intensity (I_{SPTA}).

The use of intensity, however, as an indicator of safety is limited, particularly where Doppler is concerned, as Doppler intensities can be considerably greater than those in B-mode imaging. The US FDA (Food and Drug Administration) sets maximum intensity levels allowed for machine output, which differ according to the application.[16]

BIOLOGICAL EFFECTS OF ULTRASOUND

Harmful effects from ultrasound have been documented in laboratory conditions. These include *thermal effects* and *mechanical effects*.

Thermal effects

These are demonstrated as a slight rise in temperature, particularly in close proximity to the transducer face, during ultrasound scanning. This local effect is usually of no significance but the operator must be aware of the phenomenon. The most significant thermal effects occur at bone–tissue interfaces and are greater with pulsed Doppler. Increases in temperature of up to 5 °C have been produced. Areas at particular risk are fetal bones and the interfaces in transcranial Doppler ultrasound scans.

Pulsed Doppler has a greater potential for heating than B-mode imaging as it involves greater temporal average intensities due to high PRF and because the beam is frequently held stationary over an area while obtaining the waveform. Colour and power Doppler usually involve a greater degree of scanning and transducer movement, which involves a potentially lower heating potential than with pulsed Doppler. Care must be taken to limit the use of pulsed Doppler and not to hold the transducer stationary over one area for too long.

Mechanical effects

Mechanical effects include cavitation and radiation pressure, are caused by stresses in the tissues and depend on the amplitude of the ultrasound pulse. These effects are greatest around gas-filled organs, such as lungs or bowel and have, in laboratory conditions, caused small, surface blood vessels in the lungs to rupture.

Potentially, these effects could be a hazard when using contrast agents that contain microbubbles.

SAFETY INDICES (THERMAL AND MECHANICAL INDICES)

In order to inform users about the machine conditions which may potentially be harmful, mechanical and thermal indices are now displayed as an output display standard (ODS) on all equipment manufactured after 1998. This makes the operator aware of the ultrasound conditions that may exceed the limits of safety and enables him/her to take avoiding action, such as reducing the power or restricting the scanning time in that area.

In simple terms the mechanical index (MI) is related to amplitude and indicates how 'big' an ultrasound pulse is, giving an indication of the chances of mechanical effects occurring. It is therefore particularly relevant in the abdomen when scanning gas-filled bowel or when using microbubble contrast agents. Gas bodies introduced by contrast agents increase the probability of cavitation.

The thermal index (TI) gives an indication of the temperature rise that might occur within the ultrasound beam, aiming to give an estimate of the reasonable worst-case temperature rise. The thermal index calculation alters, depending upon the application, giving rise to three indices: the soft tissue thermal index (TIS), the bone-at-focus index (TIB) and the bone-at-surface, or cranial index (TIC). The first of these is obviously most relevant for abdominal applications. In well-perfused tissue, such as the liver and spleen, thermal effects are less likely due to the cooling effect of the blood flow. The display of safety indices is only a general indication of the possibility of biological hazards and cannot be translated directly into real heating or cavitation potential.[17]

These 'safety indices' are limited in several ways. They require the user to be educated with respect to the implications of the values shown, and they do not take into account the duration of exposure, which is particularly important in assessing the risk of thermal damage. In addition, the TI does not take account of the patient's temperature, and it is logical to assume that increased caution is therefore required in scanning the febrile patient.

MI and TI are also unlikely to portray the optimum safety information during the use of contrast agents, in which, theoretically, heating effects and cavitation may be enhanced.[10]

OTHER HAZARDS

While most attention in the literature is focused on the possible biological effects of ultrasound, there are several other safety issues which are within the control of the operator:

- Electrical safety: All ultrasound machines should be subject to regular quality control and should be regularly checked for any signs of electrical hazards. Loose or damaged wiring, for example, is a common problem if machines are routinely used for mobile work. Visible damage to a transducer, such as a crack in the casing, should prompt its immediate withdrawal from service until a repair or replacement is effected.
- Microbiological safety: It is the responsibility of the sonographer to minimize the risks of cross-infection. Hospital-acquired infection is a serious and potentially life-threatening condition which must be minimized by careful infection control measures during and between scanning operations. Most manufacturers make recommendations regarding appropriate cleaning agents for transducers, which should be carefully followed. Sterile probe covers should be used in cases where there is increased risk of infection, such as

patients with open wounds, those on immunosuppression, or in a ward environment.

- 'Operator' safety: By far the most serious hazard of all is that of the untrained or badly trained operator. Misdiagnosis is a grave risk for those not aware of the pitfalls. Apart from the implications for the patient of subsequent, incorrect management, the operator risks litigation which is difficult or impossible to defend if he/she has had inadequate training in ultrasound.

WORK-RELATED MUSCULOSKELETAL DISORDERS

There is continuing concern about WRMSDs related to ultrasound scanning, as workloads increase, and it has been estimated that a significant proportion of sonographers who practise full-time ultrasound scanning may be affected.[7] One contributing factor is the ergonomic design of the ultrasound machines, together with the position adopted by the operator during scanning. While more attention is now being paid by ultrasound manufacturers to designs which limit WRMSDs, there are various other contributing factors that should be taken into account when providing ultrasound services. Well-designed, adjustable seating for operators, adjustable patient couches, proper staff training for manoeuvring patients and a varied work load all contribute to minimizing the potential problems to staff.

THE SAFE PRACTICE OF ULTRASOUND

It is fair to say that the safety of ultrasound is less of an issue in abdominal scanning than in obstetric or reproductive organ scanning. Nevertheless it is still incumbent upon the operator to minimize the ultrasound dose to the patient in any practicable way.

The use of X-rays is governed by the *ALARA* principle – that of keeping the radiation dose As Low As Reasonably Achievable. Although the risks associated with radiation are not present in the use of ultrasound, the general principle of keeping the acoustic exposure as low as possible is still good practice and many people still refer to *ALARA* in the context of diagnostic ultrasound (Box 1.3).

BOX 1.3 Steps for minimizing the ultrasound dose

1. Ensure operators are properly trained, preferably on recognized training programmes
2. Minimize the output (or power) level. Use amplification of the received echoes to manipulate the image in preference to increasing the transmitted power
3. Minimize the time taken to perform the exam
4. Do not rest the transducer on the skin surface when not scanning
5. Make sure the clinical indications for the scan are satisfactory and that a proper request has been received. Do not do unnecessary ultrasound examinations
6. Be aware of the safety indices displayed on the ultrasound machine. Limit the use of pulsed Doppler to that necessary to contribute to the diagnosis
7. Make the best use of your equipment – maximize the diagnostic information by manipulating the controls effectively

MEDICOLEGAL ISSUES

Litigation in medical practice is increasing and the field of ultrasound is no exception. The majority of cases involve, firstly, obstetric and, secondly, gynaecological ultrasound. Nevertheless it is prudent for the operator to be aware of the need to minimize the risks of successful litigation in all types of scanning procedures.

Patients have higher expectations of medical care than ever before and ultrasound practitioners should be aware of the ways in which they can protect themselves medicolegally. The onus is upon the defendant to prove that he or she acted responsibly and there are several helpful guidelines which should routinely be followed (Box 1.4).[13]

Depending on their profession, operators are constrained by codes of conduct of their respective colleges and/or Councils.[19] Delegation by senior medically qualified staff to non-medically qualified ultrasound practitioners is now accepted practice in the UK. It is incumbent upon the person delegating the scan (frequently a consultant radiologist) to ensure that the person to whom they delegate (practitioner or specialist registrar) is

BOX 1.4 Guidelines for defensive scanning (adapted from Meire[18])

1. Ensure you are properly trained. Operators who have undergone approved training are less likely to make mistakes
2. Act with professionalism and courtesy. Good communication skills go a long way to avoiding litigation
3. Use written guidelines or schemes of work
4. Ensure a proper request for the examination has been received
5. A written report should be issued by the operator
6. Record images to support your findings
7. Clearly state any limitations of the scan which may affect the ability to make a diagnosis
8. Ensure that the equipment you use is adequate for the job

properly trained and skilled. The operator then becomes legally accountable for his/her professional actions. The same standard of care is expected from medically and non-medically qualified staff alike.[20] To avoid liability, a practitioner must comply with the Bolam test, in which he/she should be seen to acting in accordance with practice accepted as proper by a responsible body of relevant medical people.

DEPARTMENTAL GUIDELINES/ SCHEMES OF WORK

It is good and safe practice to use written guidelines for ultrasound examinations.[3] These serve several purposes:

- They may be used to support a defence against litigation (provided, of course, that the operator can prove he/she has followed such guidelines)
- They serve to impose and maintain a minimum standard, especially within departments which may have numerous operators of differing experience levels
- They form a record of current practice.

Guidelines should ideally be:

- Written by, and have input from, those practising ultrasound in the department, (usually a combination of medically and non-medically qualified personnel) taking into account the requirements of referring clinicians, available equipment and other local operational issues
- Regularly reviewed and updated to take account of the latest literature and practices
- Flexible – to allow the operator to tailor the scan to the patient's clinical presentation and individual requirements.

The guidelines should be broad enough to allow operators to respond to different clinical situations in an appropriate way while ensuring that the highest possible standard of scan is always performed. Guidelines which are too prescriptive and detailed are likely to be ignored by operators as impractical. In cases when it is simply not possible to adhere to departmental guidelines, the reasons should be stated on the report – for example when the pancreas cannot be demonstrated due to body habitus or overlying bowel gas.

QUALITY ASSURANCE

The principles of quality assurance affect all aspects of the ultrasound service. These include staff issues (such as education and training, performance and continuing professional development), patient care, the work environment (including health and safety issues) and quality assurance of equipment. Quality assurance checks on ultrasound equipment, unlike most other aspects of an ultrasound service, involve measurable and reproducible parameters.

Equipment tests

After installation, a full range of tests and safety checks should be carried out, preferably by a qualified medical physicist, and the results recorded. This establishes a baseline performance against which comparisons may later be made.

It is useful to record an image of a tissue mimicking phantom, with the relevant settings marked on it. Such images form a reference against which the machine's subsequent performance can be assessed, and are especially useful if your machine seems to be performing poorly, or the image seems to have deteriorated.

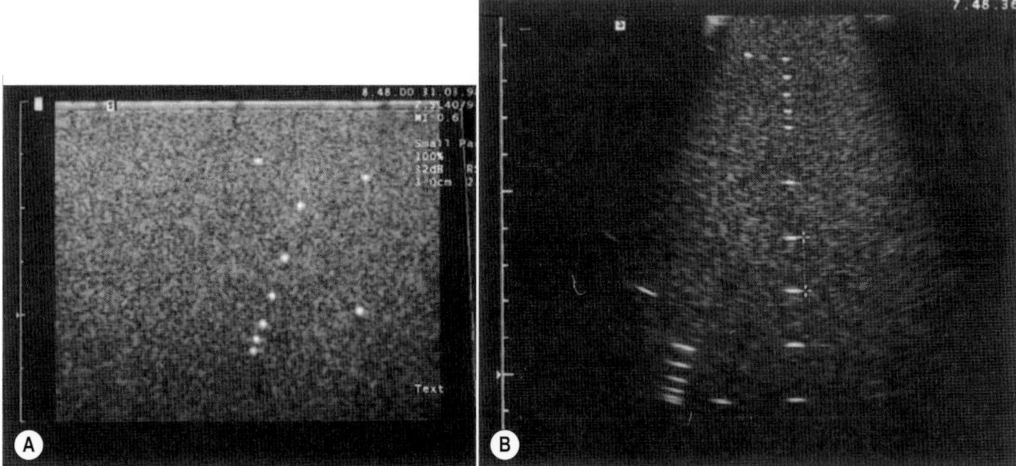

Fig. 1.12 • Tissue-mimicking phantom. (A) When using a high frequency linear array, cross-sections of the wires in the phantom are clearly demonstrated as small dots. (B) When using a curved array of a lower frequency, such as that used for abdominal scanning, the lateral resolution is seen to deteriorate in the far field as the beam diverges. The wires are displayed correctly in the near field but appear as short lines in the far field. Spacing of the wires is known, allowing caliper accuracy to be assessed.

A regular testing regimen must then be set up, to ensure the standards of quality and safety are maintained. This programme can be set up in conjunction with the operators and the medical physics department and relevant records should be kept. The use of a tissue mimicking phantom enables the sonographer to perform certain tests in a reproducible and recordable manner (Fig. 1.12).

Checks should be carried out for all probes on the machine.

Suggested equipment checks include:

- Caliper accuracy
- System sensitivity and penetration
- Axial and lateral resolution
- Slice thickness
- Grey scale
- Dead zone
- Checks on the various machine controls/ functions
- Output power
- Safety checks; electrical, mechanical, biological and thermal including a visual inspection of all probes and leads
- Imaging device checks for image quality, settings, dynamic range, functionality and electrical safety
- Biopsy guide checks
- Colour, power and spectral Doppler checks (complex, requiring specialized equipment).

Some of these checks can be regularly carried out by users in the department, for example caliper checks and biopsy guide checks. Others are more complex and are more appropriately undertaken by specialist medical physicists. All equipment should undergo regular servicing and any interim faults should naturally be reported.

References

1. Desser TS, Jedrzejewicz MS, Bradley C. Native tissue harmonic imaging: basic principles and clinical applications. Ultrasound Q 2000; 16: 40–48
2. Choudhry S, Gorman B, Charboneau JW et al. Comparison of tissue harmonic imaging with conventional US in abdominal disease. Radiographics 2000; 20: 1127–1135
3. Kim SH, Lee JM, Kim KG et al. Comparison of fundamental sonography, tissue-harmonic sonography, fundamental compound sonography, and tissue-harmonic compound sonography for focal hepatic lesions. Eur Radiol 2006; 16: 2444–2453
4. Elliott S. A user guide to compound imaging. Ultrasound 2005; 13: 112–117
5. Elliott ST. Volume ultrasound: the next big thing? Br J Radiol 2008; 81: 8–9

6. Talwalkar JA, Kurtz DM, Schoenleber SJ et al. Ultrasound-based transient elastography for the detection of hepatic fibrosis; systematic review and meta-analysis. Clin Gastroenterol Hepatol 2007; 5: 1214–1220
7. Society of Radiographers. The causes of musculoskeletal injury amongst sonographers in the UK. Society of Radiographers, London, 2002
8. UKAS. Guidelines for Professional Working Practice. UKAS, London, 1996
9. BMUS: British Medical Ultrasound Society. Guidelines for the acquisition and retention of hard copy ultrasound images. BMUS Bull 2000; 8: 2
10. ter Haar G, Duck FA, eds. The safe use of ultrasound in medical diagnosis. BMUS/BIR, London, 2000
11. EFSUMB. Clinical safety statement for diagnostic ultrasound. 2006. Available at: www.efsumb.org
12. WFUMB: World federation for ultrasound in medicine and biology symposium on safety of ultrasound in medicine: conclusions and recommendations on thermal and non-thermal mechanisms for biological effects of ultrasound. Barnett SB, ed. Ultrasound Med Biol 1998; 24: 1–55
13. EFSUMB Study Group. Guidelines for the use of contrast agents in ultrasound. Ultraschall Med 2004; 25: 249–256
14. WFUMB. Safety symposium on ultrasound contrast agents: clinical applications and safety concerns. Ultrasound Med Biol 2007; 33: 180–186
15. American Institute for Ultrasound in Medicine (AIUM). Bioeffects considerations for the safety of diagnostic ultrasound. J Ultrasound Med 1988; 7 (Suppl)
16. Food and Drug Administration, US Department of Health and Human Services. Information for manufacturers seeking marketing clearance of diagnostic ultrasound systems and transducers. Center for Devices and Radiological Health, Rockville, MD, 1997
17. Duck FA. The meaning of Thermal Index (TI) and Mechanical Index (MI) values. BMUS Bull 1997; 5: 36–40
18. Meire HB, ed. Ultrasound-related litigation in obstetrics and gynecology: the need for defensive scanning. Ultrasound Obstet Gynecol 1996; 7: 233–235
19. Health Professions Council. Standards of conduct, performance and ethics, 2003. Available at: www.hpc-uk.org/publications/standards.
20. Dimond B. Red dots and radiographers' liability. Health Care Risk Report. Clinical Negligence 2000; 10–13

The normal hepato-biliary system

2

CHAPTER CONTENTS

INTRODUCTION

Just in case you skipped the first chapter, I shall repeat an important message. The success, in terms of diagnostic information, of an abdominal ultrasound scan is dependent on numerous factors, the most important of which is the skill of the operator.

Familiarity with normal anatomy, and technical expertise in comprehensively examining an organ are essential. The latter can be obtained only by practice in a clinical environment under proper supervision. Having comprehensive medical and anatomical knowledge is necessary, but it does not enable you to scan, any more than being an air traffic controller enables you to fly an airliner (Box 2.1).

It is good practice, particularly on the patient's first attendance, to scan the whole of the upper abdomen, focusing particularly on the relevant areas, but also excluding or identifying any other significant pathology. A full abdominal survey would usually include the liver, gallbladder, biliary tree, pancreas, spleen, kidneys and retroperitoneal structures.[1] Apart from the fact that many pathological processes can affect multiple organs, a number of significant (but clinically occult) pathological processes are discovered incidentally, for example renal carcinoma or aortic aneurysm. A thorough knowledge of anatomy is assumed at this stage, but diagrams of upper abdominal sectional anatomy are included in the appendices to this chapter for quick reference (see Chapter 2 Appendices, pages 47–50.)

Box 2.1

Key points:

- Get properly trained before you attempt ultrasound diagnosis
- Understand your limitations. Know when to ask for assistance and when to refer on
- If you haven't used your left hand throughout the scan, you have not performed an optimum examination. So get properly trained – I can't emphasize this too much!
- Have an independent practitioner assess your performance. If you don't feel ready to do this you probably should not be scanning unsupervised
- Audit your practice. Liaise with multidisciplinary teams/radiology department

GENERAL POINTERS ON UPPER ABDOMINAL TECHNIQUE

- It is neither desirable nor possible to be prescriptive in ultrasound scanning, but there are some general approaches that help to get the best from the scanning procedure:
- Scan in a systematic way to ensure the whole of the upper abdomen has been thoroughly interrogated. The use of a worksheet, indicating structures to be examined, is helpful when learning.[1]
- Always scan any organ in *at least* two planes – preferably at right angles to each other. This reduces the risk of missing pathology and helps to differentiate artefact from true pathology.
- Where possible, scan in at least two patient positions. It is surprising how the available ultrasound information can be enhanced by turning your patient decubitus or erect. Inaccessible organs flop into better view and bowel moves away from the area of interest.
- Use a combination of subcostal and intercostal scanning for all upper abdominal scanning. The different angles of insonation can reveal pathology and eliminate artefact. Good technique is about finding a good acoustic window.
- Do not limit yourself to longitudinal and transverse sections. Use a variety of planes and angulations. Trace ducts and vessels along their courses. Use the transducer like a pair of eyes.
- Deep inspiration is useful in a proportion of patients, but not all. Sometimes it can make matters worse by filling the stomach with air and obscuring structures. An intercostal approach with the patient breathing gently often has far more success.
- Positioning patients supine, particularly if elderly or very ill, can make them breathless and uncomfortable. Raise the patient's head as much as necessary – a comfortable patient is much easier to scan.
- Images are a useful record of the scan and how it has been performed, but do not make these your primary task. Scan first – sweeping smoothly from one aspect of the organ to the other in two planes, then take the relevant images to support your findings.
- Make the most of your equipment (see Chapter 1). Increase the confidence level of your scan by fully utilizing all the available facilities; using Doppler, tissue harmonics, changing transducers and frequencies and manipulating the machine settings and processing options.

THE LIVER

Normal appearances

The liver is a homogeneous, mid-grey organ on ultrasound. It has the same, or slightly increased echogenicity when compared to the cortex of the right kidney. Its outline is smooth, the inferior margin coming to a point anteriorly (Fig. 2.1). The liver is surrounded by a thin, hyperechoic capsule, which is difficult to see on ultrasound unless outlined by fluid (Fig. 2.2).

The smooth parenchyma is interrupted by vessels (see below) and ligaments (Figs 2.3–2.15), and the liver itself provides an excellent acoustic window onto the various organs and great vessels situated in the upper abdomen.

The ligaments are hyperechoic, linear structures; the falciform ligament, which separates the anatomical left and right lobes, is situated at the superior margin of the liver and is best demonstrated when surrounded by ascitic fluid. It surrounds the left main portal vein (PV) and is known as the ligamentum teres as it descends towards the infero-anterior aspect of the liver (Figs 2.9, 2.15). The ligamentum venosum separates the caudate lobe from the rest of the liver (Fig. 2.6).

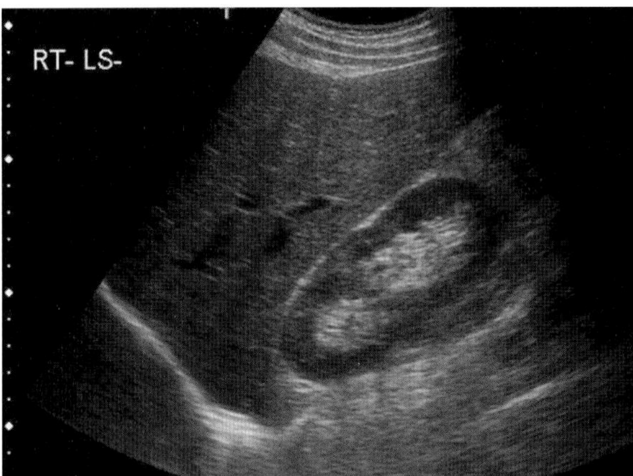

Fig. 2.1 • LS through the right lobe of liver. The renal cortex is slightly less echogenic than the liver parenchyma.

The size of the liver is difficult to quantify, as there is such a large variation in shape between normal subjects and direct measurements are notoriously inaccurate. Size is therefore usually assessed subjectively. Look particularly at the inferior margin of the right lobe which should come to a point anterior to the lower pole of the right kidney (Fig. 2.1). A relatively common variant of this is the *Reidel's lobe*, an inferior elongation of segment V1 on the right. This is an extension of the right lobe over the lower pole of the kidney, with a rounded margin (Fig. 2.16), and is worth remembering as possible cause of a palpable right upper quadrant 'mass'.

To distinguish mild enlargement from a Reidel's lobe, look at the left lobe – if this also looks bulky, with a rounded inferior edge, the liver is enlarged. A Reidel's lobe is often accompanied by a smaller, less accessible left lobe, with the overall liver volume remaining normal.

The segments of the liver

It is often sufficient to talk about the 'right' or 'left' lobes of the liver for the purposes of many

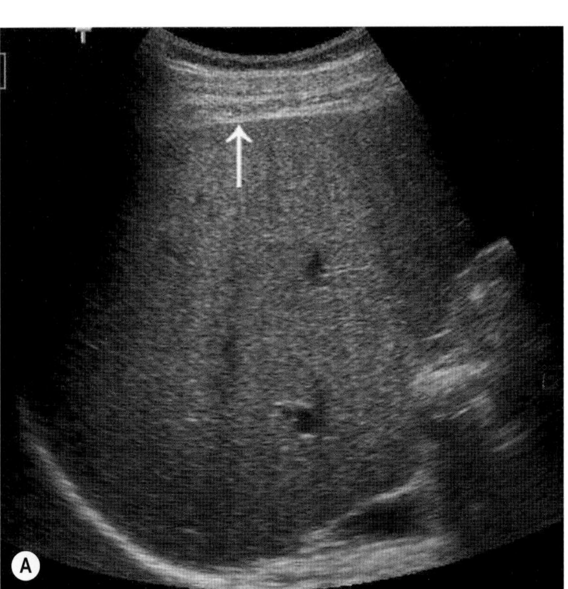

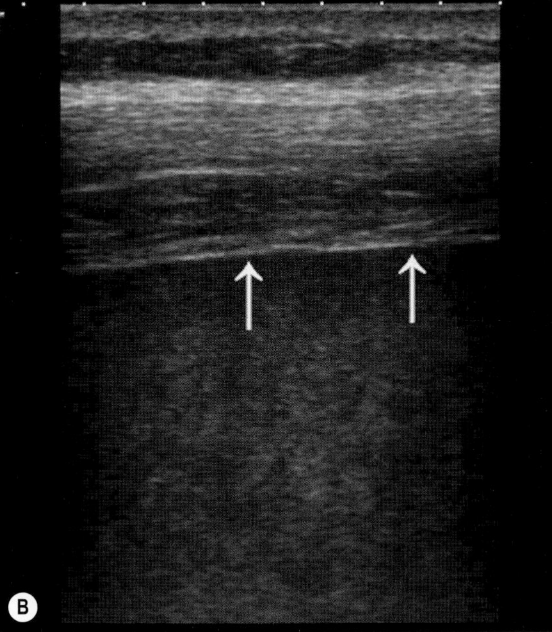

Fig. 2.2 • (A) The capsule of the liver is a thin, hyperechoic layer seen anteriorly. (B) It is much better appreciated at higher frequencies (arrows) (7.5 MHz).

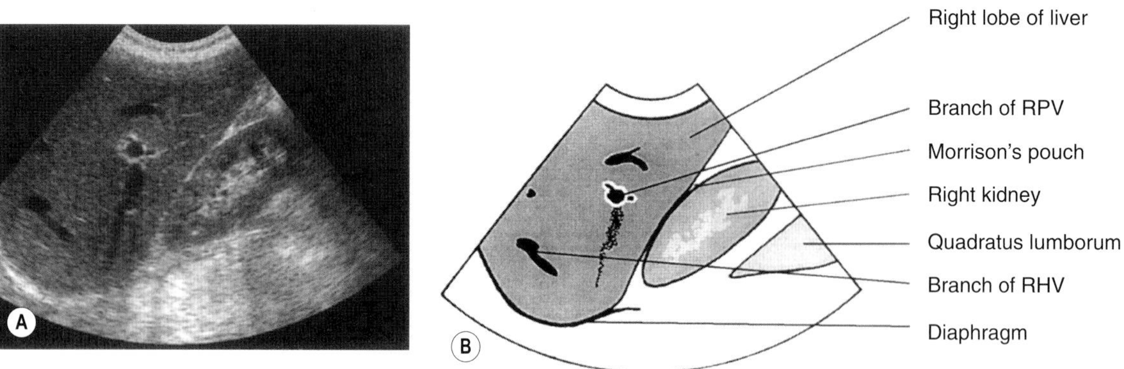

Fig. 2.3 • LS through the right lobe of liver and right kidney.

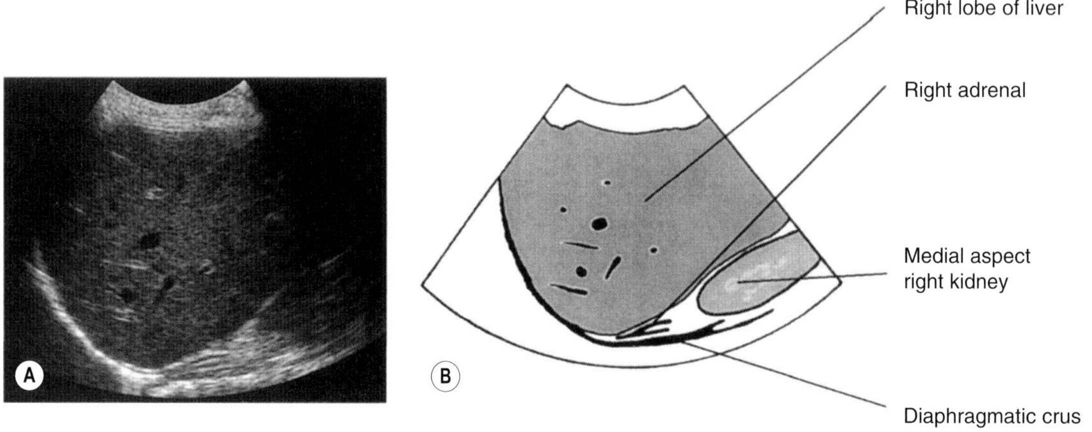

Fig. 2.4 • LS right lobe, just medial to the right kidney.

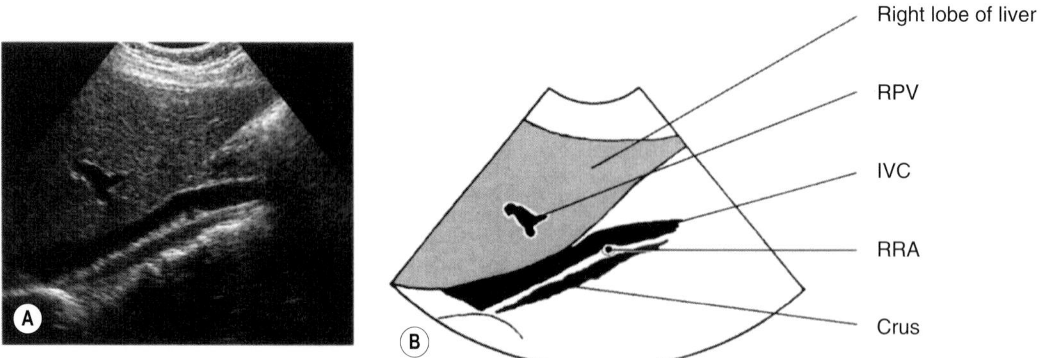

Fig. 2.5 • LS through the right lobe, angled medially towards the IVC.

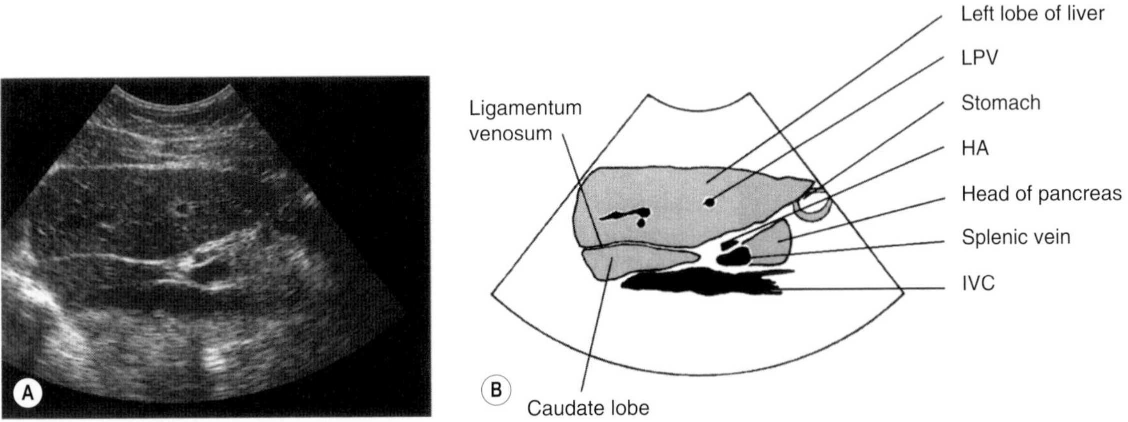

Fig. 2.6 • LS midline, through the left lobe, angled right towards the IVC.

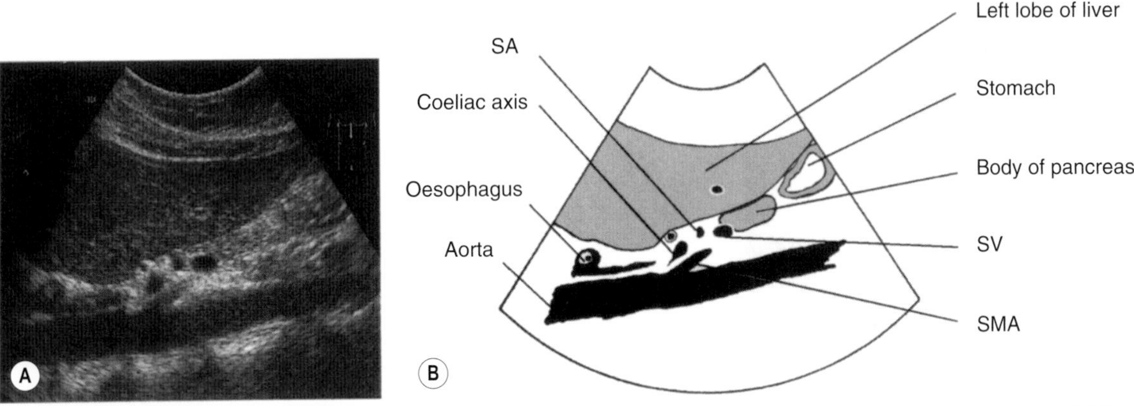

Fig. 2.7 • LS through the midline.

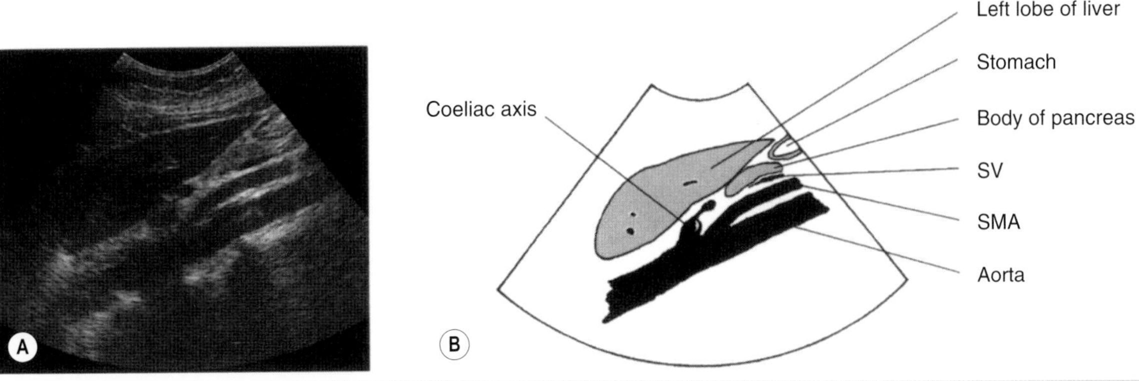

Fig. 2.8 • LS just to the left of midline.

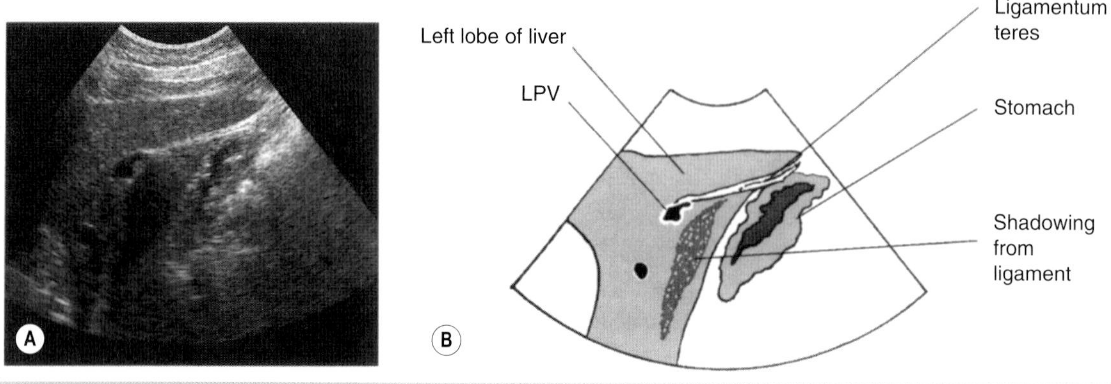

Fig. 2.9 • LS, left lobe of liver.

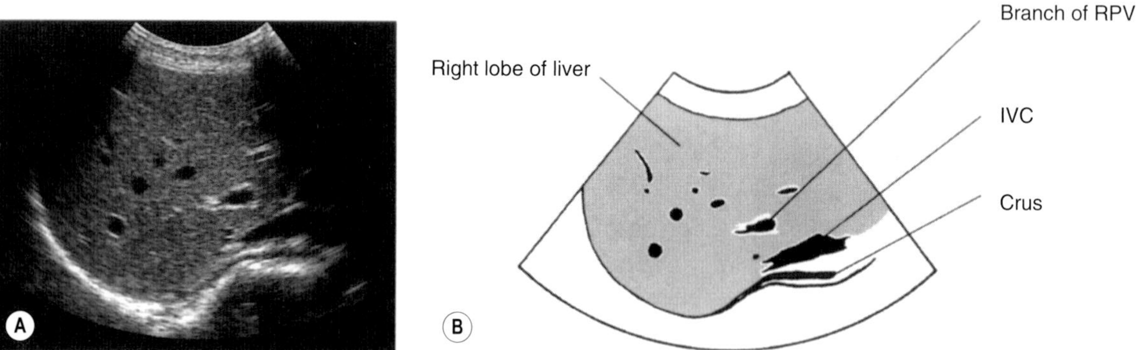

Fig. 2.10 • TS through the liver, above the confluence of the hepatic veins.

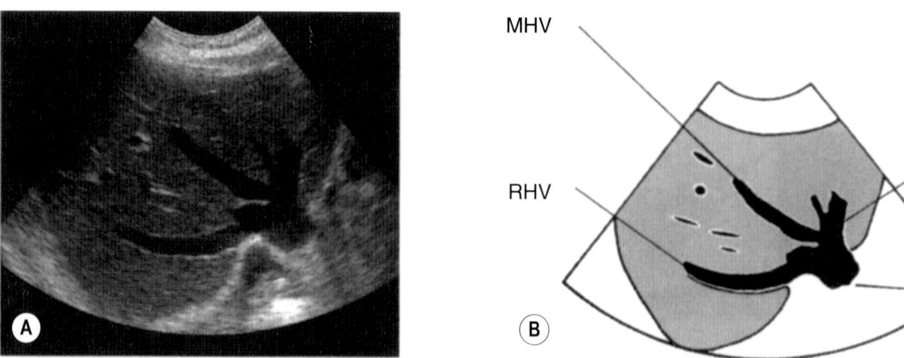

Fig. 2.11 • TS at the confluence.

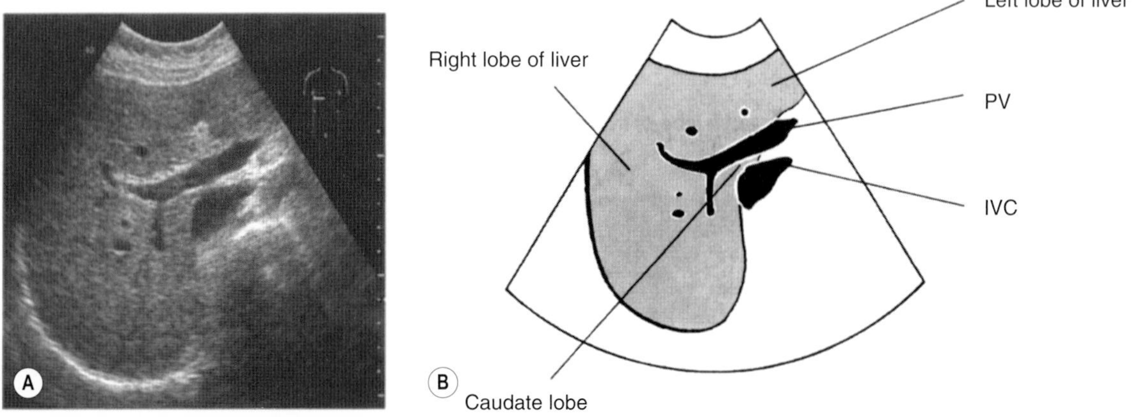

Fig. 2.12 • TS at the porta hepatis.

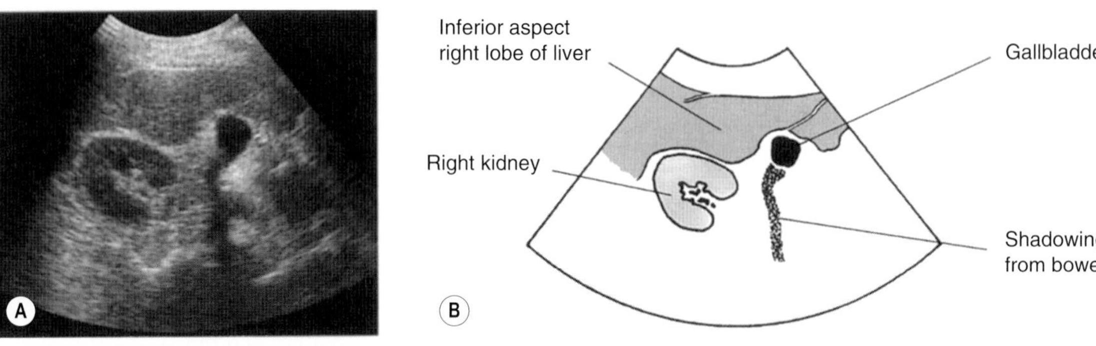

Fig. 2.13 • TS through the right kidney.

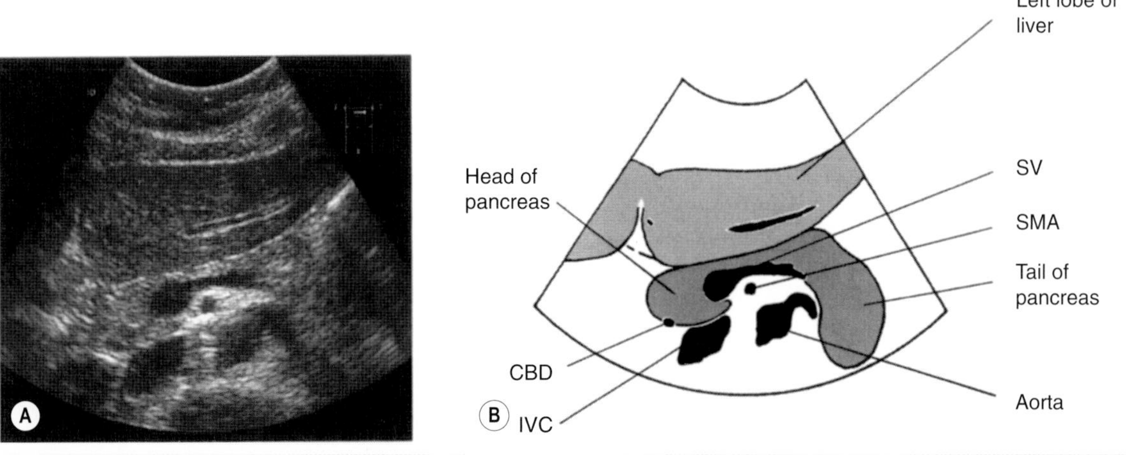

Fig. 2.14 • TS at the epigastrium.

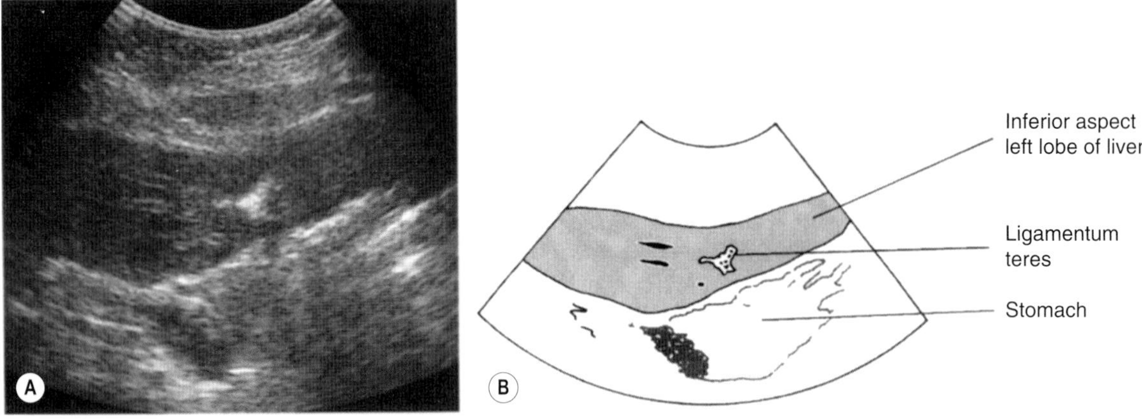

Fig. 2.15 • TS at the inferior edge of the left lobe.

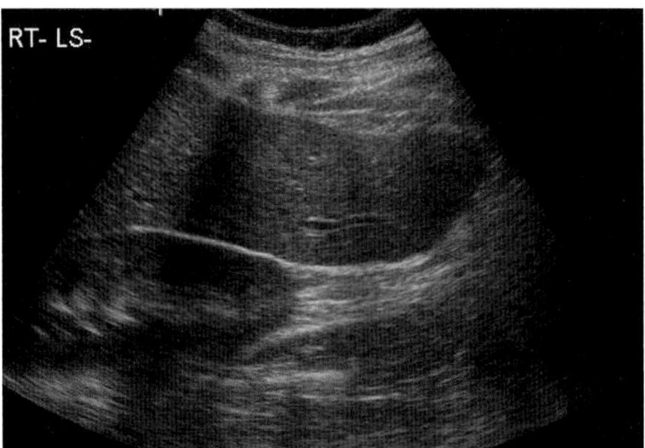

Fig. 2.16 • LS through the right lobe, demonstrating a Reidel's lobe extending below the right kidney. (Compare with the normal liver in Figure 2.1).

diagnoses. However, when a focal lesion is identified, especially if it may be malignant, it is useful to locate it precisely in terms of the surgical segments. This allows subsequent correlation with other imaging, such as computed tomography (CT) or magnetic resonance imaging (MRI), and is invaluable in planning surgical procedures.

The segmental anatomy system, proposed by Couinaud in 1900,[2] divides the liver into eight segments, numbered in a clockwise direction. They are divided by the portal and hepatic veins and the system is used by surgeons today when planning surgical procedures (Fig. 2.17). This system is also used when localizing lesions with CT and MRI.

Identifying the different segments on ultrasound requires the operator to form a mental three-dimensional (3D) image of the liver. The dynamic nature of ultrasound, together with the variation in planes of scan, make this more difficult to do than for CT or MRI. However, segmental localization of hepatic lesions by an experienced operator can be as accurate with ultrasound as with MRI.[3] Systematic scanning through the liver, in transverse section, identifies the main landmarks of the hepatic veins (Fig. 2.11) separating segments VII, VIII, IV and II in the superior part of the liver. As the transducer is moved inferiorly, the portal vein appears, below which segments V and VI are located.

Hepatic vasculature

The portal veins radiate from the porta hepatis, where the main portal vein (MPV) enters the liver (Fig. 2.18). The veins are encased by the hyperechoic, fibrous walls of the portal tracts, which make them stand out from the rest of the parenchyma. Also contained in the portal tracts are a branch of the hepatic artery (HA) and a biliary duct radicle. These latter vessels are too small to detect by ultrasound in the peripheral parts of the liver, but can readily be demonstrated in the larger, proximal branches (Fig. 2.19).

At the porta, the hepatic artery generally crosses the anterior aspect of the portal vein, with the common duct anterior to this (Fig. 2.20). In a common variation the artery lies anterior to the duct. Peripherally, the relationship between the vessels in the portal tracts is variable (Fig. 2.21).

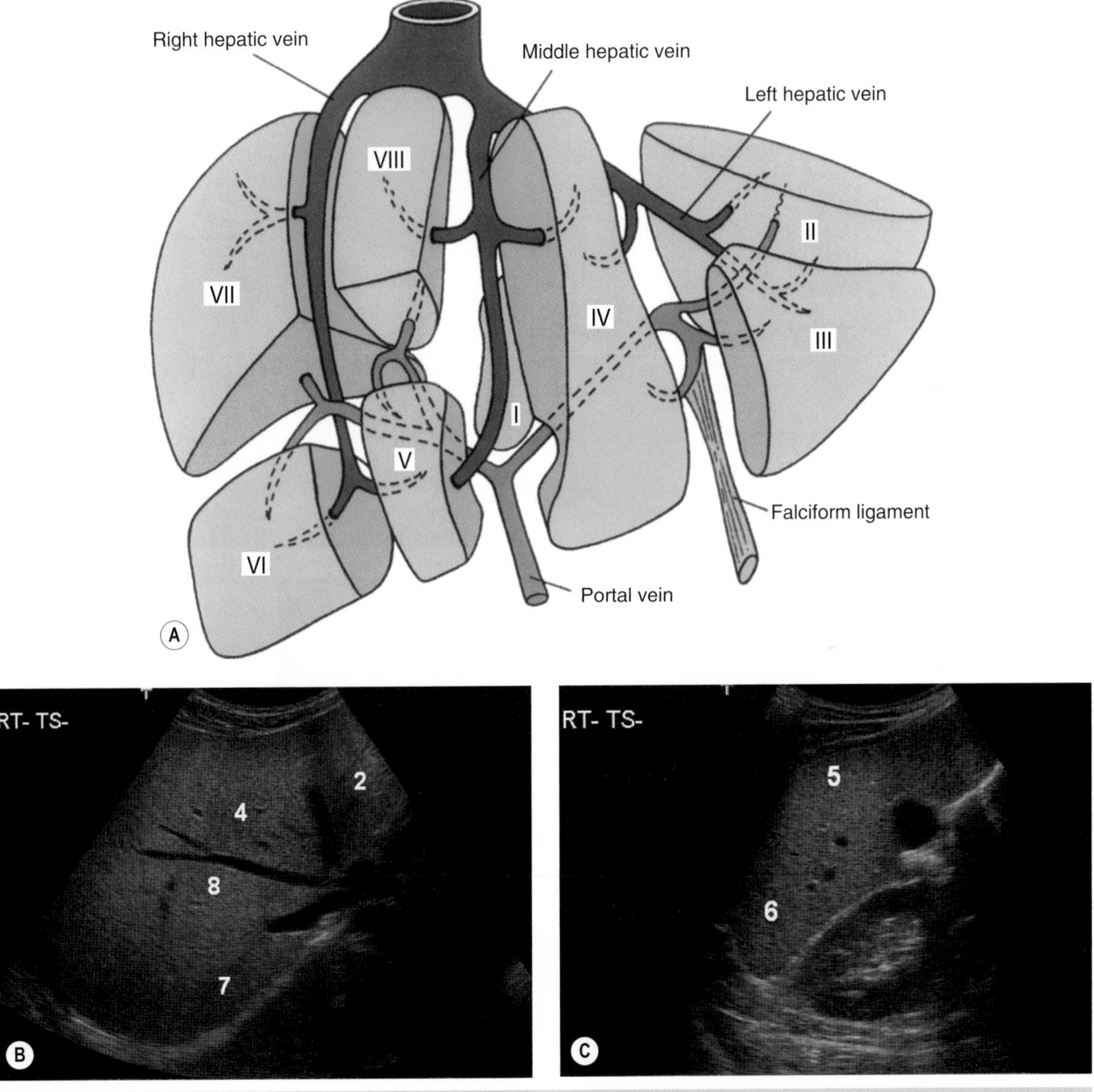

Fig. 2.17 • (A) The surgical segments of the liver (after Couinaud[1]). (B & C) Segmental anatomy in TS of the liver.

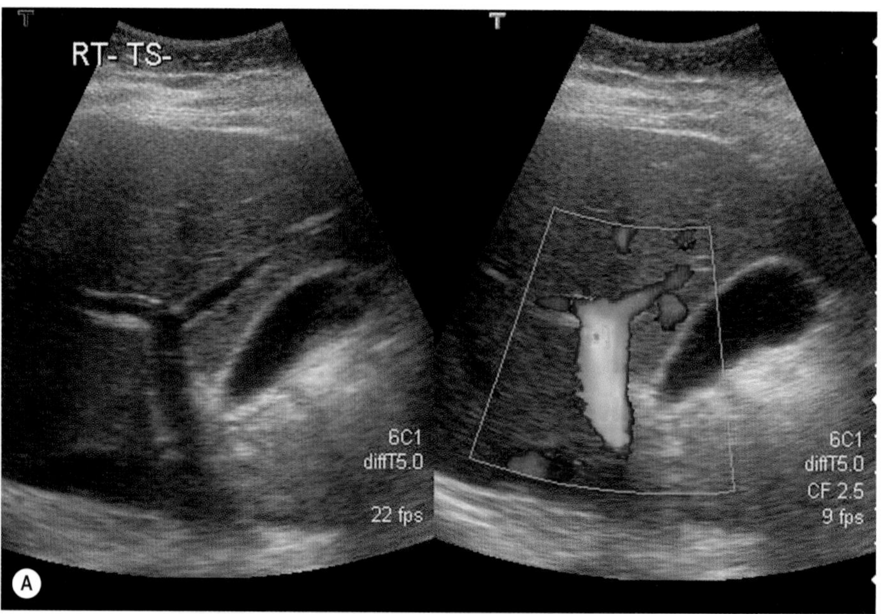

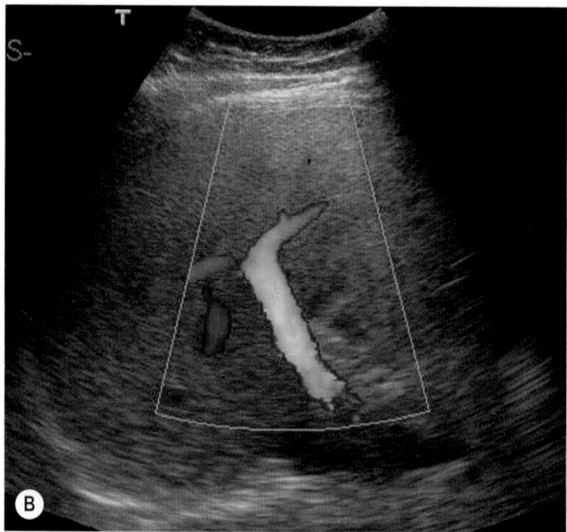

Fig. 2.18 • (A) The right and left branches of the portal vein. (B) Colour Doppler demonstrates the MPV and LPV in red, and the RPV in blue, due to the relative direction of flow to the beam.

The three main hepatic veins, left (LHV), middle (MHV) and right (RHV), can be traced into the IVC at the superior margin of the liver (Fig. 2.11). Their course runs, therefore, approximately perpendicular to the portal vessels – so a section of liver with a longitudinal image of a hepatic vein is likely to contain a transverse section through a portal vein, and vice versa. Unlike the portal tracts, the hepatic veins do not have a fibrous sheath and their walls are therefore less reflective. Maximum reflectivity of the vessel walls occurs with the beam perpendicular (Fig. 2.22).

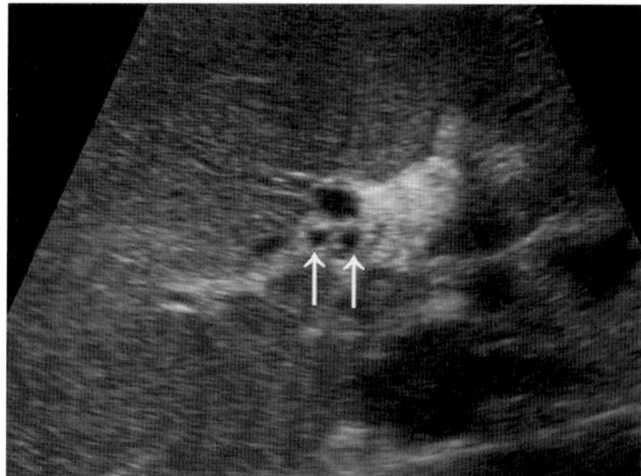

Fig. 2.19 • The portal vein radicle is associated with a branch of the hepatic artery and a biliary duct (arrows) within the hyperechoic fibrous sheath.

The anatomy of the hepatic venous confluence varies. In most cases the single, main RHV flows directly into the IVC, and the middle and left have a common trunk. In 15–35% of patients the LHV and MHV are separate. This usually has no significance to the operator. However, it may be a significant factor in planning and performing hepatic surgery, especially tumour resection, as the surgeon attempts to retain as much viable hepatic tissue as possible with intact venous outflow[4] (Fig. 2.23).

Haemodynamics of the liver

Pulsed and colour Doppler are important tools in understanding and diagnosing the extent of many disease processes. Doppler of the portal venous and hepatic vascular systems gives information on the patency, velocity and direction of flow. The appearance of the various spectral waveforms relates to the downstream resistance of the vascular bed (see Chapter 1).

Doppler should always be used in conjunction with the real-time image and in the context of the patient's presenting symptoms. Used in isolation

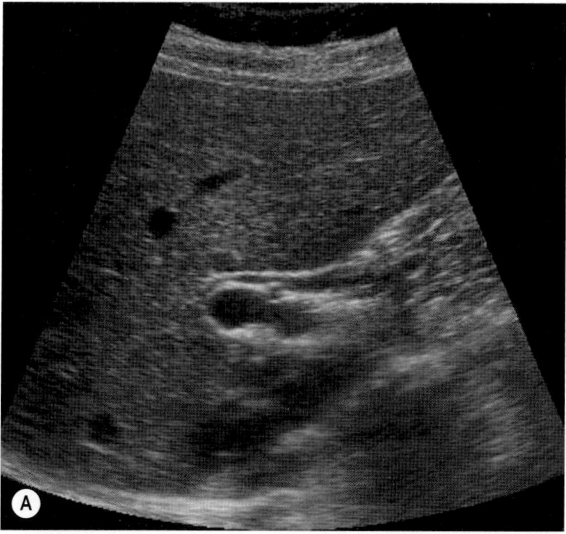

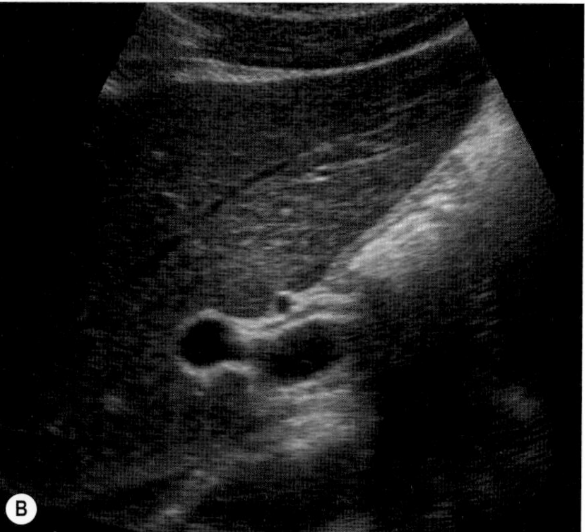

Fig. 2.20 • (A) The porta hepatis. (B) A variant with the hepatic artery anterior to the duct.

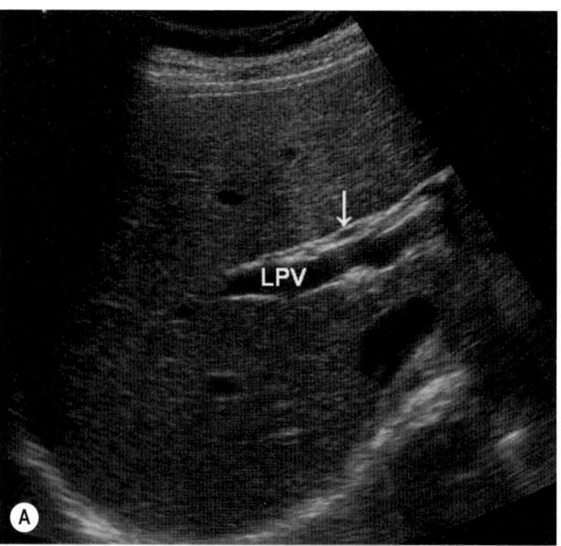

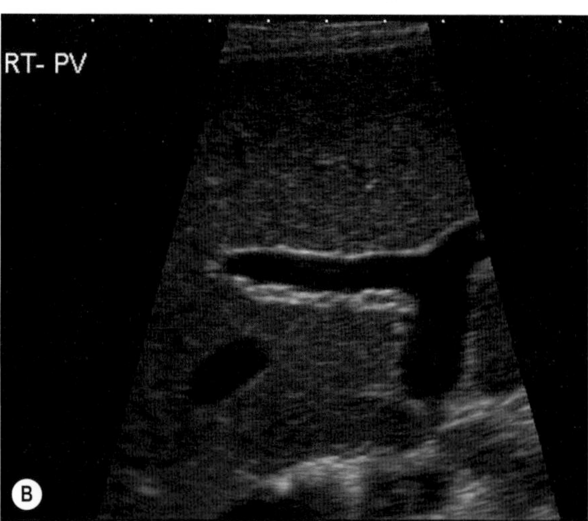

Fig. 2.21 • The relationship of the biliary duct to the portal vein varies as the vessels become more peripheral. In (A) the duct (arrow) lies anterior to the left portal vein, in (B) the duct is posterior to the RPV.

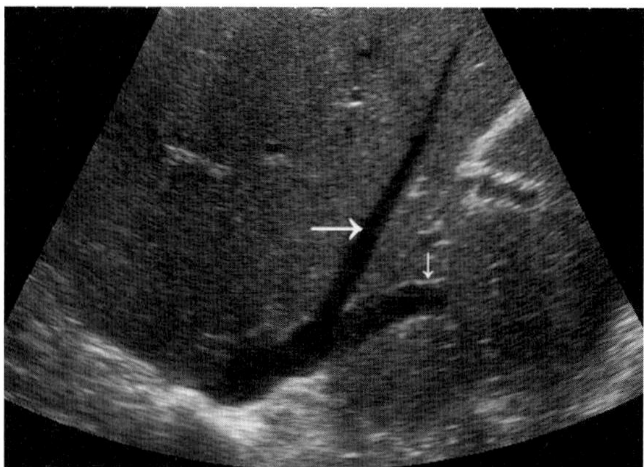

Fig. 2.22 • Hepatic vein walls are less prominent than PV tract walls (large arrow). When the beam is perpendicular to the wall, as in this branch of the LHV (small arrow) it is reflective.

it can be highly misleading. Familiarity with the normal Doppler spectra is an integral part of the upper abdominal ultrasound scan.

THE PORTAL VENOUS SYSTEM

Colour Doppler is used to identify blood flow in the splenic and portal veins (Figs 2.24, 2.25). The direction of flow is normally hepatopetal, i.e. towards the liver. The main, right and left portal branches can best be imaged by using a right oblique approach through the ribs, so that the course of the vessel is roughly towards the transducer, maintaining a low angle (<60°) with the beam for the best Doppler signal.

The normal portal vein diameter is highly variable but does not usually exceed 16 mm in a resting state on quiet respiration.[5] The diameter increases with deep inspiration and also in response to food and to posture changes. An increased diameter may also be associated with portal hypertension in chronic liver disease (see Chapter 4). An absence of postprandial increase in diameter is also a sign of portal hypertension.

The normal portal vein waveform is monophasic (Fig. 2.26) with gentle undulations which are due to respiratory modulation and cardiac activity. This characteristic is a sign of the normal, flexible nature of the liver and may be lost in some fibrotic diseases.

The mean portal vein velocity is normally between 12 cm/s and 20 cm/s[6] but the normal range is wide. (A low velocity is associated with portal hypertension. High velocities are unusual, but can be due to anastomotic stenoses in transplant patients.)

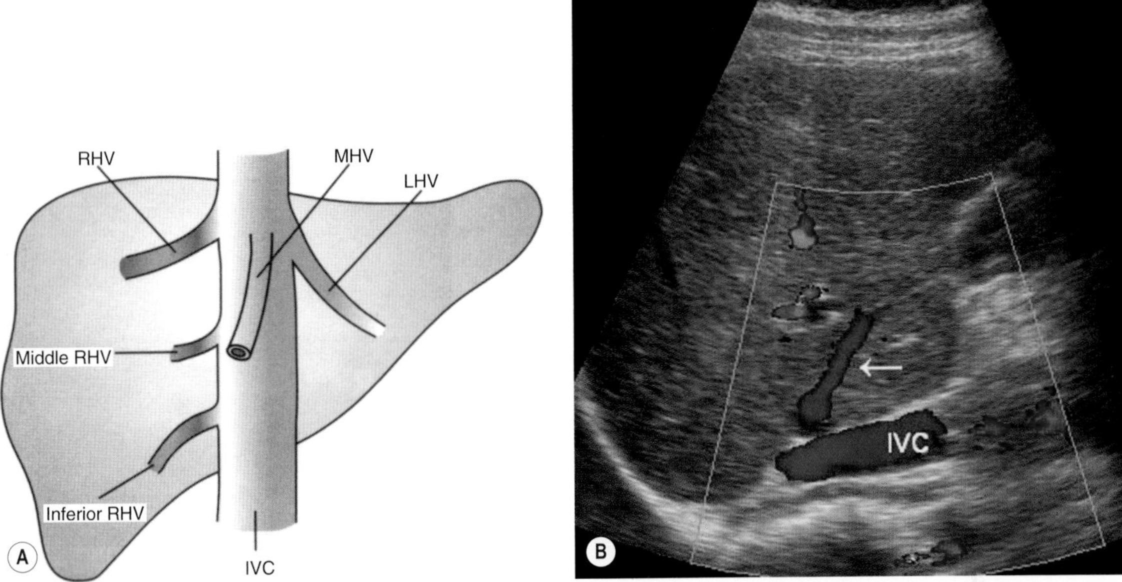

Fig. 2.23 • (A) Configuration of the hepatic venous system. (B) Inferior middle hepatic vein (arrow) draining into the IVC.

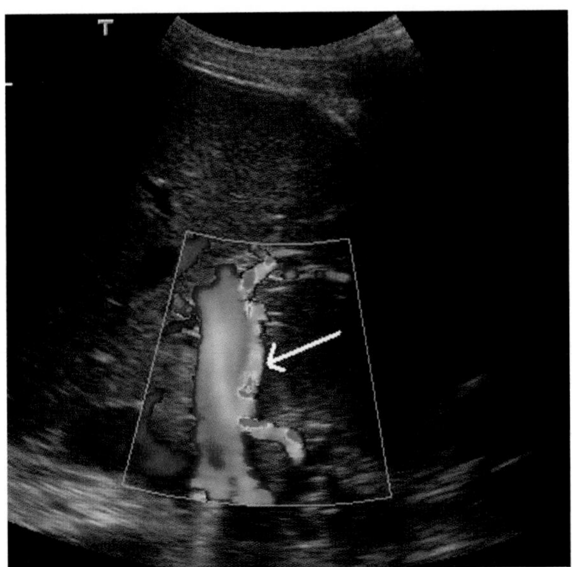

Fig. 2.24 • Main portal vein at the porta hepatis demonstrating hepatopetal flow. The higher velocity hepatic artery lies adjacent to the MPV (arrow).

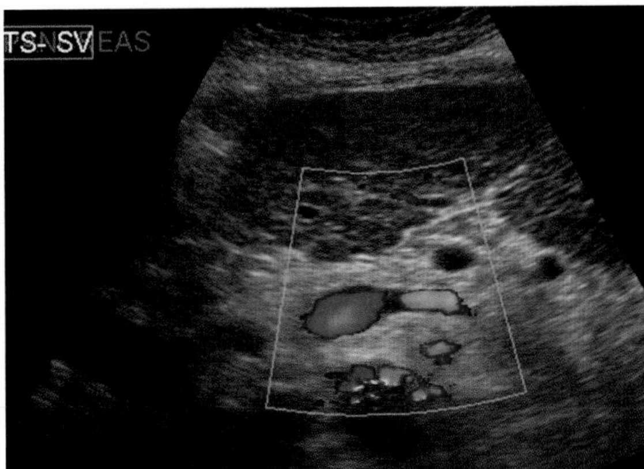

Fig. 2.25 • TS through the epigastrium demonstrating the normal splenic vein with flow towards the liver. Note the change from red to blue as the vessel curves away from the transducer.

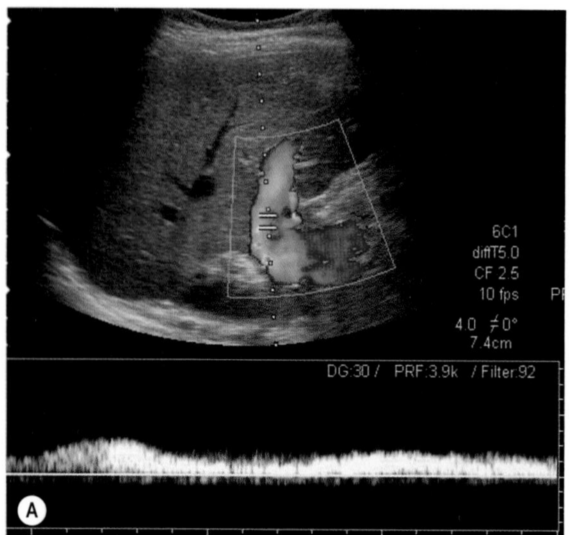

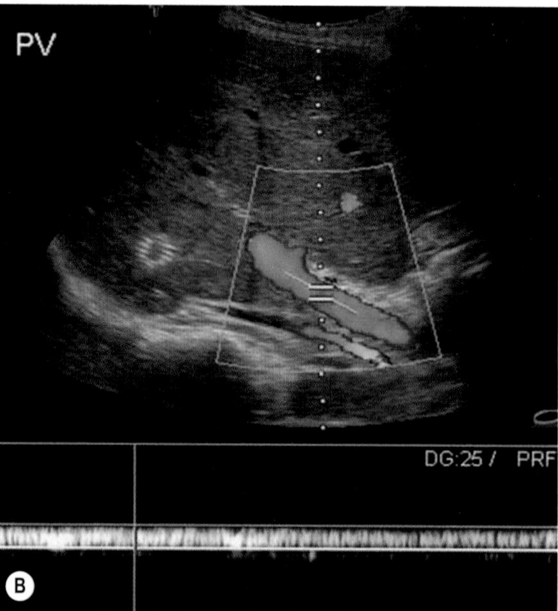

Fig. 2.26 • Normal PV waveform. (A) Respiratory modulations are evident. (B) PV velocity can be measured by using the angle corrector line in the spectral sampling box to indicate direction of flow.

The hepatic veins

The hepatic veins drain the liver into the IVC, which leads into the right atrium. Two factors shape the hepatic venous spectrum; the flexible nature of the normal liver, which can expand easily to accommodate blood flow, and the close proximity of the right atrium, which causes a brief 'kick' of blood back into the liver during atrial systole (Fig. 2.27). This causes the spectrum to be triphasic. The veins can be seen on colour Doppler to be predominantly blue with a brief red flash during atrial contraction.

Various factors cause alterations to this waveform – heart conditions, liver diseases and extrahepatic conditions which compress the liver, such as ascites. Abnormalities of the hepatic vein waveform are therefore highly unspecific and should be taken in context with the clinical picture. As you might expect, the pulsatile nature of the spectrum decreases towards the periphery of the liver, remote from the IVC.

The hepatic artery

The main hepatic artery arises from the coeliac axis and carries oxygenated blood to the liver from the aorta. Its origin makes it a pulsatile vessel and the relatively low resistance of the hepatic vascular bed means that there is continuous forward flow throughout the cardiac cycle (Fig. 2.28). In a normal subject the hepatic artery may be elusive on colour Doppler due to its small diameter and tortuous course. Use the MPV as a marker, scanning from the right intercostal space to maintain a low angle with the vessel. The hepatic artery is just anterior to this and of a higher velocity (i.e. it has a paler colour of red on the colour map, see Fig. 2.24).

THE GALLBLADDER

The normal gallbladder is best visualized after fasting, to distend it. It should have a hyperechoic, thin wall (<2 mm) and contain anechoic bile (Fig. 2.29). Measure the wall thickness in a longitudinal section of the gallbladder, with the calipers perpendicular to the wall itself. (A transverse section may not be perpendicular to the wall, and can overestimate the thickness.)

After fasting for around 6 hours, the gallbladder should be distended with bile into an elongated pear-shaped sac. The size is too variable to allow direct measurements to be of any use, but a tense,

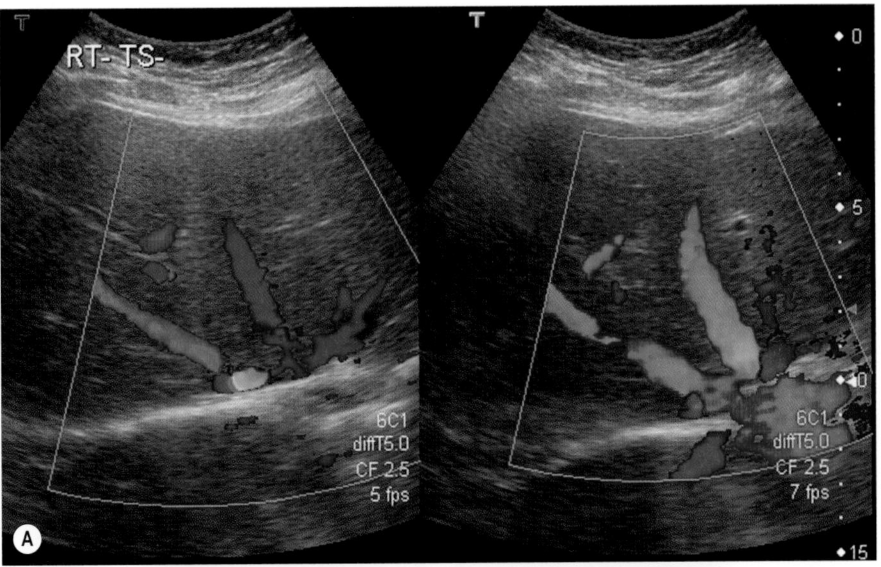

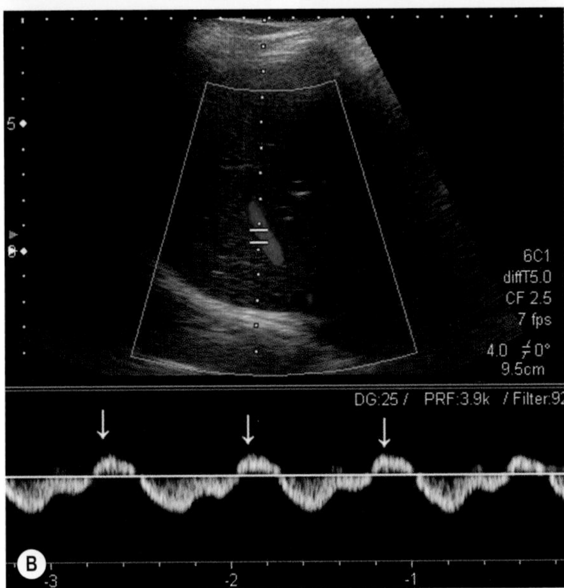

Fig. 2.27 • (A) The confluence of the right, middle and left hepatic veins with the IVC. Flow is predominantly hepatofugal – indicated by the blue colour in the left hand image, but briefly reverses under the influence of atrial systole – indicated in red in the right hand image. (B) This is demonstrated by the normal triphasic waveform. Atrial systole appears as hepatopetal flow (arrows).

rounded shape can indicate pathological, rather than physiological dilatation. Because the size, shape and position of the gallbladder are infinitely variable, so are the techniques required to scan it. There are, however, a number of useful pointers to maximize visualization of the gallbladder:

- Use the highest frequency possible – 5.0 Mhz or higher is especially useful for anterior gallbladders.
- Use a high line density to pick up tiny stones or polyps. (Reduce the sector angle and the frame rate if possible.) Make sure

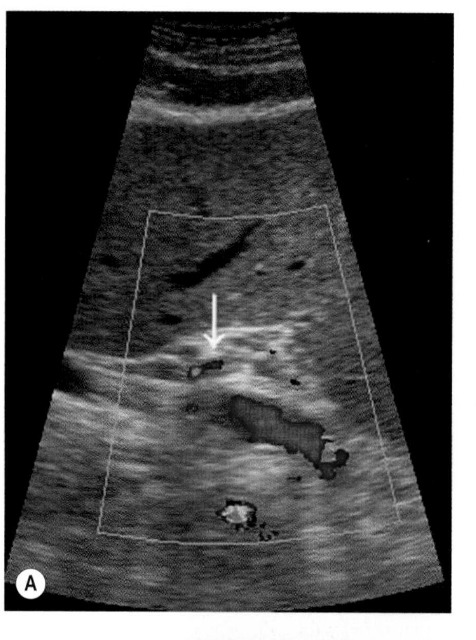

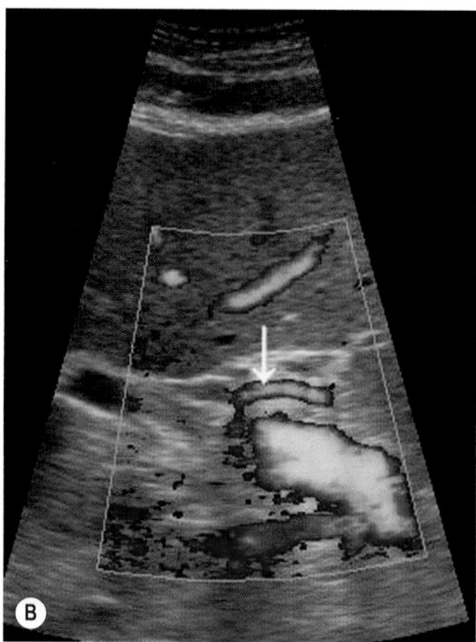

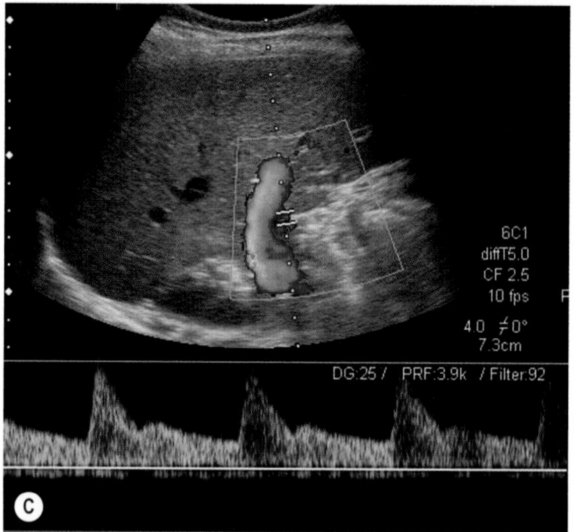

Fig. 2.28 • (A) The hepatic artery may be difficult to locate with colour Doppler, especially if the vessel is perpendicular to the beam. (B) Power Doppler is less angle-dependent and demonstrates the artery (arrow). (C) The normal HA waveform demonstrates a relatively high velocity systolic peak with good forward end-diastolic flow (EDF).

the focal zone is set over the back wall of the gallbladder to maximize your chances of identifying small stones (see Chapters 1 and 3).

- Alter the TGC to eliminate or minimize anterior artefacts and reverberation echoes inside the gallbladder, particularly in the near field.
- Use tissue harmonic imaging to reduce artefact within the gallbladder and sharpen the image of the wall (particularly in a large abdomen).
- Always scan the gallbladder in at least two planes (find the gallbladder's long axis, incorporating the neck and fundus; sweep from side to side, then transversely from

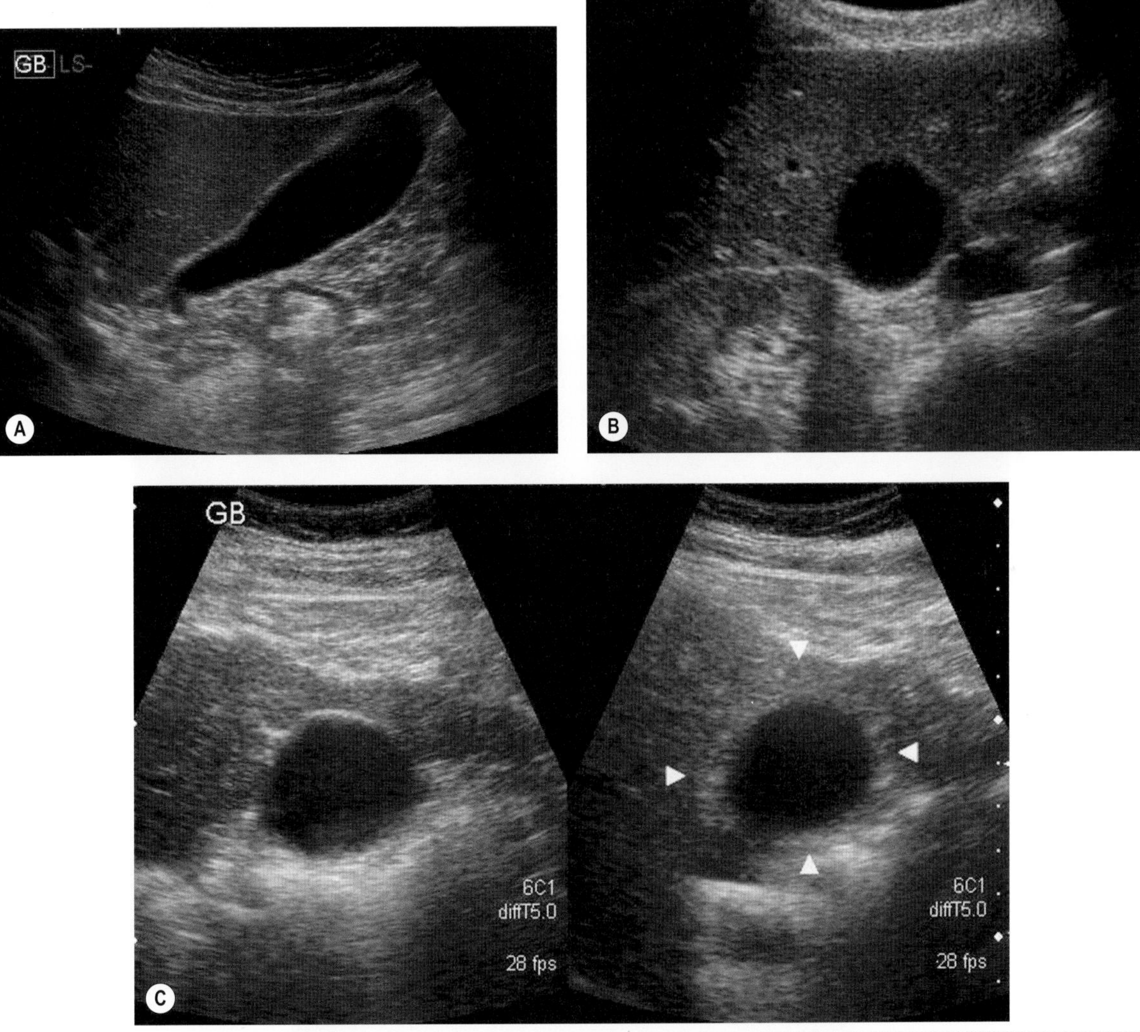

Fig. 2.29 • The gallbladder: (A) LS, (B) TS. (C) False appearance of wall thickening is apparent on the right hand image (arrowheads) when the angle of insonation is not perpendicular to the gallbladder wall. The left hand image shows that the wall is normal.

neck to fundus) and two patient positions. You will almost certainly miss pathology if you do not.

- The gallbladder may be 'folded' (the so-called Phrygian cap). To interrogate its contents fully, unfold it by turning the patient decubitus (right side raised), almost prone or erect (Fig. 2.30).
- Bowel gas over the fundus can also be moved by various patient positions.

Normal variants of the gallbladder

The mesenteric attachment of the gallbladder to the inferior surface of the liver is variable in length. This gives rise to large variations in position; at one end of the spectrum the gallbladder, attached only at the neck, may be fairly remote from the liver, even lying in the pelvis; at the other the gallbladder fossa deeply invaginates the liver and the gallbladder appears to lie 'intrahepatically' enclosed on all sides by liver tissue.

The presence of a true septum in the gallbladder is rare. A folded gallbladder frequently gives the impression of a septum but this can be distinguished by positioning the patient to unfold the gallbladder. Occasionally a gallbladder septum completely divides the lumen into two parts. True gallbladder duplication is a rare entity (Fig. 2.31) and it is important not to mistake this for a gallbladder with a pericholecystic collection in a symptomatic patient. Occasionally the gallbladder is absent altogether.

Pitfalls in scanning the gallbladder

- If the gallbladder cannot be found:
  - Check for previous surgery – evidence of laparoscopic surgery may be difficult to see in the darkened scanning room

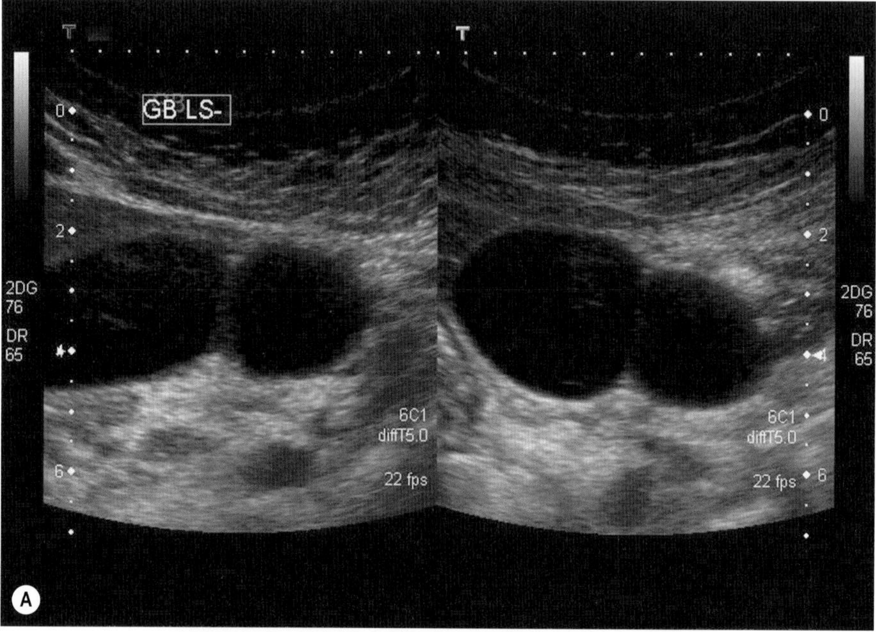

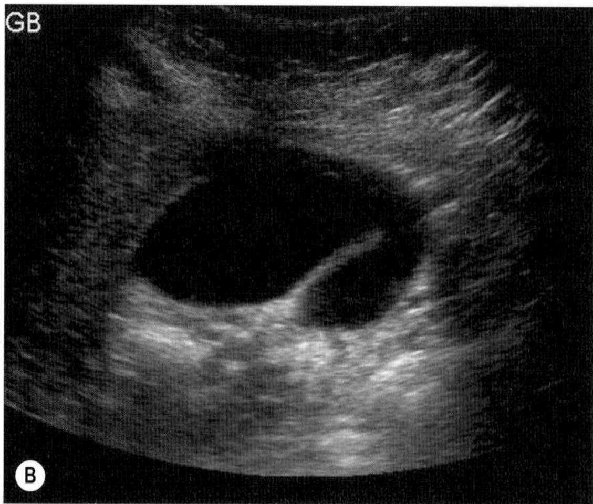

Fig. 2.30 • (A) A folded gallbladder is difficult to examine with the patient supine, and the fold may mimic a septation. (B) Scanning from a different angle (coronally) demonstrates the true nature of the folded gallbladder.

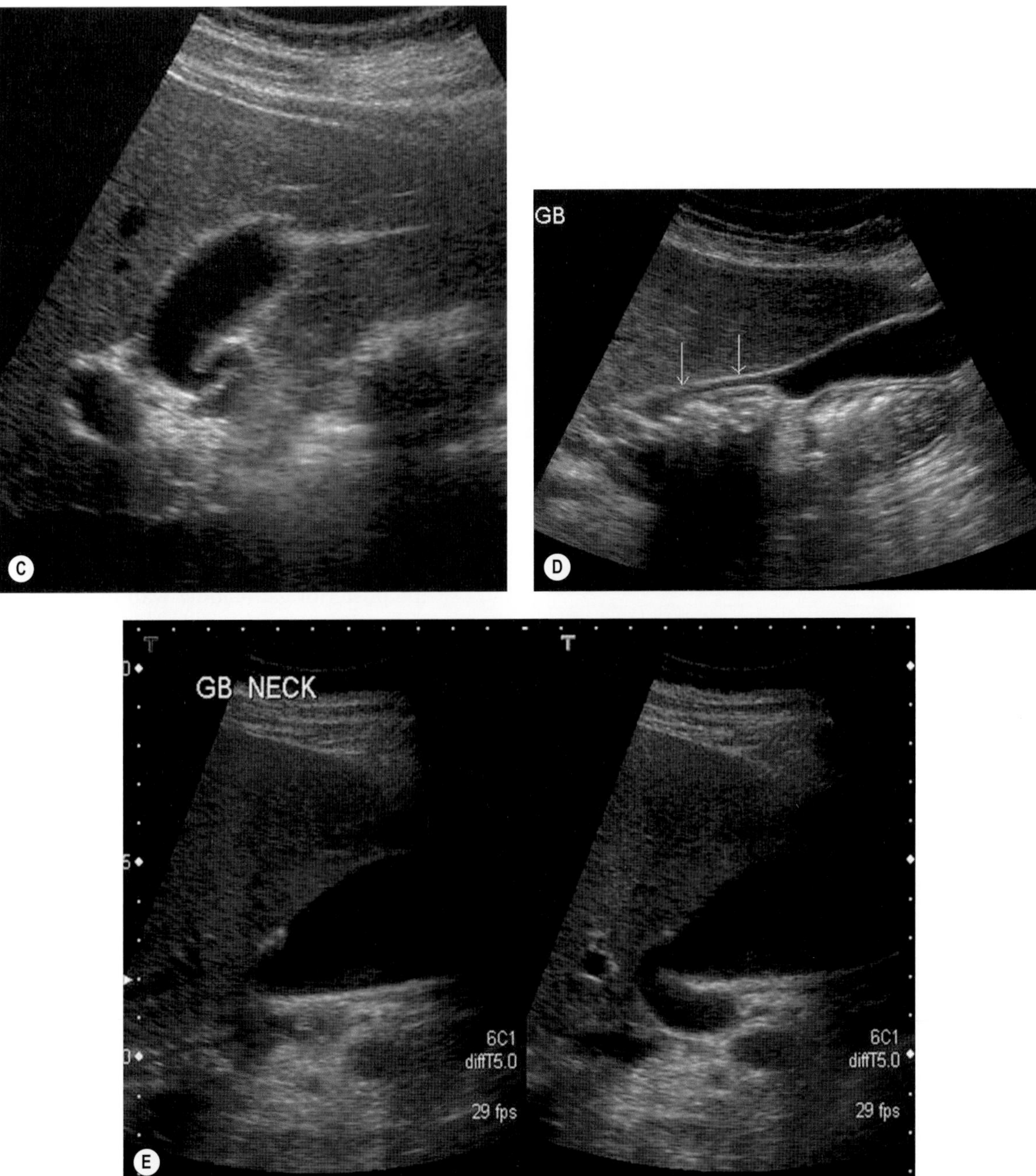

Fig. 2.30, cont'd • (C) Many gallbladder necks can be tortuous, potentially hiding pathology. (D) Turning the patient decubitus, right side raised, unfolds the gallbladder, enabling the neck to be fully examined (arrows). (E) The unwary operator may miss the neck of gallbladder altogether (left hand image) if not aware that it is folded back (right hand image); always ensure the technique used is comprehensive, rather than simply aimed at getting images.

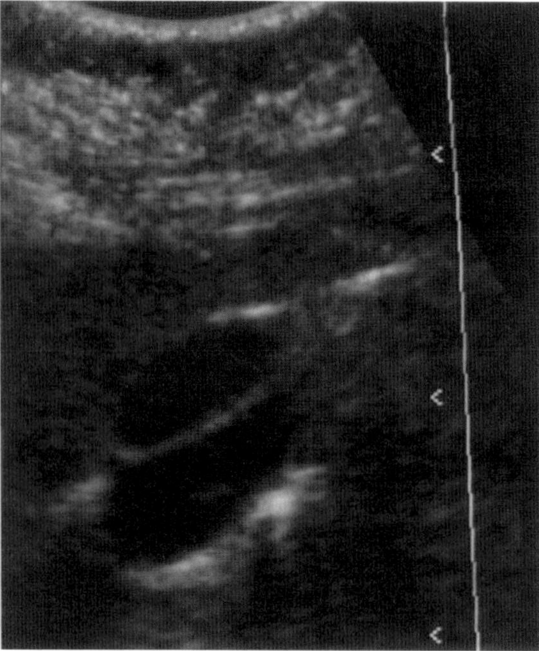

Fig. 2.31 • Double gallbladder: an incidental finding in a young woman.

- Check the patient has fasted
- Look for an ectopic gallbladder – positioned low in the pelvis for example
- Check that near-field artefact has not obscured an anterior gallbladder – a particular problem in very thin patients.

If you still cannot find it, ensure the scanner frequency and settings are optimized, find the porta hepatis and scan just below it in transverse section. This is the area of the gallbladder fossa and you should see at least the anterior gallbladder wall if the gallbladder is present (Fig. 2.32).

- A contracted, stone-filled gallbladder, producing heavy shadowing, can be difficult to identify due to the lack of any contrasting fluid in the lumen.

True agenesis of the gallbladder is rare.[7]

- Duodenum mimicking gallbladder pathology:
  - The close proximity of the duodenum to the posterior gallbladder wall often causes it to invaginate the gallbladder. Maximize your machine settings to visualize the posterior gallbladder wall separate from the duodenum and turn

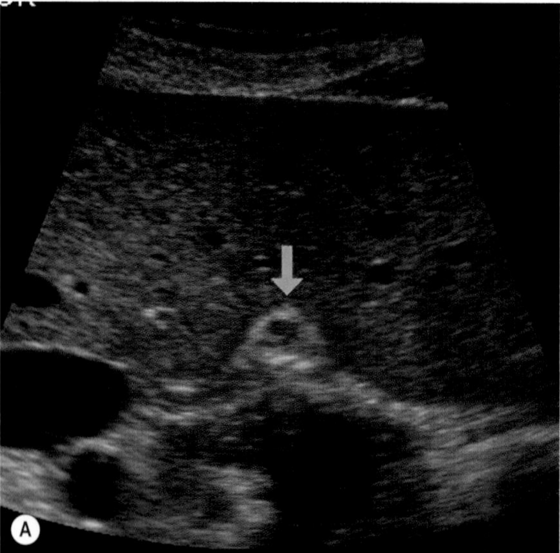

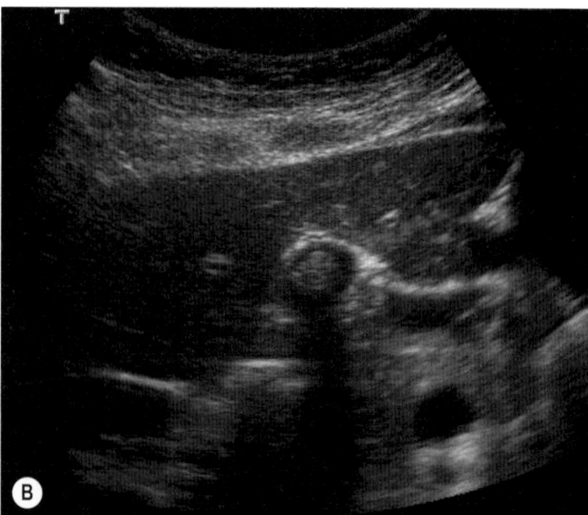

Fig. 2.32 • (A) A postprandial, contracted gallbladder located in the gallbladder fossa on TS. (B) A contracted, stone-filled gallbladder in TS.

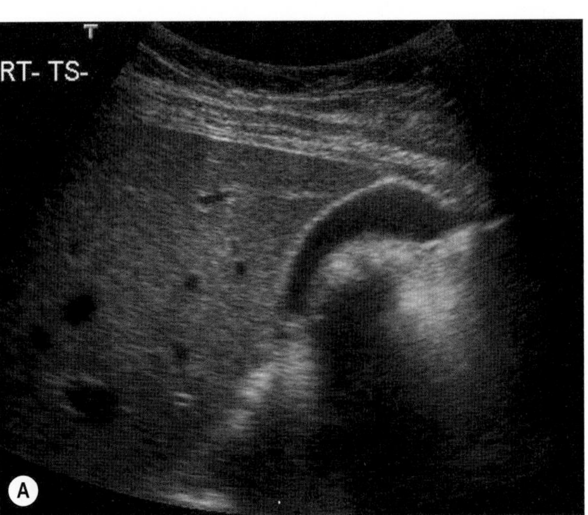

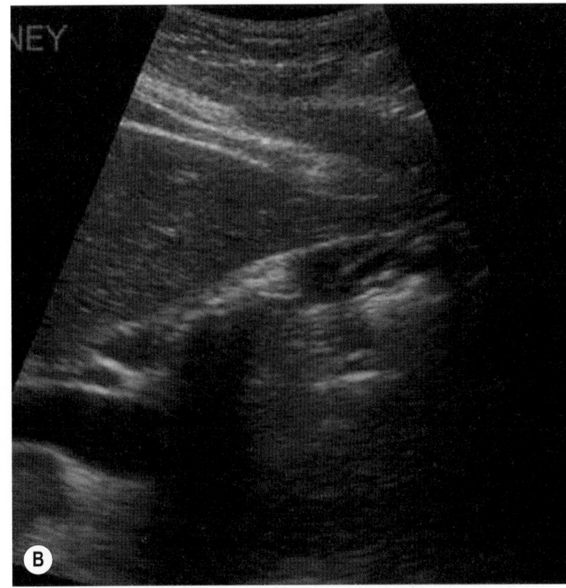

Fig. 2.33 • (A & B) The duodenum frequently invaginates the posterior wall of the gallbladder and may mimic stones if the machine settings are not correctly manipulated.

the patient to cause the duodenal contents to move
    - Other segments of fluid-containing gastrointestinal tract can also cause confusion. (Fig. 2.33).
- Stones that do not shadow:
    - This is likely to be due to poor settings, rather than any lack of stone reflectivity
    - Ensure they are stones and not polyps by positioning the patient erect and watching them move with gravity (beware – polyps on long stalks also move around)
    - The stones may be smaller than the beamwidth, making the shadow difficult to display. Make sure the focal zone is set at the back of the gallbladder
    - Increase the line density, if possible, by reducing the field of view
    - Scan with the highest possible frequency to ensure the narrowest beamwidth
    - Reduce the TGC and/or power to make sure you have not saturated the echoes distal to the gallbladder (see Chapter 3).
- Beware the folded gallbladder ...:
    - You may miss pathology if the gallbladder is folded and the fundus lies underneath bowel. Always try to unfold it by positioning the patient (Fig. 2.30)
    - A fold in the gallbladder may mimic a septum. Septae are comparatively rare and have been overreported in the past due to the presence of folding
- Pathology or artefact?
    - Sometimes the gallbladder may contain some echoes of doubtful significance, or be insufficiently distended to evaluate accurately. A rescan, after a meal followed by further fasting, can be useful. This can flush out sludge, redistending the gallbladder with clear bile. It may also help to clarify any confusing appearances of adjacent bowel loops.

THE BILE DUCTS

The common duct can be easily demonstrated in its intrahepatic portion just anterior and slightly to the right of the portal vein. A cross-section of the main hepatic artery can usually be seen passing between the vein and the duct (Figs 2.20a, 2.34) although a small proportion of hepatic arteries lie anterior to the duct (Fig. 2.20b). At this point it is usually referred to as the common duct, although

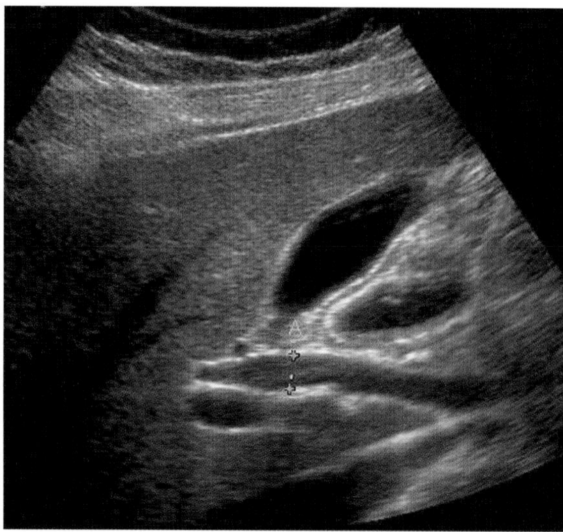

Fig. 2.34 • Normal CBD at the porta hepatis. The lower end is frequently obscured by shadowing from the duodenum. The duct should be measured at its widest portion.

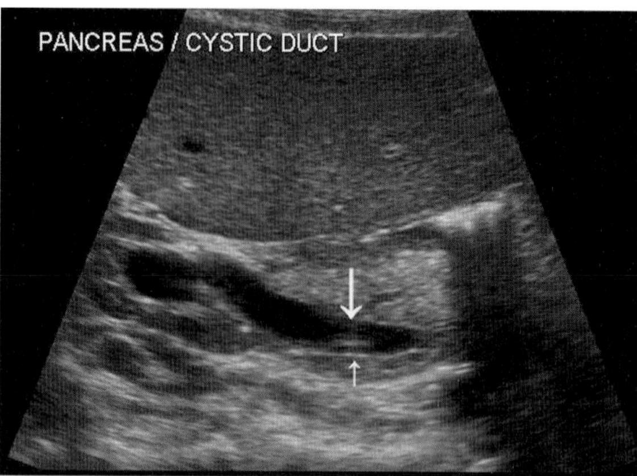

Fig. 2.35 • Visualization of the lower end of the duct often requires the operator to persevere with technique and patient positioning. The normal duct (large arrow) is seen in the head of pancreas. The cystic duct (small arrow) is just visible posterior to the CBD, in an example of an abnormally low insertion, often associated with pancreatitis.

it may, in fact, represent the right hepatic duct[8] rather than the common *bile* duct, because we cannot tell at what point it is joined by the cystic duct.

The extrahepatic portion of the duct is less easy to see as it is often obscured by overlying duodenal gas. Good visualization of the duct usually requires perseverance on the part of the operator. It is insufficient just to visualize the intrahepatic portion of the duct, as early obstruction may be present with a normal calibre intrahepatic duct and dilatation of the distal end (Fig. 2.35).

Bile duct measurements

The internal diameter of the common duct is usually taken as 6 mm or less. It is age dependent, however, and can be 8–9 mm in an elderly person, due to degeneration of the elastic fibre in the duct wall. Ensure this is not early obstruction by thoroughly examining the distal common bile duct (CBD) or rescanning after a short time interval.

The diameter can vary quite considerably, not only between subjects, but along an individual duct. The greatest measurement should be recorded, in longitudinal section. Never measure the duct in a transverse section (for example at the head of pancreas); it is invariably an oblique plane through the duct, which will overestimate the diameter. Intrahepatically, the duct diameter decreases. The right and left hepatic ducts are just visible, but more peripheral branches are usually too small to see.

Patients with a cholecystectomy who have had previous duct dilatation frequently also have a persistently dilated, but non-obstructed, duct (Fig. 2.36). Be suspicious of a diameter of 10 mm or more as this is associated with obstruction due to formation of stones in the duct.

Techniques

The main, right and left hepatic ducts tend to lie anterior to the portal vein branches, however, as the biliary tree spreads out, the position of the duct relative to the portal branches is highly variable. Do not assume that a channel anterior to the portal vein branch is always a biliary duct – if in doubt, use colour Doppler to distinguish the bile duct from the portal vein or hepatic artery.

The proximal bile duct is best seen either with the patient supine, using an intercostal approach from the right, or turning the patient oblique, right side raised. This projects the duct over the portal vein which is used as an anatomic marker.

Scanning the distal duct usually requires more effort. Right oblique or decubitus positions are

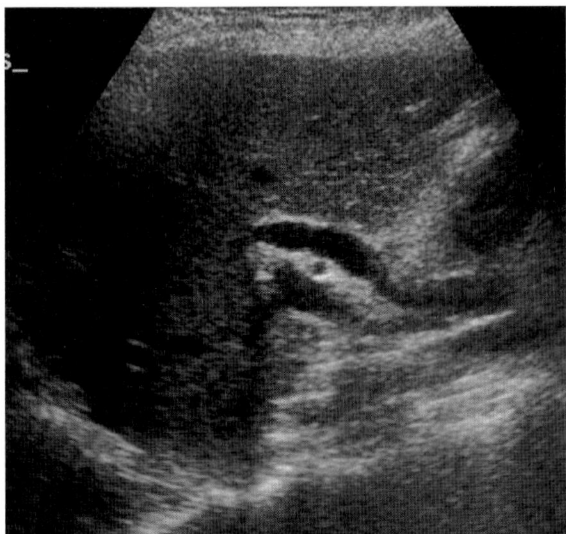

Fig. 2.36 • A persistently, mildly dilated duct post-cholecystectomy (8.5 mm). The duct is baggy, rather than under any pressure, and there is no intrahepatic duct dilatation.

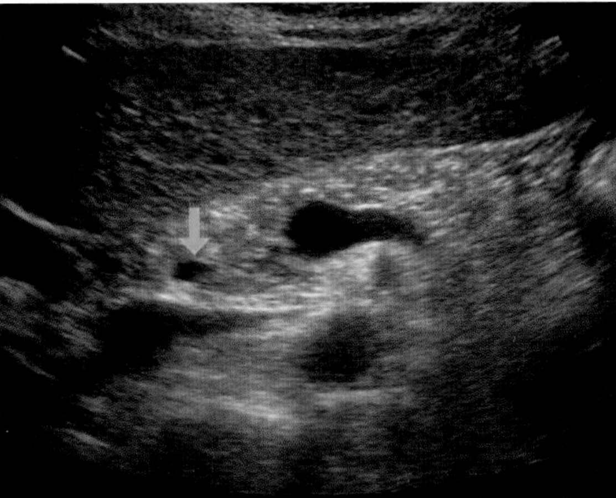

Fig. 2.37 • The common bile duct (arrow) seen in the head of pancreas on TS.

useful. Gentle pressure to ease the duodenal gas away from the duct can also be successful. Sometimes, filling the stomach with water (which also helps to display the pancreas) and allowing it to trickle through the duodenum does the trick. Try also identifying the duct in the pancreatic head (Fig. 2.37) and then tracing it retrogradely, towards the liver. Asking the patient to take deep breaths is occasionally successful, but may make matters worse by filling the stomach with air. It is definitely worth persevering with your technique, particularly in jaundiced patients.

SOME COMMON REFERRAL PATTERNS FOR HEPATO-BILIARY ULTRASOUND

There is an almost infinite number of reasons for performing abdominal ultrasound. Some of the more common referrals are discussed below.

Jaundice

Jaundice is a frequent cause of referral for abdominal ultrasound. It is therefore essential for the sonographer to have a basic understanding of the various mechanisms in order to maximize the diagnostic information from the ultrasound scan. The causes and ultrasound appearances of jaundice are dealt with more fully in Chapters 3 and 4, but an overview is included here.

Jaundice, or *hyperbilirubinaemia,* is an elevated level of bilirubin in the blood. It is recognized by a characteristic yellow colouration of the skin and sclera of the eye, often accompanied by itching if prolonged.

Bilirubin is derived from the haem portion of haemoglobin. Red blood cells are broken down in the liver into haem and globin, releasing their bilirubin which is non-soluble. This is termed *unconjugated bilirubin.* This is then taken up by the liver cells and converted to a water-soluble form – *conjugated bilirubin,* which is excreted via the biliary ducts into the duodenum to aid fat digestion.

By knowing which of these two types of bilirubin is present in the jaundiced patient, the clinician can narrow down the diagnostic possibilities. Ultrasound then further refines the diagnosis (Fig. 2.38).

Jaundice can fall into one of two categories:

- *Obstructive* (sometimes called posthepatic) – in which the bile is prevented from draining out of the liver because of obstruction to the biliary duct(s).
- *Non-obstructive* (prehepatic or hepatic) – in which the elevated bilirubin level is due to haemolysis (the breakdown of the red

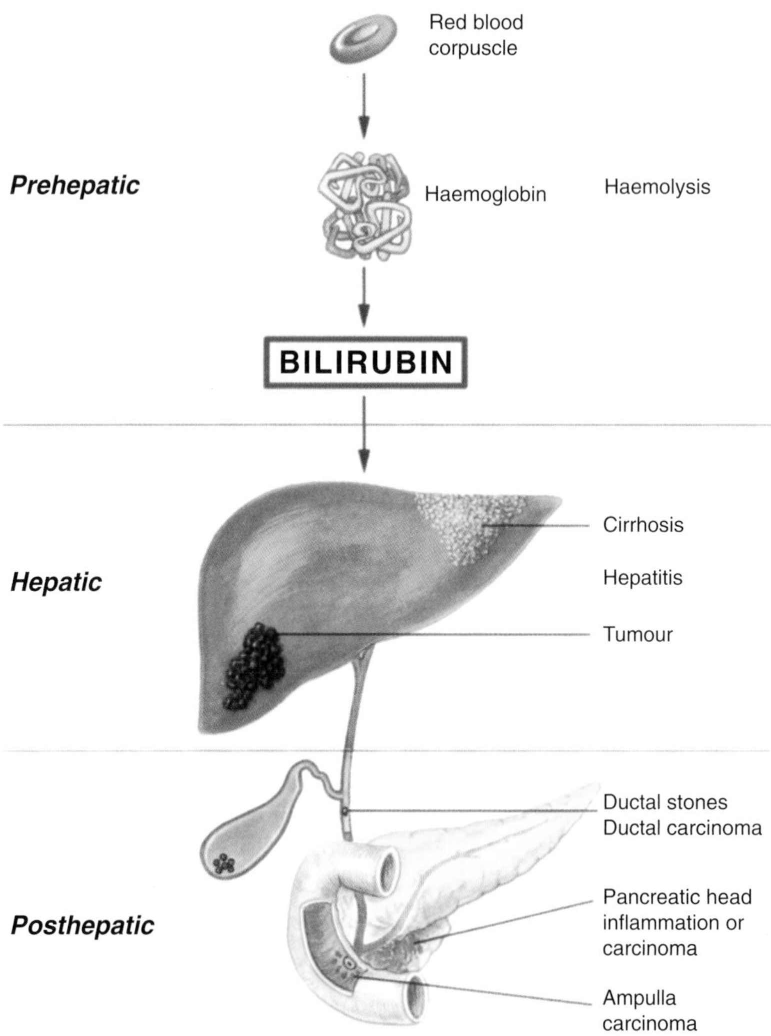

Fig. 2.38 • Some common causes of jaundice.

blood cells) or a disturbance in the mechanism of the liver for uptake and storage of bilirubin, such as in inflammatory or metabolic liver diseases.

Naturally, the treatment of jaundice depends on its cause (Table 2.1). Ultrasound readily distinguishes obstructive jaundice, which demonstrates some degree of biliary duct dilatation, from non-obstructive, which does not.

Abnormal liver function tests

Altered or deranged liver function tests (LFTs) are another frequent cause of referral for abdominal ultrasound. Biochemistry from a simple blood test is often a primary pointer to pathology and is invariably one of the first tests performed as it is quick and easily accessible.

Most of these markers are highly unspecific, being associated with many types of diffuse and focal liver pathology. The most frequently encountered LFTs are listed in Table 2.2.

Other common reasons for referral

Vague, non-specific symptoms, such as pain, require the sonographer to perform a comprehensive and knowledgeable search. The non-invasive nature of ultrasound makes it ideal for the first line investigation.

NON-OBSTRUCTIVE	
Unconjugated hyperbilirubinaemia	Haemolysis
	Haematoma
	Gilbert's disease
Mixed hyperbilirubinaemia	Hepatitis
	Alcoholic liver disease
	Cirrhosis of all types
	Multiple liver metastases
	Drug-induced liver disease
OBSTRUCTIVE	
Conjugated hyperbilirubinaemia	Stones in the biliary duct
	Carcinoma of the duct, head of pancreas or ampulla
	Acute pancreatitis
	Other masses which compress the CBD (eg lymph node mass)
	Biliary atresia

See Chapters 3 and 4 for further information.

Table 2.1 Common causes of jaundice

Box 2.2

Always:

- Take a verbal history from the patient if possible – do not rely on the request information
- Obtain the results of any previous investigations, including previous radiology
- Consider the possibility of multiple pathologies

TEST	ASSOCIATION WITH INCREASED LEVEL
Bilirubin	Obstructive or non-obstructive jaundice. (differentiation can be made between conjugated and unconjugated bilirubin)
Alkaline phosphatase (ALP) (liver enzyme)	Non-obstructive jaundice
	Metastases
	Other focal hepatic lesions
Alpha-fetoprotein	Hepatocellular carcinoma (HCC)
Prothrombin time	Malignancy
	Diffuse liver disease (often with portal hypertension)
Gamma-glutamyl transferase	Obstructive jaundice
	Alcoholic liver disease
Alanine aminotransferase (ALT)	Fatty liver
Aspartate aminotransferase (AST) (liver enzymes)	Obstructive or non-obstructive jaundice
	Hepatitis
	Viral infections
	Other organ failure (e.g. cardiac)
Protein (serum albumin)	Lack of protein is associated with numerous liver diseases. Low levels are associated with ascites, often due to portal hypertension

Table 2.2 Common serum LFTs

Upper abdominal pain

The origin of upper abdominal pain could be linked to any of the organs and it is one of the most frequent causes of referral. The sonographer can narrow the possibilities down by taking a careful history (Box 2.2).

- Is the pain focal? This may direct the sonographer to the relevant organ, for example a thick-walled gallbladder full of stones may be tender on gentle transducer pressure, pointing to acute or chronic

cholecystitis, depending on the severity of the pain.
- Bear in mind that gallstones are a common, incidental finding which may be a red herring. Always consider multiple pathologies.
- Is the pain related to any event which may give a clue? Fat intolerance might suggest a biliary cause; pain on micturition, a urinary tract cause, for example.
- Is it accompanied by other symptoms such as a high temperature? This may be associated with an infective process such as abscess.
- Could it be bowel-related? Generalized abdominal pain could be due to inflammatory or obstructive bowel conditions and knowledge of the patient's bowel habits is helpful.
- Has the patient had any previous surgery which could be significant?

Palpable right upper quadrant mass

This could be due to a renal, hepato-biliary, bowel-related or other cause. The sonographer should gently palpate to get an idea of the size and position of the mass, and whether or not it is tender. Specifically targeting the relevant area may yield useful and unexpected results – for example a Reidel's lobe, colonic carcinoma or impacted faeces – which will help to guide the nature of further investigation and management. Remember to check the chest if you have a palpable liver edge but no obvious pathology – the liver could just be depressed by a large pleural effusion.

References

1. UK Association of Sonographers. Guidelines for professional working standards – ultrasound practice. UKAS, London, 2001
2. Couinaud C. Lobes et segments hepatiques, note sur l'architecture anatomique et chirugicale du foie. Presse Med 1954; 62: 709
3. Conlon RM, Bates JA. Segmental localisation of focal hepatic lesions – a comparison of ultrasound and MRI. Conference proceedings of BMUS, Edinburgh, 1996
4. Cheng Y, Huang T, Chen C et al. Variations of the middle and inferior right hepatic vein: application in hepatectomy. J Clin Ultrasound 1997; 25: 175–182
5. Goyal AK, Pokharna DS, Sharma SK. Ultrasonic measurements of portal vasculature in diagnosis of portal hypertension. J Ultrasound Med 1990; 9: 45
6. Gaiani S, Bolondi L, Li Bassi S et al. Effect of meal on portal hemodynamics in healthy humans and in patients. Hepatology 1989; 9: 815–819
7. Kabiri H, Domingo OH, Tzarnas CD. Agenesis of the gallbladder. Curr Surg 2006; 63: 104–106
8. Davies RP, Downey PR, Moore WR et al. Contrast Cholangiography versus ultrasonographic measurement of the 'extrahepatic' bile duct: a two-fold discrepancy revisited. J Ultrasound Med 1991; 10: 653–657

APPENDIX 2.1: LS THROUGH THE RIGHT LOBE OF THE LIVER (Fig. 2A.1)

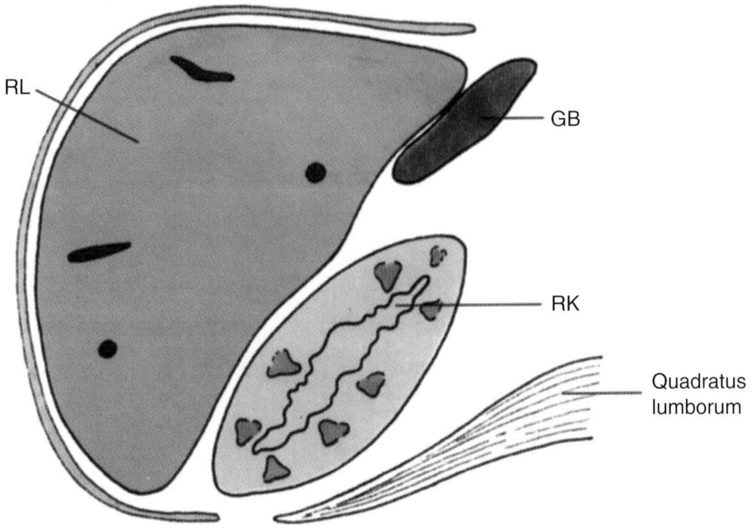

RL
GB
RK
Quadratus lumborum

Fig. 2A.1 • Appendix 2.1: LS through the right lobe of the liver.

APPENDIX 2.2: LS THROUGH THE IVC (Fig. 2A.2)

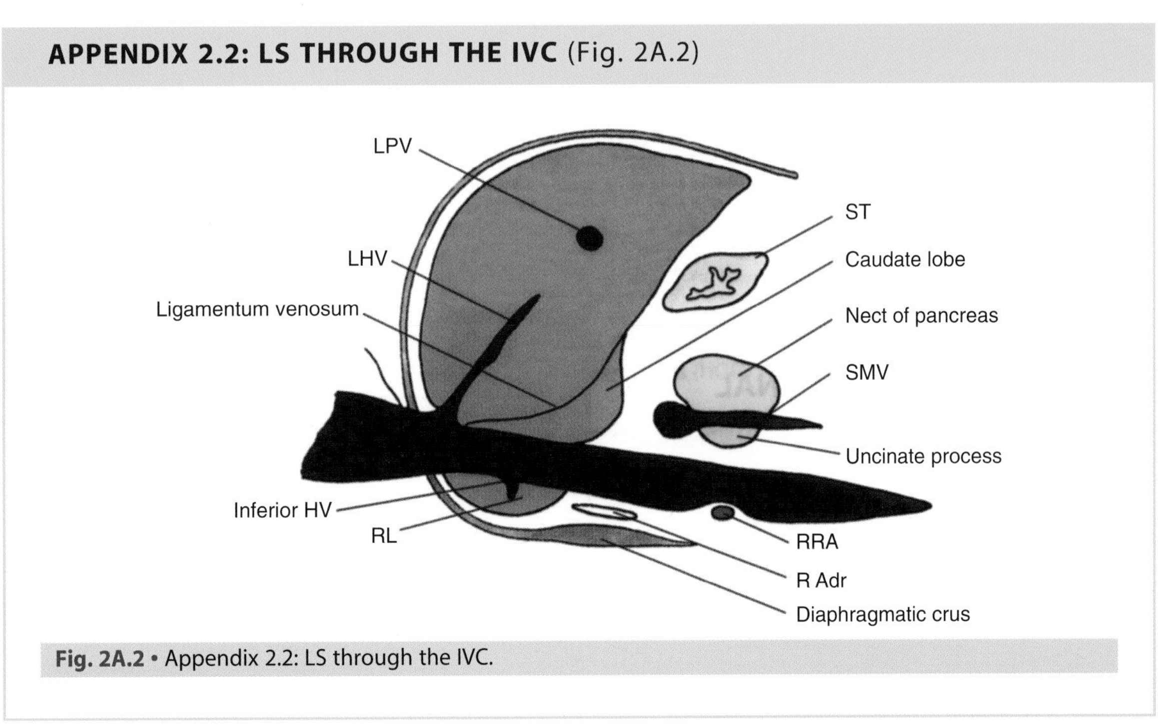

Fig. 2A.2 • Appendix 2.2: LS through the IVC.

APPENDIX 2.3: LS THROUGH THE MIDLINE, LEVEL OF THE AORTA (Fig. 2A.3)

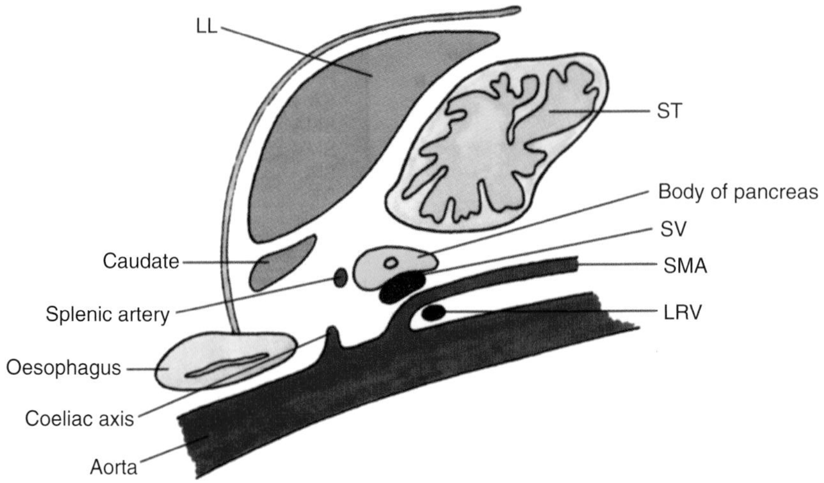

Fig. 2A.3 • Appendix 2.3: LS through the midline, level of the aorta.

APPENDIX 2.4: LONGITUDINAL OBLIQUE SECTION ALONG THE CBD (Fig. 2A.4)

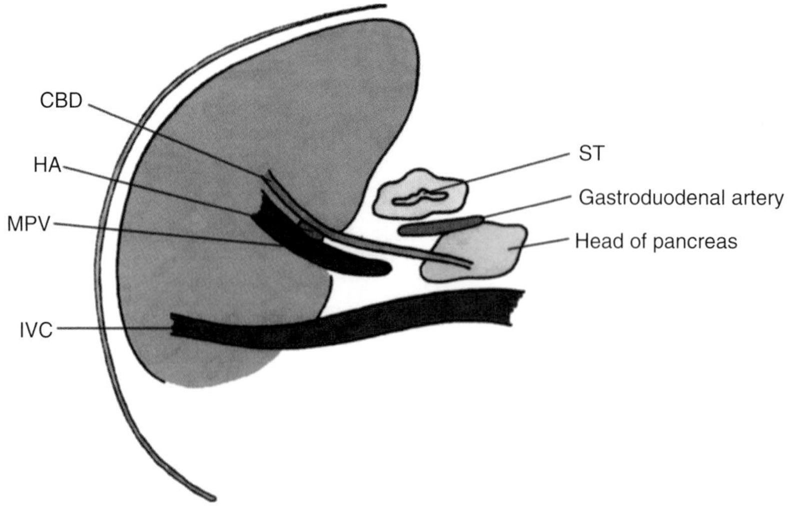

Fig. 2A.4 • Appendix 2.4: Longitudinal oblique section along the CBD.

APPENDIX 2.5: TRANSVERSE OBLIQUE SECTION THROUGH THE HEPATIC VENOUS CONFLUENCE (Fig. 2A.5)

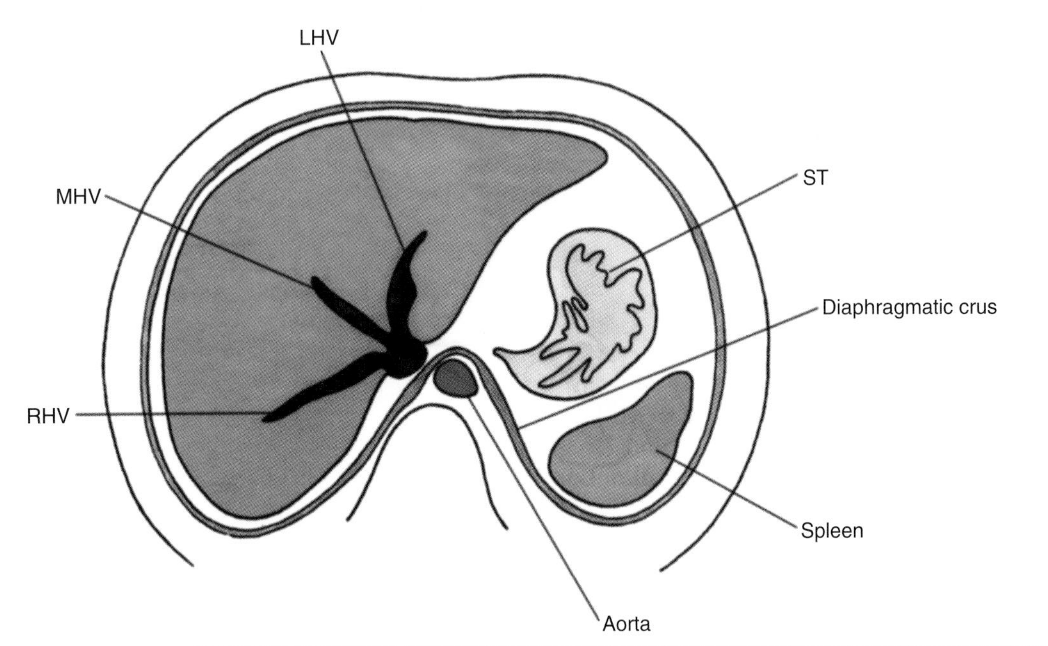

Fig. 2A.5 • Appendix 2.5: Transverse oblique section through the hepatic venous confluence.

APPENDIX 2.6: TS THROUGH THE LEVEL OF THE PORTA HEPATIS (Fig. 2A.6)

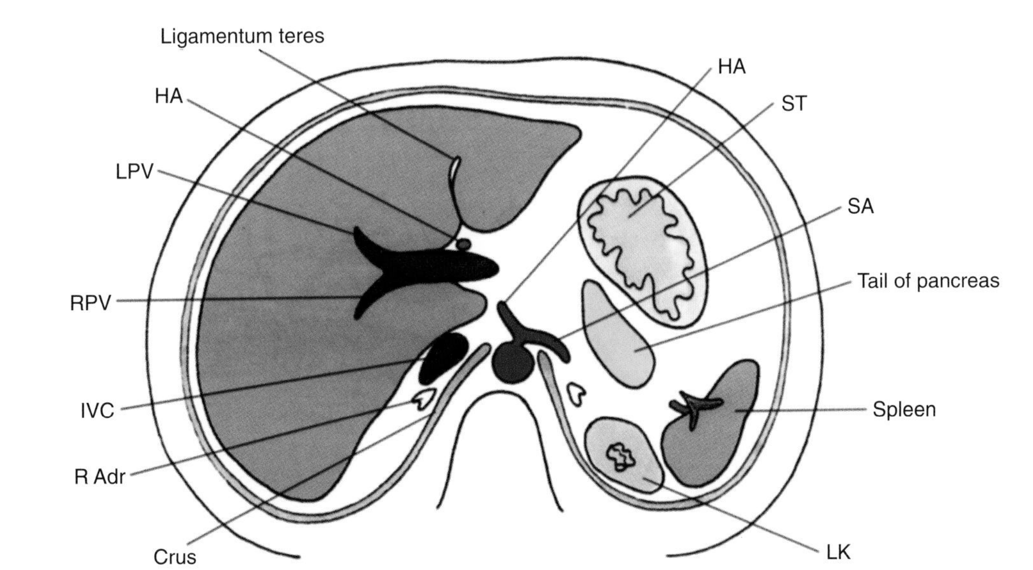

Fig. 2A.6 • Appendix 2.6: TS through the level of the porta hepatis.

APPENDIX 2.7: TS AT THE LEVEL OF THE PANCREAS (Fig. 2A.7)

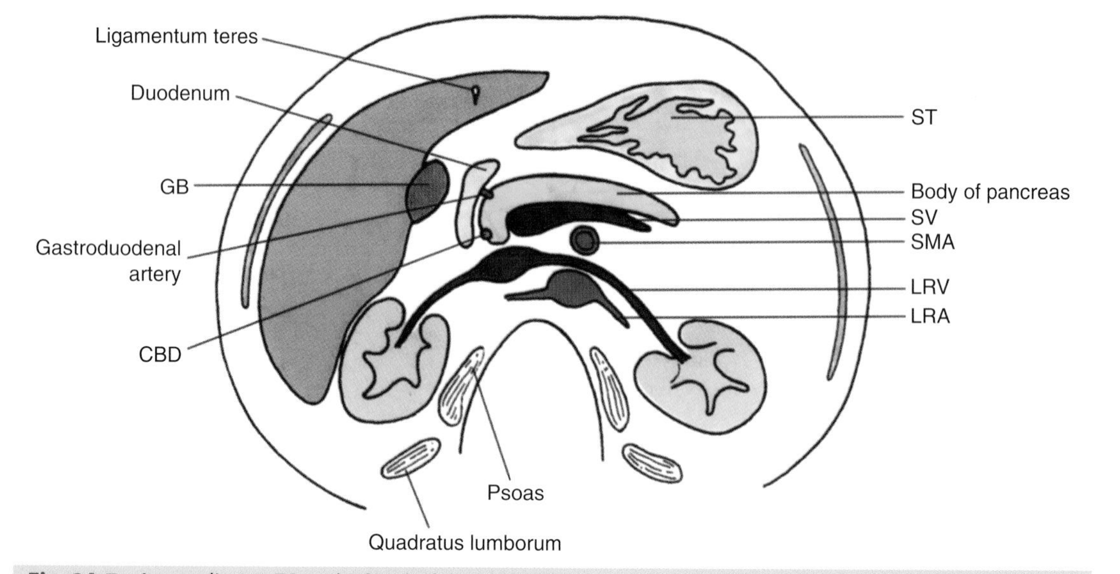

Fig. 2A.7 • Appendix 2.7: TS at the level of the pancreas.

Pathology of the gallbladder and biliary tree

3

CHAPTER CONTENTS

INTRODUCTION

Ultrasound is an essential first-line investigation in suspected gallbladder and biliary duct disease. It is highly sensitive, accurate and comparatively cheap and is the imaging modality of choice.[1] Gallbladder pathology is common and is asymptomatic in over 13% of the population.[2]

CHOLELITHIASIS

The most commonly and reliably identified gallbladder pathology is gallstones. More than 10% of the population of the UK have gallstones. Many of these are asymptomatic (Box 3.1), which is an important point to remember. When scanning a patient with abdominal pain it should not automatically be assumed that, when gallstones are present, they are responsible for the pain. It is not uncommon to find further pathology in the presence of gallstones and a comprehensive upper abdominal survey should always be carried out. However, up to 35% of patients who have gallstones require surgery to relieve symptoms (Table 3.1).[3]

Gallstones are associated with a number of conditions. They occur when the normal ratio of components making up the bile is altered, most commonly when there is increased secretion of cholesterol in the bile. Conditions that are associated with increased cholesterol secretion, and therefore the formation of cholesterol stones, include obesity, diabetes, pregnancy and oestrogen therapy. The incidence of stones also rises with age, probably because the bile flow slows down.

An increased secretion of bilirubin in the bile, as in patients with cirrhosis for example, is associated with pigment (black or brown) stones.

BOX 3.1 Gallstones – clinical features

- Often asymptomatic
- Biliary colic – RUQ pain, fatty intolerance
- +ve ultrasound Murphy's sign (if inflammation is present)
- Recurring RUQ pain in chronic cholecystitis
- Jaundice (depending on degree of obstruction)
- Fluctuating fever (if infection is present)

Ultrasound appearances

There are three classic acoustic properties associated with stones in the gallbladder; they are *highly reflective, mobile* and cast a *distal acoustic shadow*. In the majority of cases, all these properties are demonstrated (Figs 3.1–3.3).

Shadowing

The ability to display a shadow posterior to a stone depends on several factors:

1. The reflection and absorption of sound by the stone. This is fairly consistent, regardless of the composition of the stone.
2. The size of the stone in relation to the beamwidth. A shadow occurs when the stone fills the width of the beam (Fig. 3.4). This will happen easily with large stones, but a small stone may occupy less space than the beam, allowing sound to continue

Physiological	Post-prandial
Inflammatory	Acute or chronic cholecystitis
	Sclerosing cholangitis
	Crohn's disease
	AIDS
Adjacent inflammatory causes	Pancreatitis
	Hepatitis
	Pericholecystic abscesses
Non-inflammatory	Adenomyomatosis
	Gallbladder carcinoma
	Focal areas of thickening due to metastases or polyps
	Leukaemia
Oedema	Ascites from a variety of causes, including organ failure, lymphatic obstruction and portal hypertension
Varices	Varices of the gallbladder wall in portal hypertension

Table 3.1 Causes of a thickened gallbladder wall

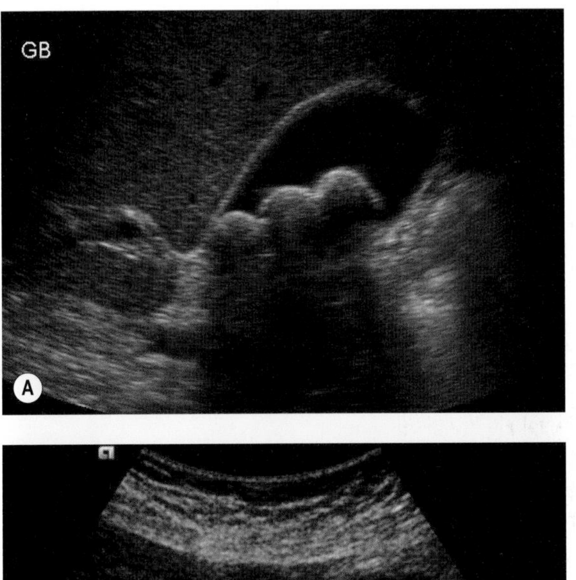

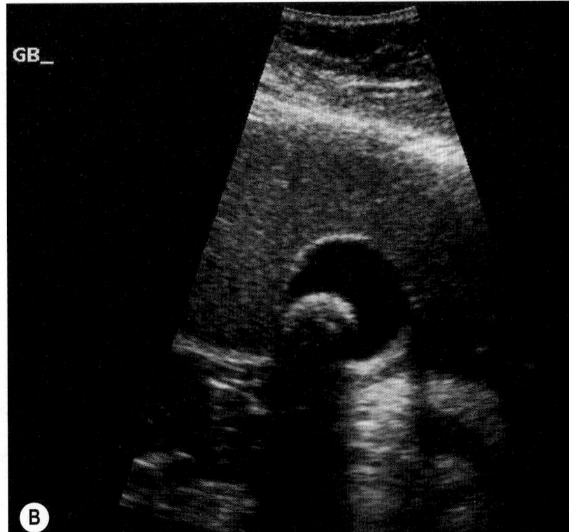

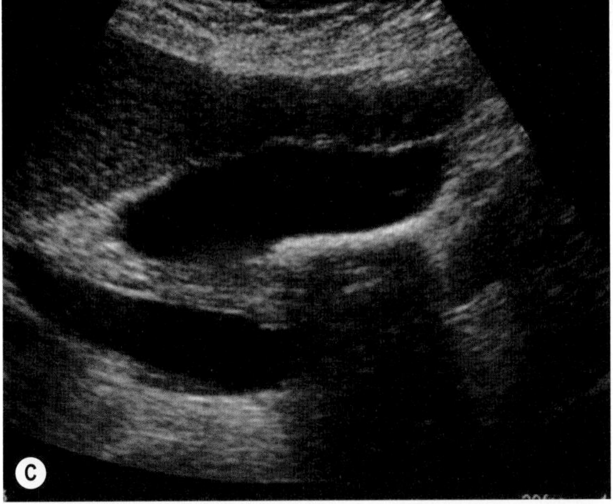

Fig. 3.1 • (A) LS and (B) TS through a gallbladder demonstrating stones with posterior acoustic shadowing. (C) Tiny stones lie together to form a block of acoustic shadow behind the gallbladder.

behind it, so a shadow is not seen. Small stones must therefore be within the focal zone (narrowest point) of the beam and in the centre of the beam to shadow (Fig. 3.5). Higher frequency transducers have better resolution and are therefore more likely to display fine shadows than lower frequencies.

3. The machine settings must be compatible with demonstrating narrow bands of shadowing. The fluid-filled gallbladder often displays posterior enhancement, or increased through-transmission. If the echoes posterior to the gallbladder are 'saturated' this will mask fine shadows. Turn the overall gain down to display this better (Fig. 3.6). Some image processing options may reduce the contrast between the shadow and the surrounding tissue, so make sure a suitable dynamic range and image programme are used.
4. Bowel posterior to the gallbladder may cast its own shadows from gas and other contents, making the gallstone shadow difficult to demonstrate (Fig. 3.7). This is a particular problem with stones in the CBD. Try turning the patient to move the gallbladder away from the bowel. The shadow cast by gas in the duodenum, which contains reverberation, should usually be distinguishable from that cast by a gallstone, which is sharp and clean.

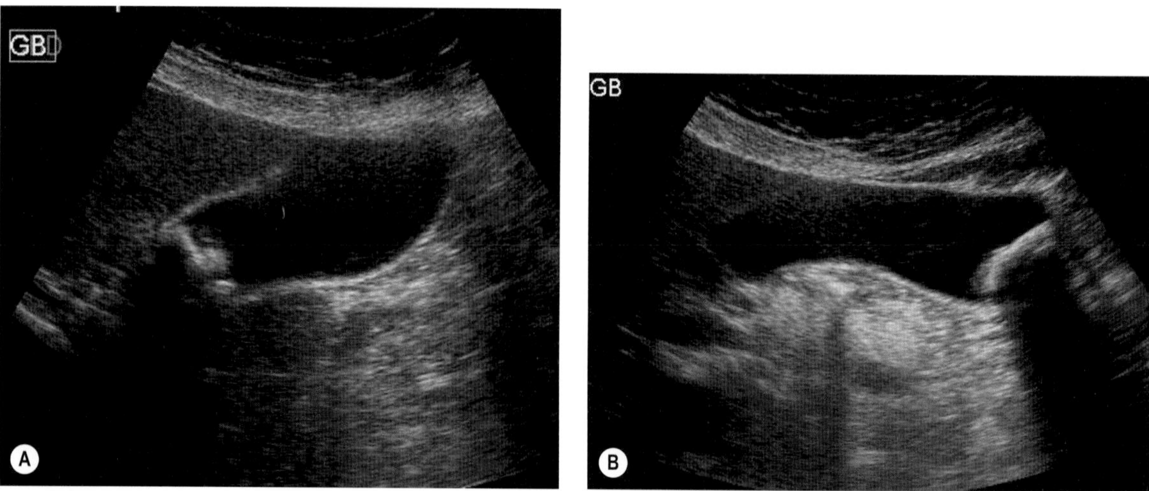

Fig. 3.2 • Gallstone mobility: (A) Shadowing from a stone in the neck of the gallbladder. (B) With the patient erect, the stone drops to the fundus of the gallbladder.

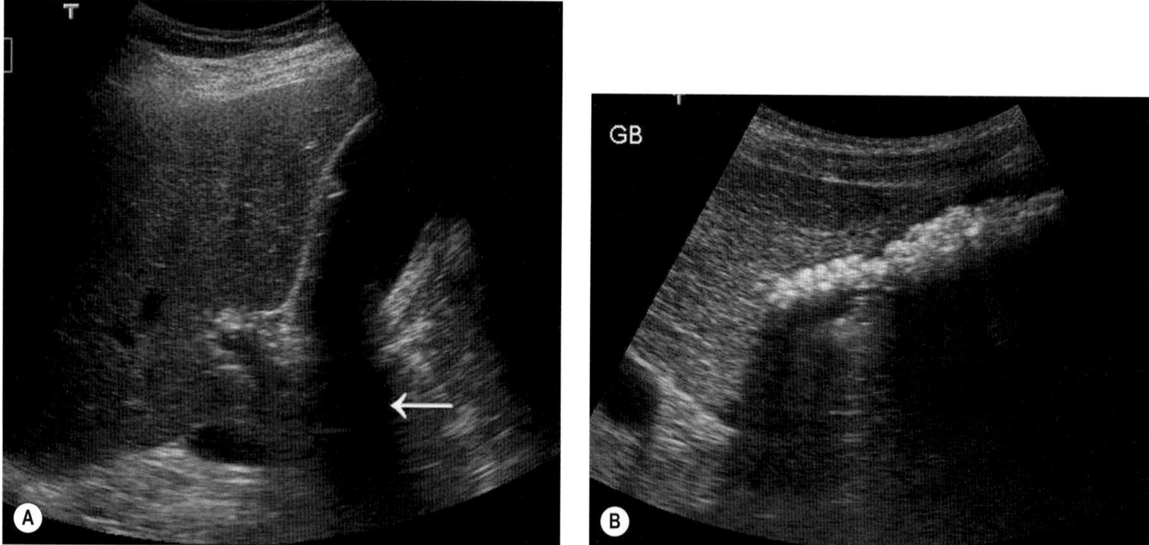

Fig. 3.3 • (A) Floating gallstones cast a shadow from the anterior gallbladder (arrow). (B) Floating stones in the gallbladder lumen, mimicking gas-filled bowel.

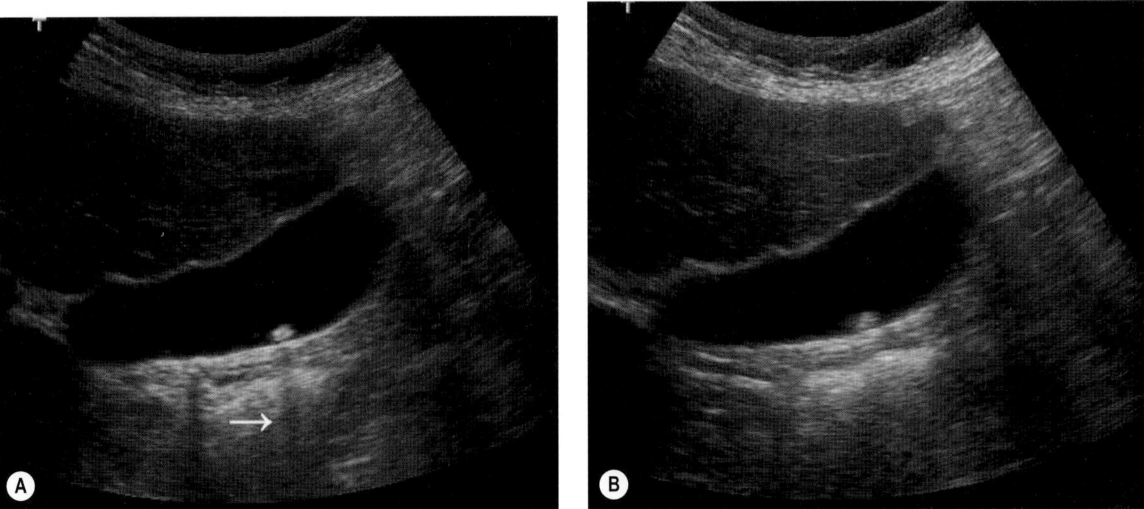

Fig. 3.4 • (A) This small stone is wider than the beamwidth, and so casts an acoustic shadow (arrow). (B) When the beam focusing is moved anterior to the gallbladder, the shadow is no longer evident as the beam is now wider than the stone.

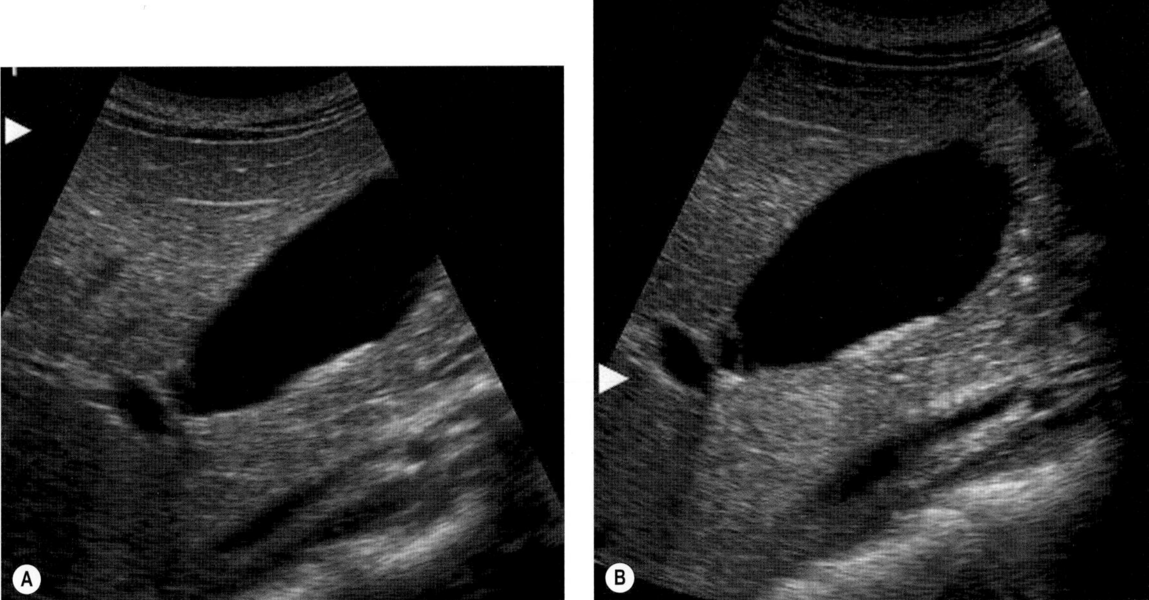

Fig. 3.5 • (A) A layer of tiny stones does not shadow when the focal zone is placed incorrectly (arrow), but the shadow is easily demonstrated (B) when the focal zone is placed at the posterior wall of the gallbladder, narrowing the beam at this point.

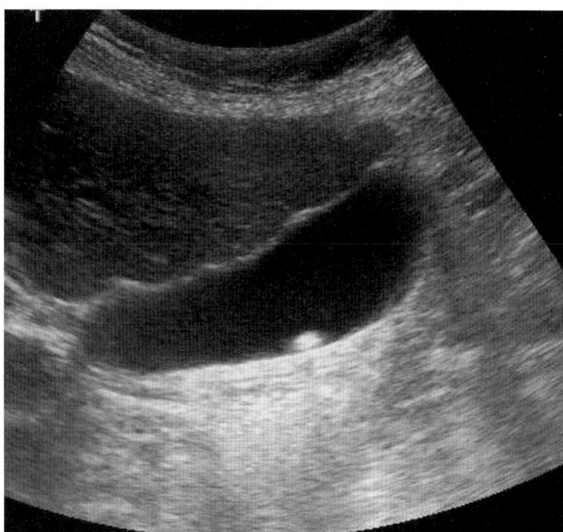

Fig. 3.6 • The shadow from the stone in Figure 3.4 is obscured by overamplification of the echoes behind the gallbladder.

Reflectivity

The reflective nature of the stone is enhanced by its being surrounded by echo-free bile. In a contracted gallbladder the reflectivity of the stone is often not appreciated because the hyperechoic gallbladder wall is collapsed over it.

Some stones are only poorly reflective, but should still cause a distal acoustic shadow.

Mobility

Most stones are gravity dependent, and this may be demonstrated by scanning the patient in an erect position (Fig. 3.2), when a mobile calculus will drop from the neck or body of the gallbladder to lie in the fundus. Some stones will float, however, forming a reflective layer just beneath the anterior gallbladder wall with shadowing that obscures the rest of the lumen (Fig. 3.3B). When the gallbladder lumen is contracted, either due to physiological or pathological reasons, any stones present are unable to move and this is also the case in a gallbladder packed with stones (Fig. 3.7D).

Occasionally a stone may become impacted in the neck, and movement of the patient is unable to dislodge it. Stones lodged in the gallbladder neck or cystic duct may result in a permanently contracted gallbladder, a gallbladder full of fine echoes due to inspissated (thickened) bile (Fig. 3.8) or a distended gallbladder due to a mucocoele (see below).

CHOLEDOCHOLITHIASIS

Choledocholithiasis develops in up to 20% of patients with gallstones.[4] Stones may pass from the gallbladder into the common duct, or may develop *de novo* within the duct. Stones in the CBD may obstruct the drainage of bile from the liver causing obstructive jaundice. Due to shadowing from adjacent duodenum ductal stones are often difficult to demonstrate, and care must be taken to visualize the lower end of the duct if possible (Fig. 3.9).

Usually CBD stones are accompanied by stones in the gallbladder and a degree of dilatation of the CBD. In these cases the operator can usually persevere and demonstrate the offending article at the lower end of the duct. However, the duct may be dilated but empty, the stone having recently passed. Stones may be seen to move up and down a dilated duct. This can create a ball-valve effect so that obstruction may be intermittent. It is not unusual to demonstrate a stone in the CBD without stones in the gallbladder, a phenomenon which is also well documented following cholecystectomy. This may be due to a single calculus in the gallbladder having moved into the duct, or stone formation, de novo, within the duct.

It is also important to remember that stones in the CBD may be present *without* duct dilatation and attempts to image the entire common duct with ultrasound should *always* be made, even if it is of normal calibre at the porta (Fig. 3.10).

Other ultrasound signs to look for are shown in Box 3.2.

Possible complications of gallstones are outlined in Figure 3.11A. In rare cases, stones may perforate the inflamed gallbladder wall to form a fistula into the small intestine or colon. A large stone passing into the small intestine may impact in the ileum, causing intestinal obstruction (Fig. 3.11B).

Biliary reflux and gallstone pancreatitis

A stone may become lodged in the distal CBD near the ampulla. If the main pancreatic duct joins the CBD proximal to this, bile and pancreatic fluid may reflux up the pancreatic duct, causing

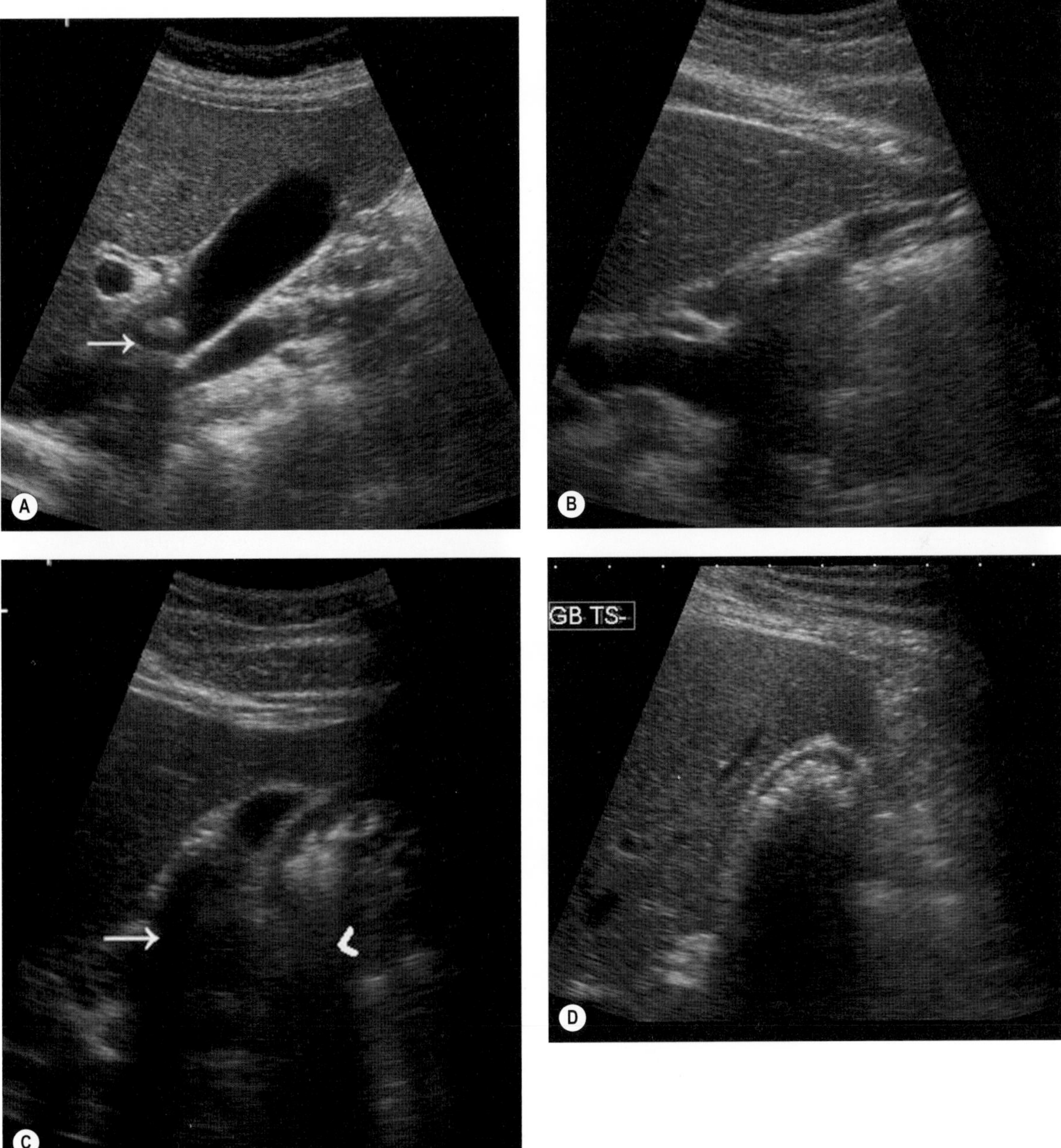

Fig. 3.7 • (A) Shadowing from the stone in the neck of the gallbladder (arrow) is less obvious due to the structures lying behind the gallbladder. (B) Shadowing from duodenum posterior to the gallbladder can obscure the shadowing from tiny stones within the gallbladder lumen. Changing patient position and angle of scanning moves the gas away from the gallbladder. (C) Shadowing from stones in the contracted gallbladder lumen (arrow) is stronger and better defined than the 'dirty' shadowing from adjacent bowel (arrowhead). (D) A contracted gallbladder full of stones casts a strong acoustic shadow from the gallbladder fossa. Note the echoes from the anterior gallbladder wall are distinct from the echoes from the stones.

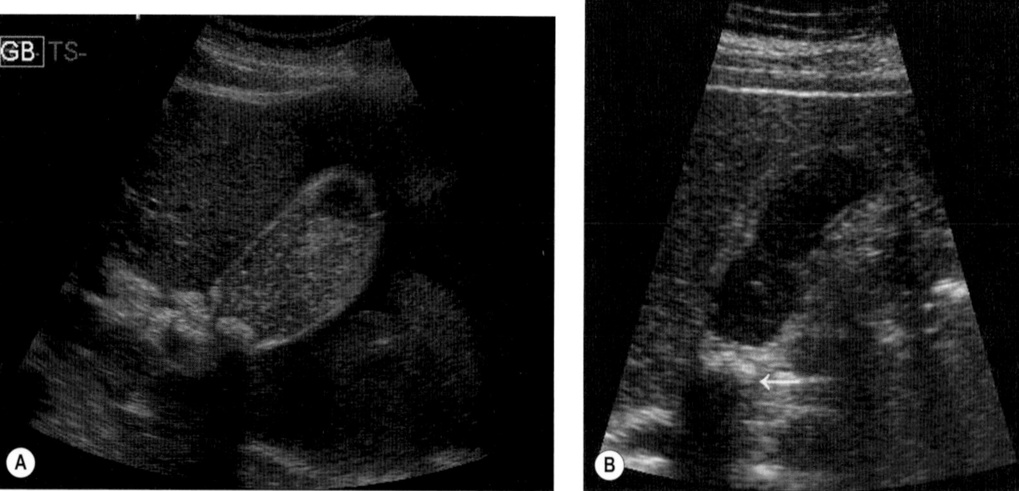

Fig. 3.8 • (A) A stone lodged in the gallbladder neck with thickened, inspissated bile filling the gallbladder lumen. (B) The gallbladder neck is curled round and a stone is lodged within it (arrow).

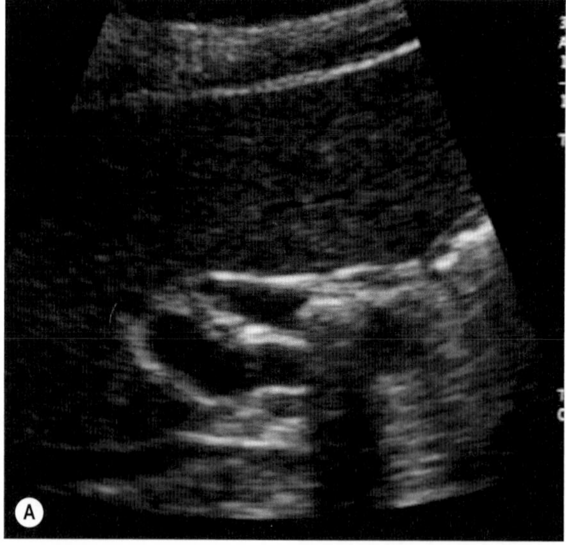

Fig. 3.9 • (A) A stone in a dilated CBD with posterior shadowing. The gallbladder was dilated but did not contain stones.

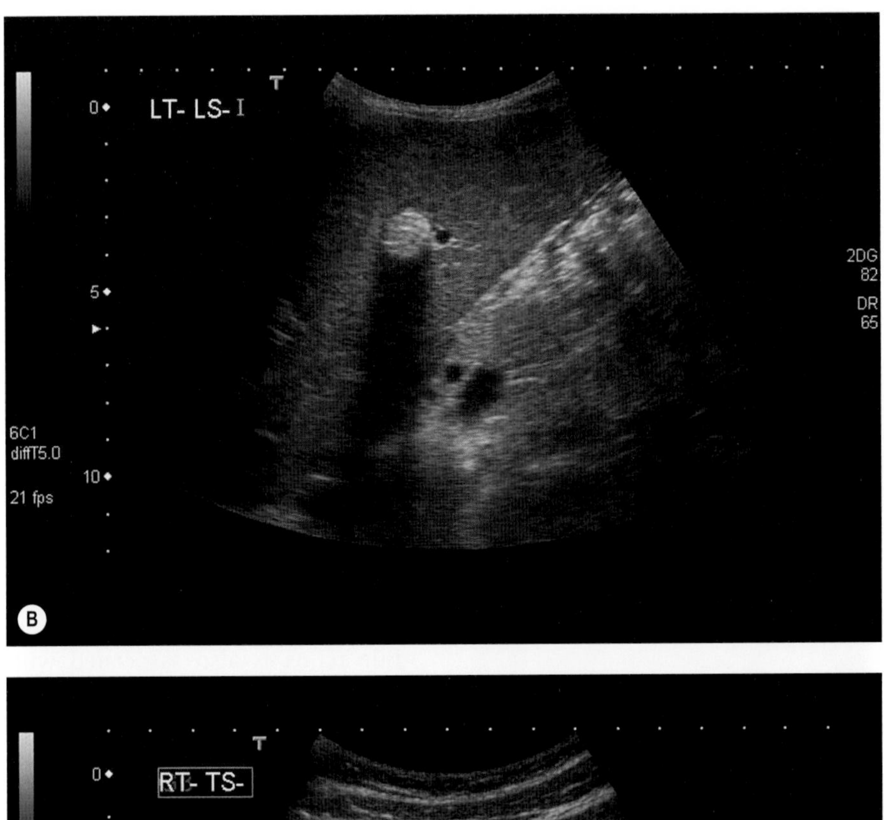

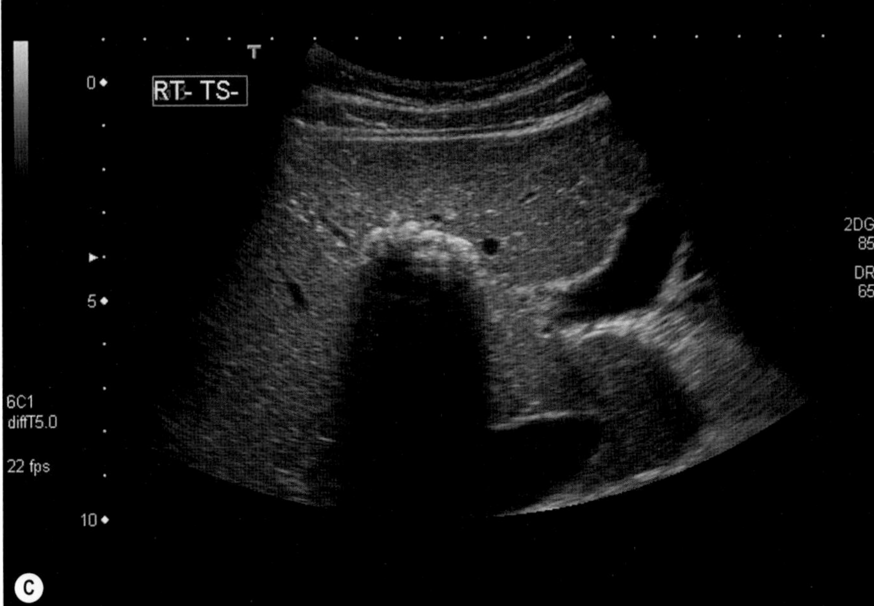

Fig. 3.9, cont'd • (B & C) Stone formation in the intrahepatic ducts.

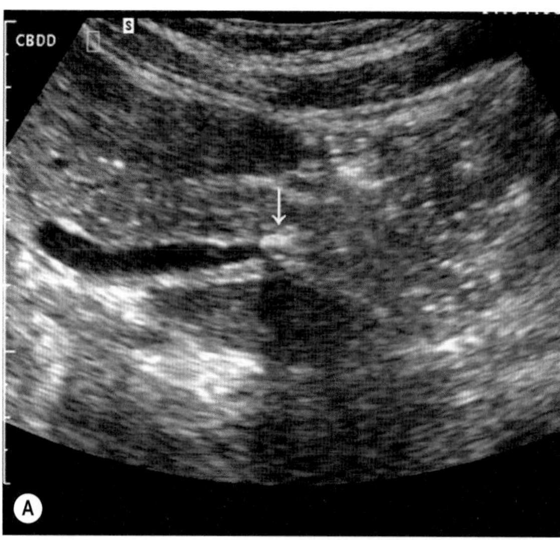

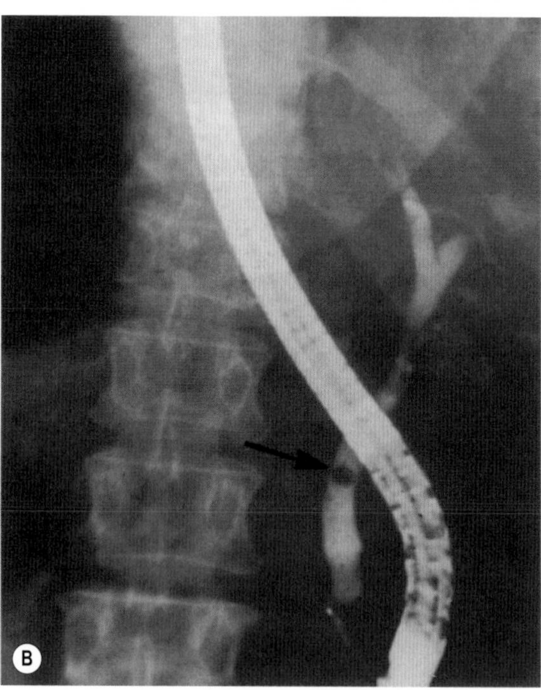

Fig. 3.10 • (A) Small stone in the CBD causing intermittent obstruction. At the time of scanning the CBD was normal in calibre. (B) ERCP of a stone in a normal calibre (5 mm) duct.

inflammation and severe pain. Reflux up the CBD may also result in ascending cholangitis, particularly if the obstruction is prolonged or repetitive. Cholangitis may result in dilated bile ducts with mural irregularity on ultrasound, but magnetic resonance cholangiopancreatography (MRCP) is usually superior in demonstrating intrahepatic ductal changes of this nature.

BOX 3.2 Gallstones – other ultrasound signs to look for

- Acute or chronic cholecystitis
- Complications of cholecystitis, e.g. pericholecystic collection
- Stone impacted in the neck of the gallbladder – mucocoele, hydrops
- CBD stones
- Biliary obstruction – dilatation of the CBD and/or intrahepatic ducts
- Pancreatitis
- Other causes of RUQ pain unrelated to stones

Bile reflux is also associated with anomalous cystic duct insertion (Fig. 3.12A, B) which is more readily recognized on MRCP than ultrasound.

Further management of gallstones

MRCP and endoscopic retrograde cholangiopancreatography (ERCP) demonstrate stones in the duct with greater accuracy than ultrasound, particularly at the lower end of the CBD, which may be obscured by duodenal gas on ultrasound[5] (Fig. 3.12C, D). ERCP is invasive, carrying a small risk of morbidity or, rarely, mortality due to perforation, infection or pancreatitis, but has the advantage of providing the therapeutic option of sphincterotomy and stone removal. This is the modality of choice when stones are known to exist in the duct, (for example following MRCP) and has supplanted surgical removal in many cases.[6]

Laparoscopic cholecystectomy is the preferred method of treatment for symptomatic gallbladder disease in an elective setting. Acute cholecystitis is also increasingly managed by early laparoscopic surgery, with a slightly higher rate of conversion to open surgery than elective cases.[7] Laparoscopic ultrasound may be used as a suitable alternative to operative cholangiography to examine the common duct for residual stones during surgery.[8] It compares well to cholangiography, with a sensitivity and specificity of 96% and 100%, and avoids any

Fig. 3.11 • (A) The possible complications of gallstones. (B) Gallstone ileus.

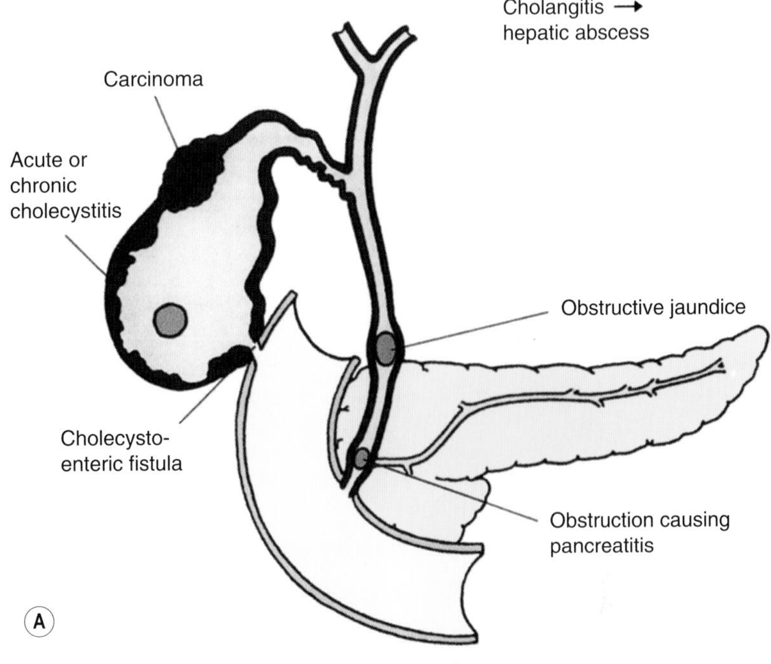

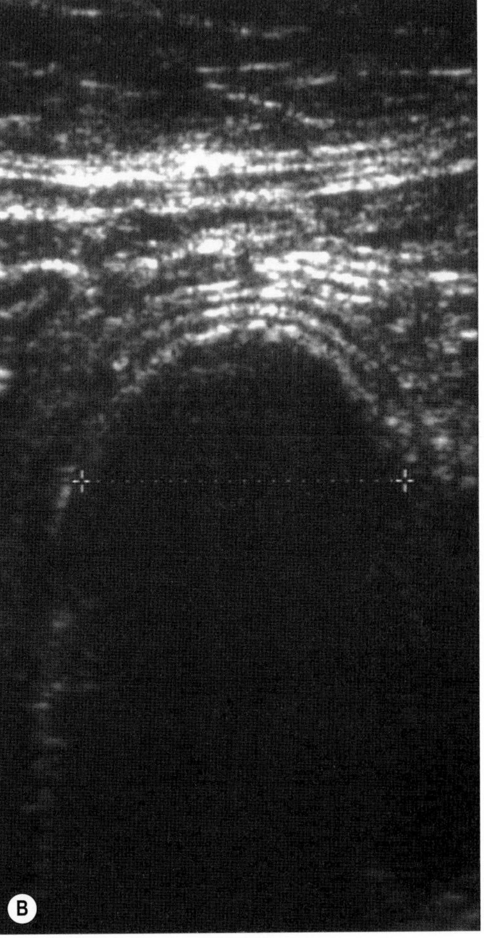

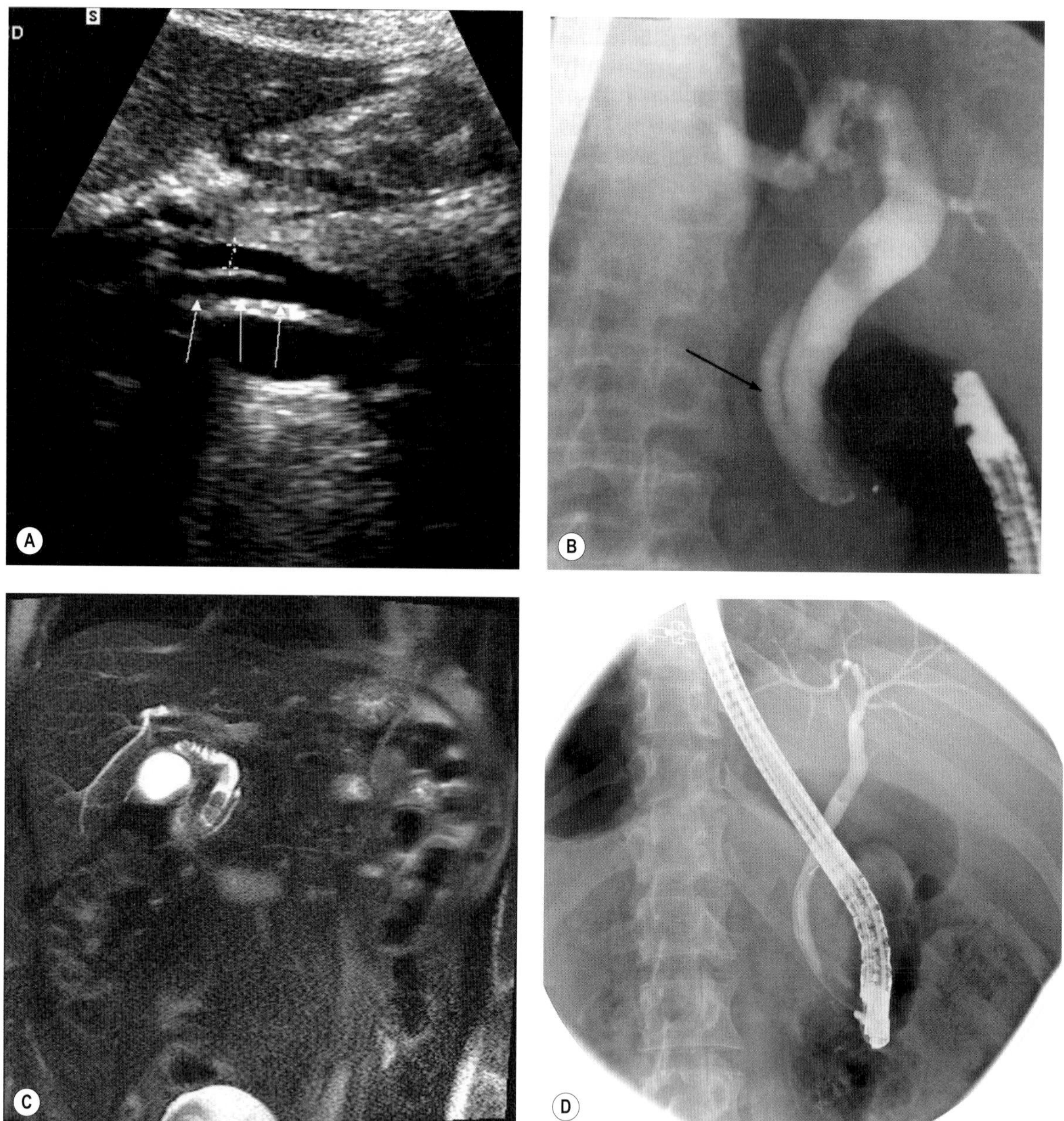

Fig. 3.12 • (A) Anomalous insertion of the cystic duct (arrows) into the lower end of the CBD. (B) Appearances of case in (A) are confirmed on ERCP. A stone is also present in the duct. (C) MRCP showing stones in the CBD. (D) ERCP can be used for therapeutic purposes, such as stone removal or stent insertion.

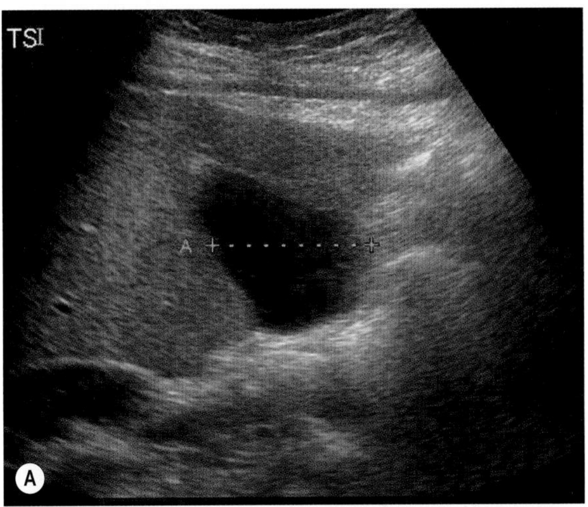

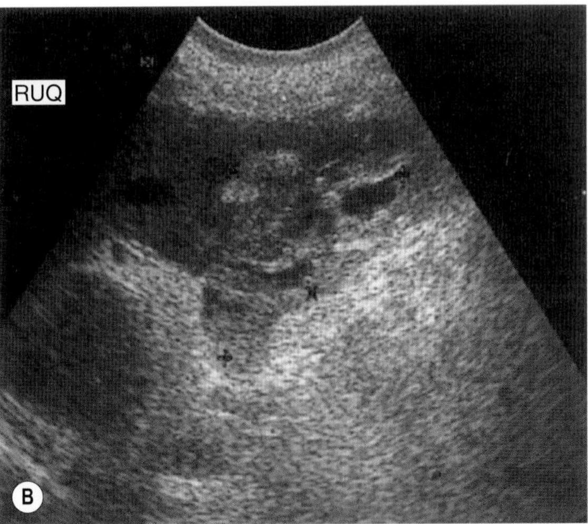

Fig. 3.13 • (A) Post-operative bile collection in the gallbladder bed. (B) Hyperechoic, irregular 'mass' in the gallbladder bed, which represents a resolving haematoma after laparoscopic cholecystectomy.

radiation dose, but has been slow to be adopted in the UK, as it requires specialized equipment and training.[9] Both ultrasound and cholescintigraphy are used in monitoring post-operative biliary leaks or haematoma (Fig. 3.13).

Other, less common options include dissolution therapy and extracorporeal shock wave lithotripsy (ESWL). However, these treatments are often only partially successful, require careful patient selection, and also run a significant risk of stone recurrence.[10]

ENLARGEMENT OF THE GALLBLADDER

Owing to the enormous variation in size and shape of the normal gallbladder, it is not possible to diagnose pathological enlargement by simply using measurements. Three dimensional techniques may prove useful in assessing gallbladder volume[11] but this is a technique which is only likely to be clinically useful in a minority of patients with impaired gallbladder emptying.

An enlarged gallbladder is frequently referred to as *hydropic*. It may be due to obstruction of the cystic duct (see below) or associated with numerous disease processes such as diabetes, primary sclerosing cholangitis, leptospirosis or in response to some types of drug. A pathologically dilated gallbladder, as opposed to one which is physiologically dilated, usually assumes a more rounded, tense appearance (Fig. 3.14).

Mucocoele of the gallbladder

If the cystic duct is obstructed – usually by a stone which has failed to pass through to the CBD – the normal flow of bile from the gallbladder is interrupted. Chronic cystic duct obstruction causes the bile to be replaced by mucus secreted by the lining of the gallbladder, resulting in a mucocoele. The biliary ducts remain normal in calibre.

If the gallbladder is dilated in the absence of duct dilatation, make a careful search for an obstructing lesion at the neck; a stone in the cystic duct is more difficult to identify on ultrasound as it is not surrounded by echo-free bile (Fig. 3.8).

Mirizzi's syndrome

Mirizzi's syndrome is a rare cause of biliary obstruction in which compression of the biliary tree is caused by a stone in the adjacent cystic duct. This usually happens in combination with a surrounding inflammatory process which compresses and obstructs the adjacent common hepatic duct, causing distal biliary duct dilatation. This is associated with a low insertion of the cystic duct into the common hepatic duct. Occasionally a fistula forms

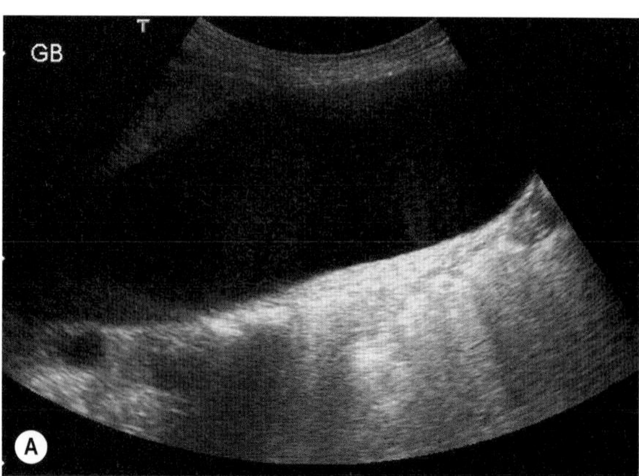

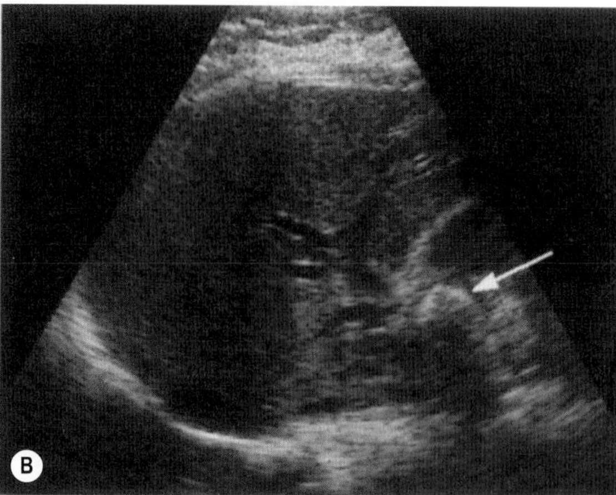

Fig. 3.14 • (A) A dilated gallbladder in a patient with obstruction of the CBD due to pancreatic carcinoma. The gallbladder is large, tense and contains low level echoes from thickened bile. (B) Mirizzi's syndrome: a large stone in the gallbladder neck compresses the adjacent bile duct causing obstruction.

between the hepatic duct and the gallbladder due to erosion of the duct wall by the stone. Ultimately this may lead to gallstone ileus – small bowel obstruction resulting from migration of a large stone through the cholecystoenteric fistula. If the condition is not promptly diagnosed, recurring cholangitis leading to secondary biliary cirrhosis may result.

On ultrasound the gallbladder is typically contracted and contains debris. A stone impacted at the neck may be demonstrated together with dilatation of the intrahepatic ducts with a normal-calibre lower common duct (Fig. 3.14). The diagnosis is a difficult one, as it is frequently not possible to rule out carcinoma. CT or MRI may assist in this distinction, and ERCP is still considered the 'gold standard' especially as it can offer therapeutic stone removal and/or stent placement.[12] Endoscopic or intraductal ultrasound, if available, have improved the diagnostic accuracy of suspected cases.[13] Although rare, it is an important diagnosis as cholecystectomy in these cases has a higher rate of operative and post-operative complications.[14]

THE CONTRACTED OR SMALL GALLBLADDER

Postprandial

The most likely cause of a contracted gallbladder is physiological, following a meal. (This may still occur despite instructions to fast and it is always worth enquiring when and what the patient has last eaten or drunk.) The normal gallbladder wall is thickened when contracted, and this must not be confused with a pathological process (Fig. 3.15).

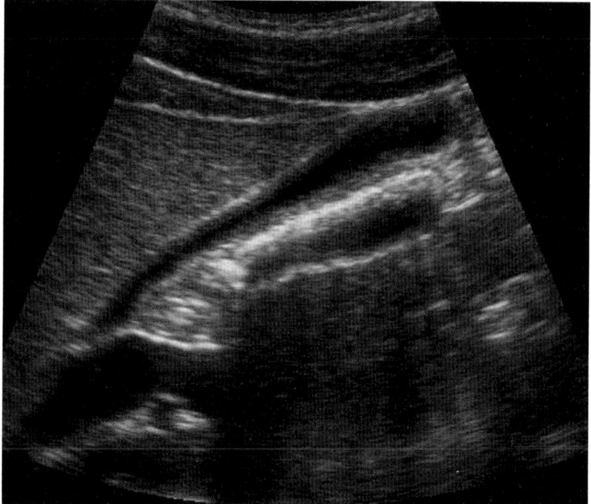

Fig. 3.15 • Normal, postprandial gallbladder with consequently thickened wall.

Pathological causes of a small gallbladder

Most pathologically contracted gallbladders contain stones. When the gallbladder cannot be

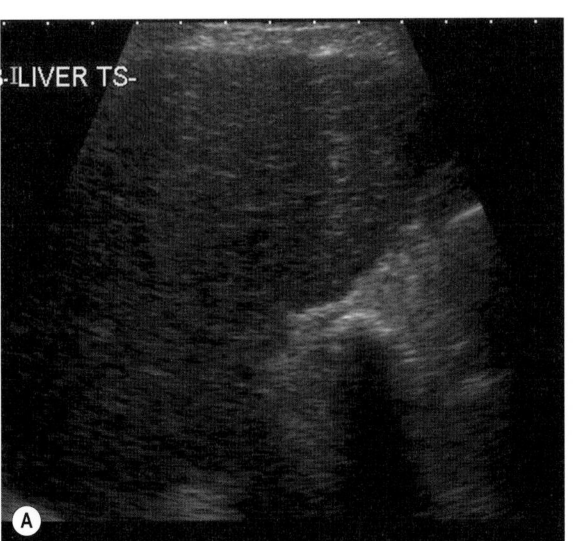

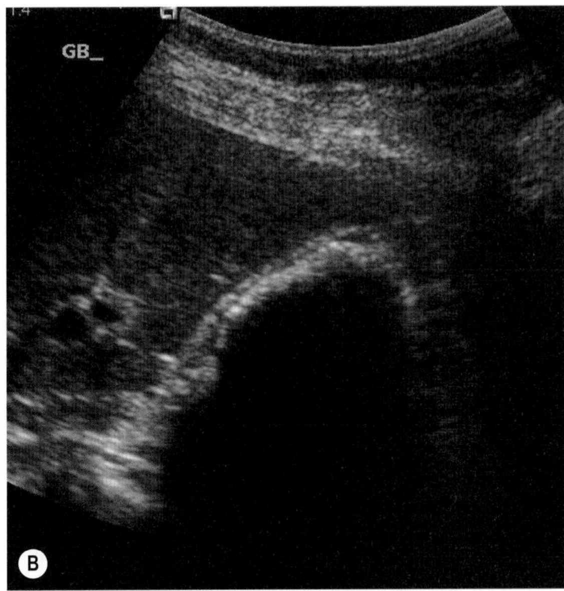

Fig. 3.16 • (A) Shadowing from the gallbladder fossa indicates a contracted gallbladder packed with stones. (B) A small layer of bile is visible between the stones and the anterior gallbladder wall.

identified, try scanning transversely through the gallbladder fossa, just caudal to the porta hepatis. Strong shadowing alerts the sonographer to the possibility of a contracted gallbladder full of stones.

The reflective surface of the stones and distal shadowing are apparent, and the anterior gallbladder wall can be demonstrated with correct focusing and good technique (Figs 3.7D, 3.16). Do not confuse the appearances of a previous cholecystectomy, when bowel in the gallbladder fossa casts a shadow, for a contracted stone-filled gallbladder.

A less common cause of a small gallbladder is the *microgallbladder* associated with cystic fibrosis (Fig. 3.17). The gallbladder itself is abnormally small, rather than just contracted. Cystic fibrosis also carries an increased incidence of gallstones because of the altered composition of the bile and bile stasis and the wall might be thickened and fibrosed from cholecystitis.

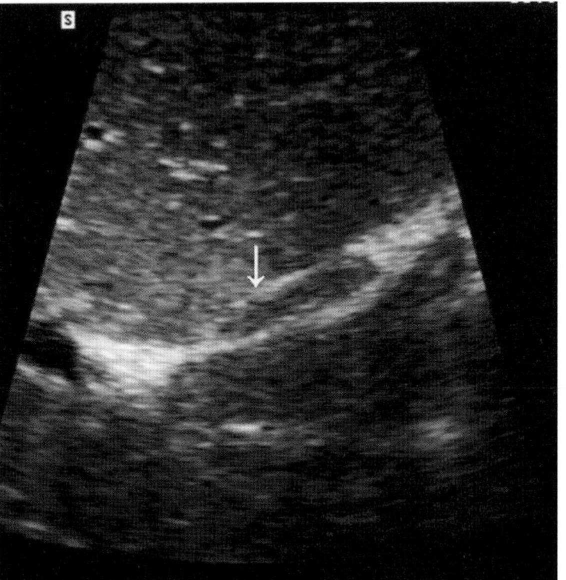

Fig. 3.17 • Microgallbladder in cystic fibrosis.

Porcelain gallbladder

When the gallbladder wall becomes calcified the resulting appearance is of a solid reflective structure causing a distal shadow in the gallbladder fossa (Fig. 3.18). (This can be distinguished from a gallbladder full of stones where the wall can usually be seen anterior to the shadowing [Fig. 3.7D]).

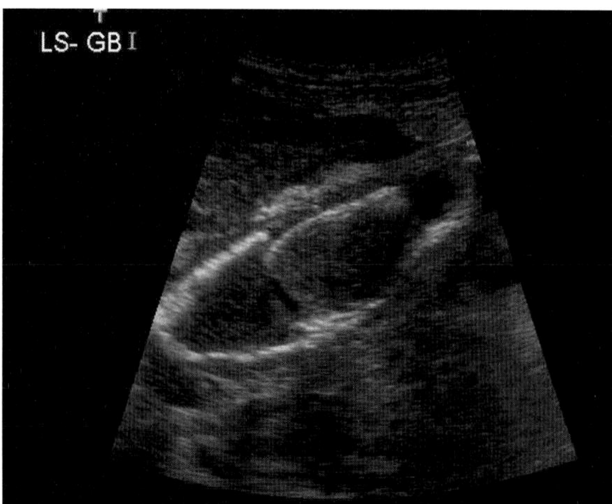

Fig. 3.18 • Porcelain gallbladder demonstrating a calcified inner layer of wall.

A porcelain gallbladder probably results from a gallbladder mucocoele – a long-standing obstruction of the cystic duct, usually from a stone. The bile inside the non-functioning gallbladder is gradually replaced by watery fluid, the wall becomes fibrotic and thickened and ultimately calcifies.

There is an association between porcelain gallbladder and gallbladder carcinoma, so a prophylactic cholecystectomy is usually performed to pre-empt malignant development.[15]

Shadowing from the calcified anterior gallbladder wall can obscure the gallbladder contents, and can mimic bowel in the gallbladder fossa. A plain X-ray also clearly demonstrates the porcelain gallbladder.

HYPERPLASTIC CONDITIONS OF THE GALLBLADDER WALL

ADENOMYOMATOSIS

This is a common, non-inflammatory, hyperplastic condition that causes gallbladder wall thickening. It occurs in around 5% of cholecystectomy specimens, and may be mistaken for chronic cholecystitis on ultrasound.

The epithelium that lines the gallbladder wall undergoes hyperplastic change – extending diverticulae into the adjacent muscular layer of the wall. These diverticulae, or sinuses (known as Rokitansky–Aschoff sinuses) are visible within the wall as fluid-filled spaces, (Fig. 3.19), which can bulge eccentrically into the lumen, and may contain echogenic material or even (normally pigment) stones.

The wall thickening may be focal or diffuse, and the sinuses may be little more than hypoechoic 'spots' in the thickened wall, or may become quite large cavities in some cases.[16] Deposits of crystals in the gallbladder wall frequently result in distinctive 'comet-tail' artefacts, due to rapid small reverberations of the sound.[17]

Focal adenomyomatosis most often occurs at the fundus (Fig. 3.19C) and may be difficult to distinguish from carcinoma. [18F]2-fluoro-2-deoxy-D-glucose positron emission tomography (FDG-PET) may be useful in the diagnosis of problem cases.[18] Often asymptomatic, it may present with biliary colic although it is unclear whether this is caused by co-existent stones. Its distinctive appearance allows the diagnosis to be made easily, whether or not stones are present.

Cholecystectomy is performed in symptomatic patients – usually those who also have stones. Although essentially a benign condition, a few cases of associated malignant transformation have been reported, usually in patients with associated anomalous insertion of the pancreatic duct.[19]

POLYPS

Gallbladder polyps are common, usually asymptomatic lesions which are incidental findings in up to 5% of the population. Occasionally they are the cause of biliary colic. They are reflective structures, projecting into the gallbladder lumen, which do not cast an acoustic shadow. Unless on a long stalk they will remain fixed on varying the patient

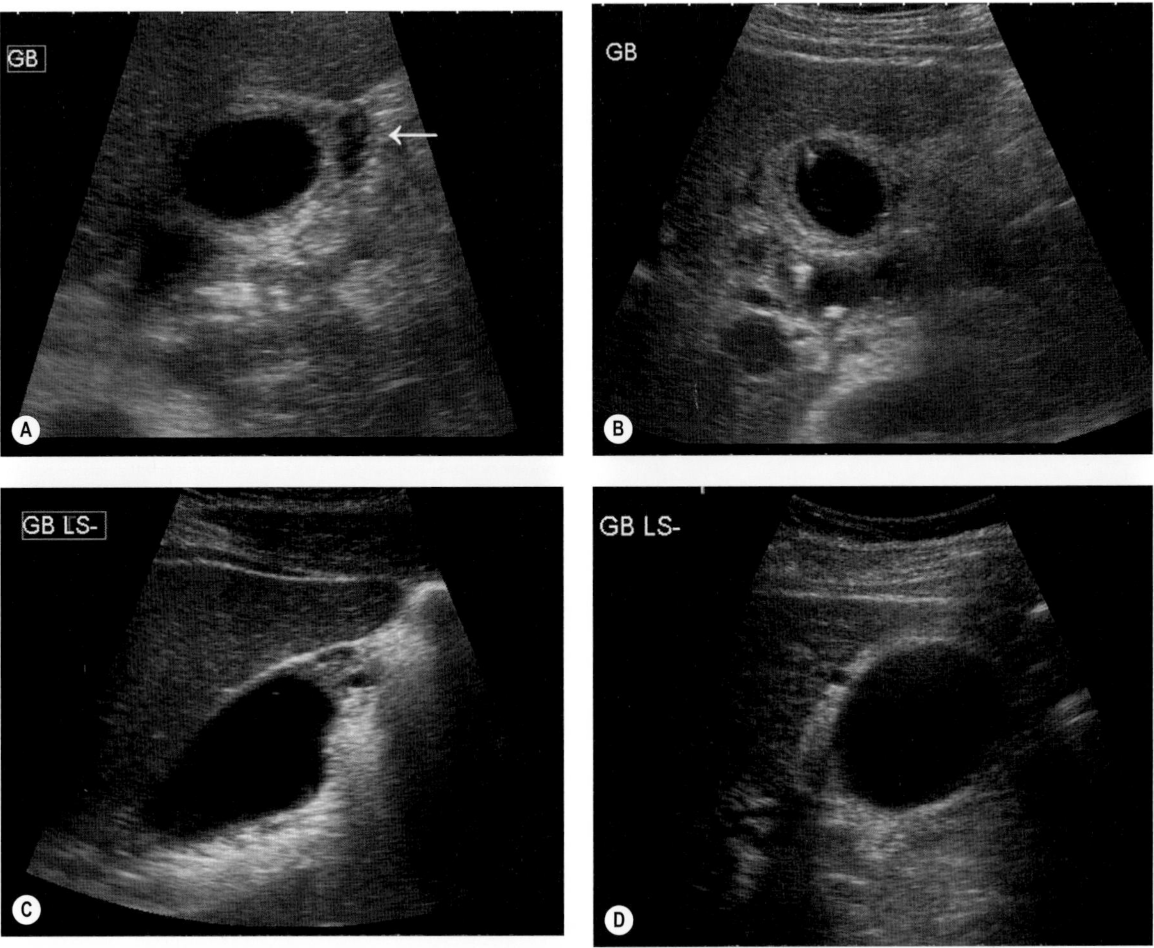

Fig. 3.19 • Adenomyomatosis: (A) TS of the gallbladder demonstrating a thickened gallbladder wall with a Rokitansky–Aschoff sinus (arrow). (B) TS of another gallbladder demonstrating a thickened hyperplastic wall with a comet-tail artefact due to crystal deposits. (C) A focal region of adenomyomatosis at the gallbladder fundus. This can sometimes be difficult to distinguish from early gallbladder carcinoma. (D) TS through the gallbladder showing a hyperplastic thickened wall with a small Rokitansky–Aschoff sinus.

position and are therefore usually distinguishable from stones (Fig. 3.20).

Several types of polyps exist, the most common being cholesterol polyps, which account for around 60% of gallbladder polyps. Others are adenomyomatosis and inflammatory polyps, both of which are also usually benign. True adenomas are less common. There is an association between larger adenomatous gallbladder polyps (>10 mm) and subsequent carcinoma, especially in patients over 50 years of age. The finding of a solitary polyp therefore poses a diagnostic dilemma, and cholecystectomy is often advised (Fig. 3.20D, E). Endoscopic ultrasound (EUS) may provide further information in such cases,[20] as it provides high-resolution images of tiny polyps and of the layers of the gallbladder wall, and there is some evidence that there is a correlation between EUS appearances and gallbladder polyp histology. Generally gallbladders in asymptomatic patients with polyps of >1 cm should undergo re-scanning to identify subsequent polyp growth and increased risk of carcinoma, and many clinicians advocate cholecystectomy to pre-empt malignant transformation.[21] In particular, gallbladder polyps in patients with primary sclerosing cholangitis (PSC) have a much greater likelihood of malignancy (40–60%).[22] Smaller polyps of less than 1 cm in diameter may also be safely monitored with ultrasound.[23]

There is some evidence to suggest that ultrasound contrast agents are useful in demonstrating tumour vascularity in potentially malignant polyps, such as adenomatous polyps[24] although so far this technique has proved non-specific, as some benign cholesterol polyps also demonstrate increased vascularity (Fig. 3.20F, G).

CHOLESTEROLOSIS

Also known as the 'strawberry gallbladder', this gets its name because of the multiple tiny nodules on the surface of the gallbladder mucosal lining.

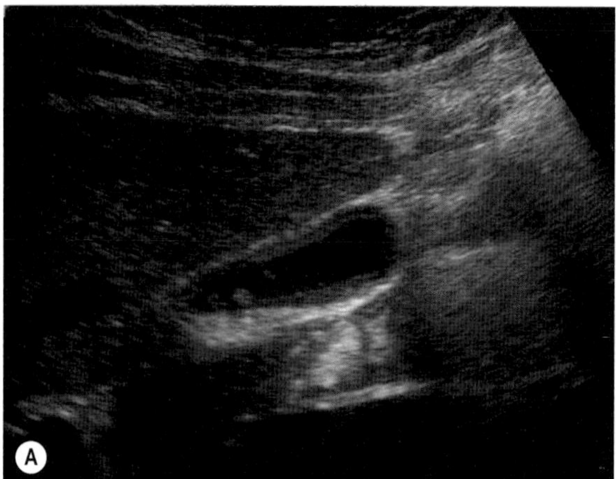

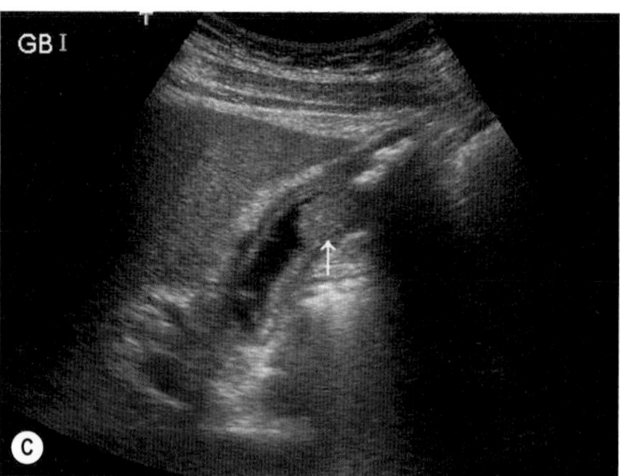

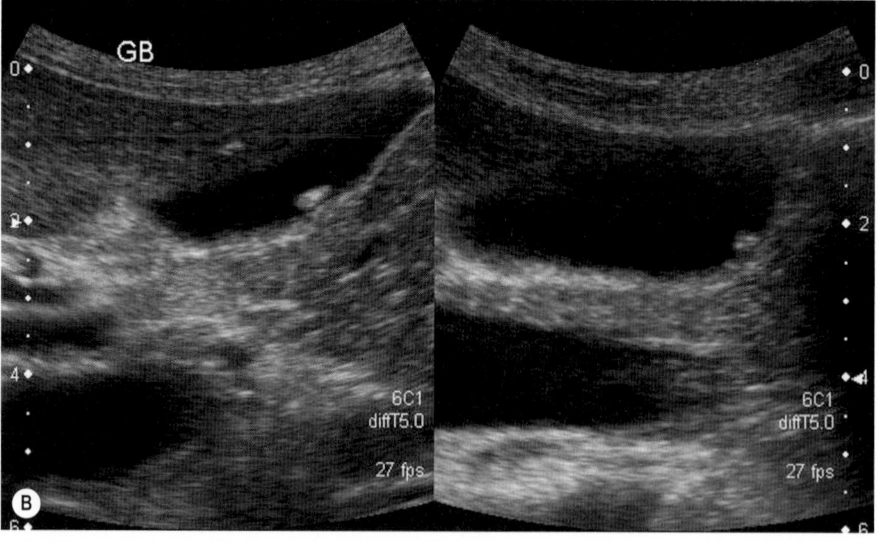

Fig. 3.20 • (A) Small polyps in the gallbladder lumen – no posterior shadowing is evident. (B) A gallbladder polyp remains in a fixed position on the gallbladder wall, despite moving the patient erect. (C) Large, sessile gallbladder polyp (arrow) in a thick-walled gallbladder. Stones are present in the gallbladder fundus.

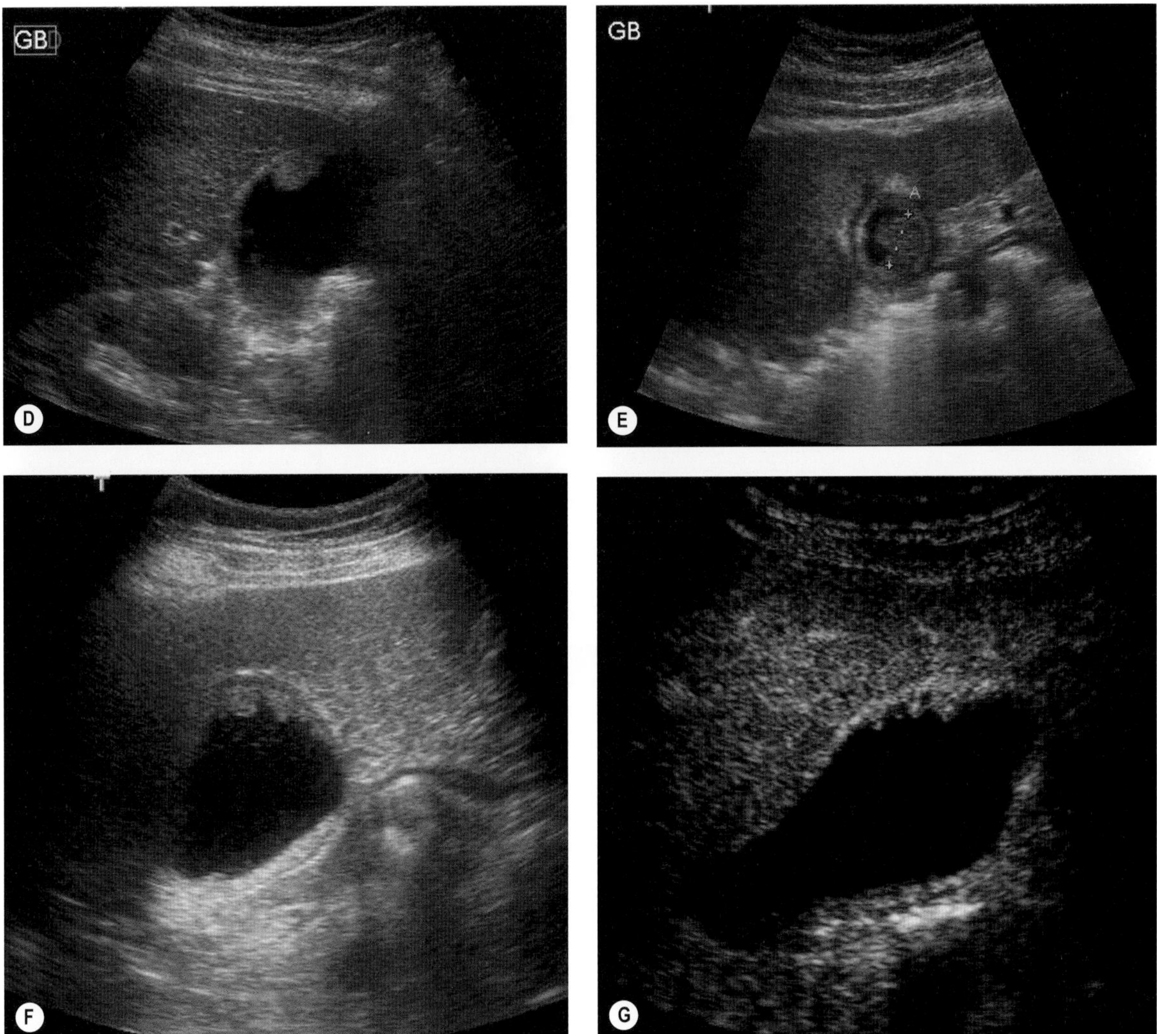

Fig. 3.20, cont'd • (D) Large, broad-based, solitary gallbladder polyp. (E) Such polyps are generally considered at greater risk of malignant transformation and patients generally undergo cholecystectomy. (F) Multiple gallbladder polyps pre-contrast and (G) post-contrast scan demonstrating take up of contrast in the polyps.

These nodules are the result of a build up of lipids in the gallbladder wall and are often not visible on ultrasound. However, in some cases, multiple polyps also form on the inner surface, projecting into the lumen, which are clearly visible on ultrasound (Fig. 3.21). Cholesterolosis may be asymptomatic, or may be accompanied by stones and consequently require surgery to alleviate symptoms of biliary colic. The finding of multiple gallbladder polyps should trigger ultrasound follow-up in the asymptomatic patient (see above).

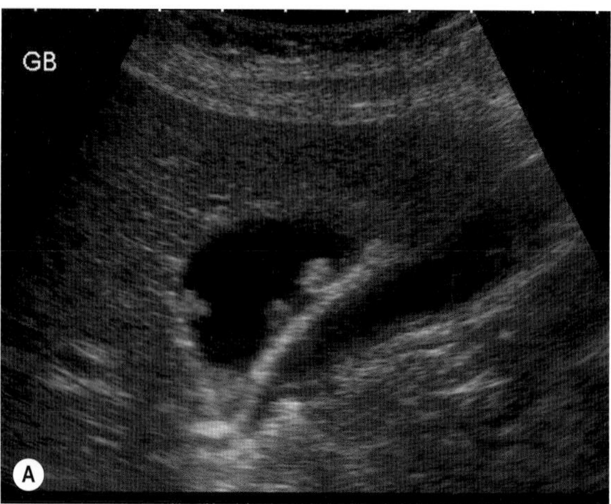

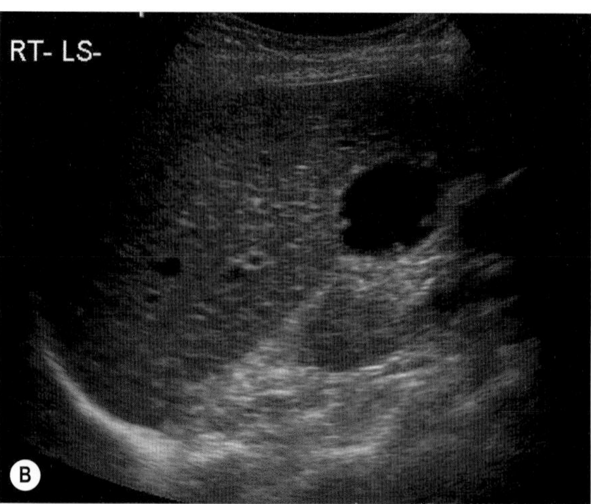

Fig. 3.21 • Cholesterolosis (A & B): multiple tiny polyps in the gallbladder.

INFLAMMATORY GALLBLADDER DISEASE

Cholecystitis is usually associated with gallstones; the frictional action of stones on the gallbladder wall causes some degree of inflammation in almost all cases. The inner mucosa of the wall is injured, allowing the access of enteric bacteria. The inflammatory process may be long-standing and chronic, acute or a combination of acute inflammation on a chronic background.

ACUTE CHOLECYSTITIS

Acute inflammation of the gallbladder presents with severe right upper quadrant (RUQ) pain localized to the gallbladder area. The pain can be elicited by (gently!) pressing the gallbladder with the ultrasound transducer – a positive ultrasound Murphy's sign. (This sign, although a useful pointer to acute inflammation, is not specific and can be frequently elicited in other conditions, such as chronic inflammatory cases.)

On ultrasound, the gallbladder wall is thickened – greater than 2 mm. This is not in itself a specific sign (Table 3.1), but characteristically the thickening in acute cholecystitis is symmetrical, affecting the entire wall, and there is an echo-poor 'halo' around the gallbladder as a result of oedematous changes (Fig. 3.22). This is not invariable, however, and focal thickening may be present, or the wall may be uniformly hyperechoic in some cases.

Pericholecystic fluid may also be present, and the inflammatory process may spread to the adjacent liver. Complications may occur if the acute inflammation progresses (see below) due to infection, the formation of pericholecystic abscesses and peritonitis.

Further management of acute cholecystitis

In an uncomplicated acute cholecystitis, analgesia to settle the patient in the short term is followed by laparoscopic removal of the gallbladder. Open surgery is reserved for the more complex cases.[25,26]

If unsuitable for immediate surgery, for example in cases complicated by peritonitis, the patient is managed with antibiotics and/or percutaneous drainage of pericholecystic fluid or infected bile from the gallbladder, usually under ultrasound guidance. This allows the patient's symptoms to settle and reduces morbidity from the subsequent elective operation. Ultrasound is also useful in guiding bedside cholecystostomy or abscess drainage prior to elective surgical treatment.[27]

Hepatobiliary scintigraphy has high sensitivity and specificity for evaluating patients with acute

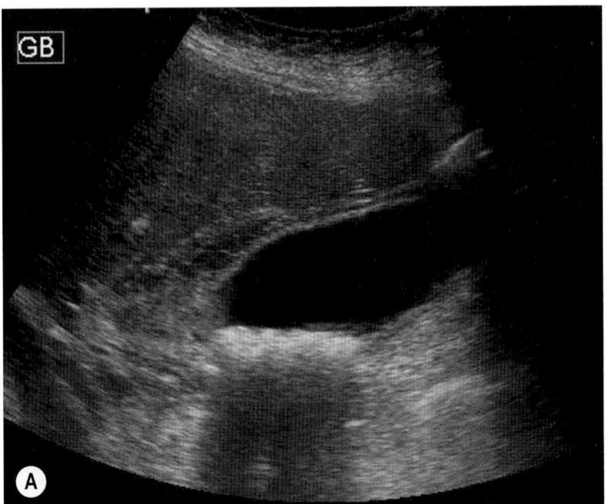

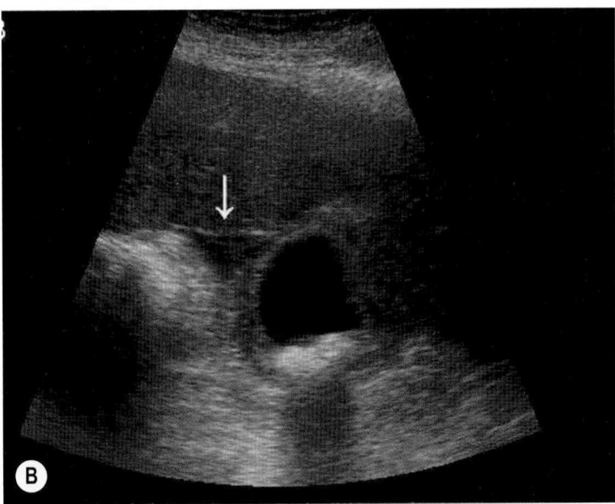

Fig. 3.22 • Acute cholecystitis: (A) The gallbladder contains stones, has an oedematous, thickened wall and is tender on scanning. (B) TS of an acutely inflamed gallbladder, with a thickened wall and stones. Pericholecystic fluid is present (arrow).

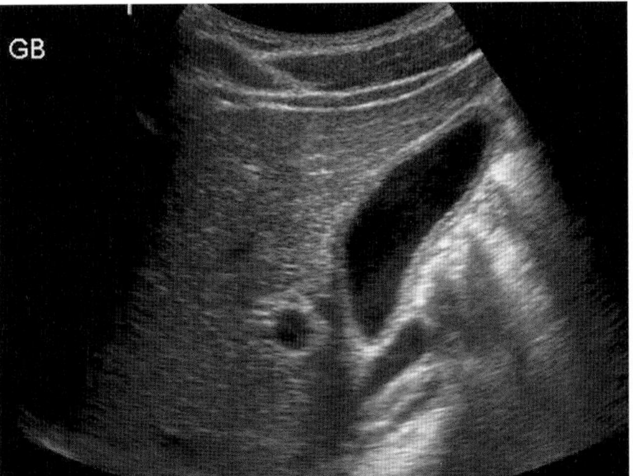

Fig. 3.23 • A normal gallbladder in a patient with hepatitis C demonstrates a thickened wall, which should not be confused with acute cholecystitis.

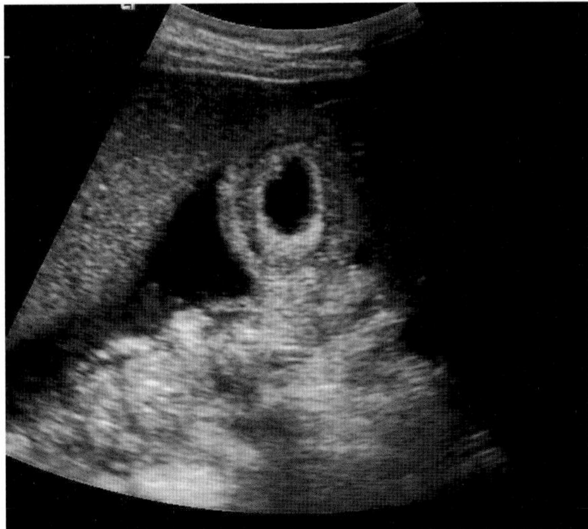

Fig. 3.24 • The gallbladder wall is oedematous due to ascites resulting from liver failure.

cholecystitis,[1] particularly if the ultrasound examination is technically difficult or equivocal, and has the advantage of being able to demonstrate hepatobiliary drainage into the duodenum. Plain X-ray is seldom used, but can confirm the presence of gas in the gallbladder.

The gallbladder may appear thick walled in the presence of adjacent inflammatory processes, such as hepatitis (Fig. 3.23). Ascites will often cause a normal gallbladder wall to look oedematous and thickened (Fig. 3.24).

CHRONIC CHOLECYSTITIS

Usually associated with gallstones, chronic cholecystitis presents with lower grade, recurring RUQ pain. The action of stones on the wall causes it to become fibrosed and irregularly thickened, frequently appearing hyperechoic (Fig. 3.25). The gallbladder may be shrunken and contracted having little or no recognizable lumen around the stones.

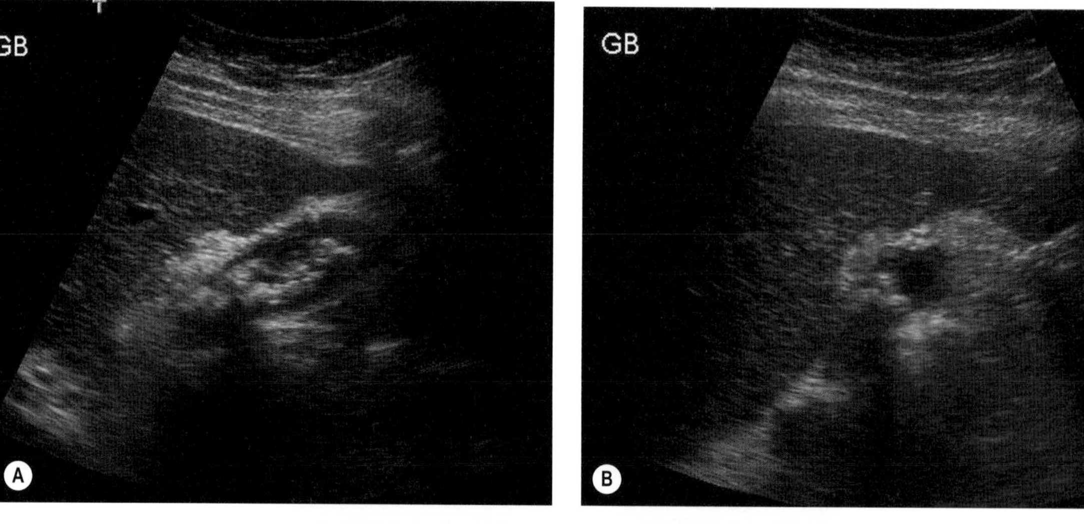

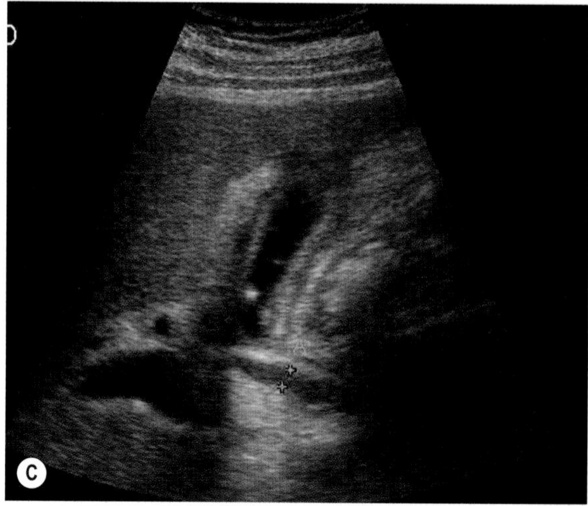

Fig. 3.25 • Chronic cholecystitis; (A) A hyperechoic, irregular, thickened wall. The gallbladder is contracted and contains numerous stones. (B) TS demonstrating irregular wall thickening with multiple stones. (C) Considerable wall thickening in chronic cholecystitis. Mildly tender on scanning.

Chronic cholecystitis may be complicated by episodes of acute inflammation on a background of the chronic condition.

Most gallbladders which contain stones show at least some histological degree of chronic cholecystitis, even if wall thickening is not apparent on ultrasound.

ACALCULOUS CHOLECYSTITIS

Inflammation of the gallbladder without stones is relatively uncommon, accounting for around 10% of cases of acute cholecystitis.[28] A thickened, tender gallbladder wall in the absence of any other obvious cause of thickening may be due to acalculous cholecystitis. Traditionally this condition is associated with patients who are already hospitalized and have been fasting, including post-trauma patients, those recovering from surgical procedures and diabetic patients. It is brought about by bile stasis leading to a distended gallbladder and subsequently decreased blood flow to the gallbladder. This, especially in the weakened post-operative state, can lead to infection. However, it also occurs

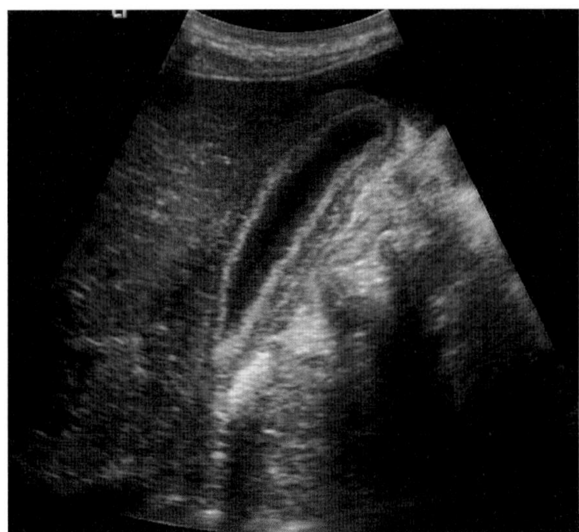

Fig. 3.26 • Acalculous cholecystitis. The gallbladder wall is markedly thickened and tender on scanning.

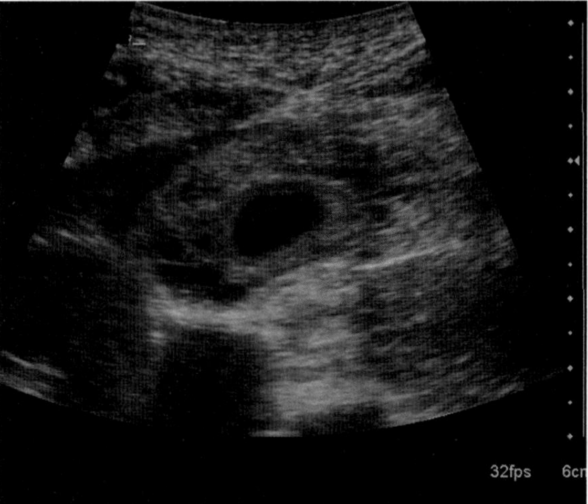

Fig. 3.27 • Acute-on-chronic cholecystitis. A patient with known gallstones and chronic cholecystitis presents with an episode of acute gallbladder pain. The wall is considerably more thickened and hyperechoic than on previous scans, and is now tender on scanning.

in otherwise healthy patients with no history of acute illness or trauma.[28]

Because no stones are present, the diagnosis is more difficult and may be delayed. Patients with acalculous cholecystitis are therefore more likely to have severe pain and fever by the time the diagnosis is made, increasing the incidence of complications such as perforation.

The wall may appear normal on ultrasound in the early stages, but progressively thickens, (Fig. 3.26). Biliary sludge is usually present and a pericholecystic abscess may develop in the later stages. A positive Murphy's sign may help to focus on the diagnosis, but in unconscious patients the diagnosis is a particularly difficult one.

In patients already critically ill with their presenting disease, or following surgery, there is a role for ultrasound in guiding percutaneous cholecystostomy at the bedside to relieve the symptoms.[29]

Chronic acalculous cholecystitis implies a recurrent presentation with typical symptoms of biliary colic, but no evident stones on ultrasound. Patients may also demonstrate a low ejection fraction during a cholecystokinin-stimulated hepatic iminodiacetic acid (HIDA) scan. The symptoms are relieved by elective laparoscopic cholecystectomy in most patients, with similar results to those for gallstone disease[30] (although some are found to have biliary pathology at surgery which might explain the symptoms – such as polyps, cholesterolosis or biliary crystals/tiny stones, in addition to chronic inflammation).

COMPLICATIONS OF CHOLECYSTITIS

Acute-on-chronic cholecystitis

Patients with a long-standing history of chronic cholecystitis may experience (sometimes repeated) attacks of acute inflammation. The gallbladder wall is thickened, as for chronic inflammation, and may become focally thickened with both hypo- and hyperechoic regions. Stones are usually present (Fig. 3.27).

Gangrenous cholecystitis

In a small percentage of patients, acute gallbladder inflammation progresses to gangrenous cholecystitis. Areas of necrosis develop within the gallbladder wall, the wall itself may bleed and small abscesses form (Fig. 3.28). This severe complication of the inflammatory process requires immediate cholecystectomy.

The gallbladder wall is friable and may rupture, causing a pericholecystic collection and possibly

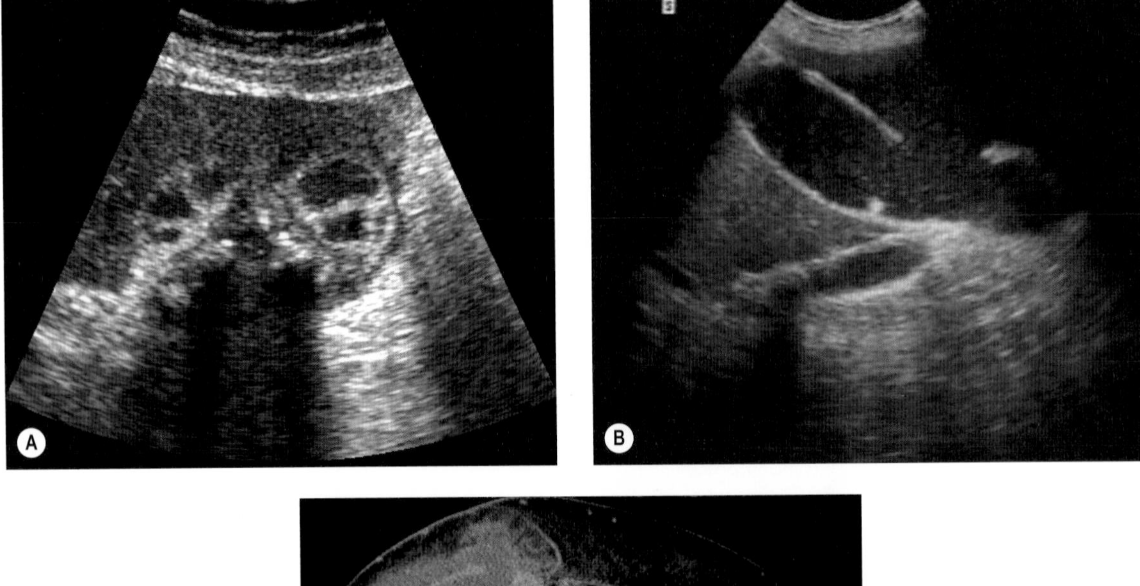

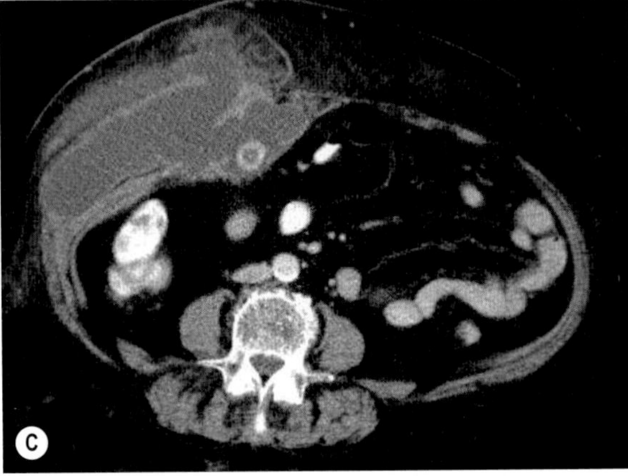

Fig. 3.28 • Gangrenous cholecystitis: (A) The gallbladder wall is irregularly thickened and an intramural abscess has formed on the anterior aspect. (B) The gallbladder has perforated and a large pericholecystic bile collection has formed. (C) CT of case in (B), showing perforation of the gallbladder.

peritonitis. Inflammatory spread may be seen in the adjacent liver tissue as a hypoechoic, ill-defined area. Loops of adjacent bowel may become adherent to the necrotic wall, forming a cholecystoenteric fistula. This condition is rare, but tends to be associated with older patients, often with a background of diabetes or cardiovascular disease, and carries increased morbidity and mortality.[31]

The wall is asymmetrically thickened and areas of abscess formation may be demonstrated. The damaged inner mucosa sloughs off, forming the appearance of membranes in the gallbladder lumen. The gallbladder frequently contains infected debris. The presence of a bile leak may also be demonstrated with hepatobiliary scintigraphy, using technetium^{99M}, which is useful in identifying a bile collection which may otherwise be obscured by bowel on ultrasound.

Emphysematous cholecystitis

This is a form of acute gangrenous cholecystitis in which the inflamed gallbladder may become infected, particularly in diabetic patients, with gas-forming organisms. Both the lumen and the wall of the gallbladder may contain air, which is highly reflective, but which casts a 'noisy' less definite shadow than that from stones. Discrete gas bubbles

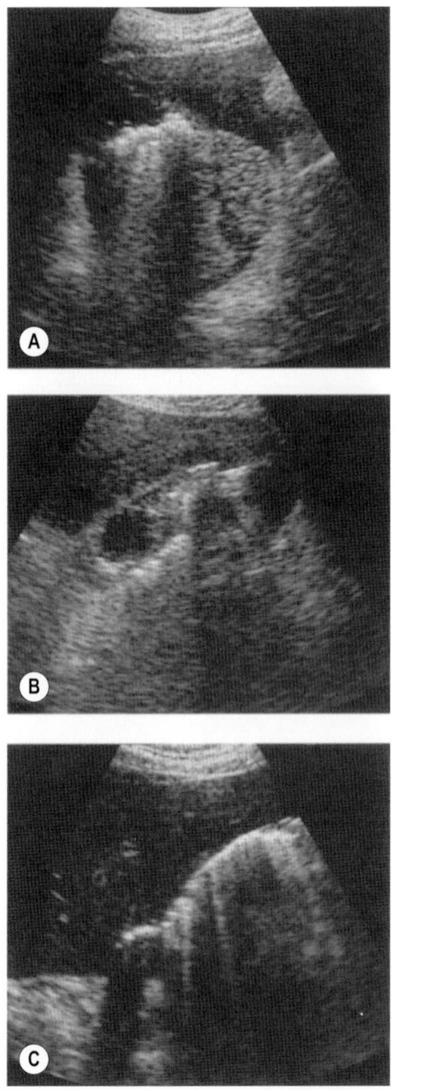

Fig. 3.29 • Emphysematous cholecystitis. (A & B) TS and LS with gas and debris in the gallbladder lumen. (C) Gas in the gallbladder lumen completely obscures the contents.

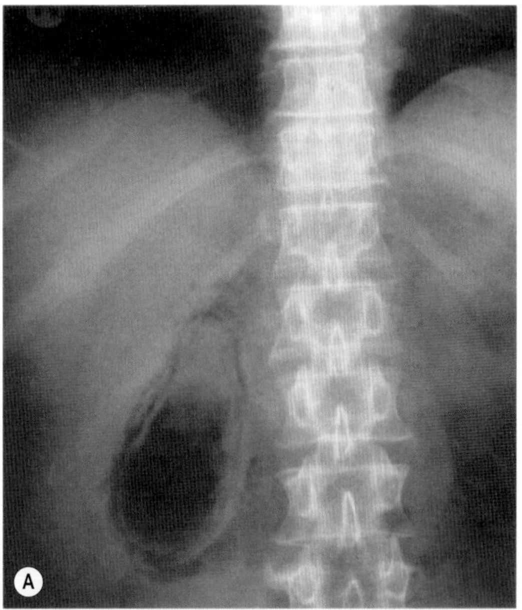

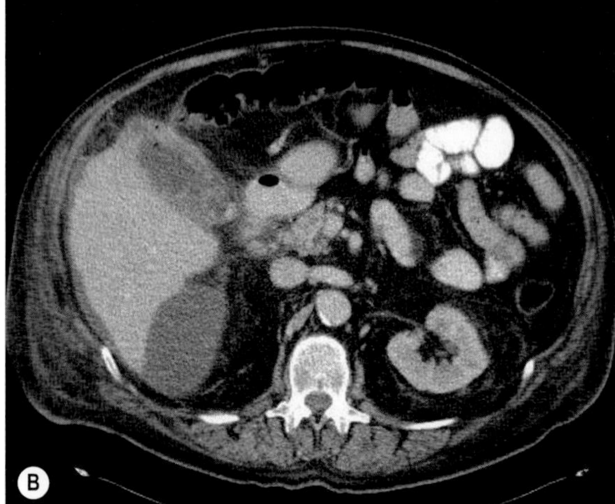

Fig. 3.30 • Emphysematous cholecystitis (A) X-ray demonstrating gas in the gallbladder in emphysematous cholecystitis. (B) CT shows small gas bubbles in the wall of the gallbladder.

have been reported on ultrasound within the gallbladder wall,[32] and may also extend into the intrahepatic biliary ducts.[33] The air rises to the anterior part of the gallbladder, obscuring the features behind it (Fig. 3.29). This effect may mimic air-filled bowel on ultrasound.

Emphysematous cholecystitis has traditionally had a much higher mortality rate than other forms of cholecystitis, requiring immediate cholecystectomy. However, improvements in ultrasound resolution, and in the early clinical recognition of this condition, suggest that it is now being diagnosed earlier and may be managed more conservatively. The gas in the gallbladder may be confirmed on a plain X-ray (Fig. 3.30), but ultrasound is more sensitive in demonstrating the earlier stages.

Gallbladder empyema

Empyema is a complication of cholecystitis in which the gallbladder becomes infected behind an obstructed cystic duct. Fine echoes, caused by pus, are present in the bile (Fig. 3.31). These patients may initially present with the usual features of acute cholecystitis, but may then progress to become very ill with fever and acute pain. Localized perforation of the gallbladder wall may cause leakage of infected bile to form a pericholecystic gallbladder collection with subsequent peritonitis. Ultrasound may be used to guide bedside drainage (Fig. 3.31D–F) to allow the patient's symptoms to settle before surgery is attempted.[34]

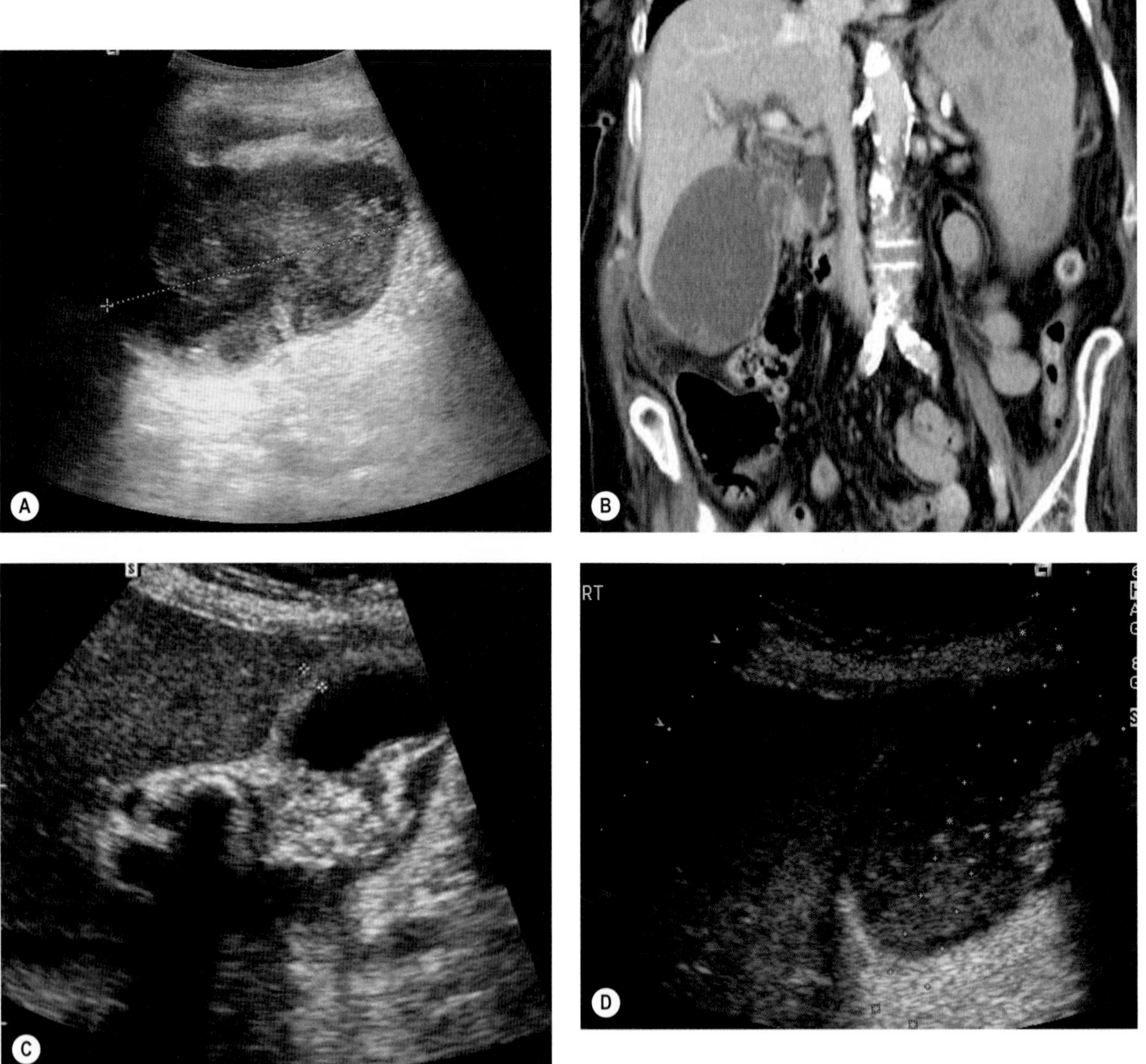

Fig. 3.31 • Gallbladder empyema. (A) Dilated tender gallbladder full of pus. (B) CT of case in (A). (C) Another case of gallbladder empyema with stones blocking the neck of the gallbladder. (D) A gallbladder empyema is about to undergo ultrasound-guided drainage.

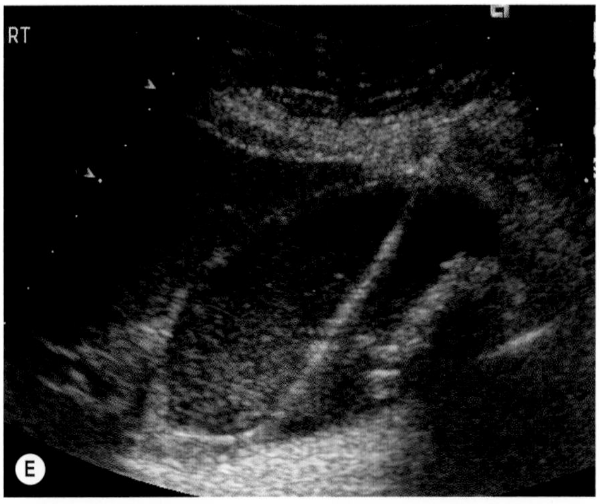

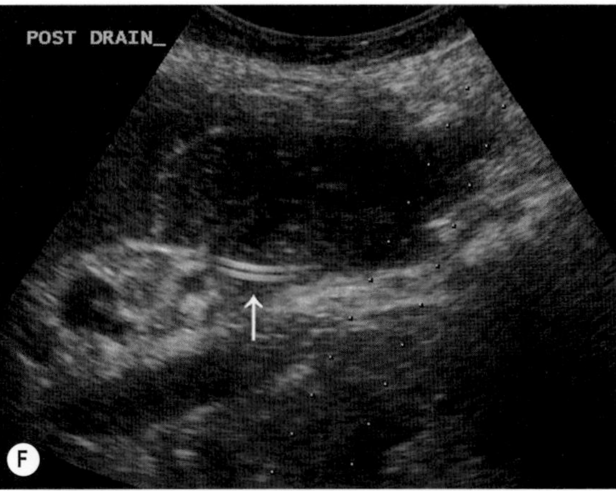

Fig. 3.31, cont'd • (E) The guidewire is inserted. (F) A drain (arrow) has been inserted into another case of gallbladder empyema under ultrasound guidance.

OBSTRUCTIVE JAUNDICE AND BILIARY DUCT DILATION

Obstruction of the biliary tree most commonly occurs around the distal (lower) end of the common duct, and almost always results in dilatation of the bile ducts within the liver. In a small number of cases it is possible to have an obstruction which fails to dilate the biliary tree, and it is also possible for the biliary tree to be dilated but not obstructed. However, the majority of cases of biliary duct dilatation are caused by obstruction of the common duct (Table 3.2), the most common causes being stones or a neoplasm of the bile duct, ampulla or head of pancreas. Up to 20% of patients with gallbladder stones will develop choledocholithiasis.[4]

The patient with obstructive jaundice may present with upper abdominal pain, abnormal LFTs (see Chapter 2) and, if the obstruction is not intermittent, the sclera of the eye and the skin adopt a yellow tinge.

Assessment of the level of obstruction

It is possible for the sonographer to work out where the obstructing lesion is situated by observing which parts of the biliary tree are dilated (Fig. 3.32):

- Dilatation of the CBD (i.e. that portion of the duct below the cystic duct insertion) implies obstruction at its lower end.

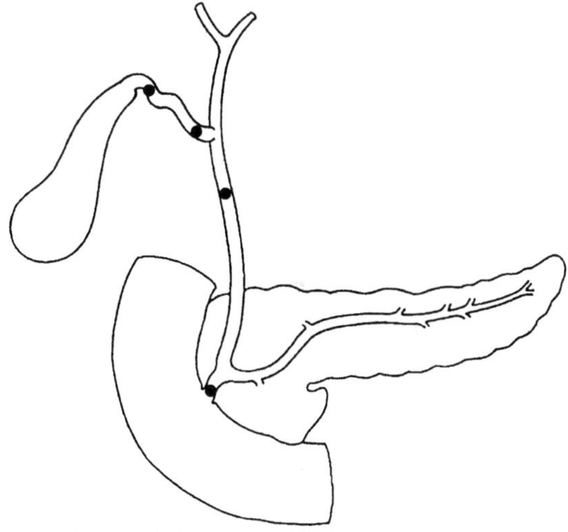

Fig. 3.32 • Sites of possible gallstone obstruction.

- Dilatation of both biliary and pancreatic ducts implies obstruction distally, at the head of the pancreas or ampulla of Vater. This is more likely to be due to carcinoma of the head of pancreas, ampulla or acute pancreatitis than a stone. However, it is possible for a stone to be lodged just distal to the confluence of the biliary and pancreatic ducts.
- Dilatation of the gallbladder alone (i.e. without ductal dilatation) is usually caused by obstruction at the neck or cystic duct (Fig. 3.8).

Intrinsic	Stones
	Carcinoma of the ampulla of Vater
	Cholangiocarcinoma
	Stricture (associated with chronic pancreatitis)
	Biliary atresia/choledochal cyst
	Post liver transplantation bile duct stenosis (usually anastomotic)
	Parasites
	Age-related or post-surgical mild CBD dilatation
Extrinsic	Carcinoma of the head of pancreas
	Acute pancreatitis
	Lymphadenopathy at the porta hepatis
	Other masses at the porta, e.g. hepatic artery aneurysm, gastrointestinal tract mass
	Intrahepatic tumours (obstructed distal segments)
Diffuse hepatic conditions	Sclerosing cholangitis
	Caroli's disease

Table 3.2 Causes of biliary duct dilatation

To assess whether the gallbladder is pathologically dilated may be difficult on ultrasound. The dilated gallbladder will have a rounded, bulging shape due to the increase in pressure inside it.

A gallbladder whose wall has become fibrosed from chronic cholecystitis due to stones will often lose the ability to distend, so the biliary ducts can look grossly dilated despite the gallbladder remaining 'normal' in size, or contracted.

Early ductal obstruction

Beware of very early common duct obstruction, before the duct becomes obviously dilated. The duct may be mildly dilated at the lower end, just proximal to a stone, but normal in its intrahepatic portion. Likewise intermittent obstruction by a small stone at the lower end of the duct may be non-dilated by the time the scan is performed (Fig. 3.10).

A significant ultrasound feature in the absence of any other identifiable findings is that of thickening of the wall of the bile duct. This not only represents an inflammatory process in the duct wall, which may be found in patients with small stones in a non-dilated duct, but is also associated with sclerosing cholangitis.[35]

It is sometimes technically difficult in some patients (particularly those with diffuse liver disease) to work out whether a tubular structure on ultrasound represents a dilated duct or a blood vessel. Colour Doppler will differentiate the dilated bile duct from a branch of hepatic artery or portal vein (Fig. 3.33), provided that the vein is not thrombosed, of course.

It is not useful to use colour Doppler routinely in order to locate the CBD; the angle of insonation is frequently perpendicular to the beam, so the vein may display no colour signal, confusing the operator further. In addition, the application of colour Doppler reduces the line density and image resolution – exactly the opposite of what you require when searching for a small duct.

Diagnosis and assessment of the cause of obstruction

The numerous causes of biliary dilatation are summarized in Table 3.2. Frequently, ultrasound diagnoses the obstruction, but does not identify the cause. This is a case for perseverance by the operator, as the lower end of the CBD is visible in the majority of cases once overlying duodenum has been moved away (Figs 3.9, 3.10, 3.34). However, ultrasound is not generally regarded as a reliable tool for identifying ductal stones, and is frequently unable to diagnose ductal strictures, especially those from benign causes. In the absence of a definite diagnosis of stones, MRCP is an effective, non-invasive technique in the diagnosis of CBD stones and strictures[5,36] (Fig. 3.34F), avoiding the need for the more invasive ERCP.

The use of ERCP, although diagnostically highly accurate, is usually reserved for occasions when

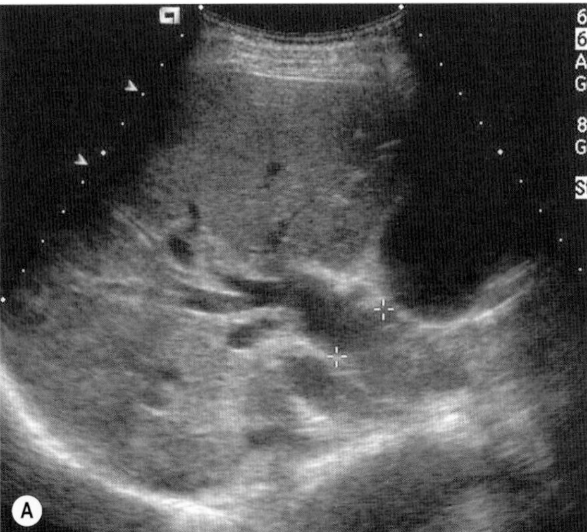

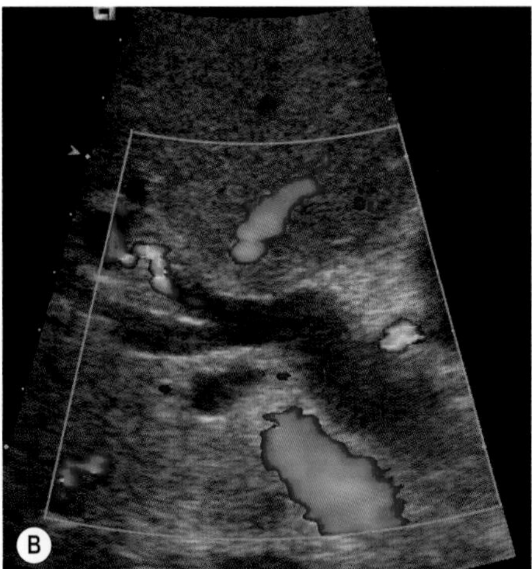

Fig. 3.33 • (A & B) Dilated biliary ducts do not demonstrate flow on colour or power Doppler, differentiating them from portal vessels.

therapeutic stone removal or stent insertion may be required, as it is an invasive procedure with attendant risks of pancreatitis, cholangitis and, rarely, perforation of the bile duct or duodenum.[37,38] Complications occur in up to 8% of patients undergoing ERCP, with a mortality rate of up to 0.5%,[39] so the technique should ideally be reserved for those requiring therapeutic intervention.

EUS also has an accuracy in detecting CBD stones comparable with ERCP, while avoiding the risks associated with radiation and biliary instrumentation. It is not yet as readily available as ERCP, and requires specialist skills and equipment with a significant learning curve.[40] CT and MRI are useful for staging purposes if the obstructing lesion is malignant. Cholangiocarcinomas spread to the lymph nodes and to the liver – and small liver deposits are particularly difficult to recognize on ultrasound if the intrahepatic biliary ducts are dilated.

In hepatobiliary scintigraphy, technetium^{99M}-labelled derivatives of iminodiacetic acid are excreted in the bile and may help to demonstrate sites of obstruction, e.g. in the cystic duct – or abnormal accumulations of bile, e.g. choledochal cysts. The technique is also useful in demonstrating postoperative bile leaks.[41]

Courvoisier's law, to which there are numerous exceptions, states that if the gallbladder is dilated in a jaundiced patient, then the cause is *not* due to a stone in the common duct. The reasoning behind this is that gallstones cause a degree of wall fibrosis from chronic cholecystitis which would prevent it from distending. In fact there are many exceptions to this 'law', which include the formation of stones in the duct, without gallbladder stones, and also obstruction by a pancreatic stone at the ampulla.

- Do not assume that obstructive jaundice in a patient with gallstones is due to a stone in the CBD. The jaundice may be attributable to other causes.
- Do not assume that obstructive jaundice cannot be due to a stone in the CBD if the gallbladder does not contain stones. A solitary stone can be passed into the duct from the gallbladder, or stones can form within the duct.

Management of biliary obstruction

Management of biliary obstruction obviously depends on the cause and the severity of the condition. Radiological imaging may be used for both diagnostic and therapeutic purpose. The first line of investigation tends to be ultrasound. Patients may then be directed either for further imaging, such as MRCP or CT, to clarify the diagnosis, or may proceed straight to therapeutic intervention.

Removal of stones in the CBD may be performed by ERCP with sphincterotomy. Elective, laparoscopic cholecystectomy may take place if gallstones are present in the gallbladder.

Laparoscopic ultrasound is a useful adjunct to surgical exploration of the biliary tree and its accuracy in experienced hands equals that of X-ray cholangiography. Its potential has been slow to be realized in many centres, as it requires training and has a steep learning curve. However the lack of ionizing radiation, together with its accuracy in experienced hands, has allowed it to replace fluoroscopic cholangiography in some centres.[42]

EUS can also be used to examine the CBD, avoiding the need for laparoscopic exploration of the duct. It is highly accurate in diagnosing ductal stones, particularly in experienced hands,[43] and may be more sensitive than MRCP in the detection

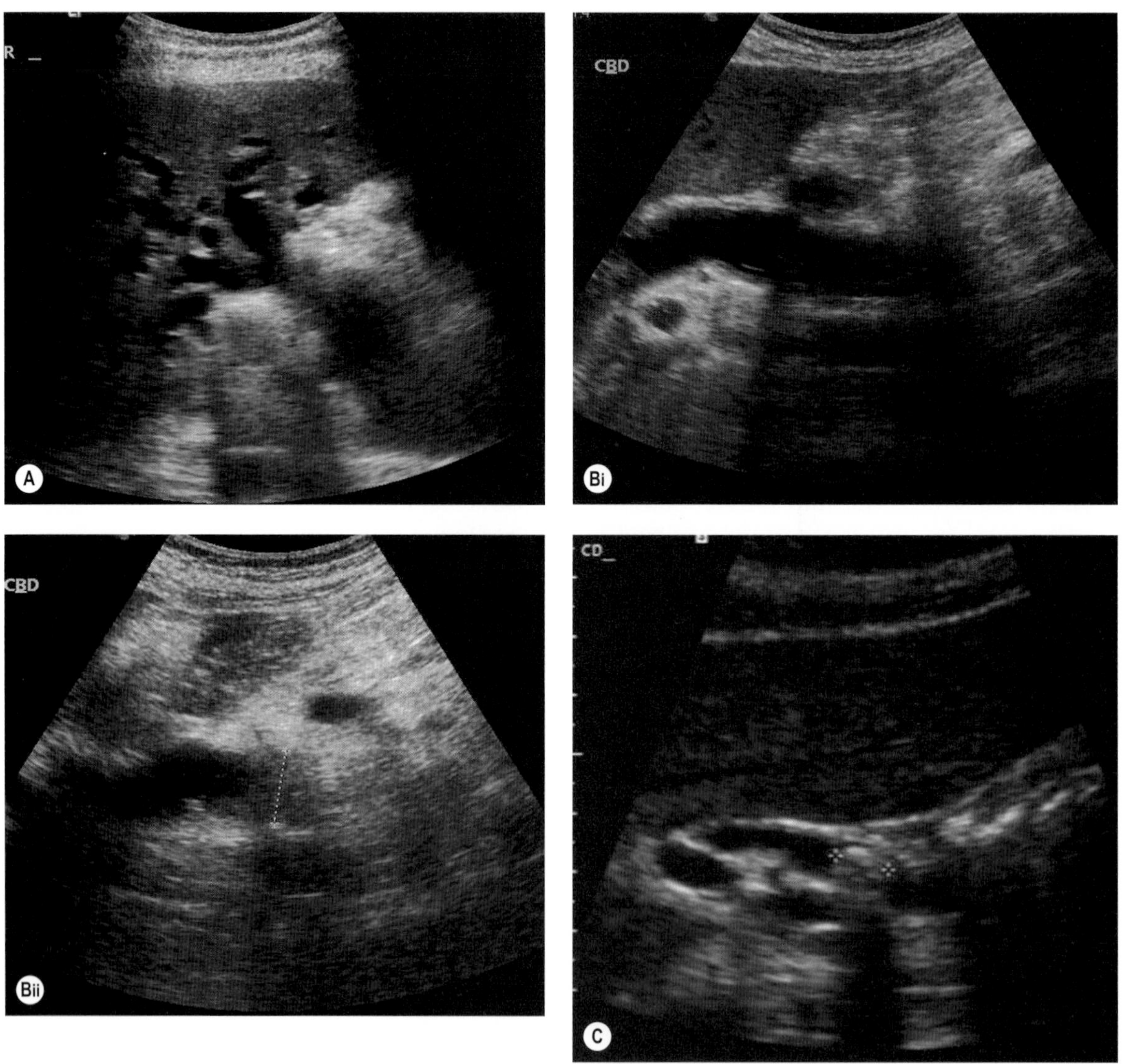

Fig. 3.34 • (A) Duodenal gas obscures the cause of obstruction at the lower end of this dilated CBD. (B) Patient positioning can move bowel gas away from the duct (Bi), demonstrating the cause of obstruction (Bii) – a carcinoma of the ampulla confirmed on EUS. (C) A mildly dilated CBD with a stone (calipers).

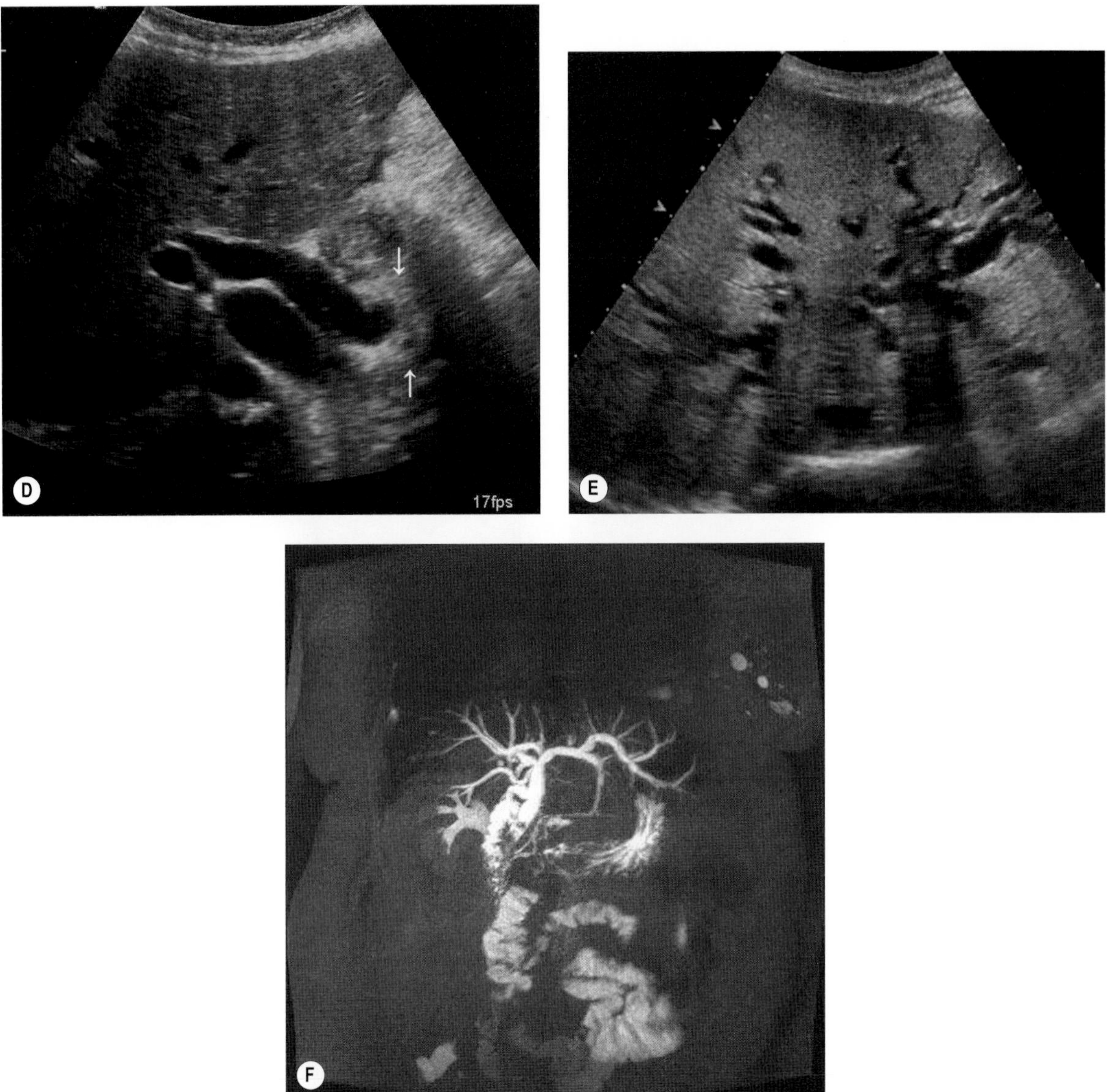

Fig. 3.34, cont'd • (D) Dilated CBD caused by a lymph node mass at the porta hepatis (arrows). (E) Intrahepatic bile duct dilatation. (F) MRCP demonstrates a stone in the lower end of the duct.

of small ductal stones, (depending on the MRCP slice thickness),[44] but its invasive nature means it is usually reserved for cases when MRCP is negative in patients where the probability of stones or an obstructing lesion remains high.

The treatment of malignant obstruction is determined by the stage of the disease. Accurate staging is best performed using CT and/or MRI. If surgical removal of the obstructing lesion is not a suitable option because of local or distant spread or other comorbidity, palliative stenting may be performed endoscopically to relieve the obstruction and decompress the ducts (Fig. 3.35). The patency of the stent may be subsequently monitored with ultrasound by assessing the degree of duct dilatation.

Clinical suspicion of early obstruction should be raised if the serum alkaline phosphatase is

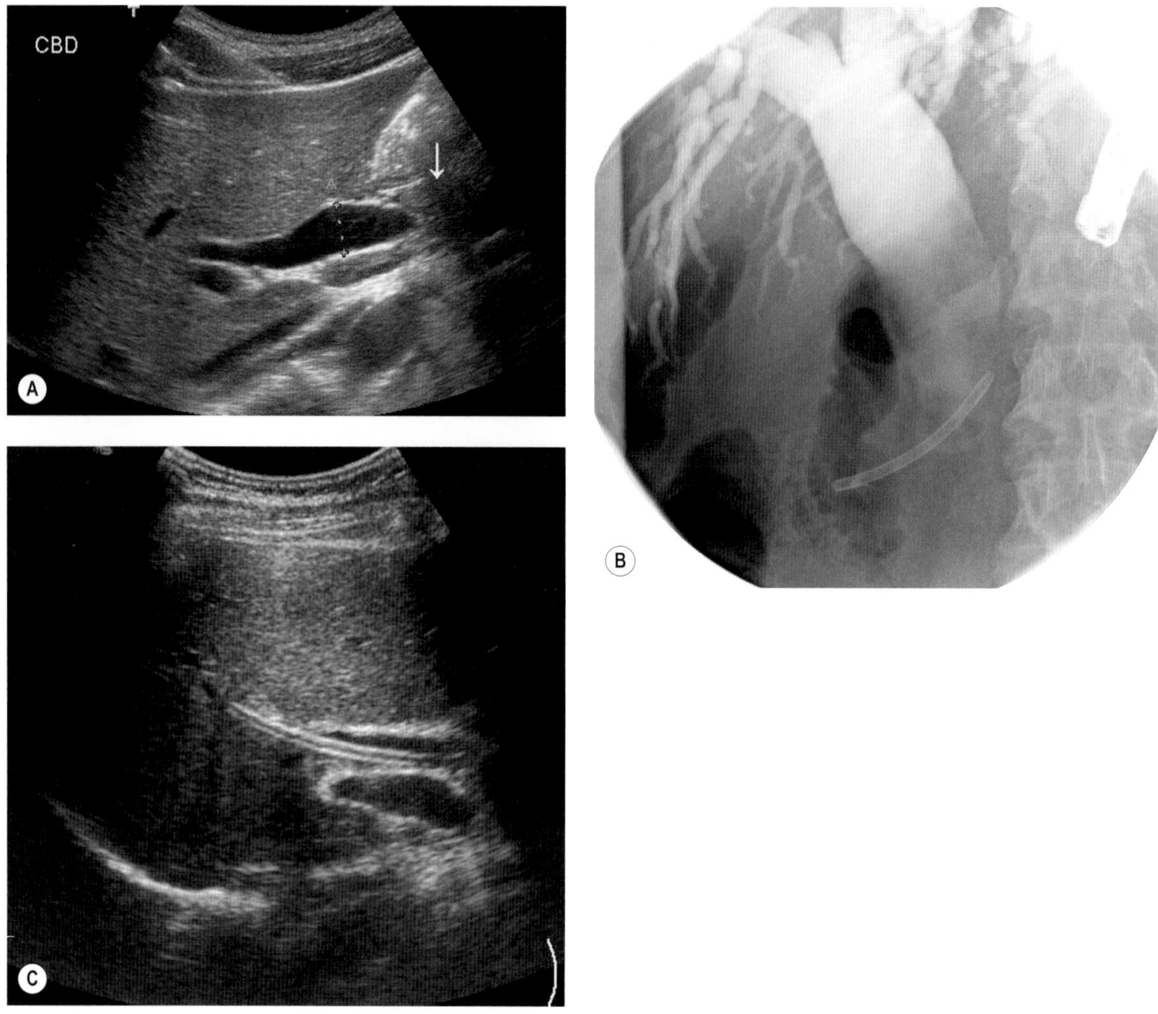

Fig. 3.35 • (A) This dilated CBD (calipers) is obstructed by a mass at the lower end (arrow) in the head of pancreas. (B) ERCP demonstrates a tight, malignant stricture from an ampullary carcinoma. A palliative stent is positioned. (C) Stent in the CBD of a patient with a cholangiocarcinoma. Decompression of the dilated biliary tree has been achieved and ultrasound can be used to monitor the patency of the stent.

elevated (often more sensitive in the early stages than a raised serum bilirubin). In the presence of ductal dilatation on ultrasound, further imaging, such as CT, MRCP or EUS, may then refine the diagnosis.

Intrahepatic tumours causing biliary obstruction

Focal masses that cause segmental intrahepatic duct dilatation are usually intrinsic to the duct itself, e.g. cholangiocarcinoma. It is also possible for a focal intrahepatic mass, whether benign or malignant, to compress an adjacent biliary duct, causing subsequent obstruction of that segment. This is not, however, a common cause of biliary dilatation and occurs most usually with hepatocellular carcinomas.[45] Most liver metastases deform, rather than compress, adjacent structures and biliary obstruction only occurs if the metastases are very large and/or invade the biliary tree. An HCC or metastatic deposit at the porta hepatis may obstruct the common duct by squeezing it against adjacent extrahepatic structures.

Benign intrahepatic lesions rarely cause ductal dilatation, but occasionally their sheer size obstructs the biliary tree.

Choledochal cysts

Most commonly found in children, this is associated with biliary atresia, in which the distal 'blind' end of the duct dilates into a rounded, cystic mass in response to raised intrahepatic pressure. Choledochal cysts in adults are rare, and tend to be asymptomatic unless associated with stones or other biliary disease. They tend to be associated with an anomalous insertion of the CBD into the pancreatic duct, which allows pancreatic enzymes to reflux into the bile duct resulting in inflammation and weakening of the duct wall forming a choledochal cyst[46] (Fig. 3.36).

Less commonly the dilatation is due to a non-obstructive cause in which the biliary ducts themselves become ectatic and can form diverticulae. This may be due to a focal stricture of the duct which causes reflux and a localized enlargement of the duct proximal to the stricture. (See also 'Caroli's disease' below.)

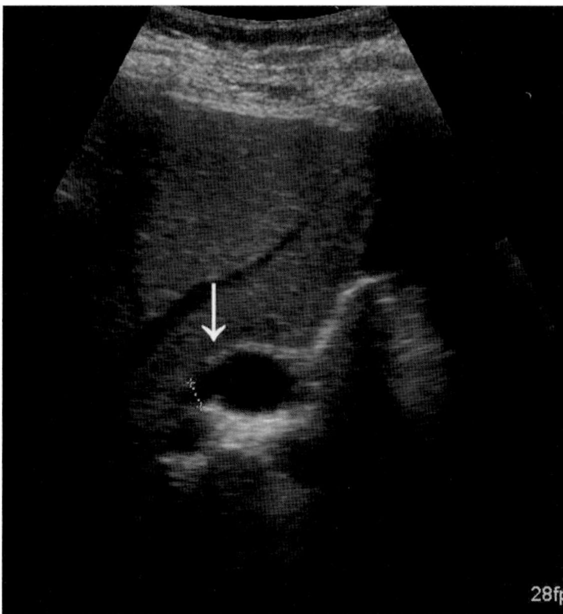

Fig. 3.36 • A small choledochal cyst (arrow) at the porta can be seen communicating with the biliary tree (calipers).

Complications of choledochal cysts include cholangitis, formation of stones and progression of the condition to secondary biliary cirrhosis, which may be associated with portal hypertension.

It may be difficult to differentiate a choledochal cyst, particularly if solitary, from other causes of hepatic cysts. The connection between the choledochal cyst and the adjacent biliary duct may be demonstrated with careful scanning, but further imaging including MRCP is frequently required.

Cholangitis

Cholangitis is an inflammation of the biliary ducts. It most commonly occurs secondary to obstruction where stasis of bile in the biliary tree may lead to infection and acute inflammation of the ducts. Other causes of cholangitis include strictures or stenosis of ducts, post-ERCP or duct manipulation, AIDS cholangiopathy, parasitic infections such as recurrent pyogenic cholangitis (oriental cholangiohepatitis) which is endemic in South East Asia, and sclerosing cholangitis. (See also 'Primary sclerosing cholangitis' below.)

Duct dilatation may be present, depending on the aetiology of the cholangitis. In severe cases the duct walls appear thickened and irregular and debris can be seen in the larger ducts (Fig. 3.37). Care should be taken to differentiate ductal wall thickening from tumour invasion, and further imaging may be necessary to exclude malignancy.

Bacterial cholangitis is the most common form, due to ascending bacterial infection from the duodenum or portal vein. Bacterial cholangitis is also associated with biliary enteric anastomoses and may be complicated by abscesses if the infection is progressive and untreated. Small abscesses may be difficult to diagnose on ultrasound, as they are frequently isoechoic and ill-defined in the early stages, and biliary dilatation makes evaluation of the hepatic parenchyma notoriously difficult.

Contrast CT may identify small abscesses not visible on ultrasound, and MRCP or ERCP demonstrate mural changes in the ducts.

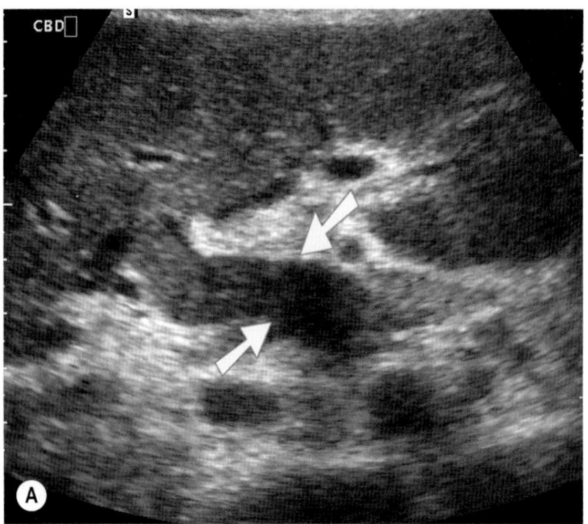

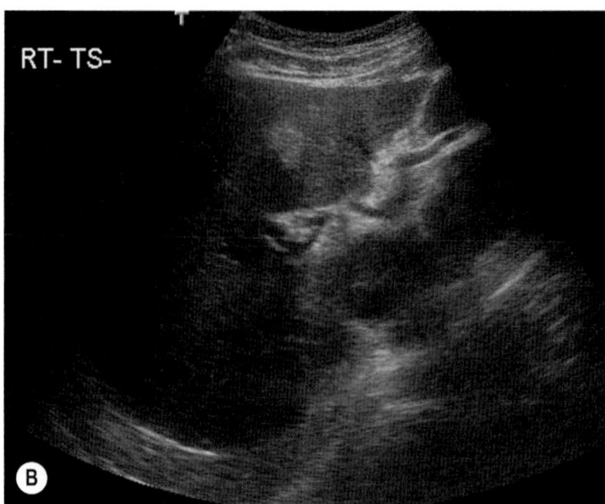

Fig. 3.37 • (A) Cholangitis with debris present in the dilated CBD (arrows). (B) Hyperechoic, thickened and inflamed portal tracts in a patient with chronic cholangitis.

BILIARY DILATATION WITHOUT JAUNDICE

Post-surgical CBD dilatation

In patients who have had cholecystectomy associated with previous dilatation of the CBD it is common to find a persistent (but non-significant) mild dilatation of the duct post-operatively. The serum alkaline phosphatase and bilirubin levels should be normal in the absence of pathology. Because stones may be found in the duct post-operatively, it is important to differentiate non-obstructive from truly obstructive dilatation in a symptomatic patient (Fig. 3.38A). If in doubt, the patient may be rescanned at a suitable interval to assess any increase in ductal diameter.

Focal obstruction

Intrahepatic tumour, such as cholangiocarcinoma, may obstruct a segment of the biliary tree whilst the remainder of the liver and biliary tree appears normal. Focal duct dilatation should trigger the operator to examine the proximal area of dilatation for a possible mass. Such tumours may be present before jaundice is clinically apparent.

Pitfalls

Patients with cirrhosis and portal hypertension may have dilated hepatic arteries, which can mimic the appearances of dilated ducts (Fig. 3.38B, C). Colour or power Doppler will readily differentiate between these, as the bile duct lacks a Doppler signal. However, care must be taken to use an appropriate angle of insonation to display the Doppler signal in the blood vessels, as both duct *and* patent vessels may display no colour if perpendicular to the sound beam.

Pneumobilia (air in the ducts) casts a distal acoustic shadow, and may therefore obscure ductal dilatation.

OBSTRUCTION WITHOUT BILIARY DILATATION

Early obstruction

It is possible to scan a patient at the time of recent onset of obstruction from a stone before the ducts have had time to dilate, leading to a false negative diagnosis. If clinical suspicion persists, a rescan is frequently useful in these cases.

Occasionally, stones have a ball-valve effect in the duct, causing intermittent obstruction which may not demonstrate ductal dilatation on the ultrasound scan.

Fibrosis of the duct walls

A number of chronic pathological conditions cause the walls of the ducts to become fibrotic and stiff.

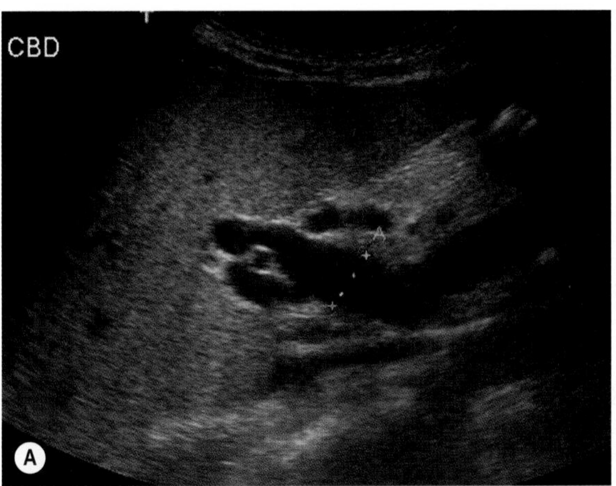

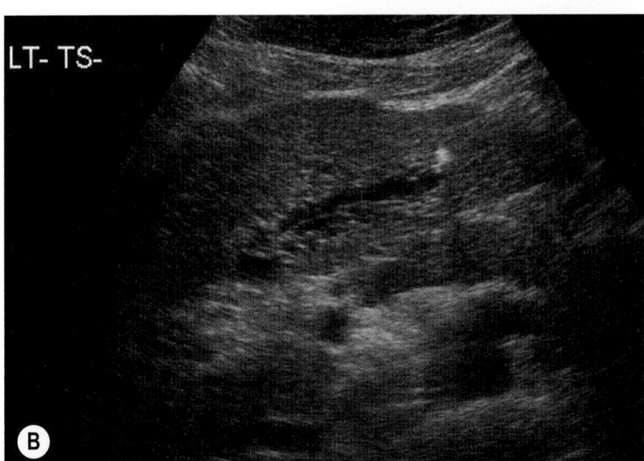

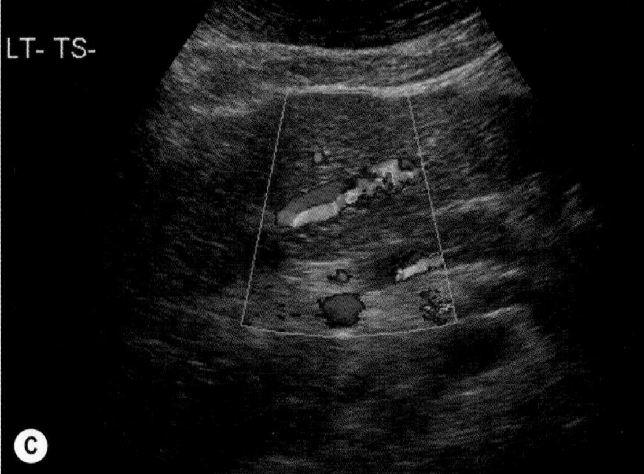

Fig. 3.38 • (A) Biliary dilatation following laparoscopic cholecystectomy due to a surgical clip across the CBD. (B) The appearance of dilated ducts is a pitfall in patients with portal hypertension. (C) Colour Doppler reveals the dilated 'tube' is actually an enlarged artery, not a duct.

These include PSC (see below) hepatitis and other chronic hepatic diseases leading to cirrhosis. The liver itself becomes rigid, and this prevents biliary dilatation. In such cases, the lack of dilated bile ducts does not necessarily imply an absence of obstruction.

OTHER BILIARY DISEASES

Primary sclerosing cholangitis

PSC is a rare form of chronic, cholestatic hepatobiliary disease in which the walls of the bile ducts become inflamed, causing narrowing. It predominantly affects young men (with a 2:1 male to female ratio) and is characterized by multiple biliary strictures and bead-like dilatations of the ducts. The aetiology of PSC remains unclear, but it is associated with inflammatory bowel disorders or may be idiopathic.

Clinical features include jaundice, itching and fatigue. Twenty-five percent of patients also have gallstones, which complicates the diagnosis; 70% of patients affected also have ulcerative colitis. Progressive gradual fibrosis causes strictures and eventually obliterates the biliary tree. Untreated, this leads to hepatic failure. PSC has a strong association with cholangiocarcinoma, and it is this, rather than hepatic failure, which may lead to death. In the absence of malignancy, however, hepatic transplantation has a 70–90% 5-year survival rate,[47] although recurrence of the disease is a recognized complication.[48]

Ultrasound appearances

The ultrasound appearances in PSC may be normal, particularly in the early stages, or may demonstrate a coarse, hyperechoic liver texture. Ductal strictures may cause downstream dilatation in some segments (Fig. 3.39), and in some cases there is marked biliary dilatation, but in the majority of patients the biliary ducts are prevented from dilatation by the surrounding fibrosis, and so appear unremarkable on ultrasound. MRCP is superior at demonstrating intrahepatic ductal strictures (Fig. 3.40). Mural thickening, particularly in the CBD, may be demonstrated with careful scanning[49] (Fig. 3.40A) and may be the only ultrasound sign. Ultrasound also demonstrates the effects of portal hypertension in advanced disease. The gallbladder may also have a thickened wall and can be dilated.[50]

Due to the association between PSC and cholangiocarcinoma, which may be multifocal, a careful search must be made for mass lesions. Because the ultrasound appearances may be those of a coarse, nodular liver texture it is difficult to identify small cholangiocarcinomas. Ultrasound contrast may help to highlight suspected lesions (Fig. 3.41), but MRI is the next investigation of choice to stage the disease. The diagnosis is an important one, because the patient's prognosis and management are affected by the presence of cholangiocarcinoma. If no masses are identified, the prognosis is favourable and patients may benefit from the endoscopic removal of stones to relieve symptoms, endoscopic stenting of main duct strictures to relieve jaundice and subsequent liver transplantation to pre-empt the formation of carcinoma. However, if carcinoma is already present, 5-year survival falls to 10%.

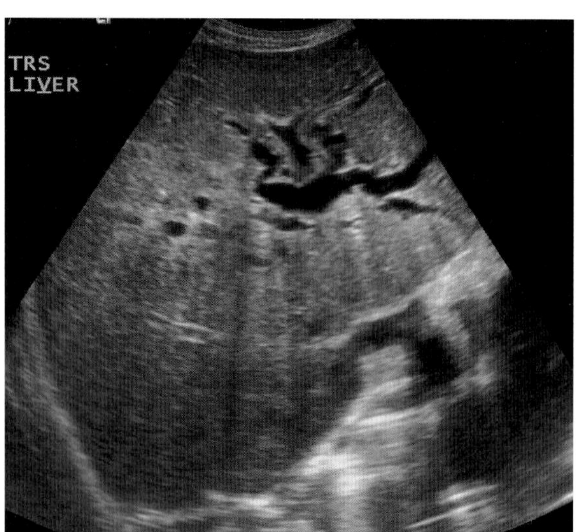

Fig. 3.39 • Localized biliary dilatation due to a ductal stricture in a patient with PSC.

Primary biliary cirrhosis

Primary biliary cirrhosis (PBC) is another example of a cholestatic disease that gradually obliterates the biliary tree and leads ultimately to cirrhosis. It is discussed more fully in Chapter 4.

Caroli's disease (congenital intrahepatic biliary dilatation)

This is a rare, congenital condition in which the bile ducts are irregularly dilated with diverticulae-like projections. These diverticulae may become infected and may separate off from the biliary duct, forming choledochal cysts (Fig. 3.42). In most cases, the entire hepatobiliary system is affected to some degree. Sufferers may present in early childhood, with symptoms of portal hypertension[51] or may remain well until adulthood, presenting with cholangitis. It is generally thought to be an autosomal recessive, inherited condition, and the prognosis is poor. Medical control of associated portal hypertension with varices can improve the quality of life.

In a few cases, the disease is confined to one or two segments of the liver, in which case a cure can be effected with hepatic resection.[52] The extrahepatic biliary tree is often unaffected.

The ultrasound appearances are of usually widespread intrahepatic duct dilatation, with saccular and fusiform biliary ectasia. Because it is also associated with biliary stone formation, the diagnosis is often not clear. The dilatation is also associated with cholangitis, and signs of infection may be present in the form of debris within the ducts, or even abscess. Sometimes frank choledochal cysts can be located.

Advanced disease is associated with portal hypertension and, in some cases, cholangiocarcinoma.[53] The presence of multiple cystic spaces on imaging must not be confused with multi- or polycystic disease, and the identification of a

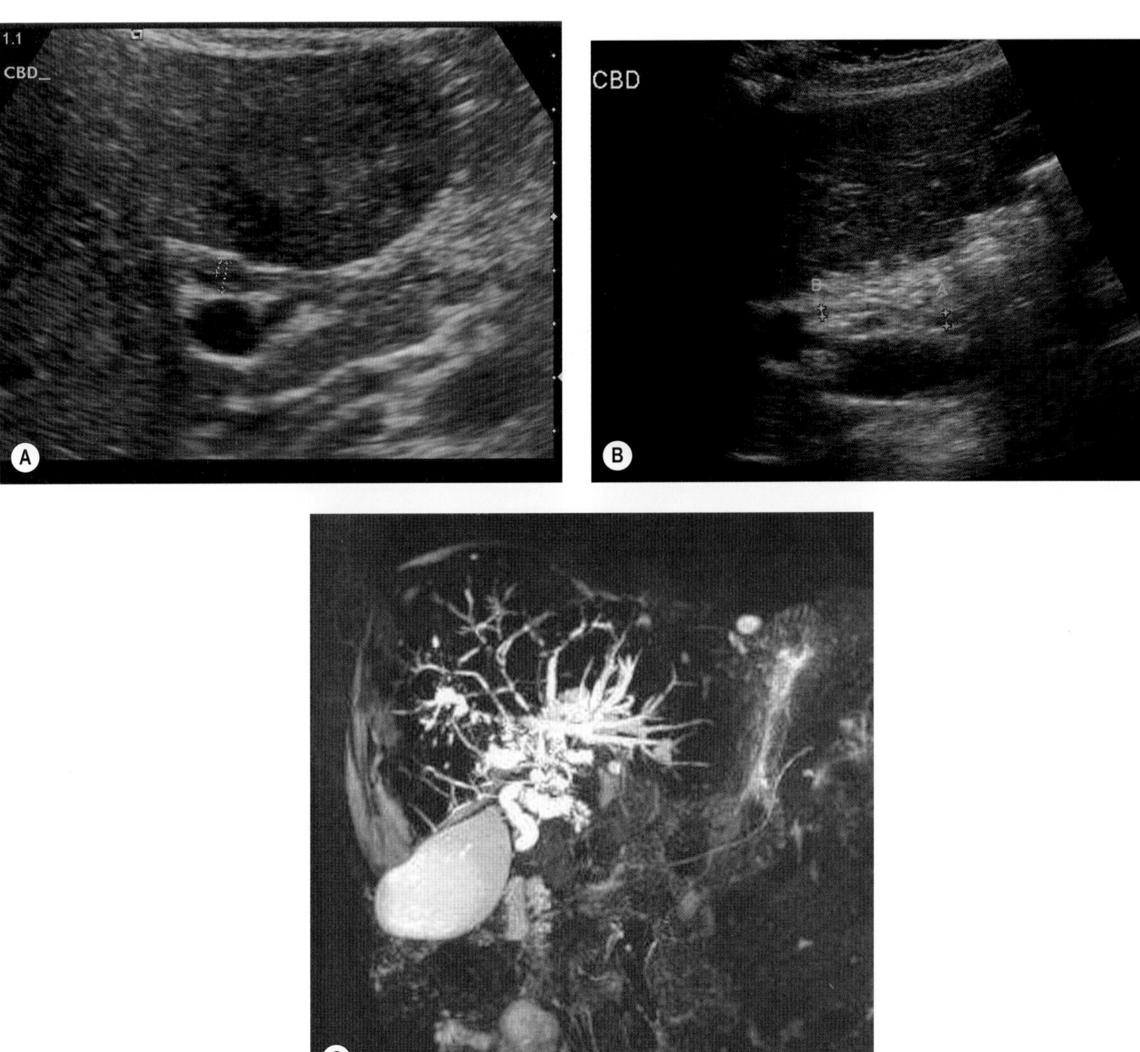

Fig. 3.40 • PSC: (A) Mural thickening in this normal-calibre CBD is typical of PSC (proven on biopsy). (B) Another case of PSC demonstrating thickening of a very narrow duct (calipers) and strictures in the CBD. (C) MRCP demonstrating numerous bile duct strictures in PSC.

communication between the cysts and the biliary tree with CT or MRI is an important factor in making the diagnosis.[54]

Parasites

Parasitic organisms, such as the *Ascaris* worm and liver fluke are extremely rare in the UK. However, they are a common cause of biliary colic in Africa, the Far East and South America. Hyperechoic linear structures in the gallbladder lumen, or in dilated ducts, should raise the sonographer's suspicion in patients native to, or those who have visited, these countries.[55] Impacted worms in the biliary ducts may also mimic other ductal masses and they are a rare cause of obstructive biliary dilatation (Fig. 3.43).

Patients may present with acute cholangitis or abdominal pain and vomiting. Endoscopic management is frequently highly effective.[56]

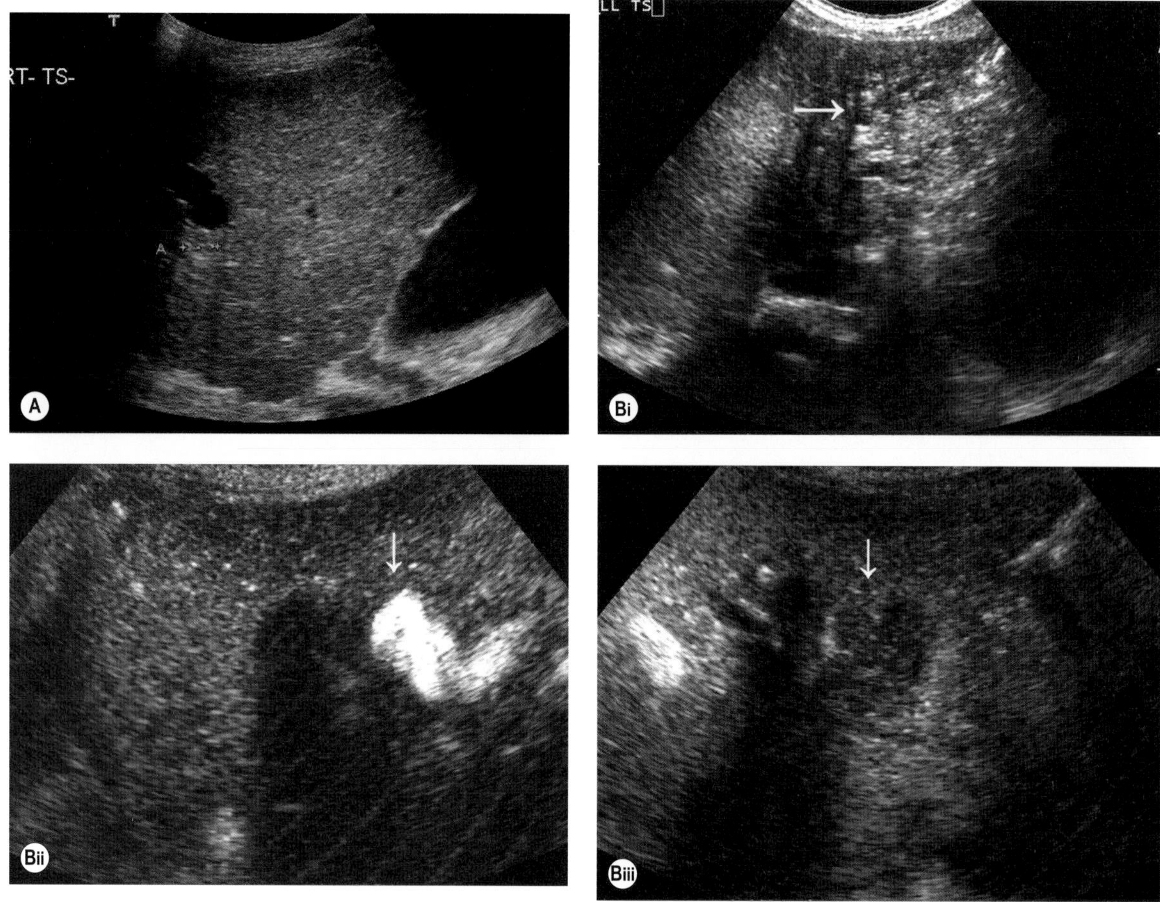

Fig. 3.41 • (A) Focally dilated bile ducts are a clue to the tiny cholangiocarcinoma (calipers) in this patient with PSC. (Bi) A cholangiocarcinoma is suspected due to focally dilated intrahepatic ducts (arrow) but not visualized on ultrasound. (Bii) CEUS demonstrates arterial enhancement of the lesions (arrow) with (Biii) sinusoidal phase hypoenhancement.

ECHOGENIC BILE

Biliary stasis and bile crystals

Fine echoes in the bile within the gallbladder are not uncommon on an ultrasound scan. This is commonly due to the inspissation of bile following prolonged starving – for example following surgery (Fig. 3.44). These appearances disappear after a normal diet is resumed and the gallbladder has emptied and refilled. Echogenic bile occurs when the solutes in the bile precipitate, often due to hypomotility of the gallbladder, and can commonly be seen following bone marrow transplantation, and in patients who have undergone prolonged periods (4–6 weeks) of total parenteral nutrition.[57]

Prolonged biliary stasis may lead to inflammation and/or infection, particularly in post-operative patients and those in immunosuppression. Its clinical course varies from complete resolution to progression to gallstones. However, following the resumption of oral feeding, the gallbladder may contract and empty the sludge into the biliary tree causing biliary colic, acute pancreatitis and/or acute cholecystitis.[58] For this reason, cholecystectomy may be considered in symptomatic patients with biliary sludge.

The fine echoes may form a gravity dependent layer and may clump together, forming 'sludge' balls (Fig. 3.44B). To avoid misdiagnosing sludge balls as polyps, turn the patient to disperse the

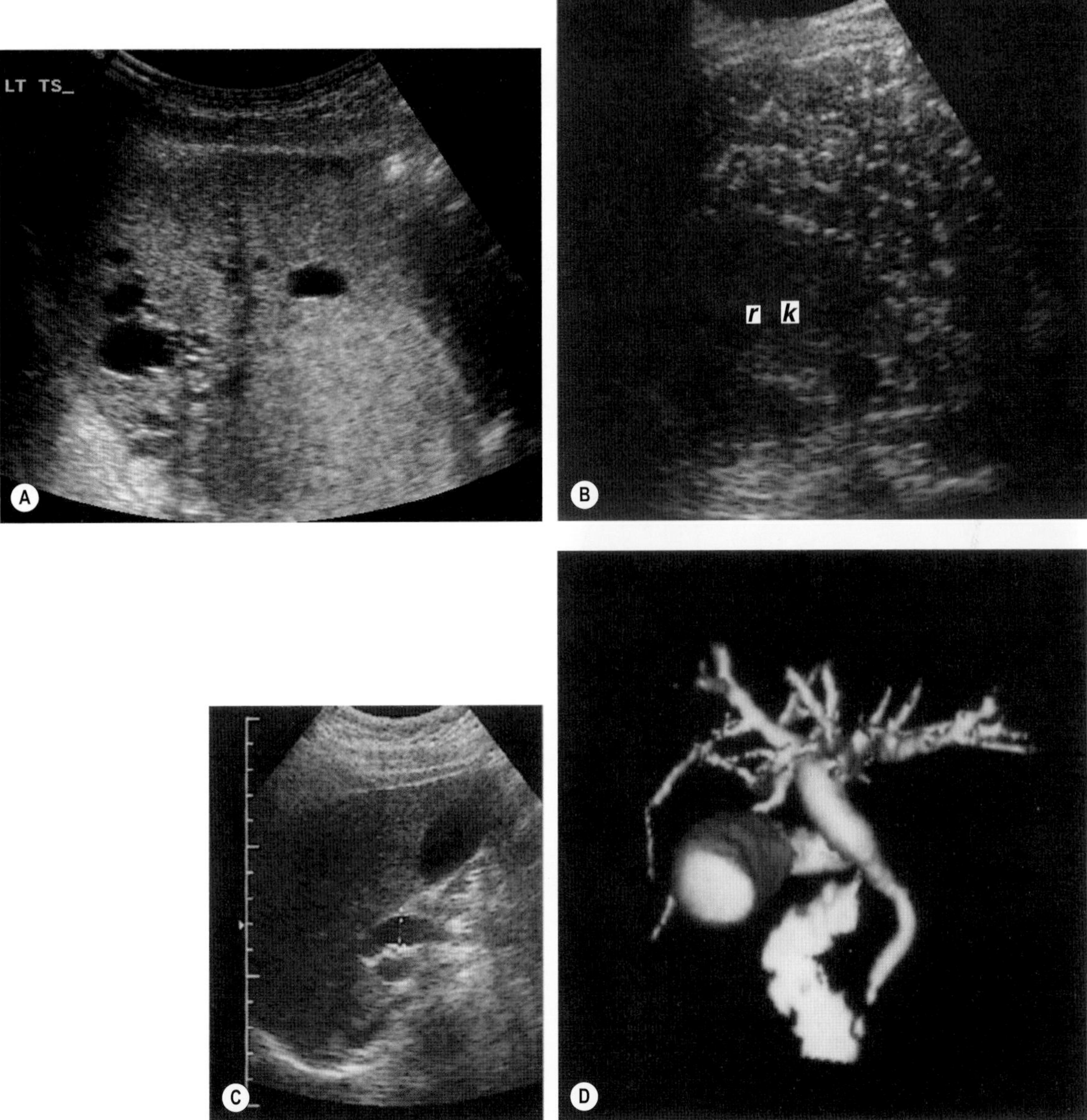

Fig. 3.42 • Caroli's disease. (A) Small cysts in the liver represent saccular bile duct dilatations in Caroli's disease. (B) TS of a different patient with end-stage disease. The grossly abnormal liver texture contrasts with the right kidney. (C) A small section of focal CBD dilatation persisted in a symptomatic patient, with normal calibre distal CBD. This was confirmed on ERCP and thought to be a dyskinetic segment, causing biliary reflux, but was later diagnosed as a mild form of Caroli's. (D) 3D CT reconstruction of the case in (C), confirming the ultrasound appearances. Note the tiny ectatic 'pouchings' of the intrahepatic ducts characteristic of Caroli's.

echoes or rescan after the patient has resumed a normal diet.

Biliary stasis is associated with an increased risk of stone formation.[59] Occasionally, echogenic bile persists even with normal gallbladder function (Fig. 3.45). It is likely that there is a spectrum of biliary disease in which gallbladder dysmotility and subsequent saturation of the bile leads to the formation of crystals in the bile and also in the gallbladder wall. Some of the particles become quite large, forming microlithiasis, and this is likely to be an intermediate stage in stone formation.[60] Pain and biliary colic may be present prior to stone formation. Biliary crystals, or 'microlithiasis' (usually calcium bilirubinate granules), have a strong association with acute pancreatitis,[61] and their presence in patients who do not have gallstones may therefore be highly significant.

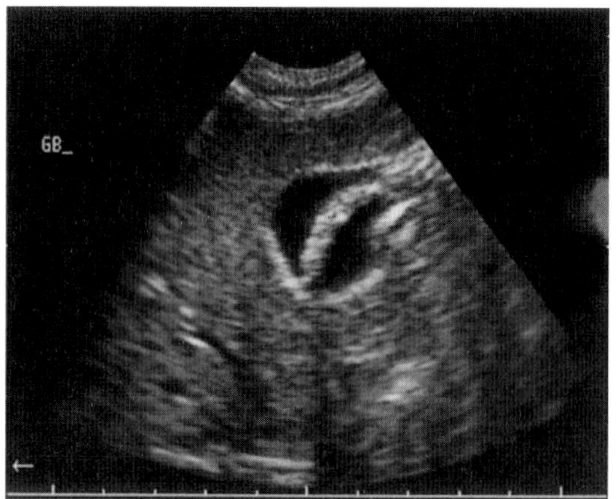

Fig. 3.43 • *Ascaris* worm in the gallbladder.

Obstructive causes of biliary stasis

Pathological bile stasis in the gallbladder is due to obstruction of the cystic duct (from a stone, for example) and may be demonstrated in a normal-sized or dilated gallbladder. The bile becomes viscous and hyperechoic. The biliary ducts remain normal in calibre. Eventually the bile turns watery and appears echo-free on ultrasound; this is known as a mucocoele (see above).

Bile stasis within the ducts occurs either as a result of prolonged and/or repetitive obstruction or as a result of cholestatic disease such as PBC (Chapter 4) or PSC. This can lead to cholangitis.

Haemobilia

Blood in the gallbladder can be the result of gastrointestinal bleeding or other damage to the gallbladder or bile duct wall – for example iatrogenic trauma from an endoscopic procedure or biopsy – or it may be associated with ruptured hepatic artery aneurysm.

The appearances depend upon the stage of evolution of the bleeding. Fresh blood appears as fine, low-level echoes. Blood clots appear as solid, non-shadowing structures and there may be

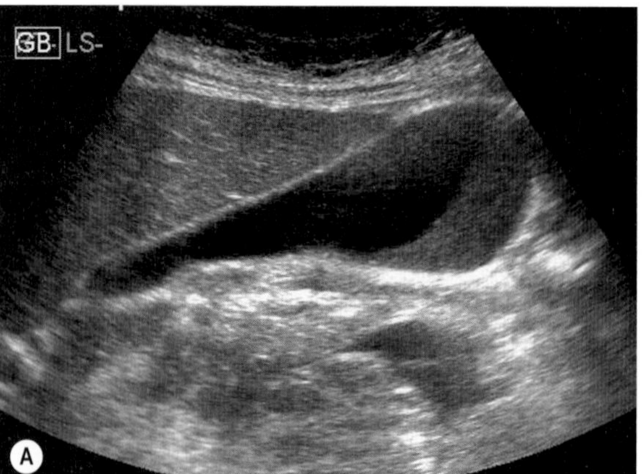

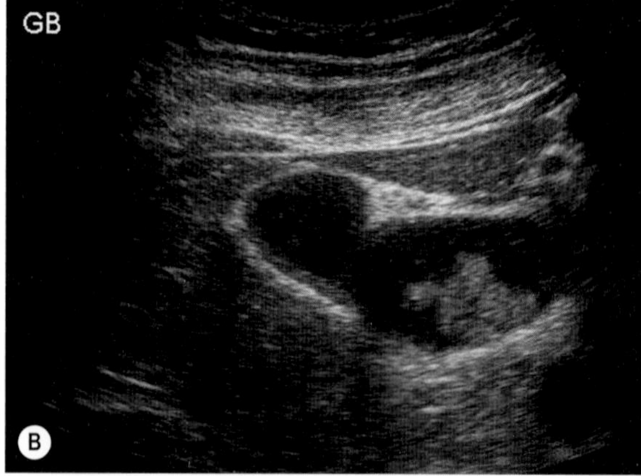

Fig. 3.44 • (A) Inspissated bile in the normal gallbladder of a fasting patient. (B) Biliary sludge in a tumefactive 'ball' can mimic a polyp. Moving the patient to disperse the sludge avoids this pitfall.

hyperechoic, linear strands.[62] A history of trauma may allow the sonographer to differentiate haemobilia from other causes of echogenic bile, particularly those associated with gallbladder inflammation, and there may be other evidence of abdominal trauma on ultrasound – such as a haemoperitoneum.

Pneumobilia

Air in the biliary tree is usually iatrogenic and frequently seen following procedures such as ERCP, sphincterotomy or biliary surgery. Although it does not usually persist, the air can remain in the biliary tree post-procedure for months, even years, and is not significant.

It is characterized by highly reflective linear echoes (Fig. 3.46), which follow the course of the biliary ducts. The air usually casts a shadow which is different from that of stones – often having reverberative artefacts and being much less well-defined or clear. This shadowing obscures the lumen of the duct and can make evaluation of the hepatic parenchyma difficult.

Pneumobilia may also be present in emphysematous cholecystitis, an uncommon complication of cholecystitis, in which gas-forming bacteria are present in the gallbladder (see above) or in cases where a necrotic gallbladder has formed a cholecystoenteric fistula. Rarely, multiple biliary stones form within the ducts throughout the liver, which can be confused with the appearances of air in the ducts.

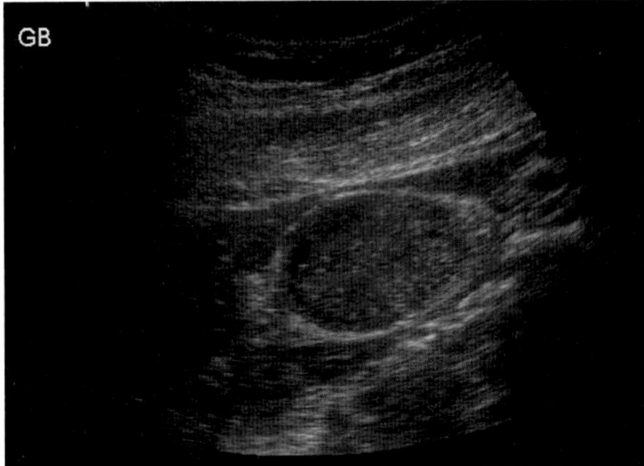

Fig. 3.45 • Biliary crystals.

MALIGNANT BILIARY DISEASE

Primary gallbladder carcinoma

Cancer of the gallbladder is usually associated with gallstones and a history of cholecystitis. Most often, the gallbladder lumen is occupied by a solid mass which may have the appearance of a large polyp. The wall appears thickened and irregular and shadowing from the stones may obscure it posteriorly. A bile-filled lumen may be absent,

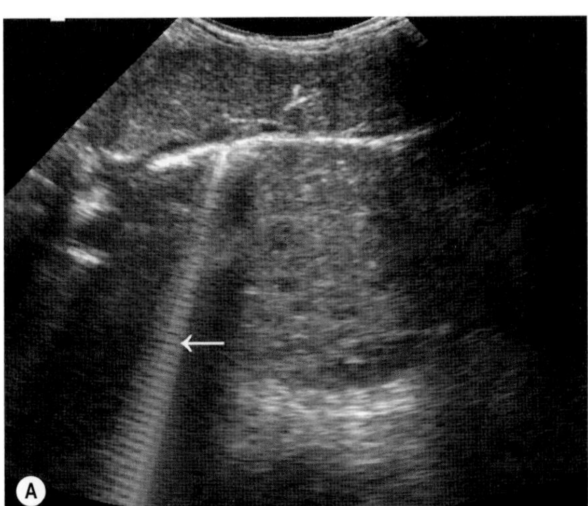

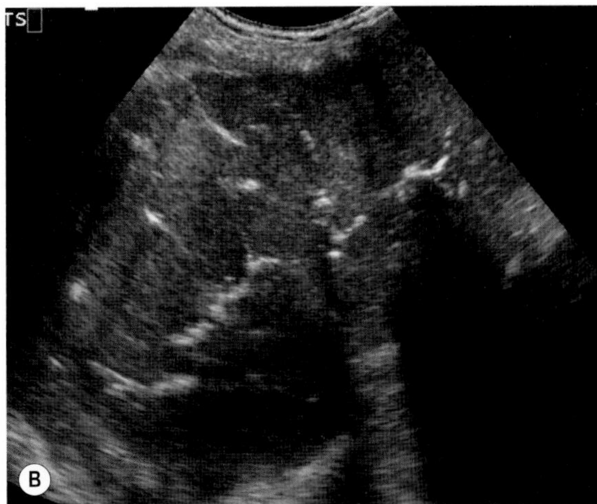

Fig. 3.46 • (A & B) Air in the biliary tree following surgery. Note the 'reverberative' shadow (arrow).

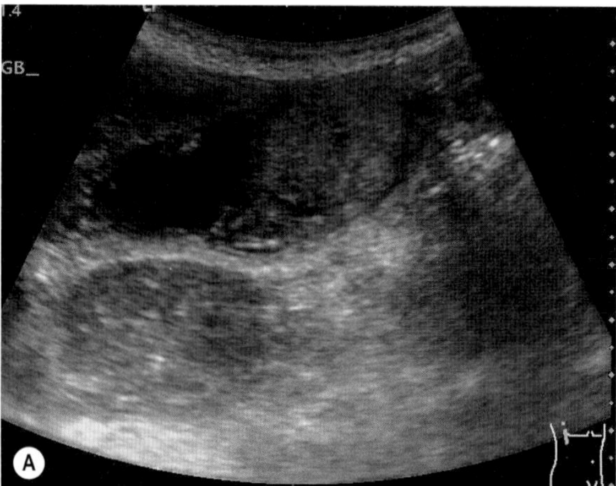

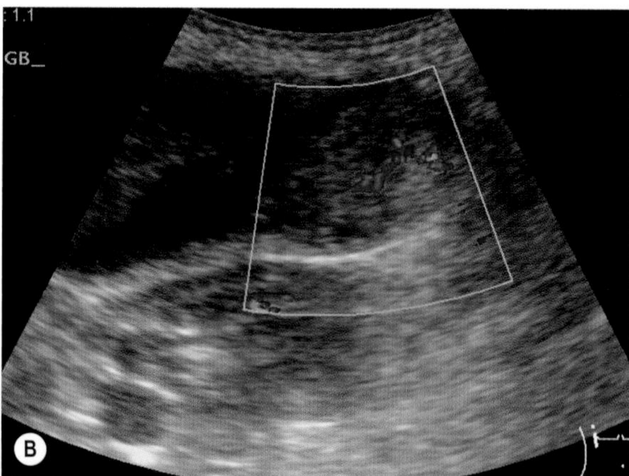

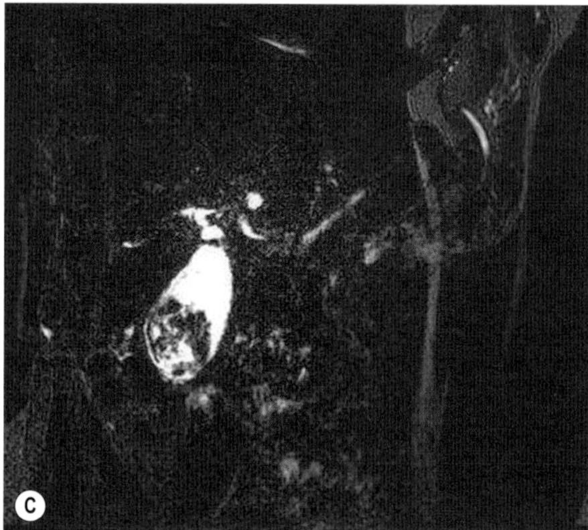

Fig. 3.47 • Gallbladder carcinoma: (A) Gallbladder containing solid material, irregular wall thickening. Stones were also present (not shown). (B) Colour Doppler shows vascularity in the solid component of the mass. (C) MRCP of gallbladder cancer.

further complicating the ultrasound diagnosis (Fig. 3.47). In a porcelain gallbladder (calcification of the gallbladder wall), which is associated with gallbladder carcinoma, the shadowing may obscure any lesion in the lumen, making detection almost impossible.

Particular risk factors for gallbladder carcinoma include large stones, polyps of over 1 cm in size, porcelain gallbladder and, occasionally, choledochal cyst due to anomalous junction of the pancreatobiliary ducts.[15]

The carcinoma itself is frequently asymptomatic in the early stages, and patients tend to present with symptoms relating to the stones. It tends to be an aggressive lesion which quickly metastasizes to the liver and portal nodes and has a very poor prognosis, with a curative surgical resection rate of around 15–20%. Ultrasound may also demonstrate local spread into the adjacent liver, but further staging with CT is invariably necessary.[63]

Cholangiocarcinoma

This is a malignant lesion arising in the wall of the bile duct. It is readily recognizable from an ultrasound point of view when it occurs in, and obstructs the common duct, as the subsequent dilatation outlines the proximal part of the tumour with bile (Fig. 3.48). However, tumours occurring intrahepatically tend to be isoechoic and notoriously difficult to detect. Cholangiocarcinoma may occur at any level along the biliary tree and is frequently multifocal.

A cholangiocarcinoma is referred to as a *Klatskin tumour* when it involves the confluence of the right and left hepatic ducts. These lesions are often difficult to detect on both ultrasound and CT, the only clue may be the proximal dilatation of the biliary ducts (Fig. 3.49). Contrast-enhanced ultrasound (CEUS) is helpful in localizing a suspected

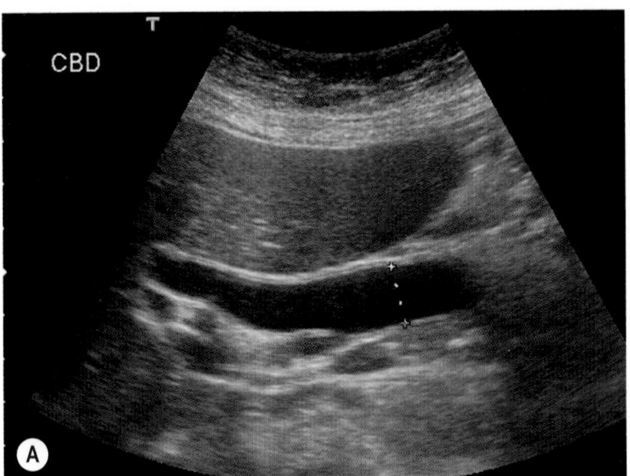

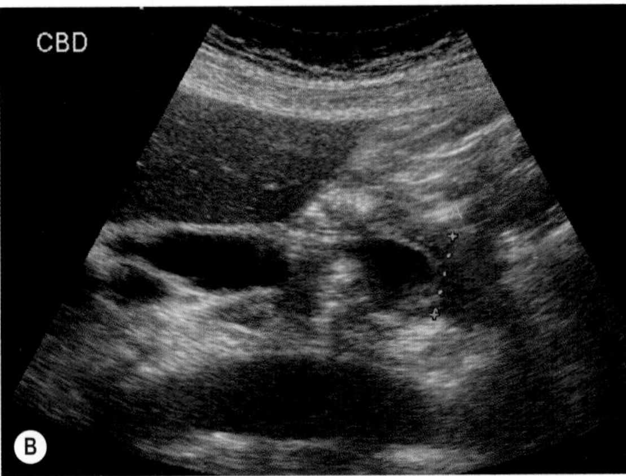

Fig. 3.48 • Cholangiocarcinoma: (A) The dilated CBD (calipers) is obstructed by a mass at the lower end, which is largely obscured by the duodenum. (B) Repositioning the patient to move the duodenal gas reveals a cholangiocarcinoma at the lower end of the duct (calipers).

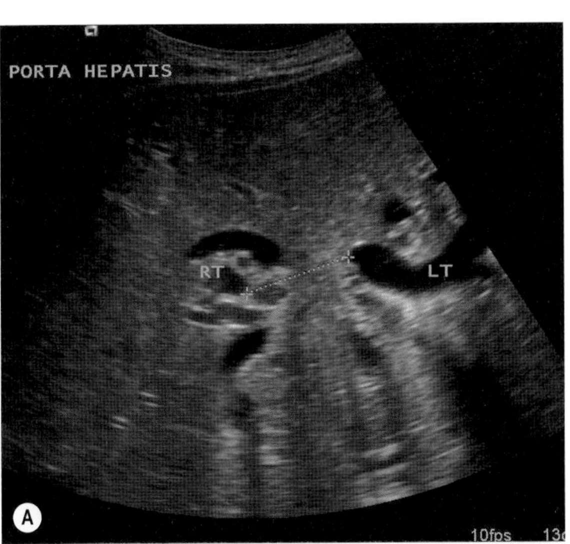

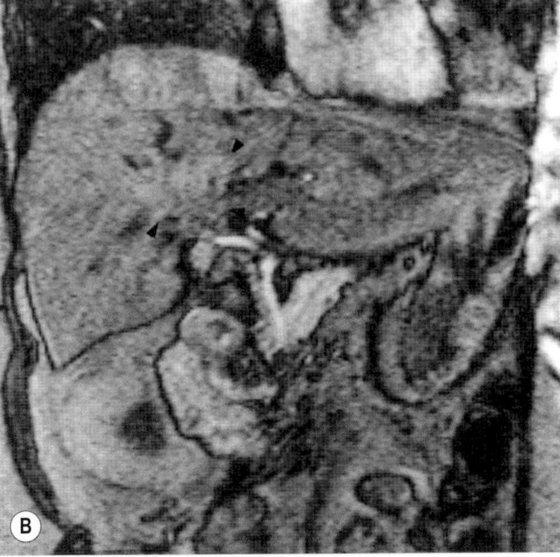

Fig. 3.49 • Cholangiocarcinoma. (A) Irregular mass at the porta (calipers) causing right and left biliary duct obstruction – a Klatskin tumour. (B) MRI of the same patient confirming the mass at the porta.

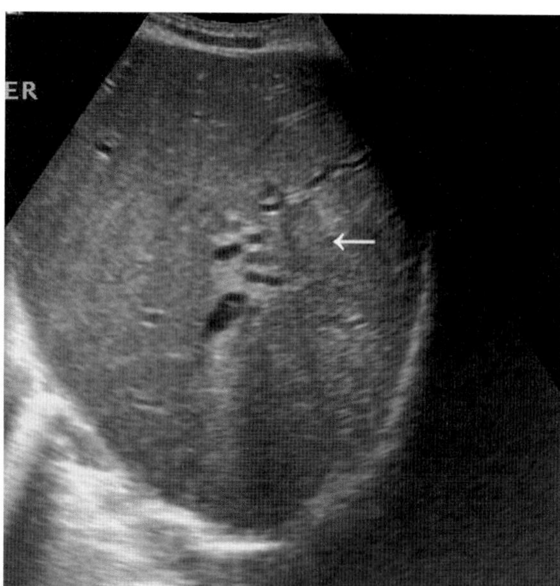

Fig. 3.50 • Focally dilated ducts in the peripheral liver are obstructed by a small intrahepatic cholangiocarcinoma (calipers).

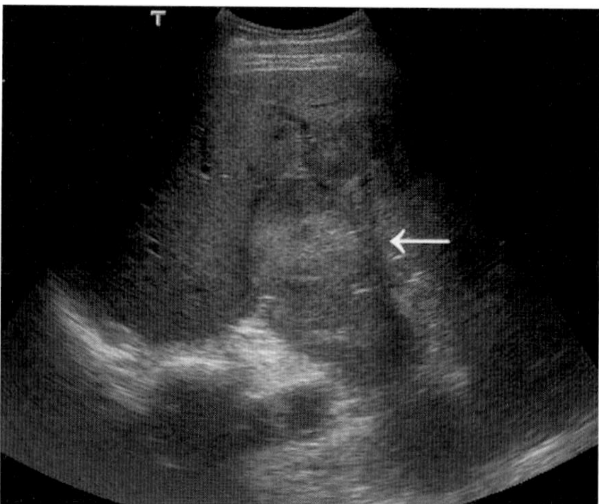

Fig. 3.51 • A large intrahepatic cholangiocarcinoma near the porta hepatis (arrow).

lesion due to arterial hypervascularity followed by hypoenhancement in the sinusoidal phase (Fig. 3.41).

Although rare, the incidence of cholangiocarcinoma seems to be increasing and it is strongly associated with PSC (see above).[64]

Multifocal cholangiocarcinoma may spread to the surrounding liver tissue and carries a very poor prognosis. In a liver whose texture is already altered by diffuse disease it may be almost impossible to identify these lesions before they become large. A pattern of dilated ducts distal to the lesion is a good clue (Figs 3.50, 3.51).

Management of the patient with cholangiocarcinoma

These patients have a poor prognosis, as the lesions usually present with jaundice due to invasion and obstruction of the duct. They spread to surrounding tissues, including the portal vein and lymph nodes, metastasize to the liver, and can be multifocal, particularly with PSC.

Staging of the disease is performed with CT or MRI. Endoscopic ultrasound can outline invasion into the biliary duct and laparoscopic ultrasound can pick up peritoneal or local spread.

Surgical resection of the tumour is becoming more successful in patients with single lesions[65] and liver transplantation in patients with PSC has a good prognosis, provided the tumour bulk is low. Palliation is frequently the only feasible option, and the insertion of a stent, either percutaneously or endoscopically, to bypass the obstructing lesion and assist drainage of the liver will relieve the symptoms and often allows the patient to return home for some months.

Other treatment options, such as chemotherapy have limited success. Despite improvements in treatment, only a minority of patients survive beyond 12 months after the initial diagnosis.[66]

Gallbladder metastases

Metastases from other primaries may occasionally be deposited within the gallbladder wall (Fig. 3.52), usually as a late presentation of the disease process. Often, other metastatic deposits, for example in the liver and lymph nodes, may raise suspicion of gallbladder metastases in an irregularly thickened gallbladder wall.

The ultrasound appearances are of focal thickening and polyp-like lesions in the wall of the gallbladder. This may mimic primary gallbladder carcinoma but knowledge of a previously diagnosed primary, for example melanoma, lung or breast carcinoma, will point towards the diagnosis.

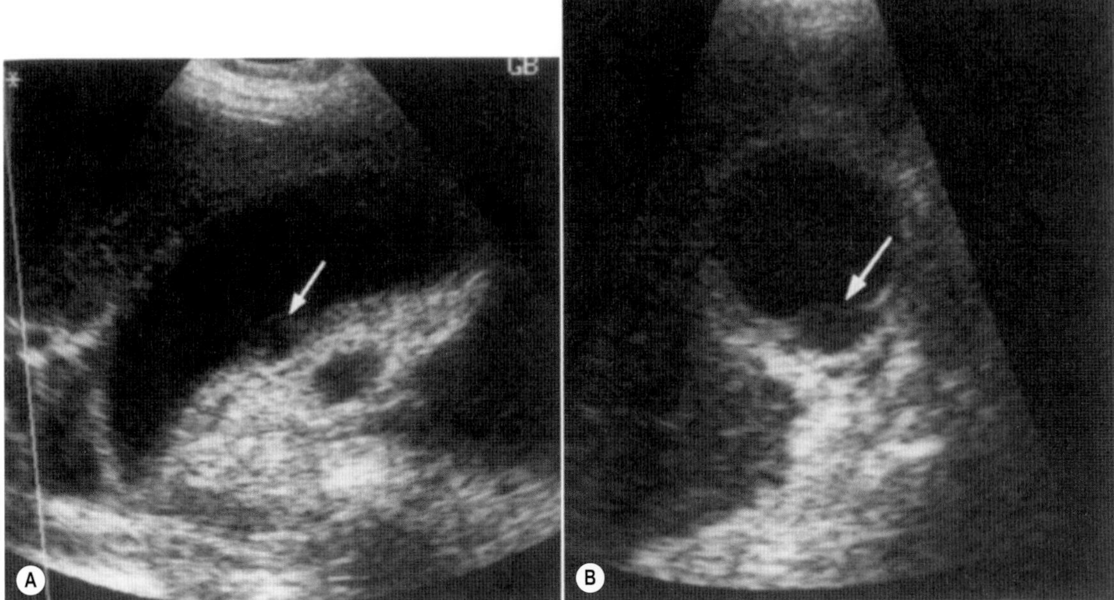

Fig. 3.52 • Metastases in the gallbladder wall: (A) LS and (B) TS from advanced ovarian carcinoma.

References

1. Shea JA, Berlin JA, Escarce JJ et al. Revised estimates of diagnostic test sensitivity and specificity in suspected biliary tract disease. Arch Intern Med 1994; 154: 2573–2581
2. Pandey M, Khatri AK, Sood BP et al. Cholecystosonographic evaluation of the prevalence of gallbladder disease: a university hospital experience. Clin Imaging 1996; 20: 269–272
3. Schirmer BD, Winters KL, Edlich RF. Cholelithiasis and cholecystitis. J Long Term Eff Med Implants 2005; 15: 329–338
4. Freitas M, Bell R, Duffy A. Choledocholithiasis: Evolving standards for diagnosis and management. World J Gastroenterol 2006; 12: 3162–3167
5. Hallal AH, Amortegui JD, Jeroukhimov IM et al. Magnetic resonance cholangiopancreatography accurately detects common bile duct stones in resolving gallstone pancreatitis. J Am Coll Surg 2005; 200: 869–875
6. Nathanson LK, O'Rourke NA, Martin IJ et al. Postoperative ERCP versus laparoscopic choledochotomy for clearance of selected bile duct calculi: a randomized trial. Ann Surg 2005; 242: 188–192
7. Liu TH, Consorti ET, Mercer DW. Laparoscopic cholecystectomy for acute cholecystitis: technical considerations and outcome. Semin Laparosc Surg 2002; 9: 24–31
8. Tranter SE, Thompson MH. Potential of Laparoscopic ultrasonography as an alternative to operative cholangiography in the detection of bile duct stones. Br J Surg 2001; 88: 65–69
9. Tranter SE, Thompson MH. A prospective single-blinded controlled study comparing laparoscopic ultrasound of the common bile duct with operative cholangiography. Surg Endosc 2003; 17: 216–219
10. Petroni ML, Jazrawi RP, Pazzi P et al. Risk factors for the development of gallstone recurrence following medical dissolution. The British-Italian Gallstone Study Group. Eur J Gastroenterol Hepatol 2000; 12: 695–700
11. Pauletzki J, Sackman M, Holl J, Paumgartner G. Evaluation of gallbladder volume and emptying with a novel three-dimensional ultrasound system: comparison with sum-of-cylinders and the ellipsoid methods. J Clin Ultrasound 1996; 24: 277–285
12. Ahlawat SK, Singhania R, Al-Kawas FH. Mirizzi syndrome. Curr Treat Options Gastroenterol 2007; 10: 102–110
13. Wehrmann T, Riphaus A, Martchenko K et al. Intraductal ultrasonography in the diagnosis of Mirizzi syndrome. Endoscopy 2006; 38: 717–722
14. Johnson LW, Sehon JK, Lee WC et al. Mirizzi's syndrome: experience from a multi-institutional review. Am Surg 2001; 67: 11–14
15. Sheth S, Bedford A, Chopra S. Primary gallbladder cancer: recognition of risk factors and role of prophylactic cholecystectomy. Am J Gastroenterol 2000; 95: 1402–1410
16. Fowler RC, Reid WA. Ultrasound diagnosis of adenomyomatosis of the gallbladder: ultrasonic and pathological correlation. Clin Radiol 1988; 39: 402–406
17. Boscak AR, Al-Hawary M, Ramsburgh SR. Adenomyomatosis of the gallbladder. Radiographics 2006; 26: 941–946

18. Koh T, Taniguchi H, Kunishima S, Yamagishi H. Possibility of differential diagnosis of small polypoid lesions in the gallbladder using FDG-PET. Clin Positron Imaging 2000; 3: 213–218
19. Tanno S, Obara T, Maguchi H et al. Association between anomalous pancreatobiliary ductal union and adenomyomatosis of the gallbladder. J Gastroenterol Hepatol 1998; 13: 175–180
20. Azuma T, Yoshikawa T, Araida T, Takasaki K. Differential diagnosis of polypoid lesions of the gallbladder by endoscopic ultrasonography. Am J Surg 2001; 181: 65–70
21. Akyürek N, Salman B, Irkörücü O et al. Ultrasonography in the diagnosis of true gallbladder polyps: the contradiction in the literature. HPB (Oxford) 2005; 7: 155–158
22. Buckles DC, Lindor KD, Larusso NF et al. In primary sclerosing cholangitis, gallbladder polyps are frequently malignant. Am J Gastroenterol 2002; 97: 1138–1142
23. Myers RP, Shaffer EA, Beck PL. Gallbladder polyps: epidemiology, natural history and management. Can J Gastroenterol 2002; 16: 187–194
24. Numata K, Oka H, Morimoto M et al. Differential diagnosis of gallbladder diseases with contrast-enhanced harmonic gray scale ultrasonography. J Ultrasound Med 2007; 26: 763–774
25. Bhattacharya D, Ammori BJ. Contemporary minimally invasive approaches to the management of acute cholecystitis: a review and appraisal. Surg Laparosc Endosc Percutan Tech 2005; 15: 1–8
26. Bellows CF, Berger DH, Crass RA. Management of gallstones. Am Fam Physician 2005; 72: 637–642
27. Foley WD, Quiroz FA. The role of sonography in imaging of the biliary tract. Ultrasound Q 2007; 23: 123–135
28. Shridhar Ganpathi I, Diddapur RK, Eugene H, Karim M. Acute acalculous cholecystitis: challenging the myths. HPB (Oxford) 2007; 9: 131–134
29. Babb RR. Acute acalculous cholecystitis: a review. J Clin Gastroenterol 1992; 15: 238–241
30. Chen PF, Nimeri A, Pham QH et al. The clinical diagnosis of chronic acalculous cholecystitis. Surgery 2001; 130: 578–581
31. Girgin S, Gedik E, Taçyildiz IH et al. Factors affecting morbidity and mortality in gangrenous cholecystitis. Acta Chir Belg 2006; 106: 545–549
32. Coffin CT, Weingardt JP, Drose JA. Sonographic appearances of emphysematous cholecystitis. JDMS 1995; 11: 204–206
33. Konno K, Ishida H, Naganuma H et al. Emphysematous cholecystitis: sonographic findings. Abdom Imaging 2002; 27: 191–195
34. Tseng LJ, Tsai CC, Mo LR et al. Palliative percutaneous transhepatic gallbladder drainage of gallbladder empyema before laparoscopic cholecystectomy. Hepatogastroenterology 2000; 47: 932–936
35. Berger J, Lindsell DRM. Case report: Thickening of the walls of non-dilated bile ducts. Clin Radiol 1997; 52: 474–476
36. Kim TK, Kim BS, Kim JH et al. Diagnosis of intrahepatic duct stones: superiority of MR cholangiopancreatography over endoscopic retrograde cholangiopancreatography. AJR Am J Roentgenol 2002; 179: 429–434
37. Calvo MM, Bujanda L, Calderon A. Role of magnetic resonance cholangiopancreatography in patients with suspected choledocholithiasis. Mayo Clin Proc 2002; 77: 407–412
38. Sakai Y, Tsuyuguchi T, Tsuchiya S et al. Diagnostic value of MRCP and indications for ERCP. Hepatogastroenterology 2007; 54: 2212–2215
39. Ong TZ, Khor JL, Selamat DS et al. Complications of endoscopic retrograde cholangiography in the post-MRCP era: a tertiary center experience. World J Gastroenterol 2005; 11: 5209–5212
40. Norton SA, Alderson D. Prospective comparison of endoscopic ultrasonography and endoscopic retrograde cholangiopancreatography in the detection of bile duct stones. Br J Surg 1997; 84: 1366–1369
41. Tripathi M, Chandrashekar N, Kumar R et al. Hepatobiliary scintigraphy. An effective tool in the management of bile leak following laparoscopic cholecystectomy. Clin Imaging 2004; 28: 40–43
42. Perry KA, Myers JA, Deziel DJ. Laparoscopic ultrasound as the primary method for bile duct imaging during cholecystectomy. Surg Endosc 2008; 22: 208–213
43. Aljebreen A, Azzam N, Eloubeidi MA. Prospective study of endoscopic ultrasound performance in suspected choledocholithiasis. J Gastroenterol Hepatol 2008; 23: 741–745
44. McMahon CJ. The relative roles of magnetic resonance cholangiopancreatography (MRCP) and endoscopic ultrasound in diagnosis of common bile duct calculi: a critically appraised topic. Abdom Imaging 2008; 33: 6–9
45. Lau WY, Leung KL, Leung TWT et al. Obstructive jaundice secondary to hepatocellular carcinoma. Surg Oncol 1995; 4: 303–308
46. Sato M, Ishida H, Konno K et al. Choledochal cyst due to anomalous pancreatobiliary junction in the adult: sonographic findings. Abdom Imaging 2001; 26: 395–400
47. Martins E, Chapman RW. Sclerosing cholangitis. Curr Opin Gastroenterol 1996; 12: 466–470
48. Alexander J, Lord JD, Yeh MM et al. Risk factors for recurrence of primary sclerosing cholangitis after liver transplantation. Liver Transpl 2008; 14: 245–251
49. Majoie CBLM, Smits NJ, Phoa SSKS et al. Primary Sclerosing Cholangitis: sonographic findings. Abdom Imaging 1995; 20: 109–113
50. Van de Meeberg PC, Portincasa P, Wolfhagen FHJ, Van Erpecum KJ. Increased gall bladder volume in primary sclerosing cholangitis. GUT 1996; 39: 594–599
51. Kawarasaki H, Sato T, Sanjo K et al. Evaluation of long-term results of Caroli's disease: 21 years' observation of a family with autosomal 'dominant' inheritance, and review of the literature. Hepato-Gastroenterology 1995; 42: 175–181

52. Benhidjeb T, Rudolph B, Muller JM. Curative partial hepatectomy in unilobar Caroli's syndrome – report of three cases with long-term follow-up. Dig Surg 1997; 14: 123–125

53. Miller WJ, Sechtin AG, Campbell WL, Pieters PC. Imaging findings in Caroli's disease. AJR Am J Roentgenol 1995; 165: 333–337

54. Levy AD, Rohrmann CA Jr, Murakata LA, Lonergan GJ. Caroli's disease: radiologic spectrum with pathologic correlation. AJR Am J Roentgenol 2002; 179: 1053–1057

55. Al Absi M, Qais AM, Al Katta M et al. Biliary ascariasis: the value of ultrasound in the diagnosis and management. Ann Saudi Med 2007; 27: 161–165

56. Misra SP, Dwivedi M. Clinical features and management of biliary ascariasis in a non-endemic area. Postgrad Med 2000; 76: 29–32

57. Chen EY, Nguyen TD. Gallbladder sludge. N Engl J Med 2001; 345: 2e

58. Ko CW, Sekijima JH, Lee SP. Biliary sludge. Ann Intern Med 1999; 131: 630–631

59. Portincasa P, Di Ciaula A, Vendemiale G et al. Gallbladder motility and cholesterol crystallization in bile from patients with pigment and cholesterol gallstones. Eur J Clin Invest 2000; 30: 317–324

60. Jüngst C, Kullak-Ublick GA, Jüngst D. Gallstone disease: Microlithiasis and sludge. Best Pract Res Clin Gastroenterol 2006; 20: 1053–1062

61. Kohut M, Nowak A, Nowakowska-Dulawa E. The frequency of bile duct crystals in patients with presumed biliary pancreatitis. Gastrointest Endosc 2001; 54: 37–41

62. Lo HW, Yuan CY. Ultrasonic spectrum of hemobilia in the bile duct and gallbladder. J Med Ultrasound 1994; 2: 77–80

63. Tsukada K, Takada T, Miyazaki M et al. Diagnosis of biliary tract and ampullary carcinomas. J Hepatobiliary Pancreat Surg 2008; 15: 31–40

64. Fevery J, Verslype C, Lai G et al. Incidence, diagnosis, and therapy of cholangiocarcinoma in patients with primary sclerosing cholangitis. Dig Dis Sci 2007; 52: 3123–3135

65. Figueras J, Llado L, Valla C et al. Changing strategies in diagnosis and management of hilar cholangiocarcinoma. Liver Transpl 2000; 6: 786–794

66. Miller G, Schwartz LH, D'Angelica M. The use of imaging in the diagnosis and staging of hepatobiliary malignancies. Surg Oncol Clin N Am 2007; 16: 343–368

Pathology of the liver and portal venous system

4

CHAPTER CONTENTS

INTRODUCTION

Ultrasound is frequently the first line of investigation for suspected liver pathology, and the decision to proceed to secondary investigative procedures, such as further radiology or histology, is determined by the findings of the initial ultrasound scan. It is used in the diagnosis, staging and monitoring of liver disorders.

Ultrasound has a much greater role, however, than that of a first line 'exclusion' test, and serves as a reliable tool for more focused, complex examinations. Developing technology and techniques now result in improved diagnostic accuracy and are increasingly obviating the need for further radiology. Ultrasound is used to both diagnose and treat conditions using ultrasound guided invasive procedures.

Intraoperative and laparoscopic ultrasound, using high frequency, direct contact techniques, set the standard for liver imaging in many cases.

FOCAL LIVER LESIONS

Focal liver lesions are common, and, once seen, require accurate characterization. In some cases – for example simple cysts – the ultrasound appearances are pathognomonic requiring no further investigation. In other cases, CEUS provides a rapid and definitive diagnosis, obviating the need for further investigation or follow-up. In other cases, ultrasound appropriately directs the patient's further management (such as further radiological imaging for staging or characterization, or biopsy).

The 'mass effect'

This term describes the effect of a focal mass – whether benign or malignant – on surrounding structures and is a useful diagnostic tool. It implies the lesion's displacing or invasive nature, i.e. the displacement of vessels and/or invasion or distortion of adjacent structures and tissues as a result of the increasing bulk of a lesion. This effect differentiates a true mass from an infiltrative process such as steatosis, or an artefact.

Masses that are large and/or closely adjacent to a vessel demonstrate the effect more readily. The mass effect does not, of course, differentiate benign from malignant masses, or help in any way to characterize the mass. It is particularly useful when the mass is isoechoic compared with normal liver (see Fig. 4.15 below). In such cases, the effect of the mass on adjacent structures may be the main clue to its presence.

BENIGN FOCAL LIVER LESIONS

SIMPLE CYSTS

One of the most frequently seen liver lesions, the simple cyst is either congenital (from abnormal development of a biliary radicle) or acquired (from trauma or previous infection). It is asymptomatic, unless large enough to cause a 'mass effect' – compressing and displacing adjacent structures – and is usually an incidental finding during the ultrasound scan. Frequently, small cysts are peripheral and therefore more likely to be missed on ultrasound than CT.

The simple cyst has three acoustic properties, which are pathognomonic: it is *anechoic*, has a *well-defined smooth capsule* and exhibits *posterior enhancement* (increased through-transmission of sound) (Fig. 4.1). Although theoretically it is possible to confuse a simple cyst with a choledochal cyst (see Chapter 3), the latter's connection to the biliary tree is usually demonstrable on ultrasound. A radioisotope HIDA scan will confirm the biliary connection if doubt exists.

COMPLEX CYSTS

Some cysts may contain a thin septum, which is not a significant finding. Occasionally haemorrhage or infection may occur in a simple cyst, giving rise to low level, fine echoes within it (Fig. 4.2). Such cysts are usually treated conservatively

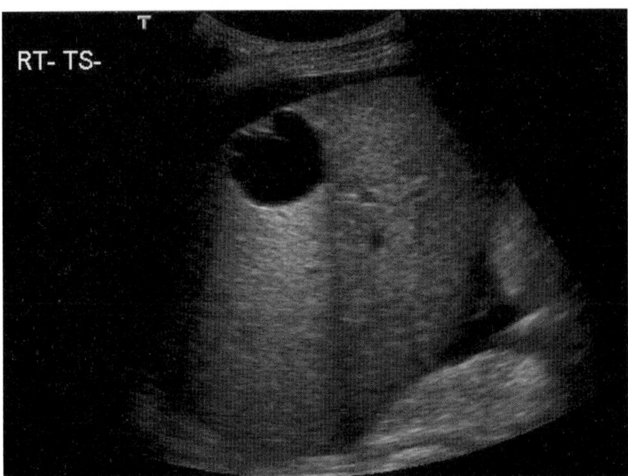

Fig. 4.1 • Typical liver cyst demonstrating a band of posterior enhancement, smooth capsule and fine septum. Note the ascites.

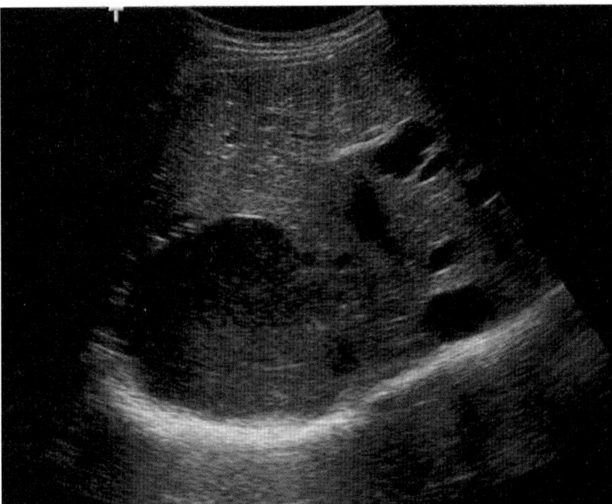

Fig. 4.2 • Large, infected hepatic cyst containing low-level echoes.

although the larger ones may be monitored with ultrasound, particularly if symptomatic. Percutaneous aspiration of larger cysts under ultrasound guidance may afford temporary decompression but is rarely performed, as they invariably recur, and there is a risk of infection. Laparoscopic fenestration (deroofing) in which part of the cyst wall is removed allowing drainage, provides a more permanent solution to large, symptomatic cysts.[1]

A rare cause of a cystic lesion in the liver is the *cystadenoma* – a benign epithelial tumour which may appear uni- or multilocular. These have a pre-

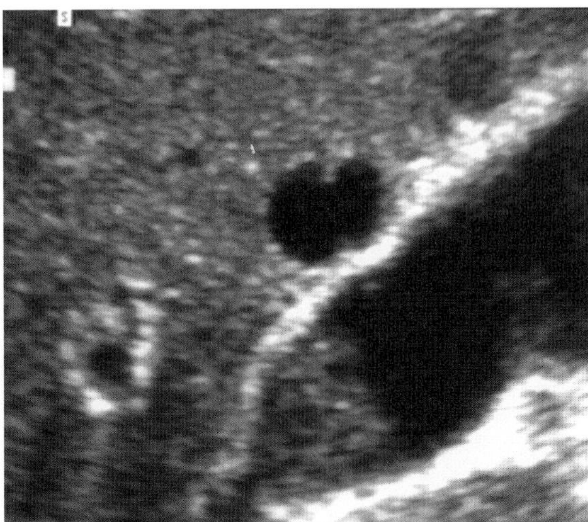

Fig. 4.3 • Small cyst adjacent to the gallbladder containing a nodule. This was a mucinous metastasis from an ovarian carcinoma.

malignant potential, rarely progressing to form a *cystadenocarcinoma*. Close monitoring with ultrasound will demonstrate gradual increase in size, changes in the appearances of the wall of the cyst, such as thickening or papillary projections, and internal echoes in some cases, which may indicate malignant change. Cystic malignant liver lesions are uncommon, and the majority represent necrotic metastases, but it is extremely important to recognize suspicious malignant features such as solid nodules or thickened walls and septations (Fig. 4.3). A diagnostic aspiration may be performed under ultrasound guidance, and the fluid may contain elevated levels of carcinoembryonic antigen (CEA) if malignant.[2] Cystadenomas are usually surgically removed due to their malignant potential (Fig. 4.4).

Rarely, cystic lesions in the liver may be due to other causes. These include pancreatic pseudocyst (within an interlobular fissure) in patients with acute pancreatitis or mucin-filled metastatic deposits in primary ovarian cancer. An AV malformation – a rare finding in the liver – may look like a septated cystic lesion. Doppler, however, will demonstrate flow throughout the structure.

POLYCYSTIC LIVER

There is a fine dividing line between a liver that contains multiple simple cysts and 'polycystic liver

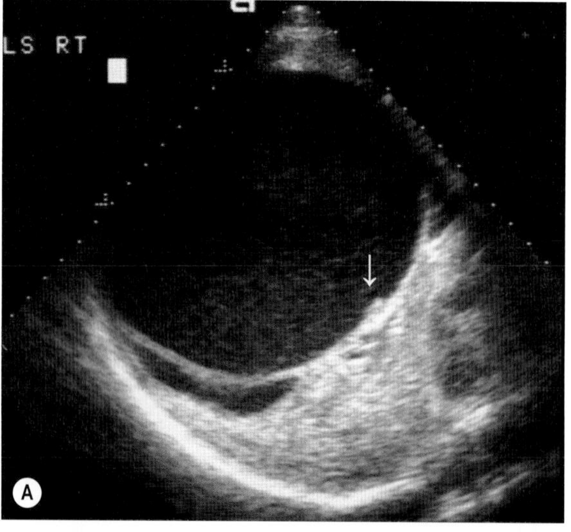

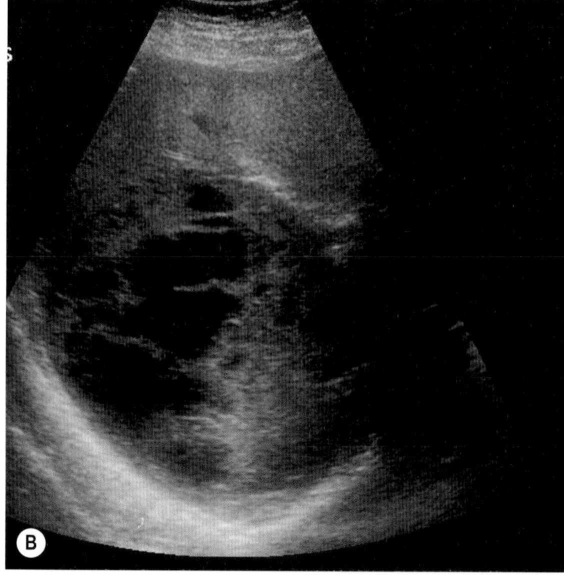

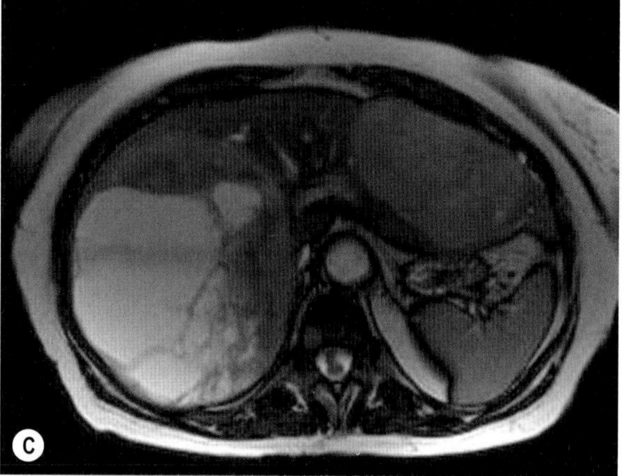

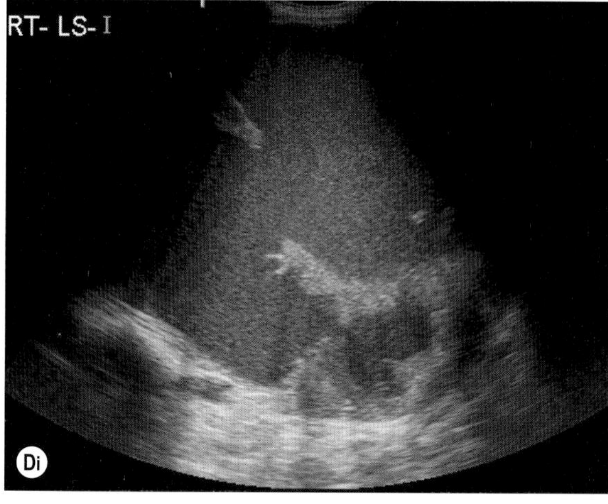

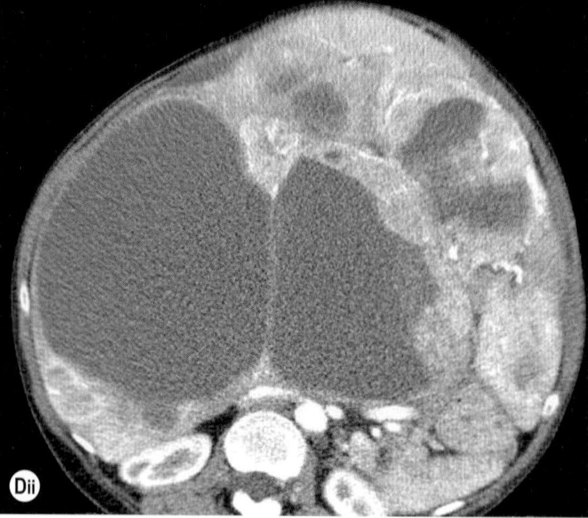

Fig. 4.4 • (A) Large cystadenoma containing echoes and a septum. The cyst was large enough to cause obstructive jaundice – the patient's presenting symptom. The diagnosis was made by ultrasound-guided aspiration. A small nodule is present (arrow) which raises the suspicion for malignancy, and the cyst subsequently developed into a cystadenocarcinoma. (B) A cystadenocarcinoma in a young woman presenting with altered LFTs, demonstrating the complex nature of the mass. (C) MRI of the case in (B). (Di) A rare primary neuroendocrine tumour of the liver, demonstrating a large complex mainly cystic lesion, diagnosed with US guided biopsy. (Dii) CT is valuable in indicating the extent of the disease.

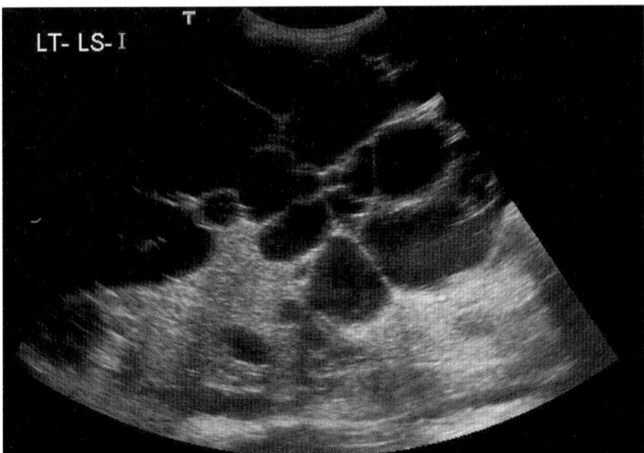

Fig. 4.5 • Multiple cysts enlarging the left lobe of liver in autosomal dominant polycystic kidney disease.

disease'. The latter usually occurs with polycystic kidneys, a common autosomal dominant condition readily recognizable on ultrasound (see Chapter 7), but rarely may affect the liver alone, sparing the kidneys (Fig. 4.5). The appearances are of multiple, often septated cysts, of varying sizes throughout the liver. The cumulative enhancement behind the numerous cysts imparts a highly irregular echogenicity to the liver texture and may make it extremely difficult to pick up other focal lesions which may be present.

The polycystic liver is usually asymptomatic, but easily palpable, and if the kidneys are also affected the abdomen can look very distended. As with cysts in the kidneys, haemorrhage or infection in a cyst can cause localized pain. Treatment of the cysts by drainage is not successful, and in rare cases, hepatic transplantation offers the only viable option in patients with intractable symptoms.

HYDATID (ECHINOCOCCAL) CYST

Hydatid disease comes from a parasite, *Echinococcus granulosus*, which is endemic in the Middle East and in sheep-farming areas but rare in the UK. The worm lives in the alimentary tract of infected dogs, which excrete the eggs. These may then be ingested by cattle or sheep and subsequently complete their lifecycle in a human. The parasite spreads via the bloodstream to the liver, where it lodges, causing an inflammatory reaction. The resulting cyst can be slow growing and asymptomatic and they may be single or multiple, depending on the degree of infestation.

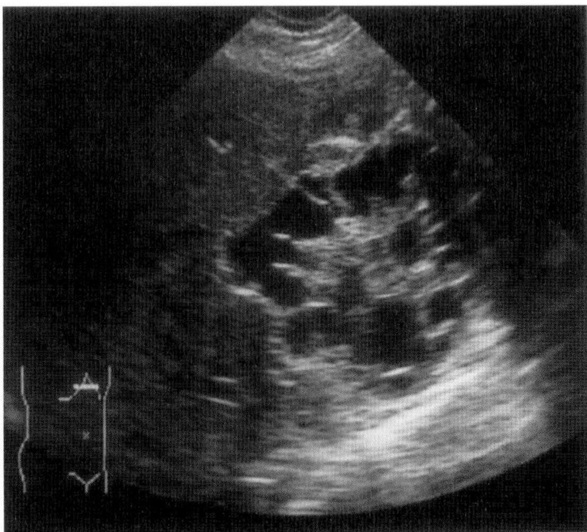

Fig. 4.6 • Hydatid cyst demonstrating surrounding daughter cysts.

Ultrasound may demonstrate a spectrum of appearances, from cystic through to solid, and the diagnosis can be made by looking carefully at the wall and contents; the hydatid cyst has two layers to its capsule, which may appear thickened, separated or detached on ultrasound. Daughter cysts may arise from the inner capsule – the honeycomb or cartwheel appearance (Fig. 4.6) and the cyst may contain floating membranes and fine sand or debris.[3] A calcified rind around a cyst is usually associated with an old, inactive hydatid lesion.

The diagnosis of hydatid, as opposed to a simple cyst, is an important one, as any attempted aspiration may spread the parasite further by seeding along the needle track if the operator is unaware of the diagnosis. Hydatids may be treated successfully using percutaneous ultrasound guided aspiration with sclerotherapy although surgical resection is necessary for some cases.[4]

ABSCESSES

Liver abscesses result from bacterial, fungal or parasitic infection. The most common are pyogenic abscesses secondary to abdominal infection – for example cholangitis (via the biliary tree), diverticulitis or appendicitis (via the portal vein). Diabetic patients and those with compromised immune response are particularly prone to such infections.

Clinical features

Patients present with fever, nocturnal sweats, often accompanied by RUQ pain and vomiting. Abnormal LFTs and anaemia can also be present. A raised white cell count and erythrocyte sedimentation rate (ESR) are a feature. The clinical history helps the sonographer to establish the nature of the focal lesion and the aetiology of the abscess. Abscesses of any type may be solitary or multiple.

Since the ultrasound appearances of abscesses can be similar to those of necrotic tumours or haematoma, the clinical picture is of particular importance in establishing the diagnosis.

Ultrasound appearances

Hepatic abscesses may display a spectrum of acoustic features. Their internal appearances vary considerably; in the very early stages there is a zone of infected, oedematous liver tissue which appears on ultrasound as a hypoechoic, solid focal lesion. As the infection develops, the liver tissue becomes necrotic and liquefaction takes place. The abscess may still appear full of homogeneous echoes from pus and can be mistaken for a solid lesion, but as it progresses, the fluid content may become apparent, usually with considerable debris within it. Because they are fluid-filled, abscesses demonstrate posterior enhancement (Fig. 4.7A). The margins of an abscess are irregular, often ill-defined and frequently thickened. The inflammatory capsule of the abscess may demonstrate vascularity on colour or power Doppler, but this is not invariable, and depends on equipment sensitivity and size of the lesion. Infection with gas-forming organisms may account for the presence of gas within some liver abscesses (Fig. 4.7B).

There are three main types of abscess.

Pyogenic abscess

These form as a result of infection entering the liver through the portal venous system. Most commonly, appendiceal or diverticular abscesses are responsible, but intrahepatic abscesses are also seen in immunosuppressed patients and following post-operative infection.

Pyogenic abscesses are frequently multiple, and the patient must be closely monitored after diagnosis to prevent rapid spread. They are still considered a lethal problem, which has increased in recent years due to increasingly aggressive surgical approaches to many abdominal neoplasms.[5]

Amoebic abscess

This is a parasitic infection which is rare in the UK, but found frequently in parts of Africa, India and the southern parts of the USA. Increasing worldwide travel means a more frequent recognition of such lesions with ultrasound,[6] and suspicion should be raised when the patient has visited these countries. It is usually contracted by drinking contaminated water and infects the colon, ulcerating the wall and subsequently being transported to the liver via the portal venous system.

About 25% of infected patients form hepatic abscesses and the infection may spread to other sites in the abdomen. Following initial ultrasound, CT is necessary to identify extrahepatic disease.

Candidiasis abscess

This is a fungal infection which may be seen in immunosuppressed patients. It is a rare cause of abscess formation and is usually bloodborne. The resulting abscesses are likely to be small but multiple on presentation.

Management of hepatic abscesses

An ultrasound guided aspiration to obtain pus for culture is useful for identifying the responsible organism. Aspiration combined with antibiotic therapy is usually highly successful for smaller abscesses, and ultrasound is used to monitor the resolution of the abscesses in the liver. Ultrasound-guided drainage is used for large lesions, and surgical removal is rarely required.

Further radiology may be indicated to establish the underlying cause and extent of infection, e.g. barium enema or CT, particularly if amoebic infection is suspected.

HAEMATOMA

A haematoma is the result of trauma (usually, therefore, via the emergency department) but the trauma may also be iatrogenic, e.g. following a

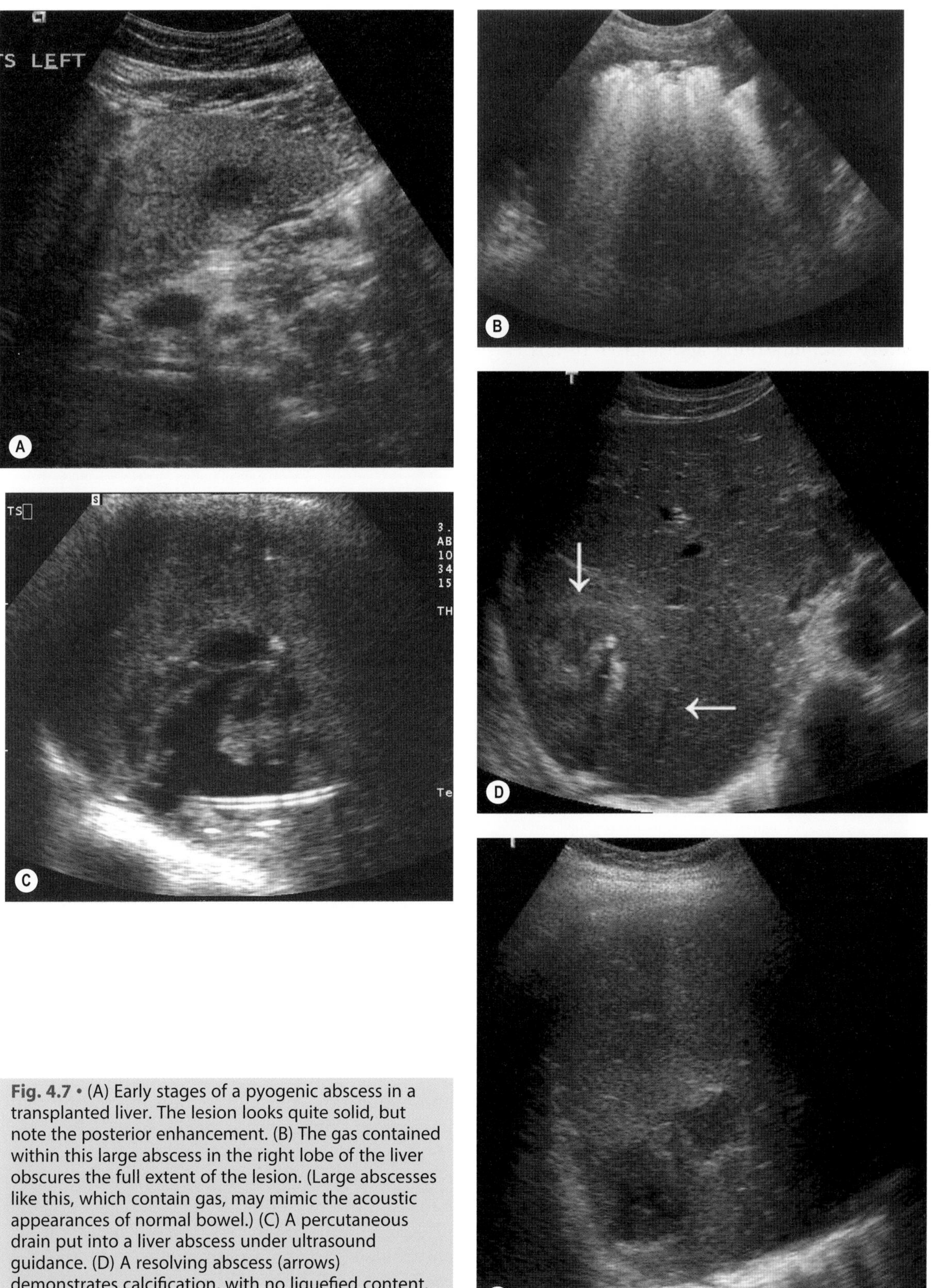

Fig. 4.7 • (A) Early stages of a pyogenic abscess in a transplanted liver. The lesion looks quite solid, but note the posterior enhancement. (B) The gas contained within this large abscess in the right lobe of the liver obscures the full extent of the lesion. (Large abscesses like this, which contain gas, may mimic the acoustic appearances of normal bowel.) (C) A percutaneous drain put into a liver abscess under ultrasound guidance. (D) A resolving abscess (arrows) demonstrates calcification, with no liquefied content. (E) Two abscesses in a patient on immunosuppression.

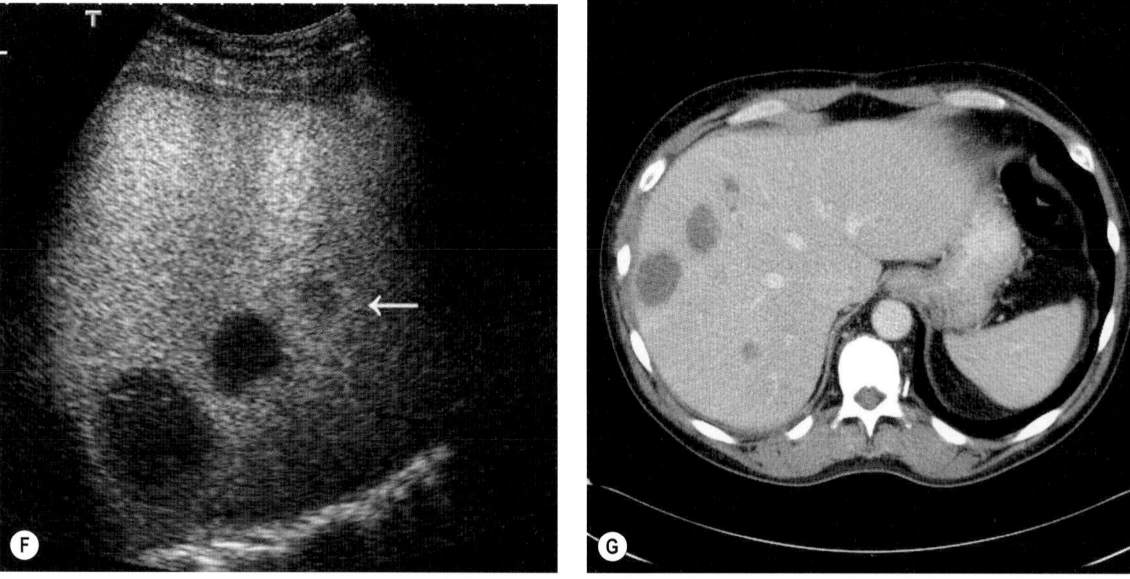

Fig. 4.7, cont'd • (F) CEUS of the case in E demonstrates a third smaller abscess (arrow) not visible pre-contrast. (G) CT confirms multiple abscesses.

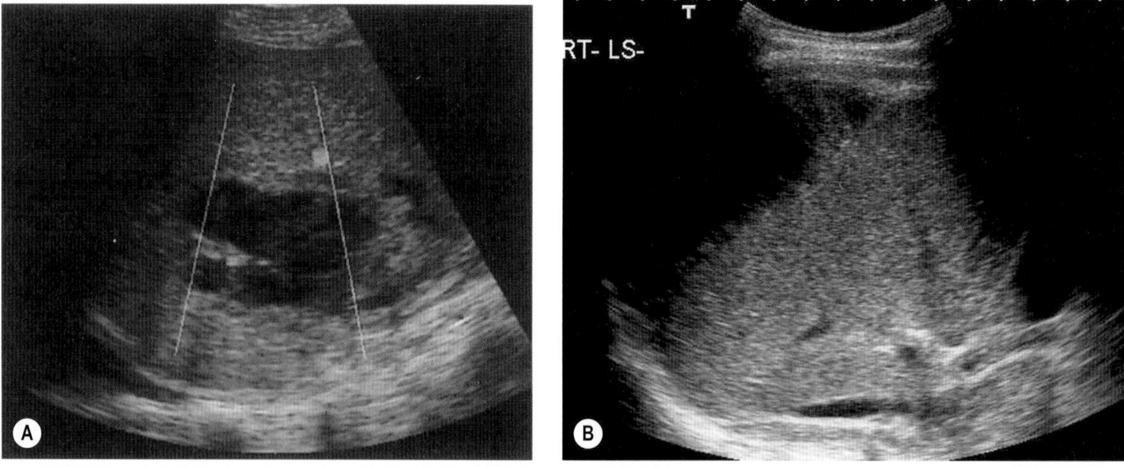

Fig. 4.8 • (A) Intrahepatic haematoma following a road traffic accident with rib fractures. The lesion is relatively fresh and contains some low level echoes. (B) A subphrenic haematoma displaces the liver inferiorly.

biopsy procedure (hence the value of using ultrasound guidance to avoid major vessels in the liver) or surgery. The liver haematoma may have similar acoustic appearances to those of an abscess but does not share the same clinical features or history (Fig. 4.8).

The acoustic appearances depend upon the timing – a fresh haematoma may appear liquid and hypoechoic, but rapidly becomes more 'solid' looking and hyperechoic, as the blood clots. As it resolves the haematoma liquefies and may contain fibrin strands. It will invariably demonstrate a band of posterior enhancement and has irregular, ill-defined walls in the early stages. Later on it may encapsulate, leaving a permanent cystic 'space' in the liver, and the capsule may calcify. Injury to the more peripheral regions may cause a subcapsular haematoma which demonstrates the same acoustic properties. The haematoma outlines the surface of the liver and the capsule can be seen surrounding it. This may be the cause of a palpable 'enlarged' liver (Fig. 4.8B).

Intervention is rarely necessary and monitoring with ultrasound confirms eventual resolution. More serious hepatic ruptures, however, causing haemoperitoneum, may require surgery. CEUS is useful in demonstrating the extent of injury and is particularly useful in the absence of a haemoperitoneum (see Chapter 10, Fig. 10.1) (Table 4.1).

SIMPLE CYST	
Anechoic, thin capsule, posterior enhancement (may contain thin septae)	Common finding, usually insignificant
	Consider polycystic disease if multiple (rarely an AV malformation may mimic a septated cyst – exclude by using colour Doppler)
COMPLEX CYST	
Thin capsule + internal echoes	Haemorrhage or infection in a cyst
	Mucinous metastasis
	Cystadenoma
Capsule thickened or complex, may also contain echoes	Hydatid cyst
	Cystadenocarcinoma
	Intrahepatic pancreatic pseudocyst (rare)
SOLID/CYSTIC LESION	
Irregular margin, internal echoes + debris/solid material	Abscess
	Haematoma
	Necrotic metastasis
	Cavernous haemangioma

Table 4.1 Cystic focal liver lesions – differential diagnoses

HAEMANGIOMA

This is the most common, solid benign tumour found in the liver. Haemangiomas are highly vascular, composed of a network of tiny blood vessels. They may be solitary or multiple. Most haemangiomas are small and found incidentally. They are rarely symptomatic but do cause a diagnostic dilemma, as they can be indistinguishable from liver metastases.

Their acoustic appearances vary; the majority are hyperechoic, rounded well-defined lesions, but they may also be hypoechoic or of mixed echogenicity. In patients with fatty livers, the haemangioma frequently looks hypoechoic relative to the background of the hyperechoic hepatic parenchyma. Larger ones can demonstrate a spectrum of reflectivity depending on their composition, and may demonstrate pools of blood and central areas of degeneration. They frequently exhibit slightly increased through-transmission, with posterior enhancement, particularly if large. This is probably due to the increased blood content compared with the surrounding liver parenchyma (Fig. 4.9).

As with many lesions, colour or power Doppler is too insensitive to pick up the slow flow in haemangiomas or to assist with lesion characterization. Microbubble contrast agents demonstrate a peripheral, globular enhancement with gradual centripetal filling to become isoechoic with the background liver in the sinusoidal phase.[7] CEUS frequently provides a definitive diagnosis at the time of scanning, reassuring the patient and obviating the need for further imaging of follow-up (Fig. 4.9).

When found in children, haemangiomas tend to be large and do produce symptoms. These masses produce shunting of blood from the aorta via the main hepatic artery and, in extreme cases, present with resulting cardiac failure. They are often heterogeneous in appearance and larger vessels within them may be identified with Doppler. Although many regress over a period of time, others may have to be embolized with coils under radiological guidance to control the symptoms.

FOCAL NODULAR HYPERPLASIA

Focal nodular hyperplasia (FNH) is the second most common solid, benign liver tumour. It is

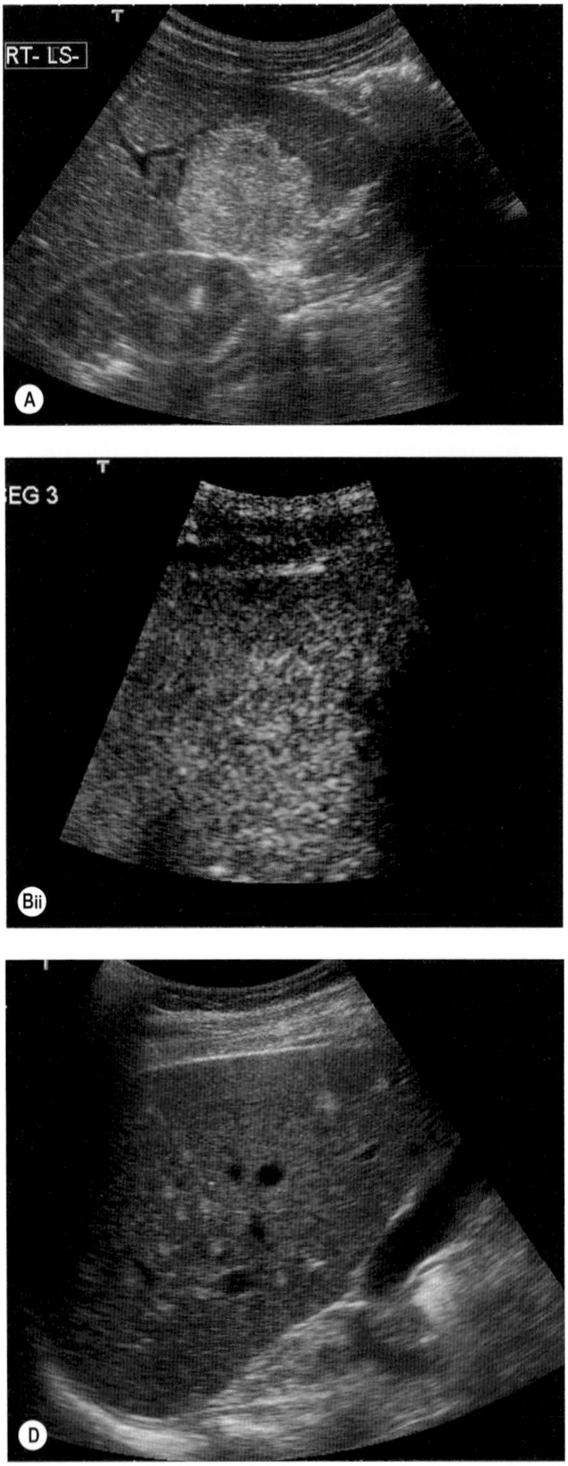

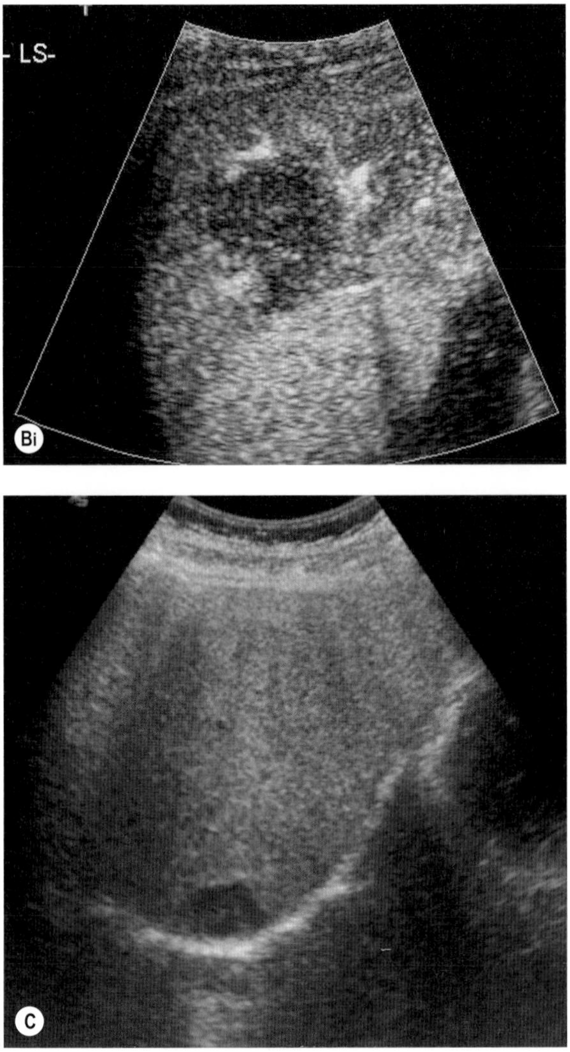

Fig. 4.9 • (A) A typical haemangioma in segment VI of the liver demonstrates hyperechogenicity with well-defined borders. (Bi) Administration of contrast demonstrates characteristic peripheral nodular enhancement in the arterial phase. (Bii) The lesion gradually takes up contrast to become isoechoic with background liver in the sinusoidal contrast phase confirming a benign haemangioma. (C) An atypical haemangioma appears hypoechoic on a background of fatty liver. CEUS confirmed its benign nature. (D) Multiple tiny haemangiomas throughout the liver.

made up of a hyperplastic proliferation of liver cells with hepatocytes, Kupffer cells, biliary and fibrous elements. It is most commonly found in young women, and is usually discovered by chance, being asymptomatic. Its ultrasound characteristics vary, from hypo-, iso- to hyperechoic compared with background liver (Fig. 4.10) and it may be multifocal. As with the haemangioma, it presents a diagnostic dilemma when found on CT or ultrasound, as its characteristics vary. As with haemangioma, CEUS is extremely helpful in characterizing incidental FNH, as it usually displays rapid arterial stellate filling, followed by centripetal enhancement with contrast uptake isoechoic with background liver in the sinusoidal phase.[8] It may, however, be difficult to differentiate from the rarer adenoma which also exhibits rapid arterialization on CEUS.[9]

Management of this benign mass is usually conservative, but surgical resection may be necessary in larger lesions.

ADENOMA

The hepatic adenoma is a benign focal lesion consisting of a cluster of atypical liver cells (Fig. 4.11). Within this, there may be pools of bile or focal areas of haemorrhage or necrosis. This gives rise to a heterogeneous, patchy echotexture. The smaller ones tend to be homogeneous with a smooth texture. Their lipid content causes a tendency to be hyperechoic, although usually less reflective than a haemangioma, and many have similar reflectivity to the surrounding liver parenchyma.

Clinical features

There is a particularly strong association between hepatic adenoma and use of the oral contraceptive, so these masses tend to present in younger women. Adenomas are also associated with glycogen storage disease and haemochromatosis.

They may cause pain, particularly if they haemorrhage, and may be palpable. If present during pregnancy, they can enlarge and rupture under the influence of oestrogen. In rare cases malignant transformation may occur[10] so surgical removal is the management of choice, although occasionally some adenomas regress if the oral contraceptive is discontinued.

FOCAL FATTY CHANGE

Not a 'lesion' as such, but included here due to its focal appearance. It may pose a diagnostic dilemma on initial ultrasound.

Focal fatty infiltration

Fatty infiltration of the liver is a common occurrence which may affect the whole, or part of the liver. It is associated with obesity and alcoholism, and can also occur in pregnancy, diabetes and with certain drugs.

The deposition of fat confined to certain focal areas of the liver is related to the blood supply to that area. Fatty infiltration increases the reflectivity of the parenchyma, making it hyperechoic. This can simulate a focal mass, such as a metastasis. Unlike a focal lesion however, it does not display any mass effect and the course of related vessels remains constant. It tends to have a characteristic straight-edged shape, rectangular or ovoid, corresponding to the region of local blood supply (Fig. 4.12). Foci of fatty change may be multiple, or may affect isolated liver segments. The most common sites are in segment IV around the porta, in the caudate lobe (segment I) and in the posterior area of the left lobe (segment III).

CEUS is useful and accurate in differentiating focal fatty change from a true lesion, as the contrast uptake is identical to background liver, and the contrast convincingly demonstrates the lack of mass effect (Fig. 4.12D) This technique usually obviates the need for further imaging in focal fatty change.

Focal fatty sparing

The reverse process may also occur, in which a diffusely fatty, hyperechogenic liver has an area which has been spared from fat deposition due to its blood supply. This area is less reflective than the surrounding liver and may mimic a hypoechoic neoplastic lesion, but as with focal fatty infiltration, it has regular outlines and shape and no mass effect. The most common sites for fatty sparing are similar to those for focal fatty infiltration; segment IV just anterior to the portal vein or gallbladder (Fig. 4.12B), segment I (the caudate lobe) and around the gallbladder fossa.

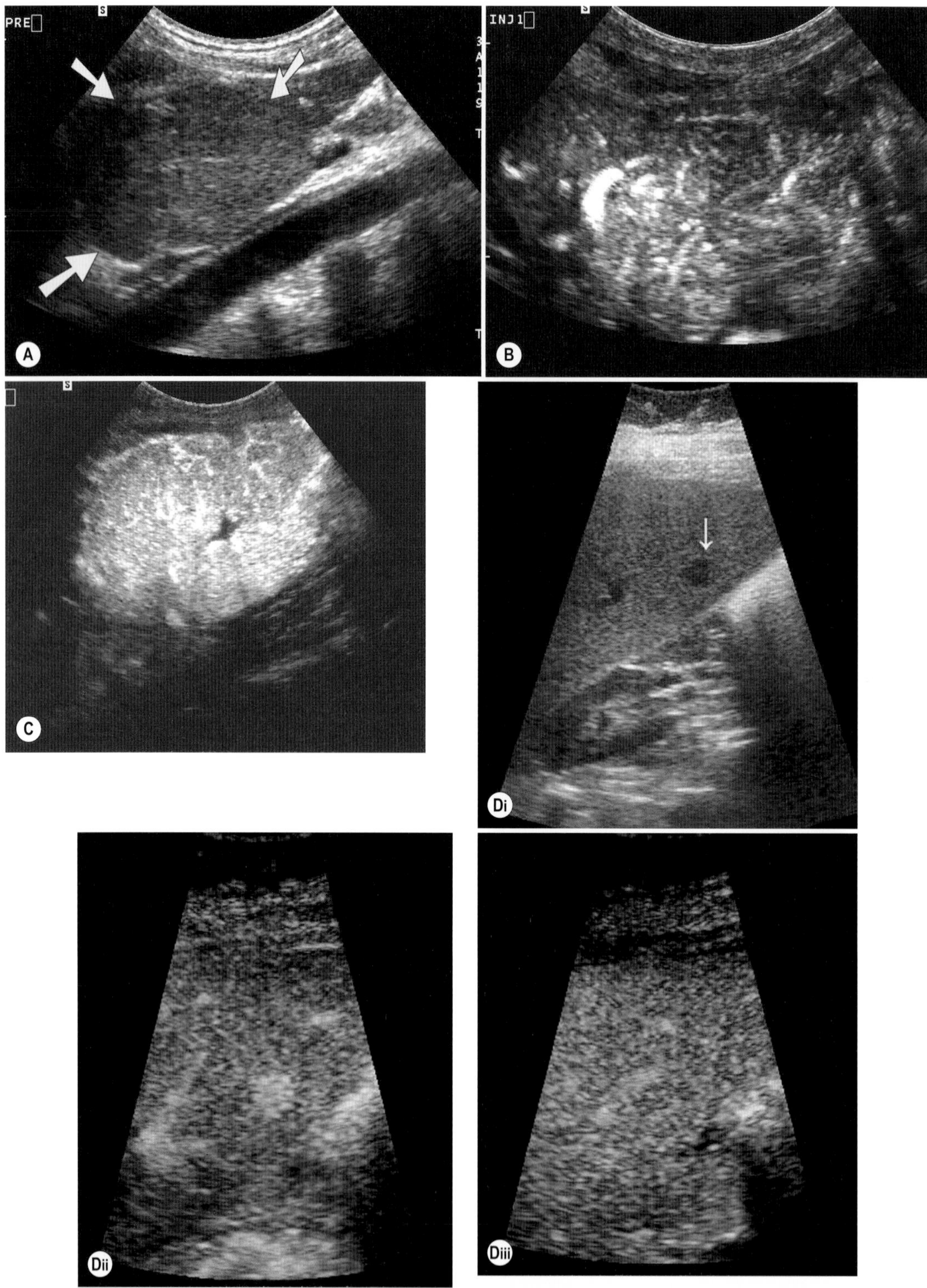

Fig. 4.10 • FNH: (A) In the left lobe (arrows). These are frequently almost isoechoic with normal liver tissue. (B) Following administration of microbubble contrast agent, FNH displays a 'spoked-wheel' pattern of vascular enhancement during the early arterial phase. (C) The same lesion seconds later, showing a central scar. (Di) A tiny FNH (arrow) (Dii) blushes rapidly in the arterial phase of contrast administration and (Diii) becomes isoechoic with background liver in the sinusoidal phase.

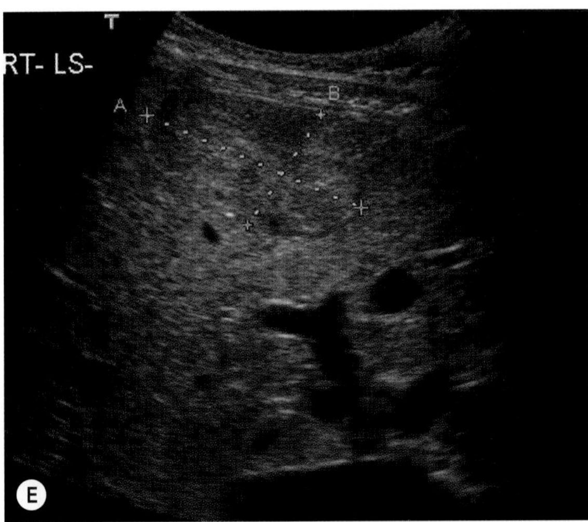

Fig. 4.10, cont'd • (E) Another example of an FNH, almost isoechoic with background liver.

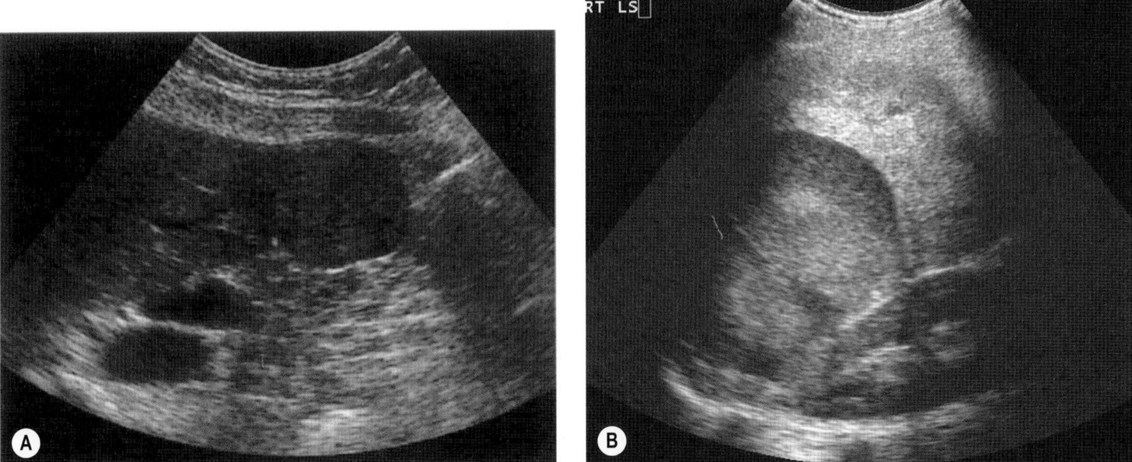

Fig. 4.11 • (A) Adenoma in segment V of the liver in a young woman on the contraceptive pill. (B) An unusual example of cystic degeneration in a large adenoma.

Unlike a true focal lesion, fatty change does not exhibit a mass effect, and normal, undisplaced vasculature can be demonstrated with colour Doppler (in the larger areas) or contrast ultrasound (particularly useful for the smaller focal areas) in both of focal fatty infiltration and fatty sparing (see also Fig. 4.19C).

Lipoma

The hepatic lipoma is a relatively rare, benign hepatic tumour which is very similar in nature and acoustic appearance to focal fatty change. It differs in that it is a discrete tumour of fatty deposition, rather than an infiltrative process, and so can exert a mass effect on surrounding vessels if large. The fat content makes the lipoma hyperechoic compared to the surrounding liver tissue.

Granuloma

Granulomas are benign liver masses which are associated with chronic inflammatory liver diseases. They have a particular association with primary biliary cirrhosis, sarcoidosis or tuberculosis. They may be multiple and small, in which case the liver often looks coarse and hyperechoic. More often they are small discrete lesions which may be hypo- or isoechoic, sometimes with a hypoechoic rim like a target, or calcified with distal shadowing (Fig. 4.13). They can undergo central necrosis.

Differential diagnoses include metastases or regenerating nodules, and their appearance on ultrasound is non-specific.

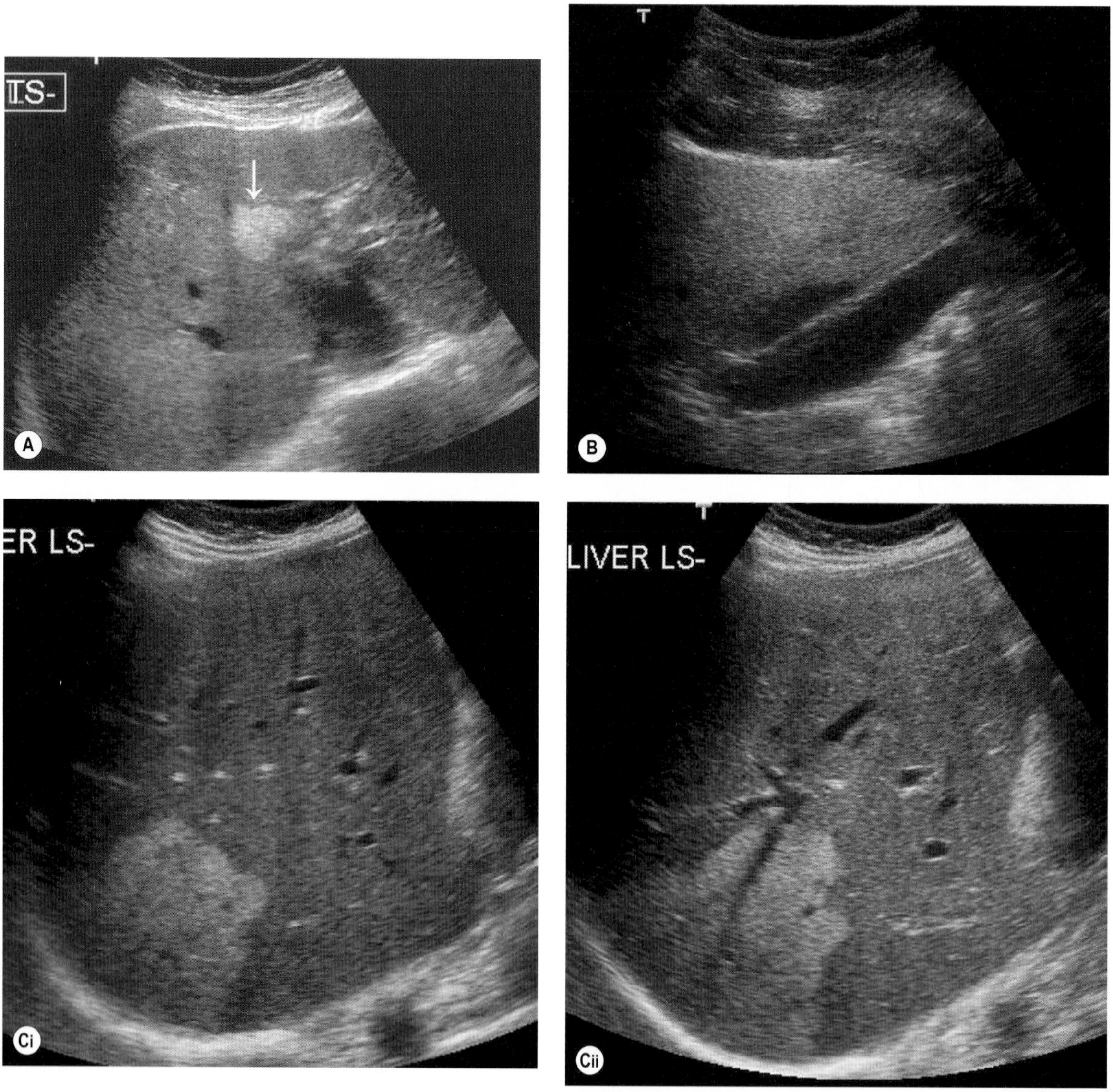

Fig. 4.12 • (A) Focal fatty change (arrow) can mimic a focal lesion. (B) Focal fatty sparing in a characteristic position just anterior to the gallbladder. (Ci) Focal fatty change in the right lobe of liver demonstrates a hepatic vein passing through it, (Cii) with no mass effect.

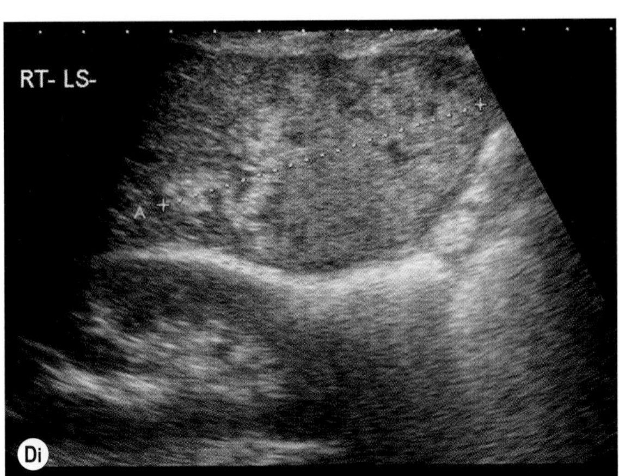

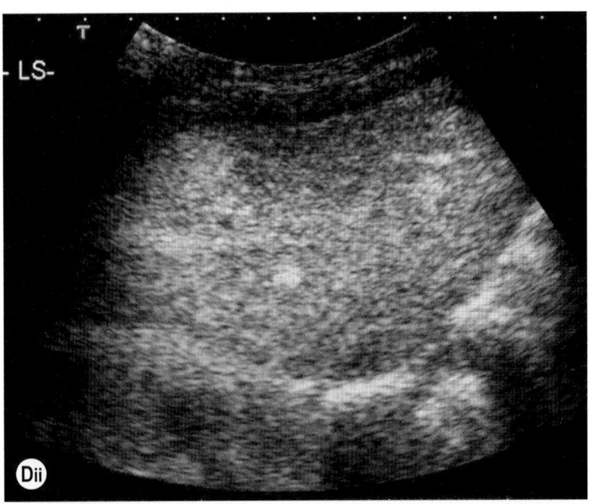

Fig. 4.12, cont'd • (Di) An irregular focal lesion in segment VI in a patient with cirrhosis is suspicious for hepatocellular carcinoma (HCC). (Dii) CEUS demonstrates normal contrast take up in the arterial, portal and sinusoidal phases, with no mass seen, confirming focal fatty change.

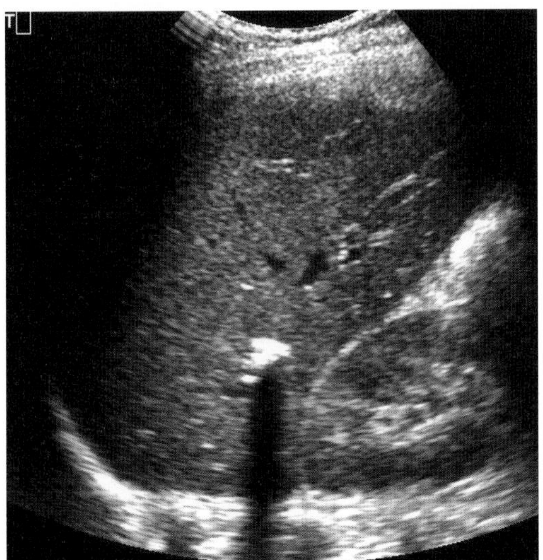

Fig. 4.13 • A calcified granuloma demonstrates acoustic shadowing.

Fig. 4.14 • Considerable deposits of calcification are seen in the liver in this patient with nephrotic syndrome.

HEPATIC CALCIFICATION

Calcification occurs in the liver as a result of some pathological processes, and may be seen following infection or parasitic infestation. It may be focal – usually the end stage of a previous abscess, haematoma or granuloma – which usually indicates that the lesion in question is no longer active. It may also be seen within some metastases. Calcification may also be linear in nature, following the course of the portal tracts. This can be associated with old tuberculosis or other previous parasitic infestations such as schistosomiasis[11] (Fig. 4.14).

Occasionally hepatic calcification is seen in children or in the fetus. This is usually not a significant finding but pre-natal infection should be excluded with a TORCH screen.

Calcification, which casts a strong and definite shadow should be distinguished from air in the biliary tree (Fig. 3.46), which casts a reverberative shadow and is usually associated with previous biliary interventions, such as ERCP, sphincterotomy or stent placement.

MALIGNANT FOCAL LIVER LESIONS

METASTASES

The liver is one of the most common sites to which malignant tumours metastasize. Secondary deposits are usually bloodborne, spreading to the liver via the portal venous system (e.g. in the case of gastrointestinal malignancies) or hepatic artery (e.g. lung or breast primaries,) or spread via the lymphatic system. Some spread along the peritoneal surfaces – for example ovarian carcinoma. This demonstrates an initial invasion of the subserosal surfaces of the liver (see Fig. 4.16A below), as opposed to the more central distribution seen with a haematogenous spread (see Fig. 4.16B below). The former, peripheral pattern is more easily missed on ultrasound because small deposits are often obscured by near-field artefact or rib shadows. It is therefore advisable for the operator to be aware of the possible pattern of spread when searching for liver metastases.

Ultrasound appearances

The acoustic appearances of liver secondaries are extremely variable (Figs 4.15, 4.16). When compared with normal surrounding liver parenchyma, metastases may be hyperechoic, hypoechoic, isoechoic or of mixed pattern. It is not possible to characterize the primary source by the acoustic properties of the metastases.

Metastases tend to be solid with ill-defined margins. Some metastases, particularly the larger ones, contain fluid as a result of central necrosis (Fig. 4.16E), or because they contain mucin, for example from some ovarian primaries. Occasionally, calcification is seen within a deposit, causing distal acoustic shadowing, and this may also develop following treatment with chemotherapy. In some diseases, for example lymphoma, the metastases may be multiple but tiny – not immediately obvious to the operator as discrete focal lesions but as a coarse-textured liver (Fig. 4.16F). This type of appearance is non-specific and could be associated with a number of conditions, both benign and malignant.

Diagnosis of focal liver lesions, such as metastases, is made more difficult when the liver texture is diffusely abnormal or when there are dilated intrahepatic ducts, because the altered transmission of sound through the liver masks small lesions. Other possible ultrasound features associated with metastases include a lobulated outline to the liver, hepatomegaly and ascites.

If the finding of liver metastases is unexpected, or the primary has not been identified, it is useful to complete a full examination to search for a possible primary carcinoma and to identify other sites of carcinomatous spread. Lymphadenopathy (particularly in the para-aortic, para-caval and portal regions) may be demonstrated on ultrasound, as well as invasion of adjacent blood vessels and disease in other extrahepatic sites including spleen, kidneys, omentum and peritoneum. CT is the usual next step, to identify a possible primary site and to stage the disease, in particular demonstrating extra-hepatic disease which is often not seen on ultrasound.

Doppler is unhelpful in characterizing liver metastases, most of which appear poorly vascular or avascular. Fundamental non-contrast ultrasound lacks sensitivity in the diagnosis of liver metastases, as many lesions are either isoechoic, or small (subcentimetre) rendering them almost invisible. The use of microbubble contrast agents radically improves both the characterization and detection of metastatic deposits on ultrasound.[12] The injection of a bolus of contrast agent when viewed using pulse-inversion demonstrates variable vascular phase enhancement in the arterial and portal phases, but the sinusoidal phase invariably lacks contrast uptake (Fig. 4.16G, H). This is a particularly useful technique as it increases the contrast resolution between metastasis and background liver, meaning that even subcentimetre lesions are reliably demonstrated.

CEUS also increases the operator's confidence in the absence of metastases, particularly in cases with altered LFTs and prior history of malignancy (Fig. 4.16J). This is useful in obviating the need for further imaging in normal livers.

Clinical features and management

Many patients present with symptoms from their liver deposits, rather than the primary carcinoma. The demonstration of liver metastases on

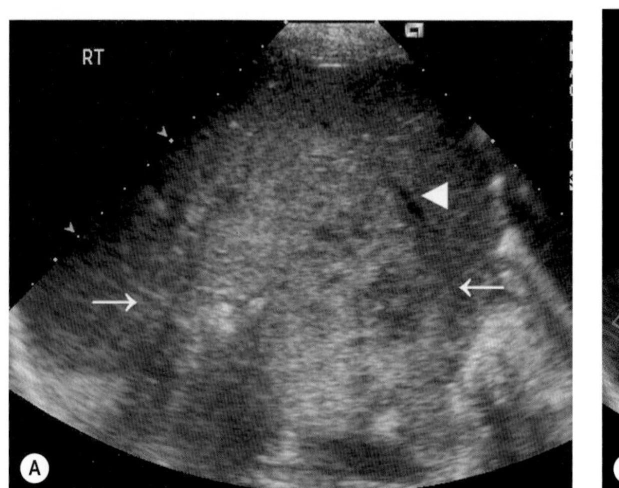

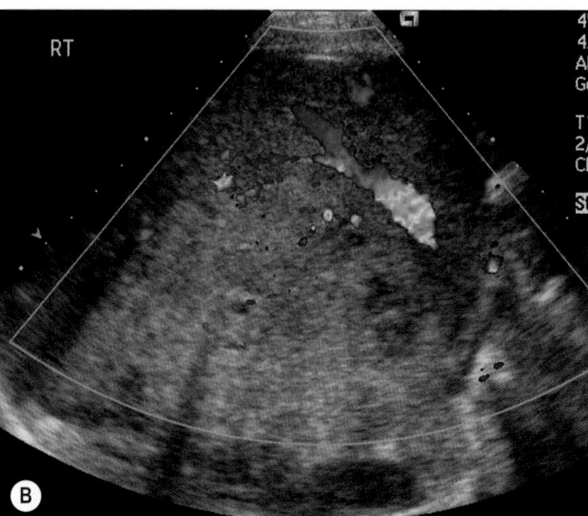

Fig. 4.15 • The mass effect (A) A large isoechoic lesion (arrows), displaces the middle hepatic vein (arrowhead). (B) Colour flow of the same case.

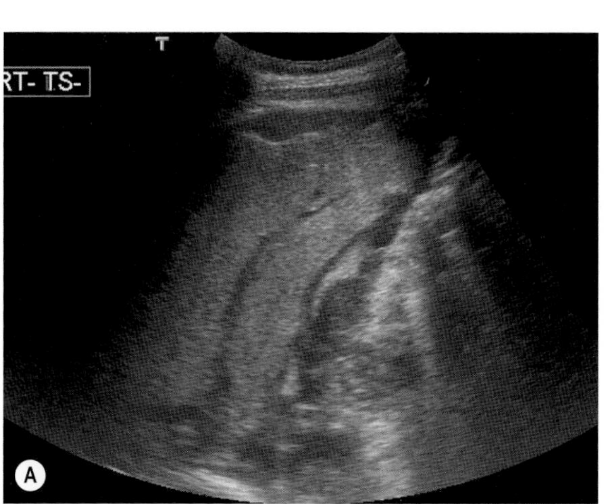

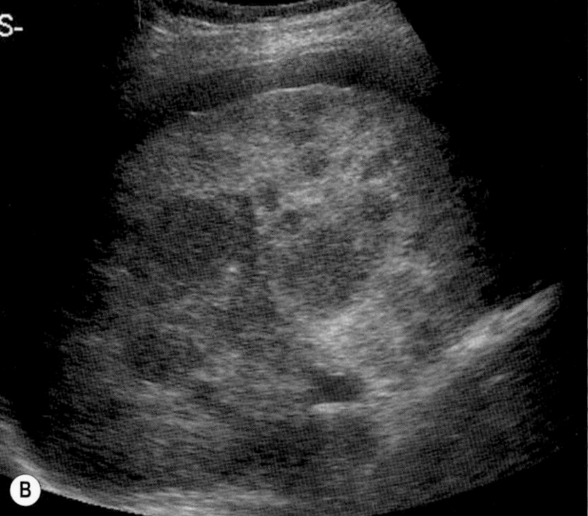

Fig. 4.16 • Examples of liver metastases: (A) Peripheral, hypoechoic secondary deposits due to peritoneal spread from a primary ovarian carcinoma. (B) Bloodborne metastases from bowel carcinoma are distributed throughout the liver.

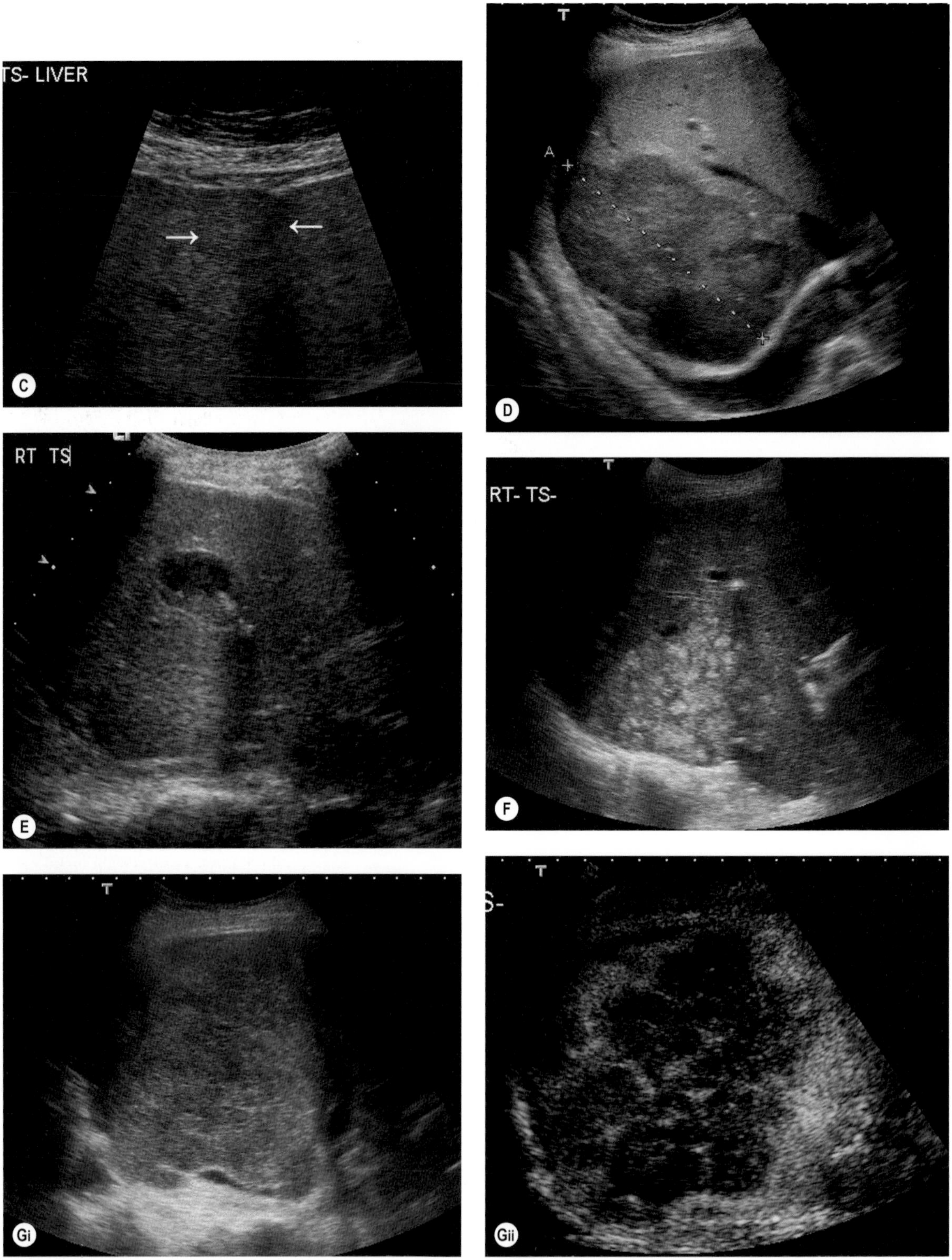

Fig. 4.16, cont'd

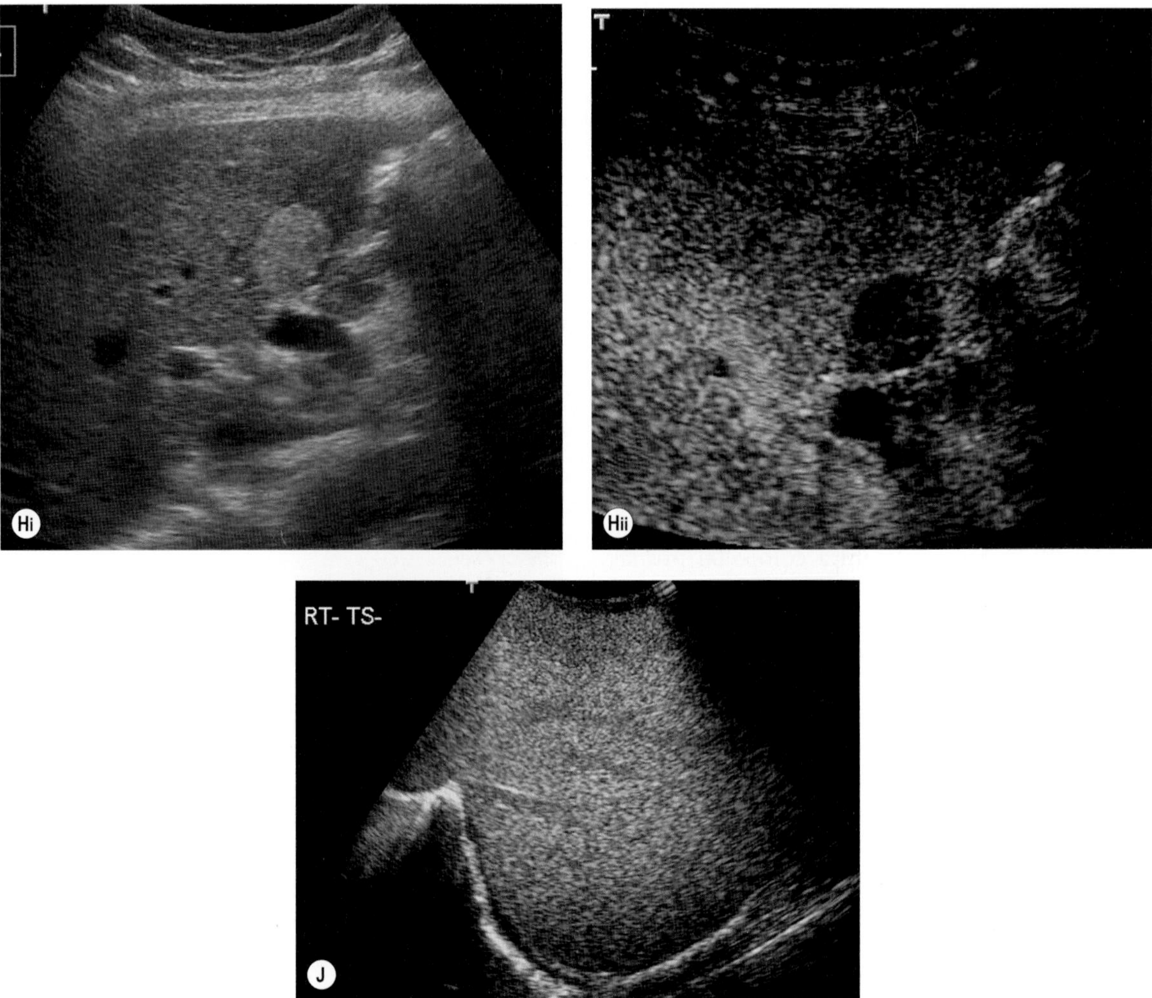

Fig. 4.16, cont'd • (C) Solitary isoechoic metastasis, confirmed on MRI. Isoechoic metastases are easy to miss, and the use of CEUS is invaluable in demonstrating them. (D) Large hyperechoic metastasis occupying segment VII of the right lobe. Note also the right pleural effusion. (E) A necrotic metastasis, demonstrating posterior acoustic enhancement. (F) Calcified metastases from breast carcinoma. (Gi, Gii), Pre- and Post CEUS. Following administration of microbubble contrast agent, numerous metastases are discovered. These appear hypoechoic in the late portal venous phase, with no contrast uptake. (Hi, Hii) Pre- and Post CEUS of a solitary metastasis in a patient who has undergone surgery for bowel carcinoma. (J) Normal CEUS in a patient at risk of liver metastases. Contrast take up is homogeneous throughout the liver in the sinusoidal phase with no evidence of lesions. CEUS greatly increases the confidence in a negative scan.

ultrasound may often prompt further radiological investigations for the primary. The symptoms of liver deposits may include non-obstructive jaundice, obstructive jaundice (which may occur if a large mass is present at the porta), hepatomegaly, right-sided pain, increasing abdominal girth from ascites and altered LFTs.

Ultrasound-guided biopsy may be useful in diagnosing the primary and complements further imaging such as X-rays and contrast bowel studies. Accurate staging of the disease is performed with CT, MRI and/or PET-CT,[13] which have improved sensitivity for identifying extrahepatic and systemic disease, such as peritoneal deposits and lymphadenopathy, and which can more accurately demonstrate adjacent spread of primary disease.

The prognosis for most patients with liver metastases has traditionally been poor, particularly if multiple, and depends to a large extent on the origin of the primary carcinoma. A regime of surgical debulking (removal of the primary carcinoma, adjacent invaded viscera, lymphadenopathy etc.) together with chemotherapy can slow down the progress of the disease. Increasingly, however, there are treatment options which result in increased, good quality survival and, in some cases, cure. This makes it important that secondary disease is diagnosed early and accurately in order to offer patients a significant chance of survival.

In an increasing number of cases, particularly those with metastases from a colorectal primary, which are less aggressive and grow more slowly, long-term survival is achieved by surgically resecting both the primary bowel lesion and then the liver deposits. The smaller and fewer the liver deposits, the better the prognosis. The success of this treatment means that tumours previously considered inoperable are now potentially curable. In such cases it is particularly useful to localize the lesions using the segmental liver anatomy prior to surgery (see Chapter 2). Intraoperative ultrasound (IOUS) is then used to confirm the preoperative appearances and examine the tumour margins to plan the line of resection (Fig. 4.17).

Other methods of treatment include chemoembolization, and radiofrequency, microwave or laser ablation often under ultrasound guidance.[14] The success of these options depends on the number and size of the lesions, and the nature of the primary. Currently, these methods are considered palliative, rather than curative, and are an option for patients who are unsuitable candidates for hepatic resection[15] (see Chapter 11).

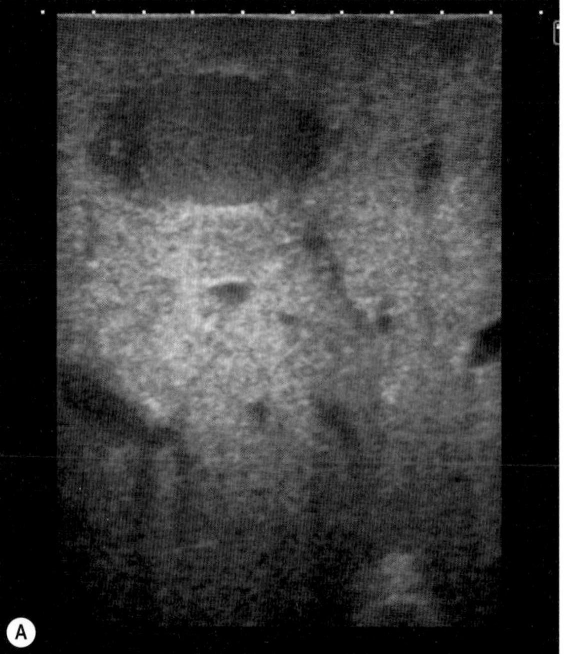

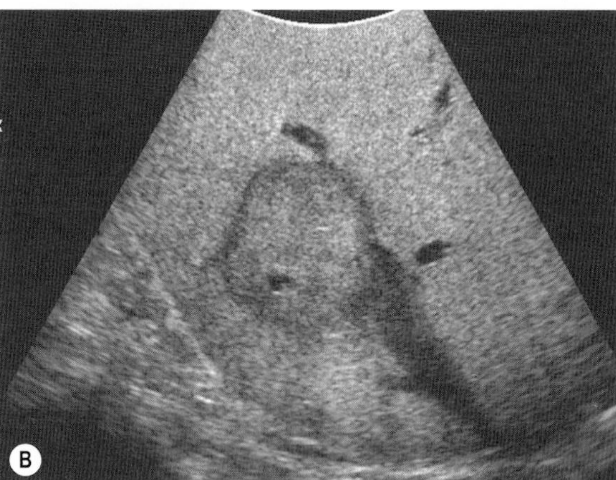

Fig. 4.17 • (A) Intraoperative ultrasound scan demonstrates a small metastasis not identified on preoperative imaging. (B) IOUS locates a metastasis prior to ultrasound-guided ablation.

Ultrasound of other relevant areas

In suspected or confirmed malignancy, the examination of the abdomen may usefully include all the sites likely to be affected. Whilst the liver is one of the most common sites for spread of the disease, it is also useful to examine the adrenals, spleen and kidneys, and to look for lymphadenopathy in the para-aortic, para-caval and portal regions.

If ascites is present, deposits may sometimes be demonstrated on the peritoneal or omental surfaces in patients with late-stage disease. These malignant plaques may also afford a useful site for ultrasound guided biopsy in order to diagnose and palliatively treat the disease.

HEPATOCELLULAR CARCINOMA

This primary carcinoma of the liver is particularly common in Africa and the Far East, and demographics show an increasing incidence in Europe and the UK. Most HCCs (over 80%) arise in diseased livers, hence the strong association with alcoholic cirrhosis and hepatitis, and one of the main reasons for ultrasound referral in such patients is to exclude focal liver lesions which could represent carcinoma. HCC is also associated with metabolic disorders and drug-related liver disease.

Clinically, small tumours are asymptomatic but cause a raised serum alpha-fetoprotein (AFP). The relationship between cirrhosis and HCC prompts screening of such patients with AFP and ultrasound. The ultrasound appearances of HCC vary from hypo- to hyperechoic or mixed echogenicity lesions (Fig. 4.18). It is often particularly difficult, if not impossible, to locate small HCCs in a

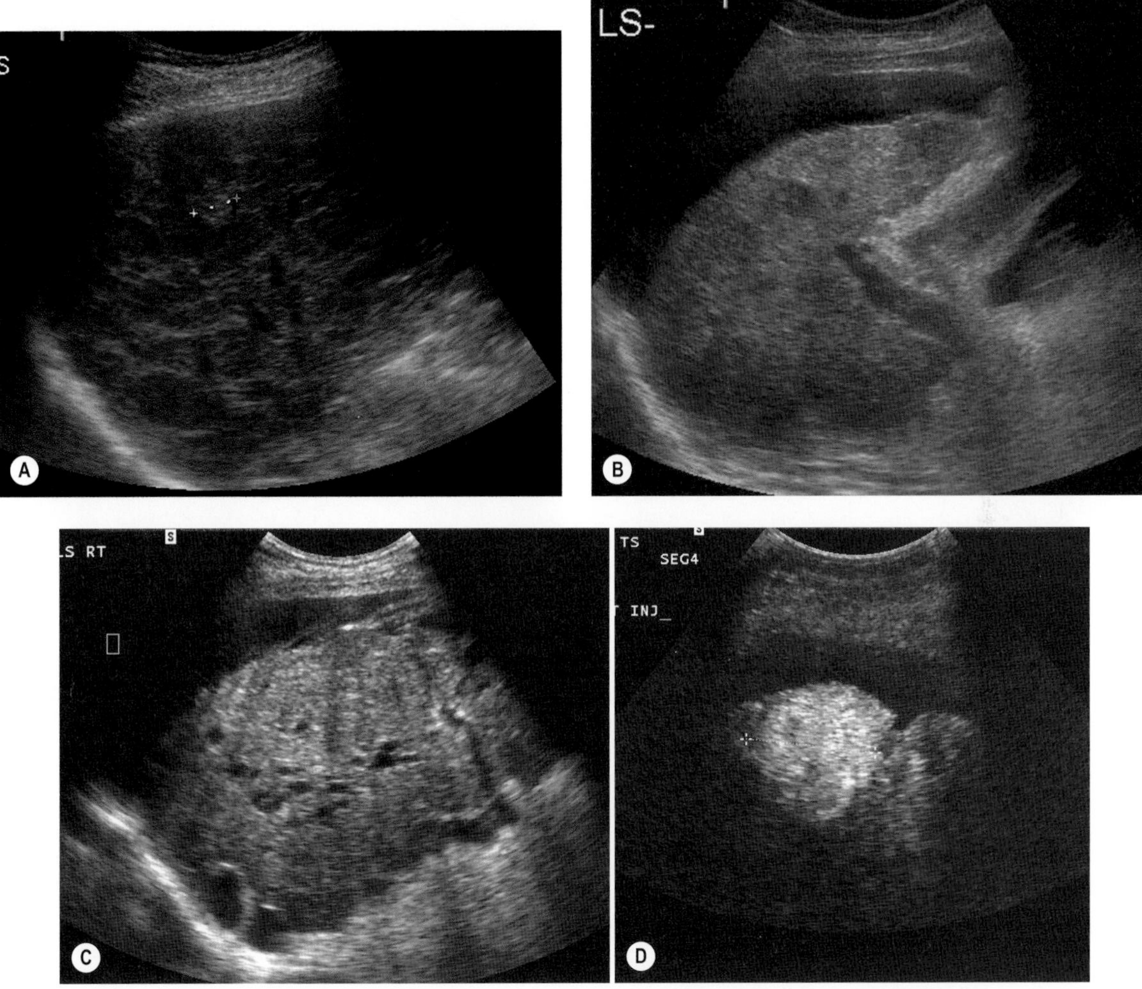

Fig. 4.18 • Hepatocellular carcinoma: (A) A small HCC (confirmed at MRI) on a background of cirrhosis. (B) Multifocal HCCs in a patient with cryptogenic cirrhosis. (C) A patient with chronic Budd–Chiari syndrome has a nodular liver with suspicion of a lesion near the anterior surface. (D) Administration of contrast in the same patient as (C) demonstrates increased uptake in the arterial phase, with hypoenhancement in the sinusoidal phase, helping to locate the lesion, and characterize it as an HCC.

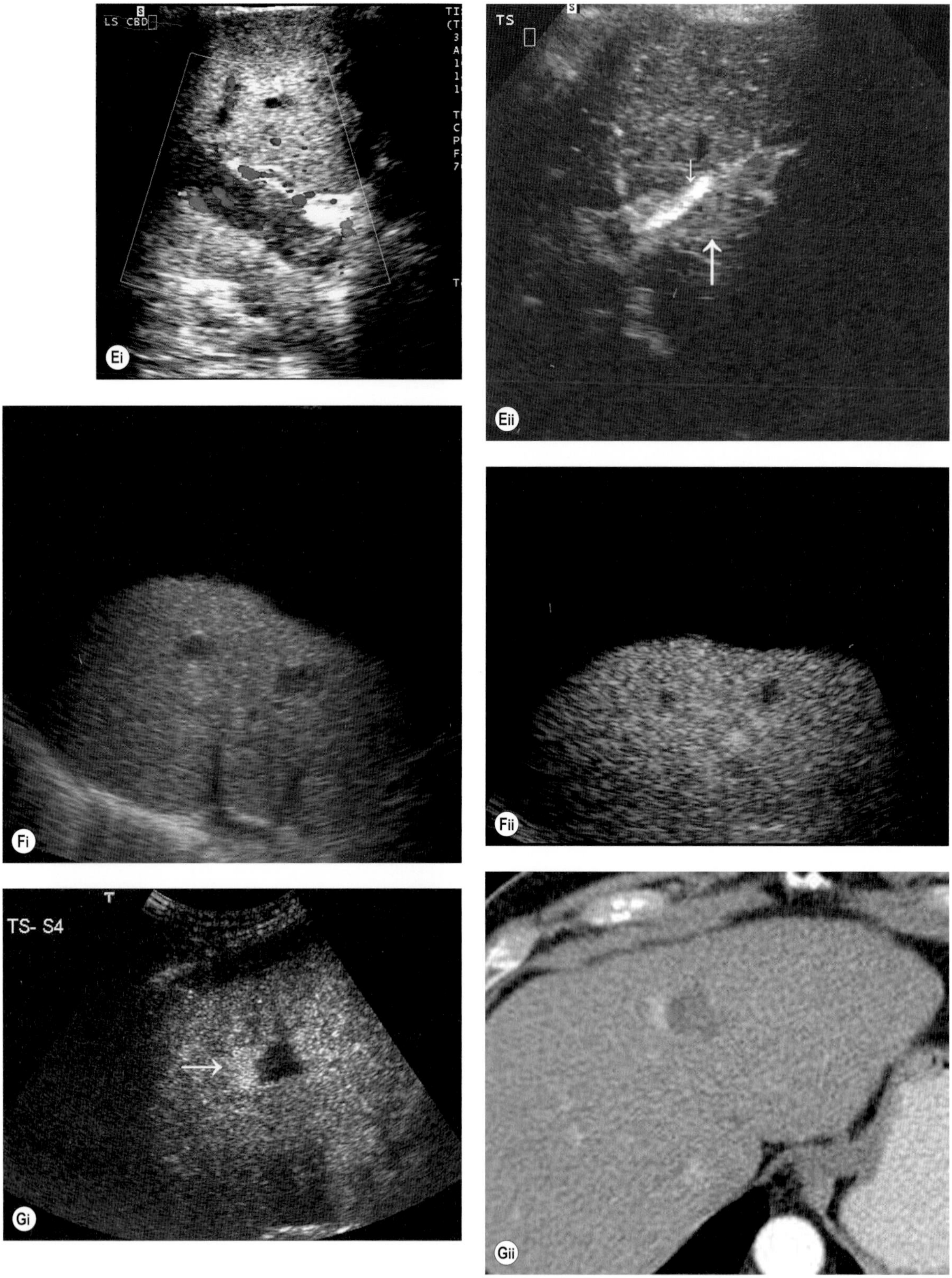

Fig. 4.18, cont'd

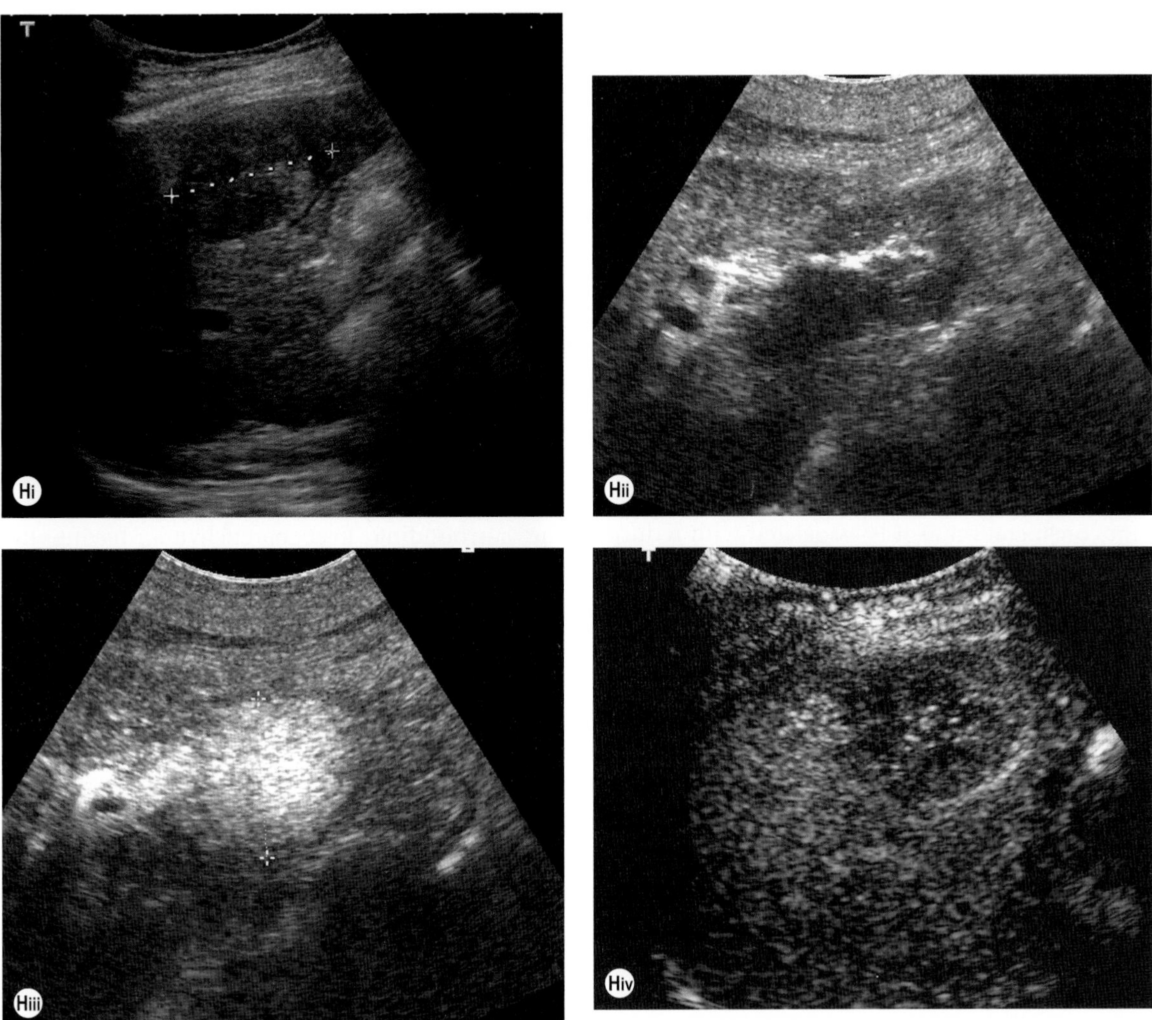

Fig. 4.18, cont'd • (Ei) Tumour thrombus in the portal vein in a patient with multifocal HCC. (Eii) CEUS of a case of invasive HCC; the PV (large arrow) shows contrast uptake due to tumour thrombus in the arterial phase. (HA = small arrow.) (Fi) Two small HCCs in a patient with cirrhosis and gross ascites. (Fii) CEUS demonstrates typical hypoenhancement in the sinusoidal phase. (Gi) CEUS in an ablated HCC. The treated lesion is almost avascular, but a rim of tumour recurrence (arrow) is present around the lesion. (Gii) CT confirms tumour recurrence and the lesion was re-ablated successfully. (H) Typical CEUS of HCC: (Hi) pre-contrast lesion, (Hii) immediate post-injection shows a tortuous feeding artery followed by (Hiii) a blush of contrast uptake. (Hiv) Sinusoidal phase shows hypoenhancement.

cirrhotic liver which is already coarse textured and nodular. MRI may be useful in these cases[16,17] as it is able to differentiate HCC from other nodules, such as dysplastic nodules, which occur frequently in the cirrhotic liver. HCCs may be solitary or multifocal.

The increase in such diseases as hepatitis C has caused the introduction of ultrasound/AFP screening programmes in many centres. This has led to the more frequent detection of early, small HCCs which can be indistinguishable on ultrasound from other, regenerative liver nodules.

Lesions of over 2 cm diameter in a cirrhotic liver have around a 90% chance of being malignant, and CEUS can demonstrate tortuous feeding arteries, the tumour blush and the hypoenhancement in the sinusoidal phase which are characteristic of HCC (Fig. 4.18H). CEUS appearances can be quite variable in HCC, however, and should be interpreted with caution.

The introduction of ultrasound screening, together with the improvement in image quality, has meant the discovery of ever smaller nodules. These frequently fail to demonstrate characteristic CEUS patterns, and MRI is the appropriate next imaging modality. The combination of MRI and CEUS when characteristic contrast patterns are present obviates the need for biopsy[18] – an important consideration as it is associated with reduced survival in patients who subsequently receive a transplant.

As with metastases, there is now a range of treatment options which can improve patient survival. Hepatic transplant is generally considered curative, and traditionally offered in the absence of malignancy. However, patients with HCCs can still be considered for a transplant, provided the malignancy is limited, and their disease may be temporarily controlled using ultrasound guided ablation if necessary.[19,20] In patients with advanced HCC, transcatheter arterial chemoembolization (TACE) may slow the progress of the tumour, and high intensity focused ultrasound (HIFU) is a further technique that is promising in improving patient survival.[21]

CHOLANGIOCARCINOMA

This primary carcinoma of the bile ducts is discussed more fully in Chapter 3. Most commonly seen affecting the main biliary ducts, it also occurs in the intrahepatic biliary tree where it infiltrates the surrounding liver parenchyma, having the appearance of a solid mass. It may be solitary or multifocal and a clue to its location is often the focal dilatation of ducts proximal to the obstructing mass. It has an association with sclerosing cholangitis, and carries a relatively poor prognosis, as it has a tendency to recur after transplantation (Table 4.2).

BENIGN	Haemangioma	Usually hyperechoic. Common incidental finding
	Focal nodular hyperplasia	Common, usually asymptomatic lesion, often in young women
	Focal fatty change	No mass effect
	Adenoma	Uncommon. Associated with contraceptive pill
	Granuloma	Associated with chronic inflammation/infection. May calcify
	Regenerating nodules	Associated with cirrhosis. Multiple lesions
	Abscess	May appear solid in the early stages. Look for posterior enhancement. Fever and pain
	Infarct	Associated with HA thrombosis in liver transplant
MALIGNANT	Metastasis	Wide spectrum of possible acoustic appearances
	HCC	Associated with cirrhosis
	Cholangiocarcinoma	Associated with cholestatic disease. Proximal biliary dilatation

Table 4.2 Common solid focal liver lesions: differential diagnoses

DIFFUSE LIVER CONDITIONS

Diseases which diffusely affect the liver may have non-specific ultrasound appearances. Suspicion is usually raised following altered liver function tests (see Chapter 1) and the diagnosis made histologically.

A number of diffuse liver conditions can cause hepatocellular (or non-obstructive) jaundice which is associated with increased levels of *unconjugated* bile in the blood. Many of these can be demonstrated with ultrasound, others cannot. The main role of ultrasound in the jaundiced patient is to exclude any obstructive cause (by the presence or absence of biliary duct dilatation) and to search for liver metastases or signs of a diffuse liver condition (Table 4.3).

FATTY INFILTRATION (STEATOSIS)

The process of accumulation of fat within the hepatic cells may be either focal (see above) or diffuse. Related to various conditions such as alcoholism, obesity and diabetes, it is associated with any process which alters liver metabolism and it is reversible in many circumstances.

Haemolysis	In which red cells are destroyed, releasing the haemoglobin (from which bilirubin is derived) into the surrounding tissue
Haematoma	Haemolytic process
Gilbert's disease	A defect in the hepatic uptake of bilirubin
Viral hepatitis, cirrhosis of all types, alcoholic or drug-induced liver disease	Destruction of the liver cells by these diseases prevents the mechanism of hepatic uptake and excretion of bilirubin. Both conjugated and unconjugated bilirubin are present
Abscess intrahepatic malignancy	Multiple and/or large lesions prevent the take up and excretion of bilirubin by the liver cells

Table 4.3 Causes of non-obstructive ('medical') jaundice

The acoustic properties of fat differ from those of normal liver tissue. The liver appears hyperechoic as the fat globules provide interfaces which are highly reflective. As the level of fat deposition increases, the level of echogenicity reaches that of the highly reflective portal tract walls. This has the effect of reducing the prominence of the portal tracts (Fig. 4.19) and making the liver appear smooth and homogeneous, with closely packed, fine echoes. The contrast between the liver and parenchyma of the right kidney is therefore increased (a particularly useful sign confirming that the correct gain settings have been used). Hepatomegaly is also a feature, though not invariably. Finally, the attenuation of fat is greater than that of normal liver tissue; this has the effect of reduced penetration in the far field – rather as if the TGC paddles or slope control had been incorrectly set. In severe cases of infiltration, most of the sound is reflected back to the transducer in the first few centimetres, creating a highly reflective near field band through which the sound is unable to penetrate.

Fatty infiltration itself is not usually a significant finding, however it often occurs in conjunction with other significant diffuse processes such as cirrhosis. Its increased attenuation reduces the ability of ultrasound to exclude other disease or focal lesions and therefore CT may be a useful adjunct. In cases of focal fatty change or sparing (see above) it may cause a diagnostic dilemma as it mimics a focal lesion. CEUS is useful in characterizing these areas (Figs 4.11, 4.19C).

Non-alcoholic steatohepatitis

Non-alcoholic steatohepatitis (NASH) or non-alcoholic fatty liver disease (NAFLD) is when fat deposition in the hepatocytes is accompanied by inflammation and fibrosis in patients who consume little or no alcohol. In contrast to 'simple' fatty liver, this process can cause irreversible damage leading to cirrhosis. Its incidence is increasing in developed countries, and it is strongly associated with obesity and diabetes.[22] It is an increasingly

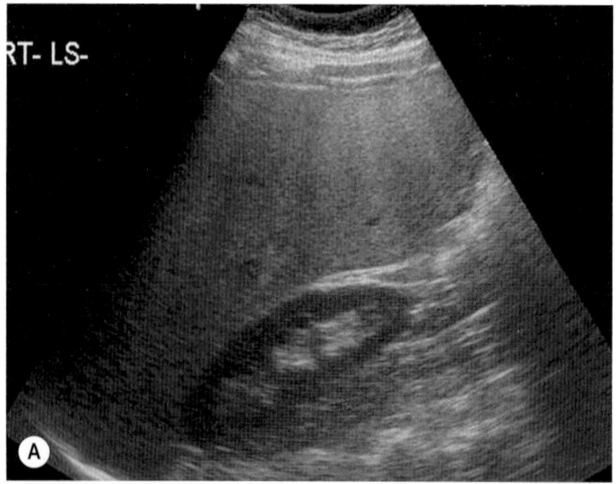

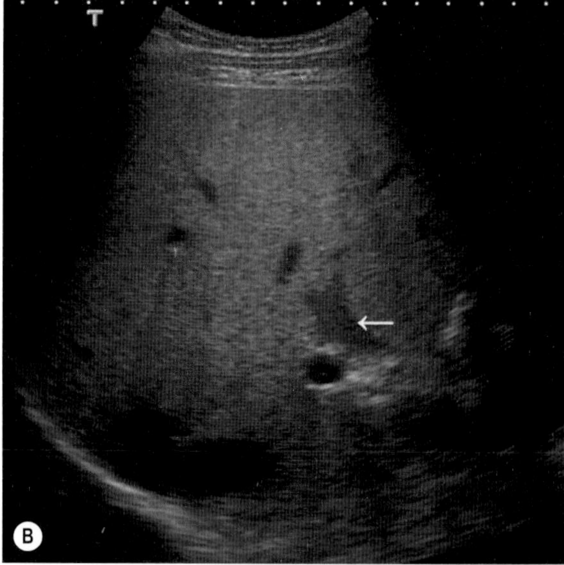

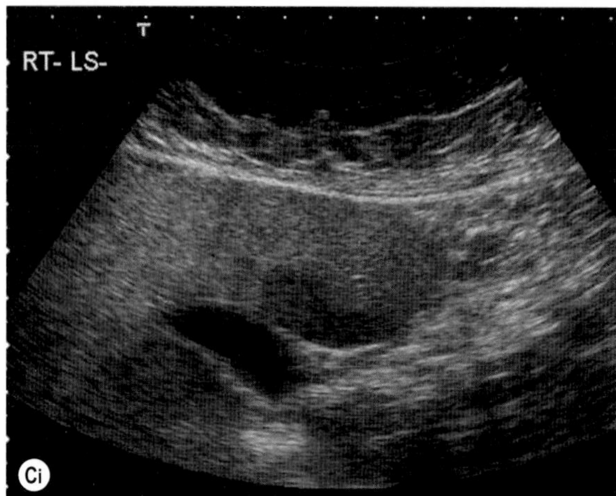

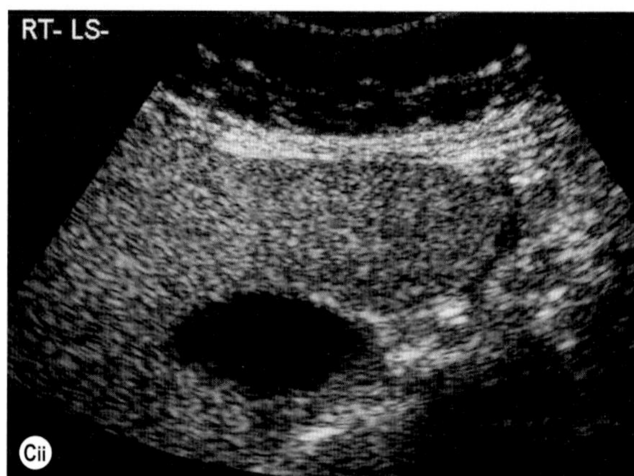

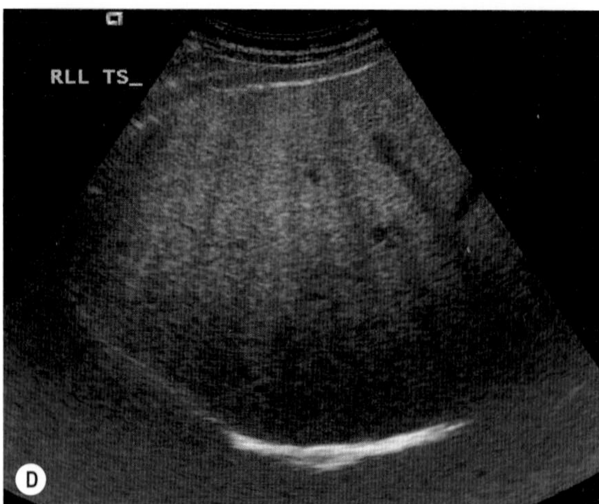

Fig. 4.19 • (A) Fatty infiltration increases the hepatorenal contrast. The portal tracts are reduced in prominence, giving a more homogeneous appearance. Attenuation is increased so that it is more difficult to penetrate to the back of the liver. (B) Fatty liver with reduced portal tract prominence and a focal area of fatty sparing (arrow). (Ci) Fatty liver in a patient taking chemotherapy following resection for bowel carcinoma. The new finding of an area of fatty sparing anterior to the gallbladder needs definitive characterization. (Cii) CEUS demonstrates contrast take up identical to background liver throughout all phases, confirming fatty sparing. (D) NASH demonstrating a coarse textured, fatty and fibrotic liver.

common reason for abnormal LFTs and referral for ultrasound (Fig. 4.19D).

CIRRHOSIS

Cirrhosis is a process associated with end-stage chronic liver disease (and not really a 'disease' in itself.) It can result from a wide range of pathological processes.

Ultrasound appearances

In cirrhosis bands of fibrous tissue are laid down in the liver parenchyma between the hepatic lobules. This distorts and destroys the normal architecture of the liver, separating it into nodules. The process may be *micronodular*, which gives a generally coarse echotexture, or *macronodular* in which discrete nodules of 1 cm and above can be distinguished on ultrasound (Fig. 4.20).

The hepatocellular damage which causes cirrhosis gives rise to *hepatic fibrosis* – a precursor of cirrhosis. The fibrosis itself may have very little effect on the ultrasound appearances of the liver, but when advanced it is more highly reflective than normal liver tissue, giving the appearance of a 'bright' liver often with a coarse texture.[16] Unlike fatty change, which is potentially reversible, fibrosis is the result of irreversible damage to the liver cells. The picture is further complicated by the association of fibrosis with fatty change, which also increases the echogenicity. The acoustic attenuation properties of fibrosis, however, are similar to normal liver – so that the ultrasound beam can penetrate to the posterior areas using normal TGC settings. Fat, on the other hand, increases both the echogenicity *and* the attenuation, preventing penetration to the far field (Fig. 4.19).

The cirrhotic liver tends to shrink as the disease progresses. However, it may be normal in size, or may undergo disproportionate changes within different lobes. In some patients the right lobe shrinks giving rise to relative hypertrophy of the caudate and/or left lobes, for example. This is likely to be due to the venous drainage of the different areas of the liver.

Nodules in cirrhosis

The nodular nature of the cirrhotic liver may give rise to diagnostic dilemma. Nodular regeneration is often present, in which the liver 'responds' to the fibrosis and architectural disturbance with the nodular regrowth of hepatocytes, visible as lumps on the ultrasound scan.

Dysplastic nodules are composed of hepatocytes which have undergone benign change. 'Low grade' nodules are non-malignant and usually small (sub centimetre) but slightly larger than the background cirrhotic nodules. These nodules may progress into 'high grade' lesions, which have an increased arterial supply, are increasingly atypical of liver cells, and are generally thought to be 'pre-malignant'. Such nodules can be monitored with imaging, and are at increased likelihood of undergoing malignant transformation to hepatocellular carcinomas, although this process is not inevitable. The use of MRI with iron oxide is useful in characterizing nodules detected on ultrasound, and in identifying early malignant change. However, a nodule of 2 cm or more on ultrasound is almost certainly (over 90% chance) malignant and requires further staging.

Haemodynamics in cirrhosis

The rigid nature of the diseased liver also causes hemodynamic changes which can be demonstrated on colour and spectral Doppler. Portal venous flow may also be compromised, due to portal hypertension (see below), associated with numerous changes on ultrasound including reduced velocity, reversed flow, partial or total thrombosis. A compensatory increase in hepatic arterial flow to the liver may also be seen as a result of portal venous compromise in portal hypertension.

The normally triphasic hepatic venous waveform become flattened and monophasic due to increased hepatic resistance. This is a non-specific sign that occurs with numerous types of chronic liver disease or any condition, either intra- or extrahepatic, which compresses the venous flow, such as polycystic liver disease or the presence of ascites.[23] Its significance to the sonographer is that the monophasic hepatofugal flow may be mistaken for reversed portal venous flow if the operator is unaware.

HCC in cirrhosis

Patients with cirrhosis are at increased risk of developing hepatocellular carcinoma, the detection of

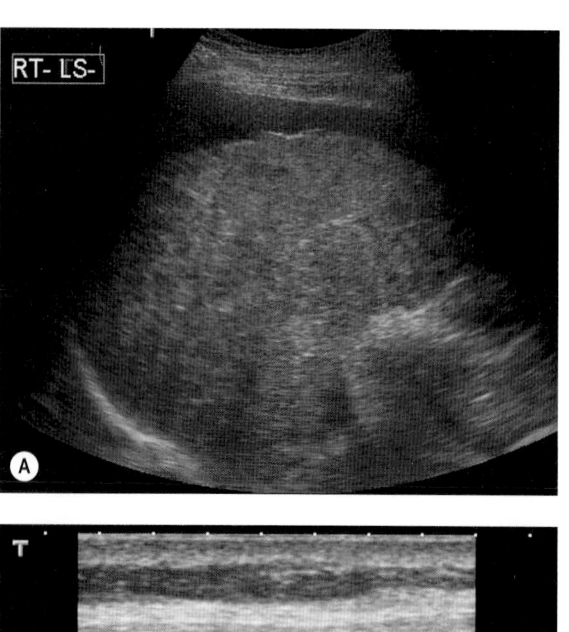

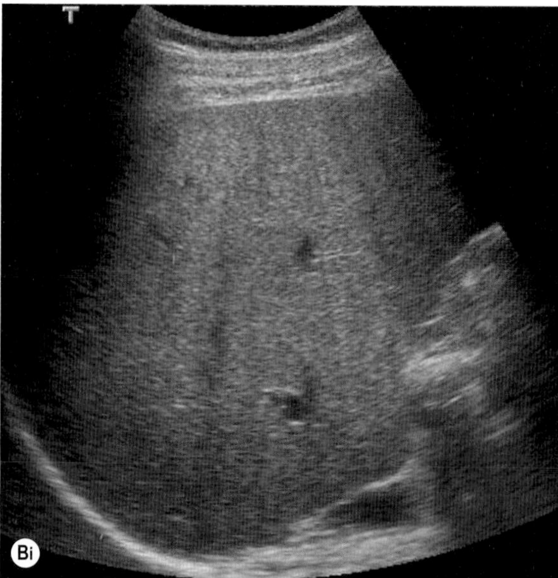

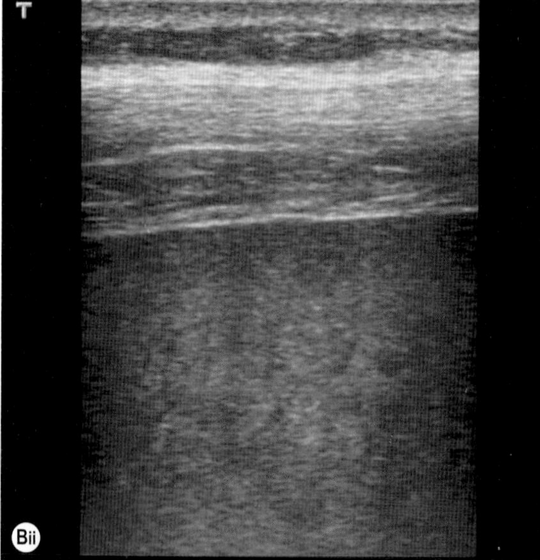

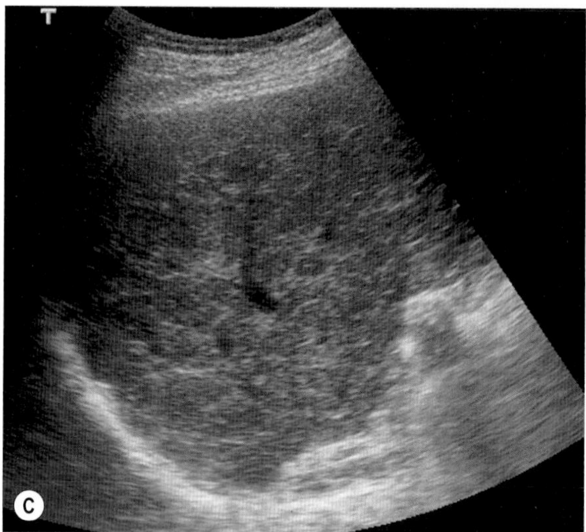

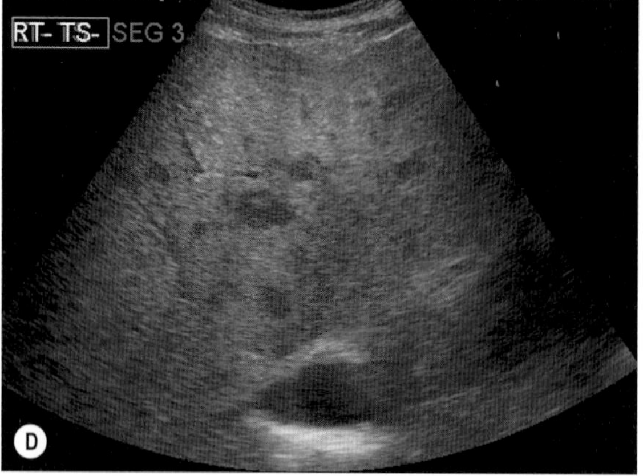

Fig. 4.20 • (A) Micronodular cirrhosis in a patient with alcoholic liver disease. Ascites outlines the lobular anterior liver surface. (Bi) Micronodular cirrhosis in hepatitis C virus. (Bii) The nodular nature of the liver is better appreciated with a high frequency probe. (C) Macronodular cirrhosis in a patient with primary biliary cirrhosis (PBC). Cirrhotic nodules are demonstrated throughout the peripheral hepatic substance with a lobulated liver outline. (D) Multiple dysplastic nodules in a patient with cirrhosis, confirmed at MRI. (The differential diagnosis would be multifocal HCC.)

which may be particularly difficult in an already nodular liver. As there are treatment options for patients with cirrhosis and HCC, some of which are curative if the malignancy is small, many institutions opt to screen cirrhotic patients with annual or 6-monthly AFP and ultrasound.[24] This remains controversial, being more cost-effective in patients with hepatitis B cirrhosis than other causes of cirrhosis, and demonstrating a doubtful overall cost effectiveness in patients with normal levels of AFP.[25] Both CT and ultrasound have a low sensitivity for detecting small focal lesions in cirrhotic livers,[17] which continue to present a diagnostic challenge, although improvements in ultrasound imaging have enabled operators to identify smaller and more subtle nodules than previously possible. The use of ultrasound contrast agents may give a characteristic pattern, confirming HCC[26] (Fig. 4.18) but HCCs can be atypical, and the technique is less useful with subcentimetre lesions, such as dysplastic nodules. MRI using iron oxide is useful in characterizing small nodules and in detecting additional, small HCCs not identified on ultrasound.[27,28]

Aetiology

Cirrhosis has numerous aetiologies:

Hepatitis

Hepatitis B (HBV) and C (HCV) viruses are infections with a worldwide distribution. Transmission of infection is by exposure to bodily fluids, unsafe injection practices, blood transfusions and mother to child infection amongst other causes. Around 25% of cases will result in severe liver damage (depending on the age at diagnosis) and death from cirrhosis and/or HCC, pose a massive health problem.

It is estimated that 3% of the world's population is now infected with HCV,[29] which is now a leading factor in the development of HCC.[30]

Alcoholic cirrhosis

The spectrum of alcoholic liver disease may take three forms; steatosis (alcoholic fatty liver), alcoholic hepatitis (often preceding cirrhosis) and finally cirrhosis. The incidence of death from alcoholic cirrhosis continues to climb in the UK.

Alcoholic liver disease may be halted or reversed in the early stages in patients who discontinue alcohol intake, with subsequent nodular regeneration of hepatic tissue (Fig. 4.20D).

PBC

PBC is an autoimmune, progressive cholestatic liver disease which presents predominantly in middle-aged females. The term 'cirrhosis' may be rather misleading for the early stages of this condition, which actually take the form of an inflammatory destruction of the intrahepatic bile ducts. These early stages of cholangitis are not, strictly speaking, cirrhotic. However as the destruction progresses, bands of fibrosis form in a process of macronodular cirrhosis (Fig. 4.20C).

Treatment of PBC involves control of the associated symptoms of portal hypertension and pruritis, but its progression is inevitable. Liver transplantation now offers a successful therapeutic option for these patients, with a 70% survival at 7 years.[31] Although the liver frequently looks normal on ultrasound in the early stages of the disease, lymphadenopathy can be demonstrated in up to 80% of PBC patients.[32]

Secondary biliary cirrhosis

Occurs as a result of chronic biliary obstruction. Causes usually include benign strictures or chronic stone impaction in the CBD causing progressive, gradual obstruction over a period of time. This causes ascending cholangitis and jaundice. The bile ducts may appear only mildly dilated on ultrasound. It is also a recognized sequel of biliary atresia in children.

Other causes

Cirrhosis may be drug-induced, particularly in patients on long term treatment or therapy, and may also result from prolonged exposure to some environmental toxins, and to parasitic infections. It is associated with many other diseases, such as cystic fibrosis, human immunodeficiency virus (HIV), diabetes, ulcerative colitis, rheumatoid arthritis, NASH, Budd–Chiari disease, primary sclerosing cholangitis (PSC) or any long-term conditions, acquired or congenital, which can affect the liver.

Congenital forms of cirrhosis exist due to metabolic disorders: Wilson's disease (deposition of copper in the liver and kidneys), glycogen storage disease (inability to break down glycogen to glucose), haemochromatosis (deposition of iron in the liver and pancreas) and others. Liver congestion from heart failure can also lead to cirrhosis in severe, prolonged cases. Up to 10% of patients have cirrhosis from no recognizable cause. This is termed cryptogenic cirrhosis (Table 4.4).

Clinical features and management

Clinical presentation depends upon the aetiology, and may involve either chronic symptoms or an acute episode. Pruritus, fatigue and jaundice, with steatorrhoea and deranged LFTs (raised alkaline phosphatase and serum bilirubin in PBC, raised ALT and AST in alcoholic disease) are generally present by the later stages. This is followed by the symptoms of portal hypertension (see below)

Normal	May appear normal, particularly in the early stages
Parenchyma	
• Changes in texture	Coarse texture (micronodular)
• Changes in reflectivity	Irregular nodular appearance (macronodular)
• Changes in size and outline	Fibrosis increases the overall echogenicity (but *not* the attenuation)
• Focal lesions	May be accompanied by fatty change, which increases both echogenicity *and* attenuation giving a hyper-reflective near field with poor penetration to the posterior liver
	Small, shrunken liver
	Nodular, irregular surface outline
	Deep fissures
	Possible disproportionate hypertrophy of left or caudate lobes
	Increased incidence of HCC
	Regenerative or dysplastic nodules (low to high grade)
Vascular	Signs of portal hypertension:
	Changes in portal vein velocity and direction
	Thrombosis (occlusive or non-occlusive)
	Varices and collaterals
	Increased hepatic arterial flow
	Flattened, monophasic hepatic venous flow on spectral Doppler (a non-specific finding)
Other signs	Ascites
	Splenomegaly
	Lymphadenopathy

Table 4.4 Summary of possible ultrasound appearances in cirrhosis

which is a poor prognostic feature associated with late-stage cirrhosis.

The process may be reversed in alcoholics who stop drinking. However, the prognosis of any cirrhotic condition is poor if malignancy is present. In severe cases, the management revolves around palliating the symptoms of portal hypertension, as bleeding from varices is a major cause of morbidity and mortality.

The degree of fibrosis and severity of cirrhosis is currently usually established histologically by biopsy. This is an invasive technique with the potential for serious complications, however these are minimized if the needle is guided into the liver under ultrasound control (see Chapter 11). *Elastography* is currently being investigated as a possible non-invasive alternative to biopsy.[33] This technique transmits ultrasonic vibrations into the liver in order to measure its 'stiffness'. The principle is that the more fibrotic the tissue, the stiffer it is, and the faster the vibration is transmitted.

Patients with cirrhosis are frequently monitored using 6-monthly ultrasound and AFP in an attempt to diagnose HCC as early as possible. Liver transplant is now an established and highly successful treatment option for cirrhosis when the symptoms can no longer be controlled with drugs, and may be considered curative in some patients. Although the success of transplant is reduced in patients with malignancy, the presence of a modest burden of HCC is no longer a contraindication to transplant.[34] However, patients waiting for suitable transplant organs may have disease which progresses, making them unsuitable for transplantation when the opportunity occurs. Palliative measures such as percutaneous ablation or surgical resection can be employed to contain the effects of malignancy in a patient otherwise suitable for transplantation. Chemoembolization may be of benefit to some patients with HCC and reasonably good liver function. In patients with advanced disease palliation of symptoms, such as sclerotherapy of varices, ascitic drainage or transjugular intrahepatic portosystemic shunt (TIPSS), may improve the quality of life.

PORTAL HYPERTENSION

Portal hypertension occurs when the pressure in the portal venous system is raised. This may happen as a result of chronic liver disease – particularly in the cirrhotic stage – when the nodular and fibrosed nature of the parenchyma impedes the flow of blood into the liver. It is significant because it causes numerous deleterious effects on the patient, many of which can be recognized on ultrasound (Table 4.4).

Raised portal venous pressure is associated with several complications. These are discussed below.

Portal vein signs

Portal vein flow is influenced by numerous factors, including prandial state, patient position, exercise and cardiac output.[35] Its velocity varies considerably in both cirrhotic and healthy subjects, and it is essential to use colour and spectral Doppler to properly investigate the portal flow.[36] The vein may appear dilated and tortuous, but not invariably. Portal venous flow may be:

- *Normal* in direction (hepatopetal) and velocity.[37]
- *Reduced in velocity*[38] (Fig. 4.21A), <10 cm/s, although there is overlap with the normal range.
- *Damped*, in which there is a lack of normal respiratory variation of both the calibre and the waveform of the splenic and portal veins. The normal spectrum has a 'wavy' characteristic, which may be lost.
- *Reversed* (hepatofugal) (Fig. 4.21B). This indicates serious liver disease. Interestingly, patients with hepatofugal PV flow are much less likely to suffer from bleeding varices, suggesting a type of 'protective' mechanism here.
- *'Balanced'* in which both forward and reverse low velocity flow is present – a condition which may precede imminent thrombosis or reversal (Fig. 4.21C).
- *Thrombosed* (Fig. 4.21D–F). Low level echoes from the thrombus may be evident but with fresh thrombus the vein may appear anechoic, as in the normal vein. The absence of power Doppler flow, provided the settings are appropriate, is a much better indicator for thrombosis than the grey-scale image. Although PV thrombosis most commonly results from portal hypertension in cirrhosis, there are many other causes,

including inflammatory or malignant conditions which may surround, compress or invade the portal and/or splenic veins (Table 4.5). Thrombosis may be occlusive or non-occlusive, and may extend into the intrahepatic portal venous system. CEUS is useful in distinguishing a patent from a non-patent vein if technical difficulties limit the Doppler information (Fig. 4.21F).

- *Hepatopetal main PV flow with hepatofugal peripheral flow* may be a sign of HCC, requiring careful scanning to identify the lesion.
- *Cavernous transformation.* A network of collateral vessels may form around a

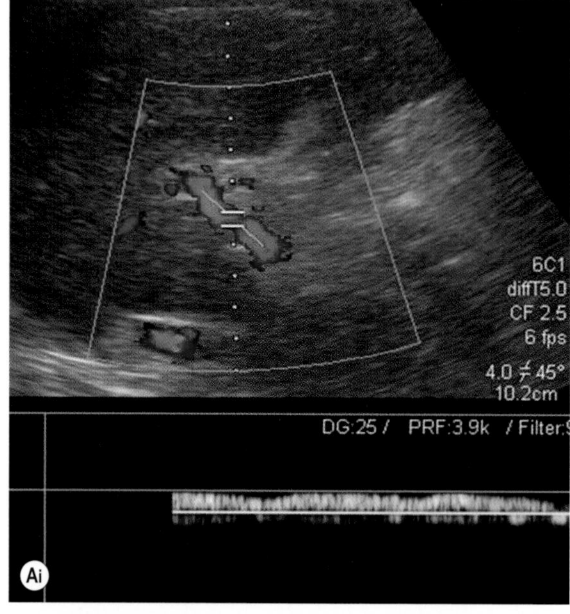

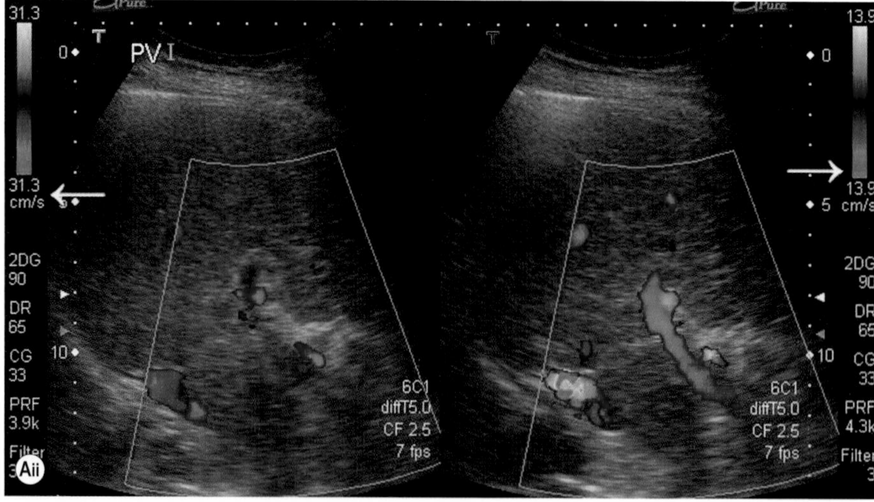

Fig. 4.21 • The MPV in portal hypertension: (Ai) PV velocity is greatly reduced, at 3 cm/s. A low PRF and increased colour gain may be necessary to demonstrate this. (Aii) The left image shows a false positive scan for PV thrombosis, as the PRF is high (arrow). The right hand image demonstrates flow in a patent vein once the PRF is reduced.

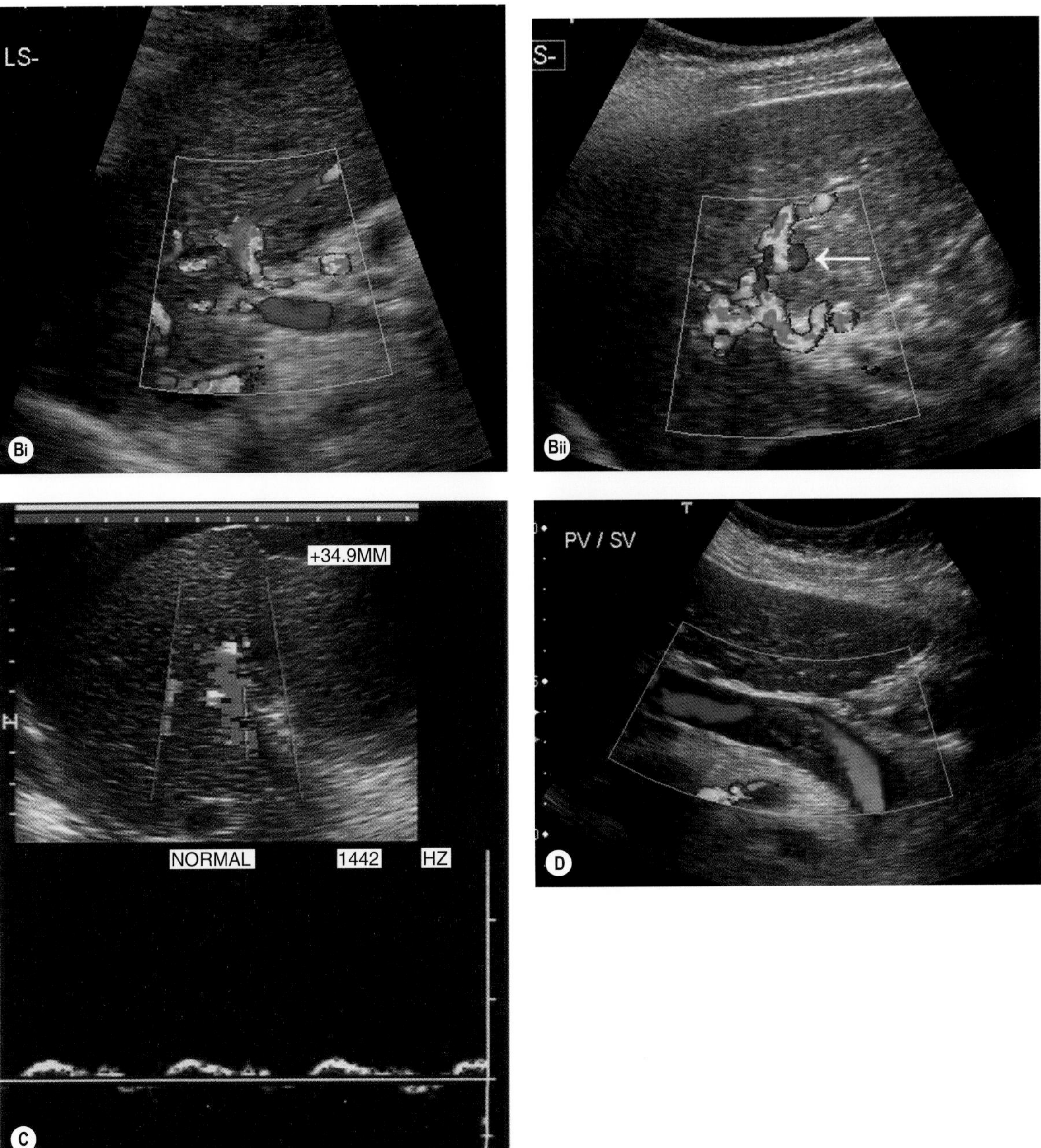

Fig. 4.21, cont'd • (Bi) Reversed PV flow in portal hypertension. (Bii) Compensatory, increased prominence of the hepatic arteries with reversed PV flow. The PRF is set to display the slow flow of the almost occluded PV (arrow) and so the high velocity arterial flow demonstrates 'aliasing'. (C) Balanced PV flow. Alternate forward and reverse low velocity flow on the Doppler spectrum. The PV colour Doppler alternates red and blue. (D) PV thrombosis. The PV is dilated and contains non-occlusive thrombus.

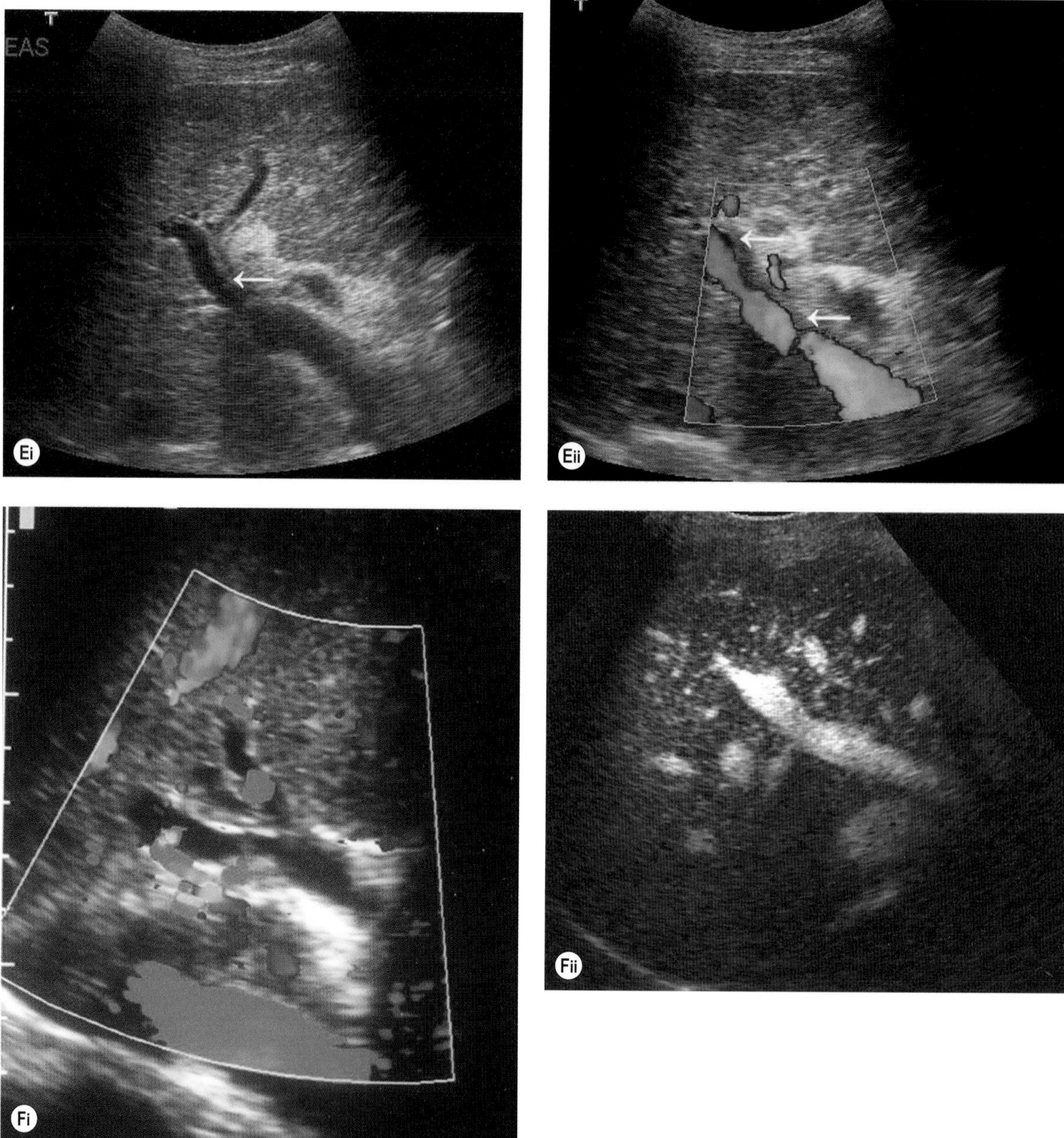

Fig. 4.21, cont'd • (Ei) The PV contains a rim of non-occlusive thrombus (arrow) on the anterior wall. (Eii) Colour flow Doppler demonstrates a corresponding lack of flow. (F) CEUS may be useful in demonstrating low velocity flow in the technically difficult PV; (Fi) False positive for PV thrombosis, despite low PRF, due to an inadequate angle to display the Doppler shift. (Fii) Contrast demonstrates a patent PV.

thrombosed main portal vein at the porta, especially if the cause of thrombosis is due to extrahepatic causes (e.g. pancreatitis) rather than diseased liver. The appearance of cavernous transformation of the PV is quite striking (Fig. 4.22A) and colour Doppler is particularly useful in its diagnosis.[39] Varices at the porta may be the cause of a false negative ultrasound in the hunt for thrombosis (see below).

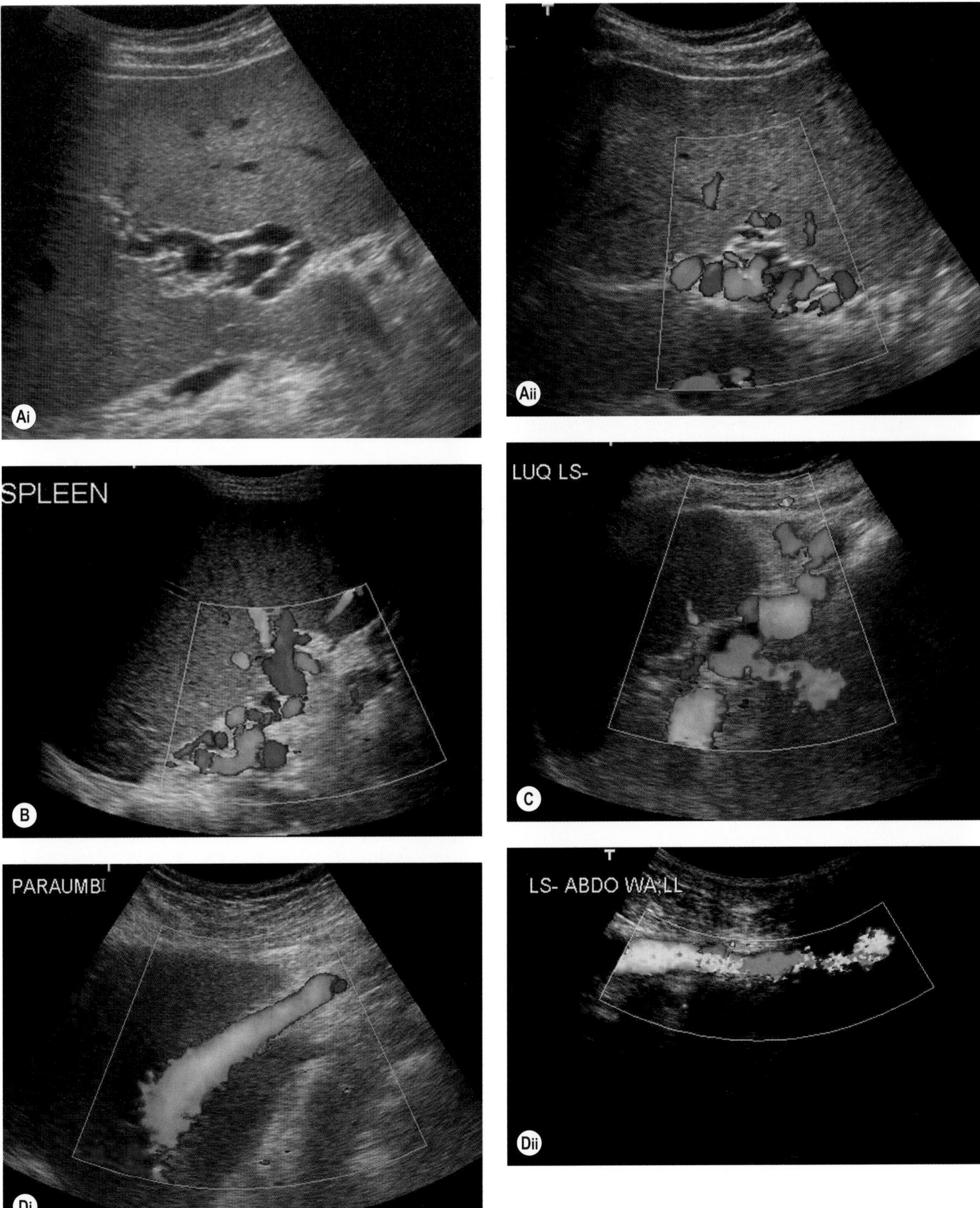

Fig. 4.22 • Portal hypertension – further signs: (A) Cavernous transformation of the PV (Ai, ii). (B) Varices are demonstrated along the inferior border of the spleen. (C) Colour Doppler demonstrates the tortuous vascular channel of a splenorenal shunt inferior to the spleen. (Di) Patent para-umbilical channel running along the ligamentum teres to the anterior abdominal wall in a patient with end-stage chronic liver disease and portal hypertension. (Dii) the vein is seen continuing inferiorly along the anterior abdominal wall.

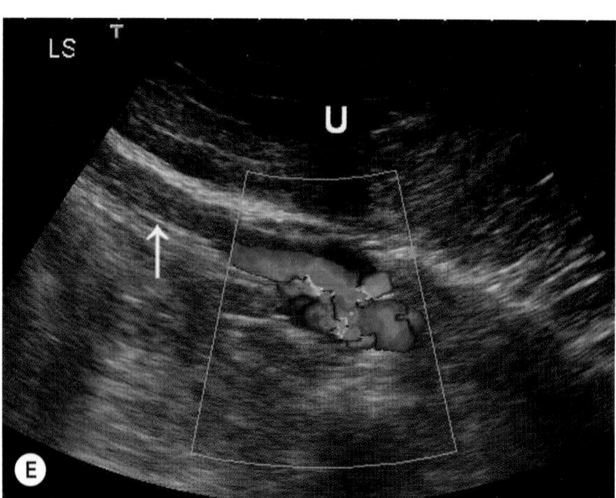

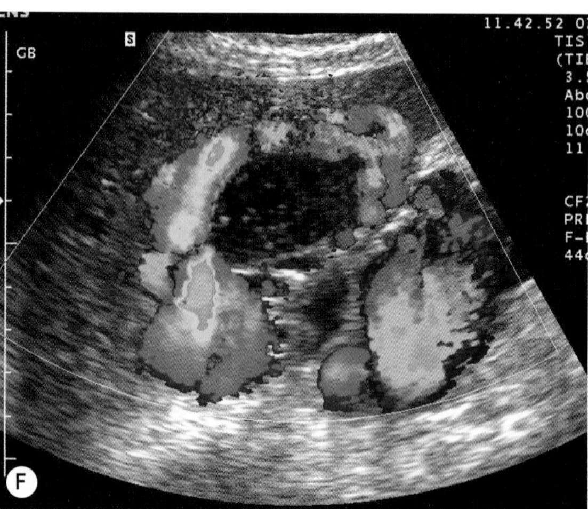

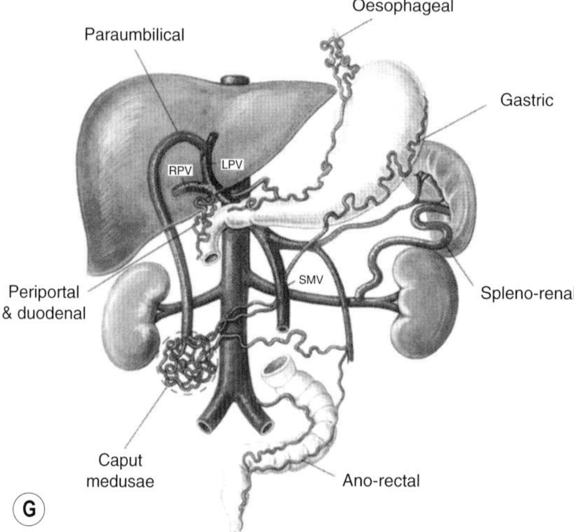

Fig. 4.22, cont'd • (E) A paraumbilical vein (arrow) culminates in a small caput medusae just beneath the umbilicus (U). (F) Varices can be seen around the gallbladder wall in a case of hepatic fibrosis with portal hypertension. (G) Collaterals in portal hypertension.

Chronic liver disease	Especially when cirrhosis is present
Inflammatory	Pancreatitis; acute cholecystitis; necrotizing enterocolitis
Malignancy	Pancreatic tumour; gastric tumour
Coagulation disorders	May be associated with Budd–Chiari syndrome

Table 4.5 Causes of portal vein thrombosis

Technique is important in the diagnosis of portal vein thrombosis. False positive results – when the patent vein is incorrectly diagnosed as thrombosed – usually result from inadequate technique. The vein axis must be less than 60° to the transducer; an intercostal approach from the right lateral aspect is frequently most successful for this. Doppler sensitivity must be set to pick up low velocity flow (a low scale, or PRF) and have the colour gain correctly set. Ultrasound contrast is useful in identifying slow flow in a vessel which is technically difficult to scan. Contrast angiography with arterioportography is considered the gold standard for assessing portal vein patency, but this technique is time-consuming and invasive and has similar results to carefully performed ultrasound.[40]

False negative results – indicating that flow is present in a vein which is actually thrombosed – are due to the detection of flow within a collateral vessel at the porta, which can be mistaken for the main portal vein.

- Ascites – a transudate from the serosal surfaces of the gut, peritoneum and liver. Small traces of ascites may be missed if the correct technique, including focal zone placement, is not employed.
- Splenomegaly – the result of back-pressure in the portal and splenic veins. The spleen can enlarge to six times its normal size, and extends both inferiorly and medially, making accurate measurement difficult.
- Varices – (Fig. 4.22), i.e. venous anastomoses from the high pressure portal system to the lower pressure systemic circulation, which shunts the blood away from the portal system. These vessels have thinner walls than normal vessels, which makes them prone to bleeding.

The common sites are:

- Gastric and lower oesophagus: oesophageal varices are particularly prone to bleeding and this is often the patient's presenting symptom. They are difficult to see on abdominal ultrasound because of overlying stomach and are better demonstrated with endoscopic techniques. Left coronal scans may demonstrate tortuous vessels at the medial aspect of the upper pole of the spleen.
- Splenorenal: an anastomosis between the splenic and left renal veins which is often seen on ultrasound as a large, tortuous vessel at the lower edge of the spleen (Fig. 4.22B, C). (These anastomoses are usually very efficient at redirecting the blood from the portal system and so these patients have a lower incidence of gastric varices and therefore a better prognosis.)
- Peraumbilical: a substantial vessel can often be seen in the liver lying in the ligamentum teres (Fig. 4.22D, E), and running down the anterior abdominal wall to a knot of vessels at the umbilicus – the so-called 'caput medusae'. (A patent para-umbilical channel of diameter 1–2 mm may occasionally be seen in normal patients.)
- Porta hepatis: varices around the main portal vein itself, especially if the latter is thrombosed (see below).
- Gallbladder wall: rarely, varices form around the gallbladder wall to bypass the main portal vein and feed into the intrahepatic portal branches (Fig. 4.22F).
- Coronary vein: a vessel may be seen arising from the portal vein near the SMV, directing blood in a cephalic direction. (Occasionally seen in normal patients.)

The extent of portosystemic collaterals is usually underestimated on ultrasound. However, a systematic approach which investigates all the possible sites can demonstrate up to 90% of collaterals[37,41] (Fig. 4.22G).

The hepatic artery may be another ultrasound clue to compromised portal venous flow. The main hepatic artery may demonstrate increased flow velocity, especially if the portal vein is thrombosed. This is a compensatory mechanism to maintain the blood flow to the liver. The main hepatic artery may appear enlarged and more 'obvious' than usual on ultrasound, and peripheral intrahepatic arterial flow (not readily demonstrated in a normal subject) may also become obvious (Fig. 4.23).

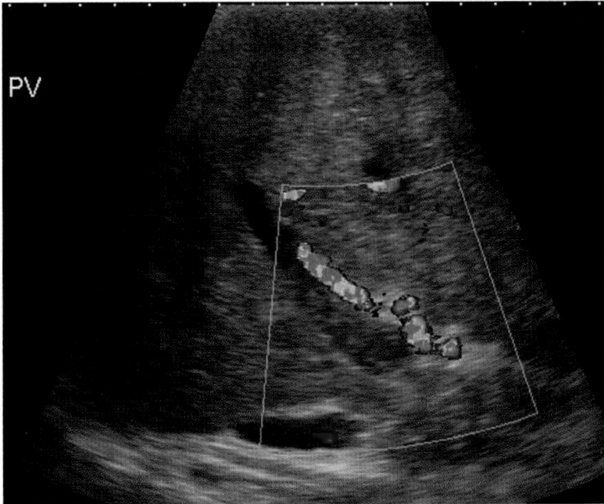

Fig. 4.23 • A thrombosed PV. High velocity compensatory arterial flow is seen anterior to the PV.

Management

The most pressing problem is often bleeding from varices, especially oesophageal varices, and patients may present with melaena or haematemesis. Management may involve medical means, endoscopic techniques (either injection sclerotherapy of oesophageal varices or 'banding' in which a ring is placed around the base of the varix causing thrombosis) compression using a Sengstaken tube with an inflated balloon, surgical or the placement of a percutaneous TIPSS (Transjugular Intrahepatic Portosystemic Shunt). All these methods are relatively temporary, and can relieve pressure in the portal venous system, controlling portal hypertensive complications in order to plan further management.

TIPSS is a percutaneous radiological intervention used to relieve the symptoms of portal hypertension including bleeding varices and refractory ascites.[42] It connects the portal vein to the (usually) right hepatic vein with an expandable metal shunt. A catheter and guide wire are passed, under X-ray control, through the jugular vein to the IVC and into the hepatic vein. A pathway is then forged with a needle through the liver parenchyma to join the portal vein with the insertion of a shunt to keep the channel open. Portal venous blood then effectively bypasses the liver, flowing straight into the hepatic vein.

Ultrasound may be used to monitor stent patency (Fig. 4.24). Shunt stenosis or occlusion is a common problem, particularly in long-term shunts, which can be detected with routine post-procedure ultrasound screening and treated with reintervention. The most common site for a stenosis is at the junction of the stent with the portal vein. The velocity of blood flow in the shunt should be between 1 m/s and 2 m/s and this should be consistent, throughout the stent. A variety of Doppler parameters can be used to detect the malfunction of the shunt. A shunt velocity of less than 50 cm/s is a sign of stenosis,[43] but this has not been reproducible in all institutions, and other factors such as a change of 50 cm/s or more from the baseline scan, a localized elevation of velocity at the stenotic site (with an upper limit of normal of up to 220 cm/s) or an increase in the velocity gradient (as the stenotic stent exhibits an increased maximum velocity and a decreased minimum velocity) are also poor prognostic signs.[44]

TIPSS is regarded as a temporary measure but can considerably improve the patient's condition pending treatment of chronic liver disease – relieving haemorrhage from varices, relieving intractable ascites and stabilizing liver function. Although the technique is highly successful in decompressing the portal circulation, it is associated with subsequent stent dysfunction and portosystemic encephalopathy. Results from stents covered with polytetrafluoroethylene, however, have shown improvements which will probably lead to an increased use of these shunts. It is increasingly used as a bridge to a liver transplant and is also used as an alternative to surgery in patients who are poor surgical risks although the diversion of blood away from the liver can result in adversely affected liver function and eventual encephalopathy.[45]

HEPATITIS

Viral hepatitis

Acute viral hepatitis may be caused by one of several viruses – A, B, C, D or E. The viruses which cause hepatitis B, C and D may also go on to chronic disease and predispose the liver to HCC in the later stages. Vaccines exist only for A and B.

Hepatitis A and E are transmitted via contaminated food or drink and are particularly prevalent in third world countries. Hepatitis B, C and D are likely to be transmitted through transfusion or sexual contact. Hepatitis C is now a particular threat to the world population, with an incidence of up to 170 million people worldwide, and rising,[46] representing a potential major problem for world health resources in the future. This epidemic is the result of numerous factors including use of infected (unscreened) blood products, high-risk sexual activity and skin penetration through injected drug use, body piercing, etc. Infection with HCV virus usually goes unnoticed until symptoms occur some years later. This time lag provides potential opportunity for infection of further individuals in the meantime, and contributes to uncertainty over the actual infection rate worldwide. It may take up to 20 years for patients to develop cirrhosis, and up to 30 years for the formation of HCC.[47]

Fulminant hepatitis, in which there is complete liver failure, is a rare complication of acute hepatitis B. Most patients with acute hepatitis recover completely, but hepatitis B, C and D may go on to develop *chronic hepatitis*. This has two forms:

- *Chronic persistent hepatitis* is a mild form of inflammation limited to the portal tracts. It is usually of comparatively little clinical significance and does not show ultrasound changes.
- *Chronic active hepatitis* is a more serious and aggressive form of the disease which causes diffuse, persistent inflammation. This may

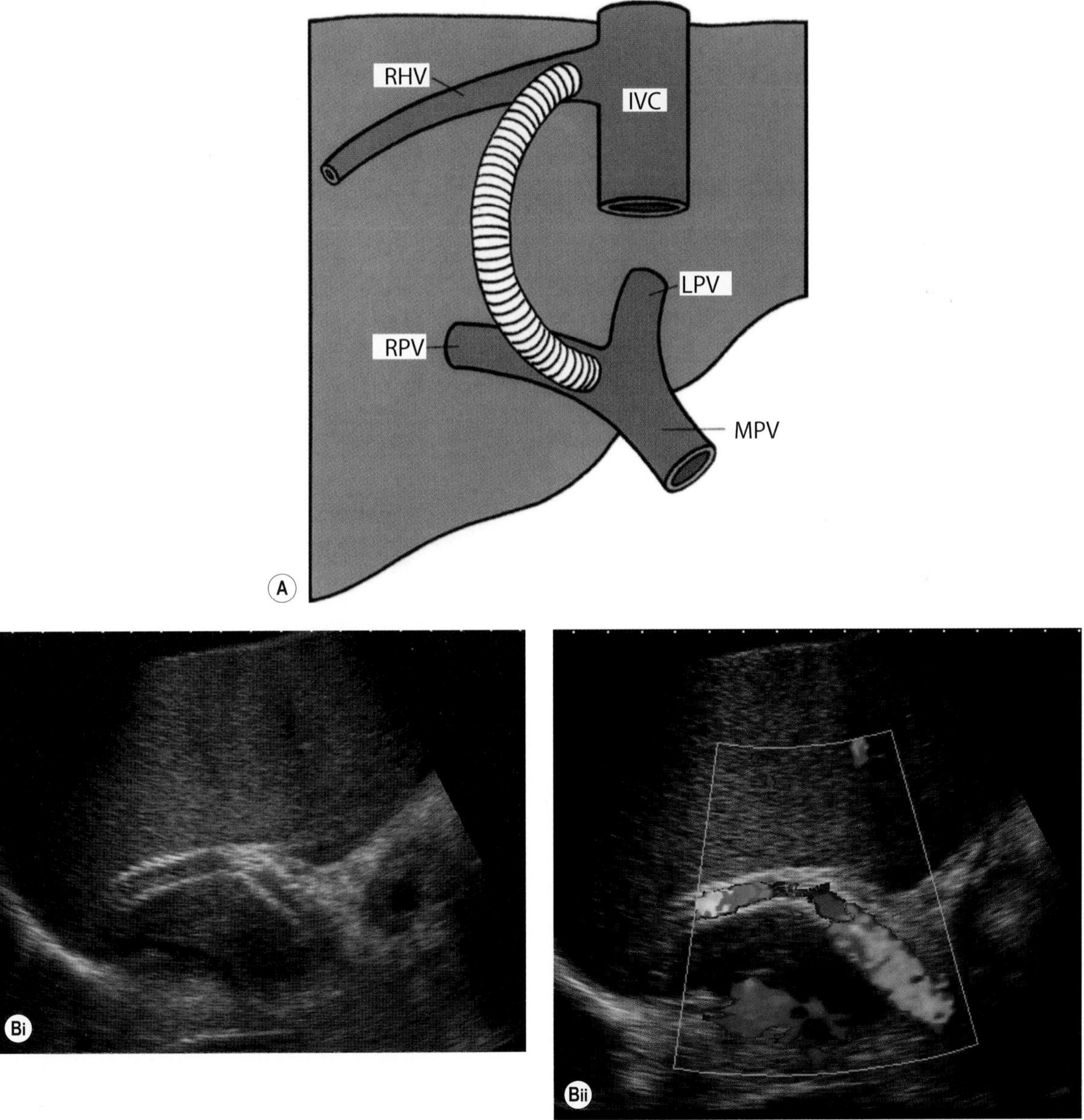

Fig. 4.24 • (A) TIPSS. (Bi) TIPSS in a patient with severe portal hypertension. (Bii) Colour Doppler demonstrates its patency, with a higher velocity in the hepatic venous end.

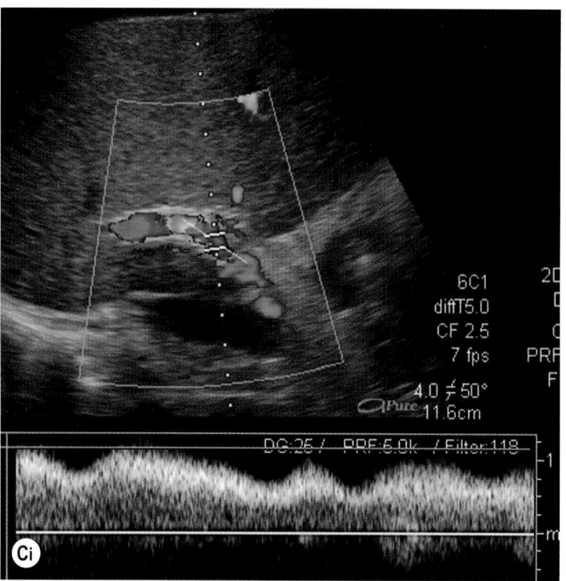

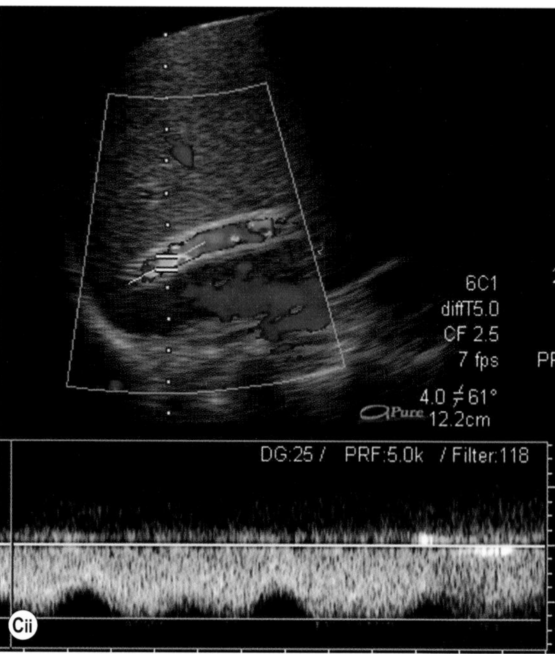

Fig. 4.24, cont'd • (C) Flow is in the correct direction with the velocity measured at the PV end (Ci) and the hepatic venous end (Cii).

eventually lead to cirrhosis, which can be associated with HCC.

Other causes of acute hepatitis

Acute hepatitis may also occur with many other conditions. The most common of these are alcoholic hepatitis (see alcoholic cirrhosis, above), infectious mononucleosis, herpes virus and cytomegalovirus. Patients with AIDS and those who are immunosuppressed are also particularly prone to hepatitis.

Clinical features

It may be asymptomatic (patients who have antibodies present, but who deny having had the disease, must have had subclinical disease at one time). Other signs include lethargy, nausea, vomiting and jaundice. The liver is enlarged and tender in the acute phase. In many cases, particularly HBV and HCV there is a considerable time lag, often of years, before symptoms and diagnosis.

The presence of hepatitis can be detected from blood tests, but the degree of liver damage must be made histologically, ideally with an ultrasound-guided biopsy.

Ultrasound appearances

The liver frequently appears normal on ultrasound. In the acute stage, if ultrasound changes are present, the liver is slightly enlarged with a diffusely hypoechoic parenchyma. The normally reflective portal tracts are accentuated in contrast (Fig. 4.25A). This 'dark liver' appearance is non-specific, and may also occur in leukaemia, cardiac failure, AIDS and other conditions.

The inflammation may start at the portal tracts working outwards into the surrounding parenchyma – so-called periportal hepatitis. In such cases, the portal tracts become less well-defined and hyperechoic. The gallbladder wall may also be thickened, and some patients demonstrate portal lymphadenopathy. If the disease progresses to the chronic stage, the liver may reduce in size, becoming nodular and coarse in appearance (Fig. 4.25).

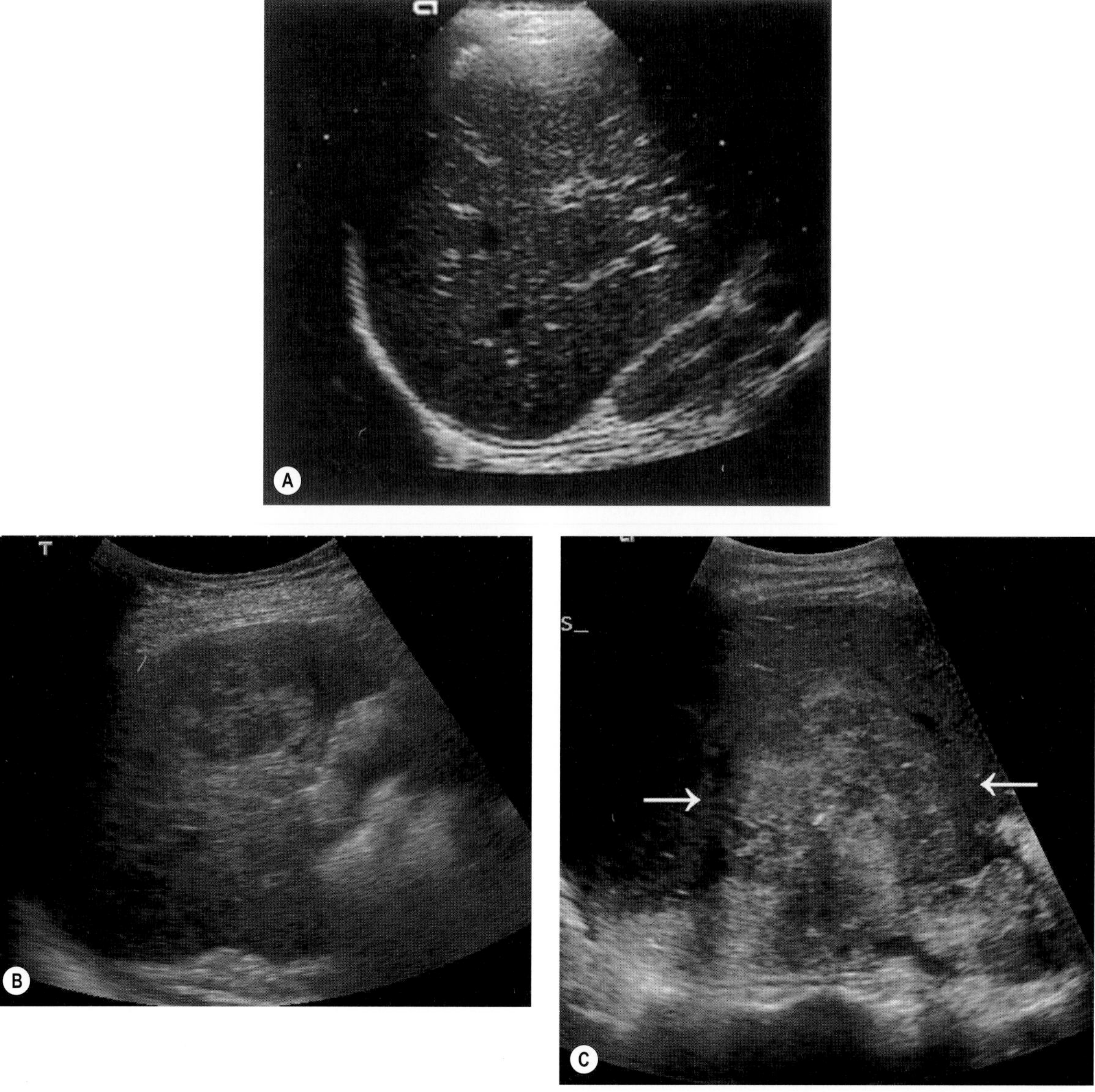

Fig. 4.25 • (A) Subtle changes of oedema in acute hepatitis; the liver is hypoechoic compared with the RK, mildly enlarged and has prominent portal tracts. (B) Chronic hepatitis with cirrhosis, demonstrating a coarse-textured, nodular liver with a large HCC, later confirmed on MRI. (C) Cirrhosis from hepatitis C, with a large, invasive HCC (arrows).

PRIMARY SCLEROSING CHOLANGITIS

This is a primary disease of the biliary ducts, most frequently found in young men. Like PBC, it is a cholestatic disease. It is discussed more fully in Chapter 3, but is included here for reference as it may often result in a coarse liver texture, similar to that seen in some forms of cirrhosis, and is associated with the formation of cholangiocarcinomas.

BUDD–CHIARI SYNDROME

Budd–Chiari is a relatively rare syndrome associated with partial or complete occlusion of the hepatic veins. There are numerous causes of hepatic vein occlusion, of which the main ones are:

- Congenital or acquired coagulation disorders, which may affect both the hepatic and portal veins, such as polycythaemia or myeloproliferative disorder
- Malignancy – primary or secondary liver tumour may invade the hepatic veins or may travel up the IVC (e.g. renal carcinoma) to occlude the hepatic vein confluence.
- Membranous web obstructing the IVC (surgically removable)
- Chronic infection or inflammatory diseases.

Ultrasound appearances

In the acute stage, the liver may enlarge. As the condition progresses, compensatory hypertrophy of any 'spared' segments occurs – usually the caudate lobe, because the venous drainage from here is inferior to the main hepatic veins. The hepatic veins may be difficult or impossible to visualize (Fig. 4.26). Dilated serpiginous collateral veins may form to direct blood away from the liver, and in some cases the portal venous flow reverses to achieve this. The spleen also progressively enlarges and, if the disease is long-standing, the liver becomes cirrhotic, acquiring a coarse texture.

Ascites may also be present, particularly if there is complete obstruction involving the IVC. The cause of IVC obstruction may be a web, which can occasionally be identified on ultrasound. If the cause is a coagulation disorder, the portal venous system may also be affected by thrombosis, causing portal hypertension.

Doppler is particularly helpful in diagnosing Budd–Chiari syndrome.[38] The hepatic veins and IVC may be totally or partially occluded; if partial, the waveforms may become flattened, losing their characteristic triphasic pattern. In some cases flow may be reversed in the IVC hepatic and/or portal veins and the presence of collateral vessels in the liver is another useful indicator on ultrasound.[48] Ultrasound may miss partial HV occlusion, but the use of contrast agents in suspected cases of Budd–Chiari syndrome may improve diagnostic accuracy.

Management

This depends upon the cause and severity of symptoms. Both medical and surgical treatments have mixed success. Severe coagulative disorders resulting in decompensated cirrhosis may have to be transplanted although there is a significant risk of recurrence. If the cause is an IVC web, this may be surgically removed. In some patients, palliative treatment with percutaneous stent placement in the hepatic veins can relieve the symptoms of ascites and varices.[49]

CYSTIC FIBROSIS

Cystic fibrosis, one of the most common chromosomal abnormalities, has historically been associated with the paediatric population. However, increasing success in the management of this condition, particularly in specialist centres, has improved the current median survival to 40 years for a child born in the 1990s.[50]

Ultrasound appearances

As the disease progresses into adulthood, signs of liver cirrhosis and portal hypertension may be demonstrated on ultrasound, although disease progression in the adult population tends to take a milder course than in the paediatric population[51] (Fig. 4.27). The liver may be steatotic, and fibrotic changes produce a coarse, hyperechoic, appearance. Patients tend to be monitored regularly with ultrasound for disease progression and signs of portal hypertension. Splenomegaly, varices, ascites and possible portal vein thrombosis may be demonstrated (see above) although splenomegaly can be present without portal hypertension in this group. Changes of fibrosis can also be seen in the pancreas.

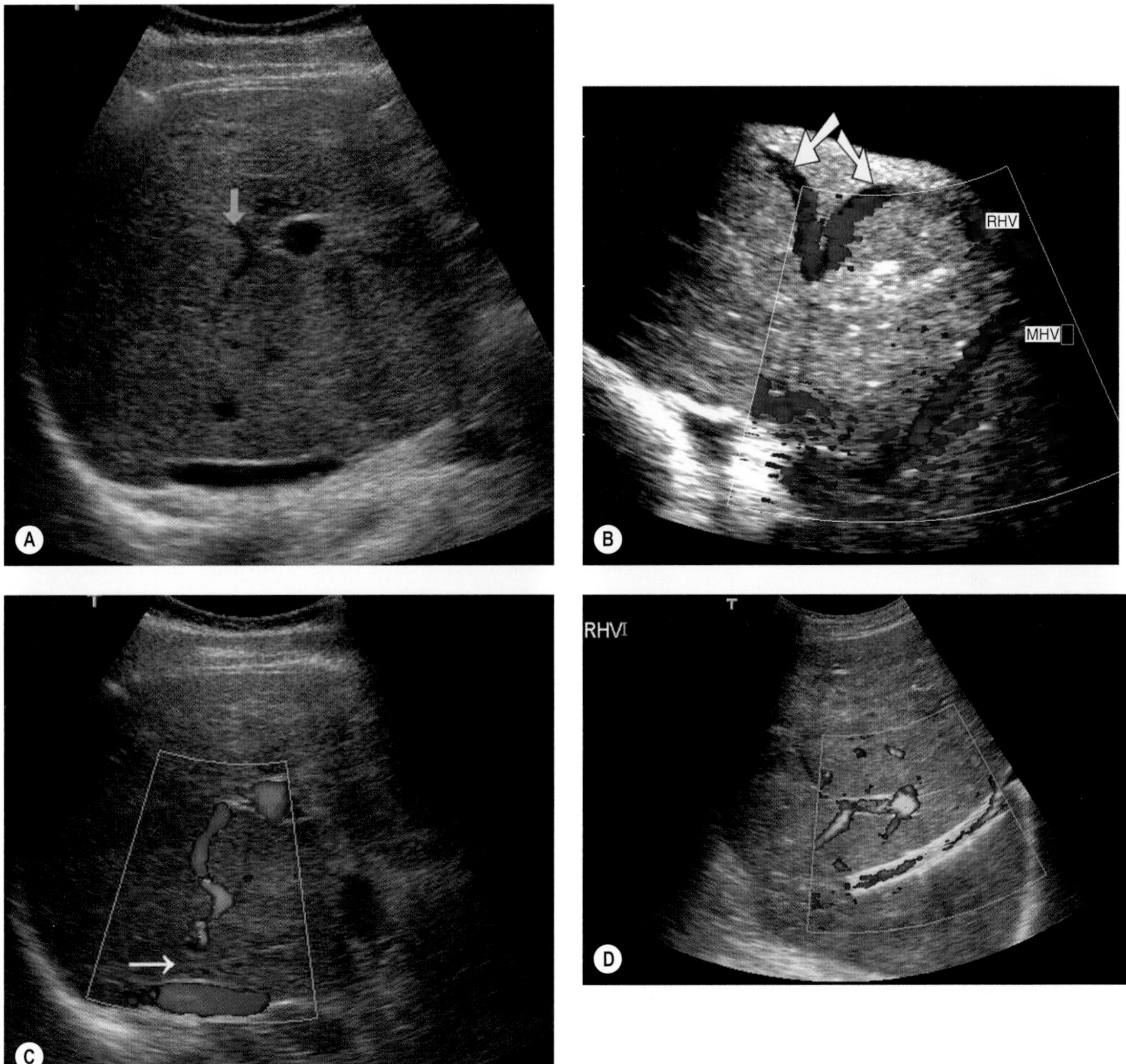

Fig. 4.26 • Budd–Chiari syndrome. (A) The MHV (arrow) is tortuous and strictured, and difficult to identify on ultrasound. (B) Large collaterals are seen (arrows) near the surface of the liver. (C) Thrombus, with lack of colour flow, in the proximal RHV (arrow). Collateral vessels are present around the HV. (D) A patent stent in the RHV restores flow and reduces ascites.

CONGESTIVE CARDIAC DISEASE

Patients with cardiac failure frequently demonstrate dilated hepatic veins in the liver, sometimes with a dilated IVC. Although this may give the sonographer the overall impression of hypoechogenicity, due to the proliferation of large, anechoic vessels, the liver texture itself tends to be of either normal echogenicity, or, in the later stages of failure, hyperechoic.

Mitral valve disease may be the cause of altered waveforms in the hepatic veins – the usual triphasic flow becomes more pronounced, with a highly pulsatile waveform (Fig. 4.28A). The portal venous waveform may sometimes be altered in cases of tricuspid valve regurgitation. The normally

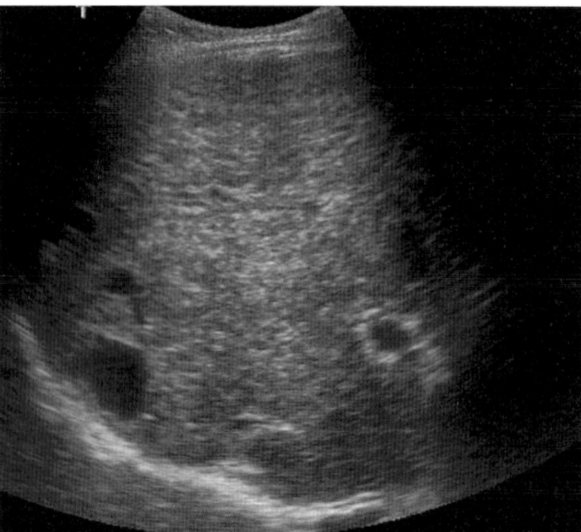

Fig. 4.27 • Marked changes in the liver of an adult patient with cystic fibrosis.

monophasic flow may become bi-directional (Fig. 4.28B). This phenomenon, associated with congestive heart failure, also occurs in cirrhosis prior to portal vein thrombosis. However, the latter 'balanced' flow is of very low velocity (Fig. 4.21C) while that due to tricuspid regurgitation is a higher velocity, more pulsatile waveform.

HIV

HIV is an increasing and significant health problem. Patients with HIV are frequently monitored with ultrasound, as they may display abdominal symptoms including fever and weight loss.A range of appearances may be present on ultrasound, including hepatomegaly and altered or coarse texture. Focal changes may occur in around 10% of HIV patients and these include lymphoma, sarcoma, tuberculous abscess and HCC. Chronic liver damage over time may result in cirrhosis with associated nodules.[52]

LIVER CONDITIONS IN PREGNANCY

Acute fatty liver

This rare condition occurs in the third trimester of pregnancy. Acute fatty deposition in the liver tissue

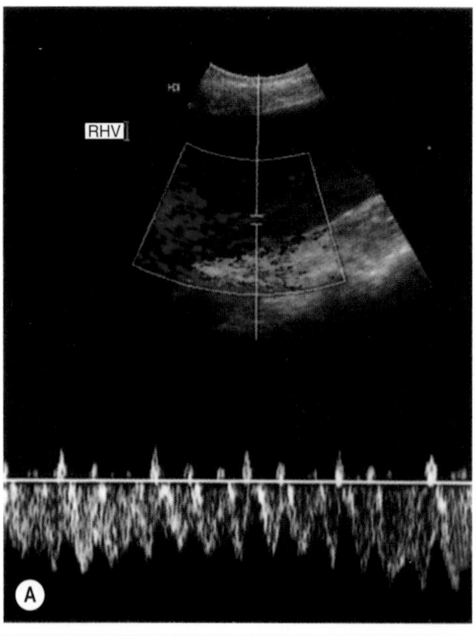

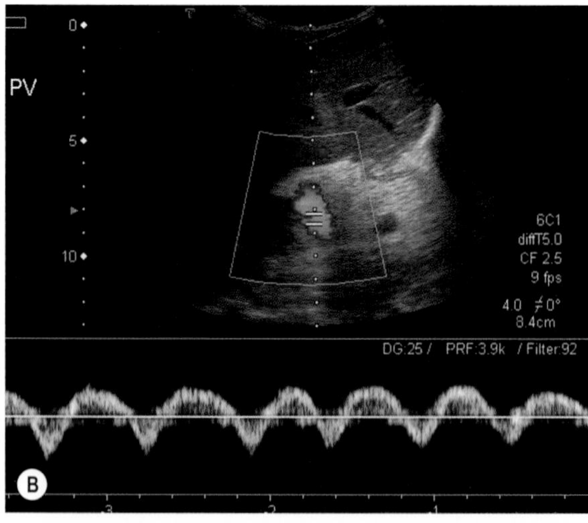

Fig. 4.28 • (A) The waveform of the hepatic vein in a patient with mitral valve disease demonstrates increased pulsatility. (B) The portal vein has an abnormal, highly pulsatile flow waveform in a patient with tricuspid regurgitation. (This is quite distinct from the low velocity 'balanced flow' of portal hypertension.)

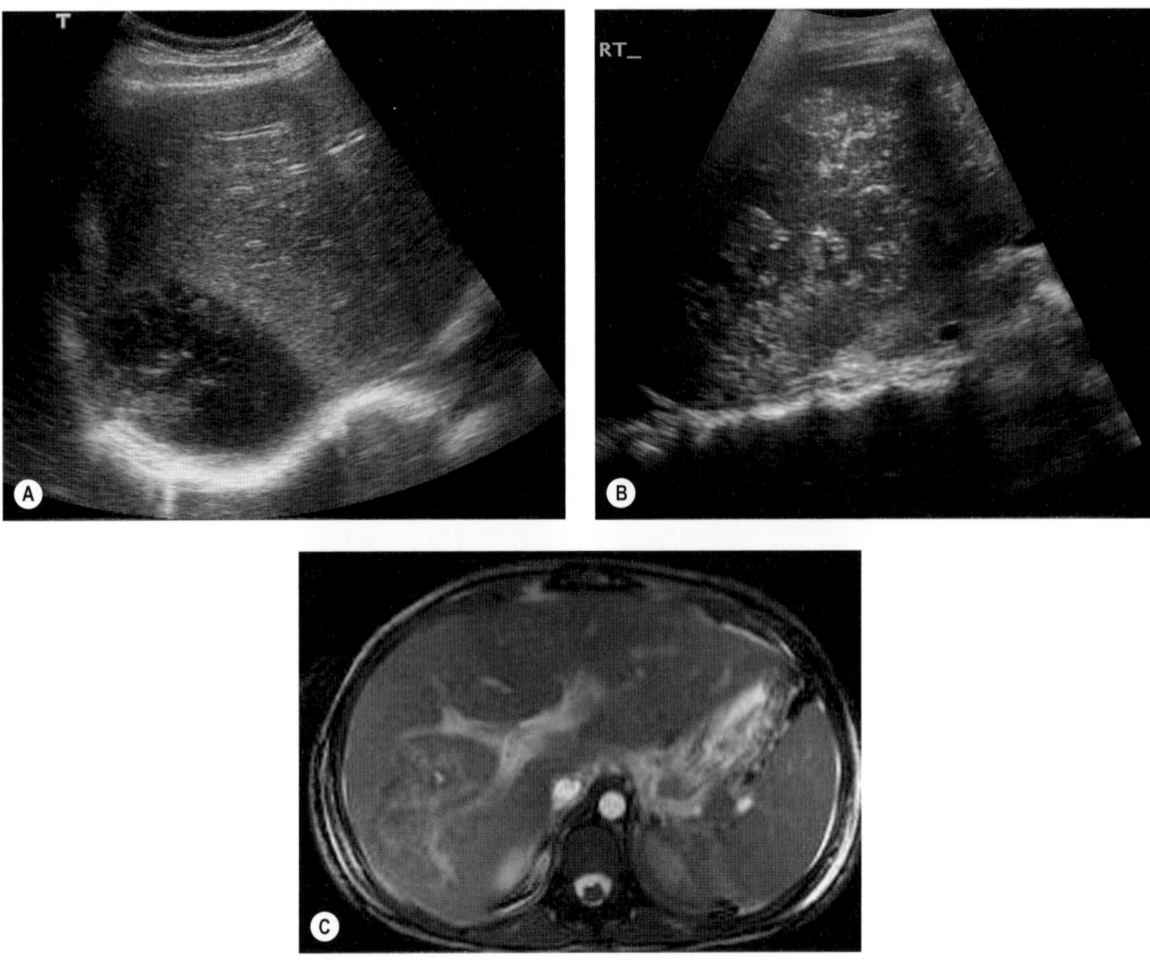

Fig. 4.29 • (A) Spontaneous subcapsular haematoma in pregnancy in a patient with HELLP syndrome. (B) Multiple areas of intrahepatic haemorrhage in HELLP. (C) MRI of the patient in (B).

can cause abdominal pain, vomiting and jaundice. The liver may appear sonographically normal or be diffusely hyperechoic, although focal areas of fatty deposition have also been reported. Acute fatty liver tends to resolve during the first month of the post-partum period, but may in rare cases progress to cause liver failure.

HELLP syndrome

HELLP syndrome is a rare complication of pregnancy occurring in up to 20% of mothers with severe pre-eclampsia.[53] Haemolytic anaemia (H), elevated liver enzymes (EL) and low platelet count (LP) cause abdominal pain, nausea and fever. Its complications may include multiple areas of spontaneous haemorrhage (either subcapsular haematoma or intraparenchymal bleeding), infarction or necrosis within the liver, which can be identified with ultrasound or MRI scanning (Fig. 4.29).

The recognition and prompt diagnosis of acute fatty liver and HELLP syndrome reduces maternal morbidity by enabling emergency caesarean section to be performed (Tables 4.6, 4.7).

Increased echogenicity	Fatty infiltration (also increases attenuation)
	Fibrosis
	Cirrhosis
	Chronic hepatitis
	Cystic Fibrosis
	HIV
Decreased echogenicity	Acute hepatitis
	AIDS or HIV
	Leukaemia
	Toxic Shock syndrome
	Can be normal, particularly in the young
Coarse or nodular texture	Cirrhosis – various aetiologies
	Regenerating nodules
	Metastases/diffuse metastatic infiltration
	Chronic or granulomatous hepatitis
	PSC, PBC
	Diffuse infective process – e.g. with AIDS or immunosuppressed patients

Table 4.6 Causes of changes in liver reflectivity

Organ failure	Chronic liver disease with portal hypertension
	Acute liver failure
	Renal failure
	Cardiac failure
Malignancy	
Inflammatory	Acute pancreatitis
	Acute cholecystitis
	Peritonitis, tuberculosis
	Crohn's disease
Budd–Chiari syndrome	
Post-operative	Blood, urine, bile or lymphatic fluid
Organ damage	Biliary perforation
	Urinary tract perforation
	Bowel perforation (e.g. in diverticulitis)
	Trauma to liver, spleen or pancreas
CAPD Fluid	Patients on peritoneal dialysis
Ruptured ectopic pregnancy	Haemoperitoneum
Gynaecological	Ruptured ovarian cyst, ovarian carcinoma, ovarian fibroma (Meig's syndrome), ovarian torsion, pelvic inflammatory disease

Table 4.7 Causes of free intraperitoneal fluid

LIVER TRANSPLANTS

Indications

Liver transplantation has now become an accepted treatment for patients with end-stage liver disease and it is also used in the treatment of fulminant hepatic failure. Improvements in both surgical techniques and immunosuppression have led to an increasing range of indications for transplantation (Table 4.8). The majority of hepatic transplants (80%) are still performed in patients with

Hepatitis C, hepatitis B	Transplantation is considered once irreversible end-stage liver failure is present, usually with complications such as portal hypertension and encephalopathy
Alcohol-related disease	
NASH	
Cryptogenic cirrhosis	
Chronic cholestatic disease (PBC, PSC, secondary biliary cirrhosis)	
HCC	Usually on a background of cirrhosis
Metabolic diseases	
Paediatric	Biliary atresia, cholestatic diseases, metabolic disorders, some malignancies
Budd–Chiari syndrome	Non-malignant occlusion of the hepatic veins, especially total venous occlusion and/or patients with cirrhosis resulting from Budd–Chiari syndrome
Fulminant hepatic failure	Due to drug (usually paracetamol) overdose, acute hepatitis, Budd–Chiari syndrome, Wilson's disease or massive hepatic trauma
Others	Rarely, transplant is undertaken for benign lesions such as polycystic disease, adenoma or large haemangiomas

Table 4.8 Indications for liver transplantation

cirrhosis, most commonly from hepatitis C and primary cholestatic disease.[54]

Lack of organ availability has, to some extent, driven the progress of alternative surgical procedures. The use of live related donor organ transplanation, in which part of the liver of a healthy (usually) related donor is transplanted into the recipient, and the use of split liver transplantation, in which the cadaveric organ is split to be transplanted into two recipients (one of which is usually paediatric) have effectively enlarged the organ pool and allowed continuing improvements in overall survival.[55] Contraindications for liver transplantation continue to dwindle. These include active extrahepatic malignancy, diffuse invasive intrahepatic malignancy and some co-morbidities which prevent major surgery.

The prognosis following transplantation is highly dependent upon both the primary disease and upon the clinical state of the patient. Patient selection is an important issue, as organs are limited. Priority for organ allocation is managed by use of the model of end-stage liver disease (MELD) score which prioritizes patients with the highest short-term mortality.[56]

Presence of malignant liver disease is not a contraindication to transplantation, provided the bulk of tumour remains relatively modest and is confined to the liver.[57] Patients with larger HCCs (>3 cm) and those with cholangiocarcinoma have a higher rate of recurrence post-transplantation, and are generally not considered for transplantation.

Pre-operative assessment

The ultrasound scan is one of many investigations leading up to transplantation. The diagnosis of liver pathology usually involves ultrasound scanning as a first line, augmented by histology and additional cross-sectional imaging. The role of ultrasound includes contributing to, or confirming, the initial diagnosis, assessing the degree of severity and associated complications of the disease and providing guidance for biopsy. An important objective is also to exclude patients for whom liver transplantation is not feasible, or of little benefit – for example those with extrahepatic malignant disease.

The pre-operative assessment focuses on the complications of liver disease, such as features of portal hypertension, the presence of suspicious liver nodules, and any other unsuspected extrahepatic conditions that may delay or compromise potential surgery. In particular, the sonographer should look for:

- *Portal vein thrombosis* – this may be a contraindication to transplantation if it is extensive, or unable to be effectively bypassed by the surgeon
- Other features of *portal hypertension* associated with chronic liver disease (see above) including spleen size and varices

- *Focal liver lesions* that may represent malignancy. These may require the administration of ultrasound contrast agents, or further imaging such as MRI for characterization
- *Extrahepatic malignancy*, in cases with an initial diagnosis of carcinoma
- Degree and scope of *vascular thrombosis* in cases of Budd–Chiari syndrome
- Any *incidental pathology* which may alter the management plan
- Doppler is, of course, essential in assessing the patency and direction of blood flow of the portal venous system, the hepatic veins, IVC and main hepatic artery. It may occasionally be possible to demonstrate arterial anomalies.

Although large numbers of patients are considered for transplantation and undergo ultrasound assessment, the majority of these will *never actually receive* a transplant. This factor has numerous implications for resources when setting up a pre-transplant ultrasound service. The introduction of live donor transplantation also has considerable service implications, including increased use of intraoperative sonography as well as other radiological services for donor and recipient, which must be factored in.

Operative procedure

Most transplants are *orthotopic* – that is the diseased liver is removed and replaced by the donor organ – as opposed to *heterotopic*, in which the donor organ is grafted in addition to the native organ (like most kidney transplants). The transplant requires five surgical anastomoses:

- Suprahepatic vena cava
- Infrahepatic vena cava
- Hepatic artery (either end-to-end, or end-to-side to aorta)
- Portal vein
- CBD (the gallbladder is removed).

IOUS is useful for assessing the size and spread of intrahepatic neoplastic growths and to assess vascular invasion in the recipient. Mapping of the hepatic vascular anatomy in living-related donors is also feasible using IOUS. IOUS with Doppler is also useful for assessing the vascular anastomoses and establishing if portal venous and hepatic arterial flow are adequate.

Post-operative assessment

Ultrasound plays a key role in the post-operative monitoring of liver transplant patients. Numerous complications are possible (Table 4.9) and many of these can be diagnosed with ultrasound. Ciclosporin immunosuppression is administered and blood levels of ciclosporin are a closely monitored balancing act; too low and the graft may reject, too high and the toxic effects of the drug may affect the kidneys.

Liver function is biochemically monitored for early signs of complications. Elevated serum bilirubin, alkaline phosphatase and/or aminotransferase levels are present with most types of graft

Infection	Abdominal infection → sepsis/intrahepatic abscess
Vascular	Anastomotic leaks → Haematoma
	Thrombosis or stenosis → ischaemia/infarction
Biliary	Bile duct stricture or stenosis leading to dilatation
	Bile leak → biloma
Rejection	Acute episodes are common in the first two weeks and are of variable severity
Other medical complications	Neurological
	Renal dysfunction
Recurrence of original disease	Hepatitis
	Cholangiocarcinoma or CC
	Budd–Chiari syndrome
	PSC
Post-transplantation lymphoproliferative disorder (PTLD)	More common in children, PTLD is associated with immunosuppression, occurring within the first year of transplantation

Table 4.9 Post-operative liver transplantation complications

dysfunction or complication and are investigated first with ultrasound.

Renal dysfunction is a further recognized complication following transplantation. This can be due to various causes, including ciclosporin nephrotoxicity, intraoperative hypotension or pre-operative renal failure.

Post-operative ultrasound appearances and complications

Post-transplant complications may be mechanical (problems with vessels or ducts) or non-mechanical (non-function, rejection, infection or recurrence of disease).

Hepatic artery

The hepatic artery is vital to graft success as it is the sole vascular supply to the biliary system. Most hepatic artery occlusions occur relatively soon after operation, before a good collateral supply is able to be established. HA thrombosis or stenosis can lead to bile duct necrosis, causing bile leaks and abscesses, or areas of infarction within the liver tissue. And it is therefore treated as an emergency requiring surgical intervention and, sometimes, retransplantation.

Failure to adequately display the hepatic artery with a good spectral trace on ultrasound is often due to inadequate technique. Ensure the artery is scanned intercostally to maintain a low vessel-to-beam angle, and that the Doppler sensitivity and filter controls are set for low velocities if arterial flow is not found.

Hepatic artery stenosis/thrombosis is still a relatively common post-transplant complication in up to 12% of adult patients and up to 40% of paediatric patients. Colour Doppler ultrasound has a sensitivity/specificity of 92%/97% for detecting hepatic artery complications[58] and X-ray angiography is rarely required. Stenosis of the artery at the site of anastomosis is detected by examining the Doppler spectrum (Fig. 4.30). The systolic upstroke tends to be delayed ('*tardus parvus*' pattern) downstream of the stenosis;[59] the acceleration time is increased (over 0.08 seconds). The appearance of the hepatic artery waveform immediately post-operatively is often one of a small spike with no EDF. This is not a significant finding and will usually develop into the more familiar waveform with forward EDF by 48 hours after transplantation.[60] Pseudoaneurysm of the hepatic artery is rare, most commonly occurring at the site of the anastomosis.

The administration of ultrasound contrast media is useful for detection of flow in difficult examinations (Fig. 4.31).

Portal vein

Portal vein complications (stenosis or thrombosis) occur in up to 13% of patients. The portal vein anastomosis is readily demonstrated in most patients, and shows turbulence associated with the anastomotic site (Fig. 4.32A), as the diameters of the donor and recipient veins invariably differ. This is not significant in itself but can indicate a clinically significant stenosis when accompanied by high velocities of greater than 100 cm/s (Fig. 4.32B). Portal vein stenosis is associated with a steadily increasing spleen size, which is why it is important to have a baseline measurement of the spleen.

Portal vein thrombosis may be occlusive or non-occlusive, and may affect both intra- and extrahepatic portal vessels. It is possible to have a blocked main portal vein with patent intrahepatic portal veins, due to collateral formation.

IVC and hepatic veins

IVC stenosis or thrombosis is uncommon, accounting for less than 3% of patients. The infrahepatic IVC anastomosis is readily seen on ultrasound (Fig. 4.33) but the near-perpendicular angle of the IVC to the beam makes it difficult to assess blood flow velocity and power Doppler, which is less angle-dependent, if often helpful in demonstrating flow in the IVC (Fig 4.33B). If the transplantation has been performed for Budd–Chiari syndrome, pay particular attention to the hepatic veins, which show a tendency to re-thrombose in some patients.

CBD

Biliary complications account for up to 19% of post-transplantation complications, most occurring in the first 3 months following the transplantation. A baseline measurement is important in order to detect small degrees of subsequent dilatation which may imply stenosis or obstruction. Even relatively minor dilatation can be significant

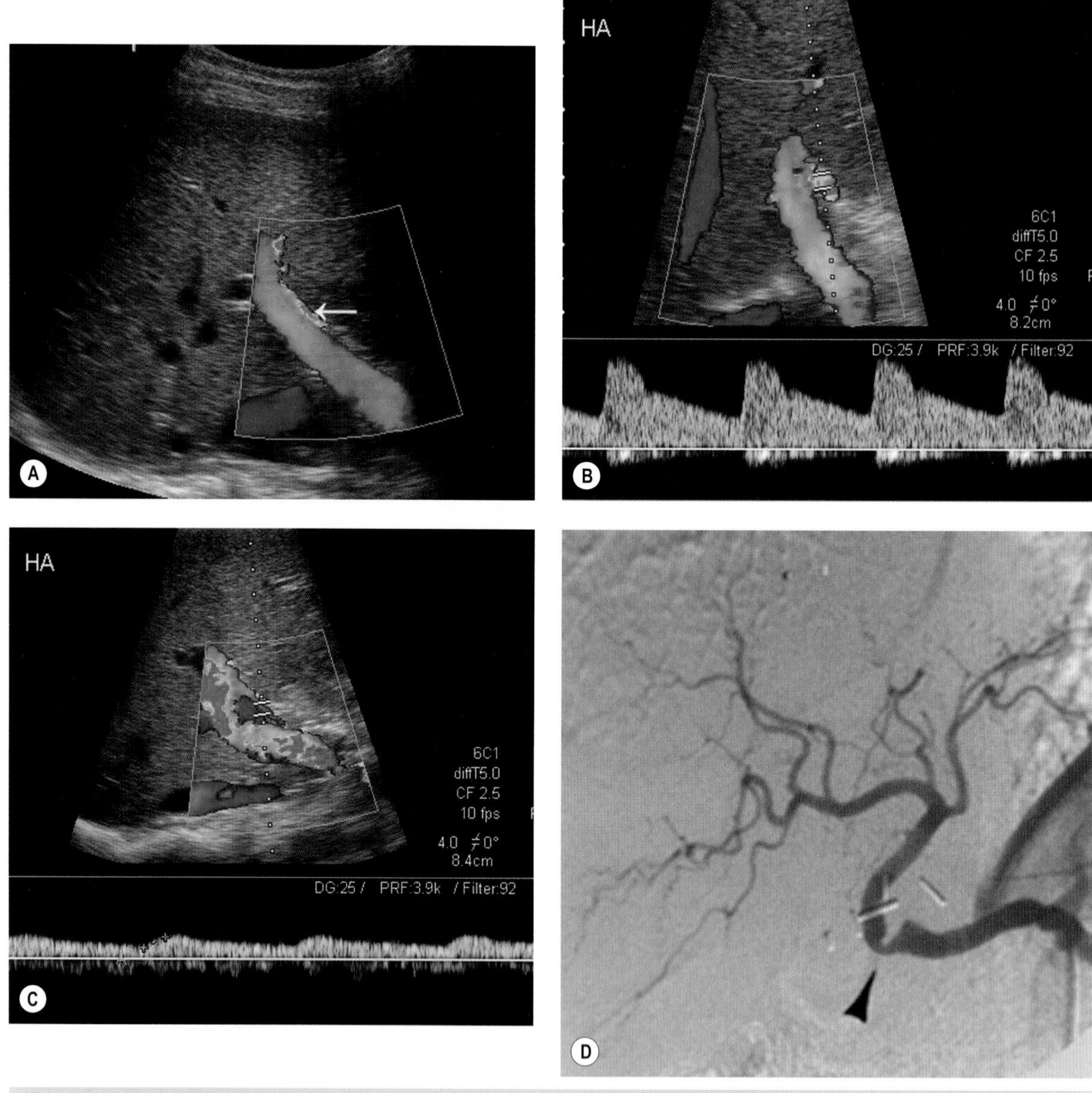

Fig. 4.30 • (A) The MHA (arrow) in a liver transplant on colour Doppler, lying anterior to the MPV. (B) Normal HA waveform post-transplantation, demonstrating a steep systolic rise with forward flow throughout the cycle. (C) Slow systolic rise (tardus parvus) and low velocity flow in hepatic artery stenosis. (D) Angiography confirms and locates the stenosis.

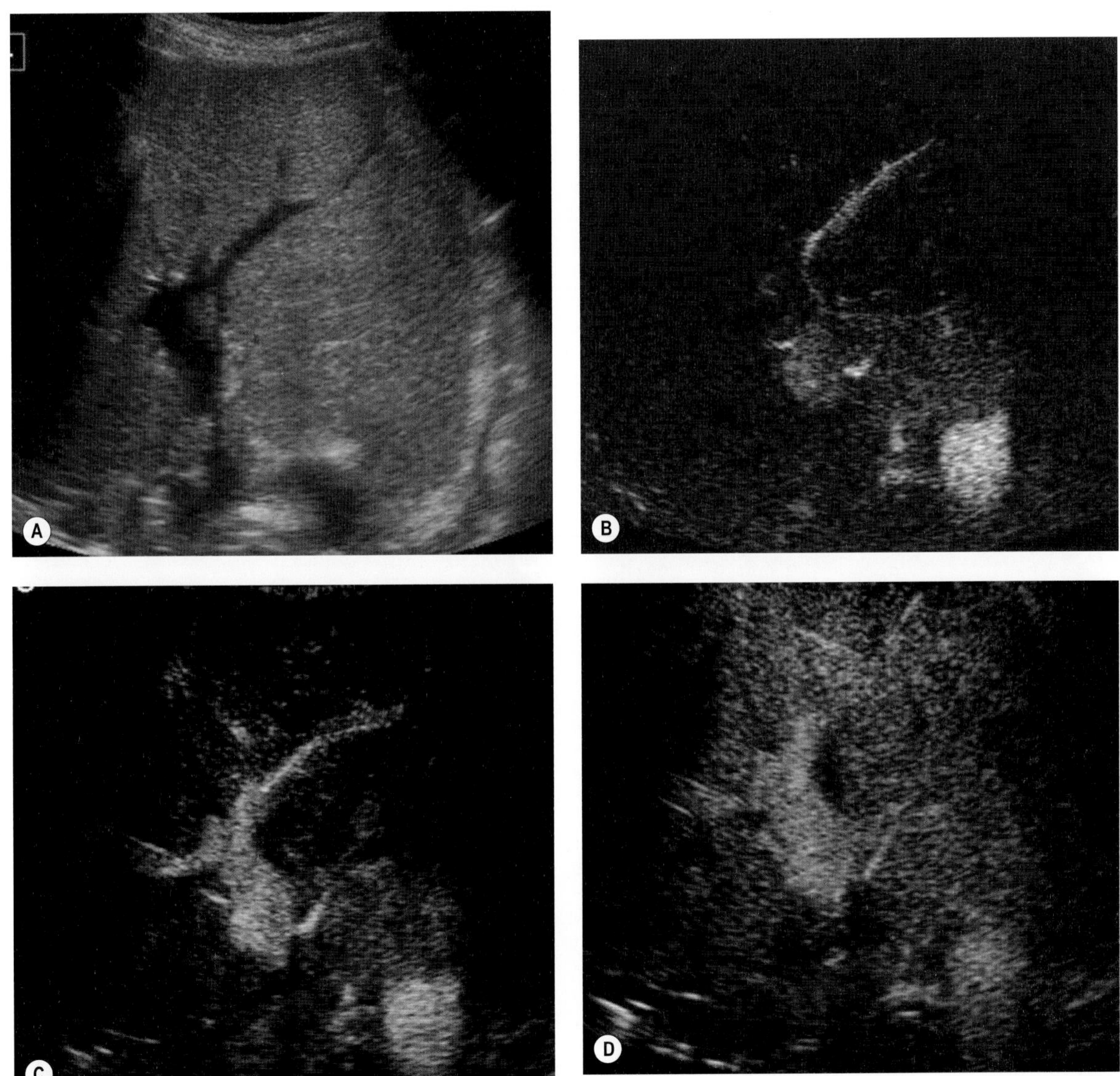

Fig. 4.31 • CEUS is useful in establishing the patency of vessels in difficult cases: (A) Colour Doppler was unable to demonstrate flow in the left HA, in a patient with clinical suspicion of thrombosis. (B) CEUS demonstrates good flow in the HA. (C) The PV phase demonstrates the left PV posterior to the artery and (D) the sinusoidal phase demonstrates good contrast take up throughout, confidently excluding the possibility of infarction.

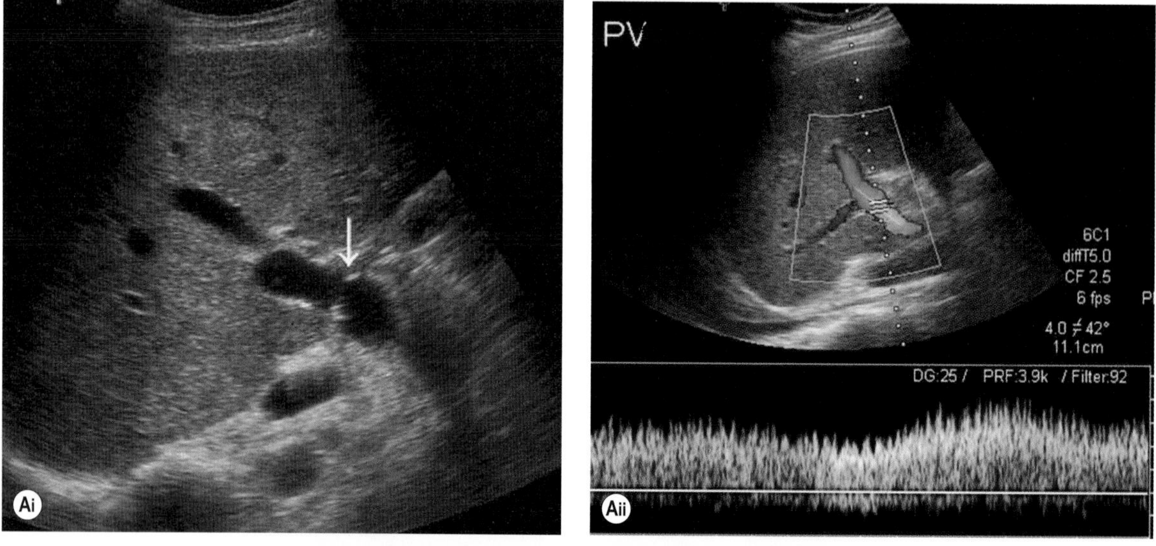

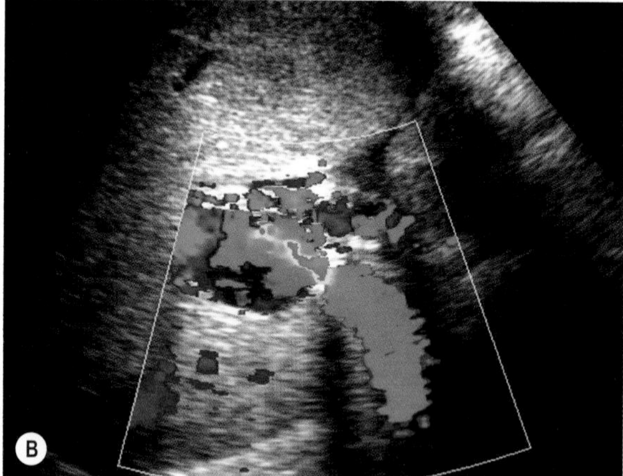

Fig. 4.32 • (Ai) The PV anastomosis (arrow) is visible post-transplantation. (Aii) The PV in a liver transplant demonstrates a turbulent waveform due to the surgical anastomosis. This is not a significant finding. (B) MPV stenosis. A high velocity jet is seen through the stenosis at the site of the anastomosis, with post-stenotic turbulence.

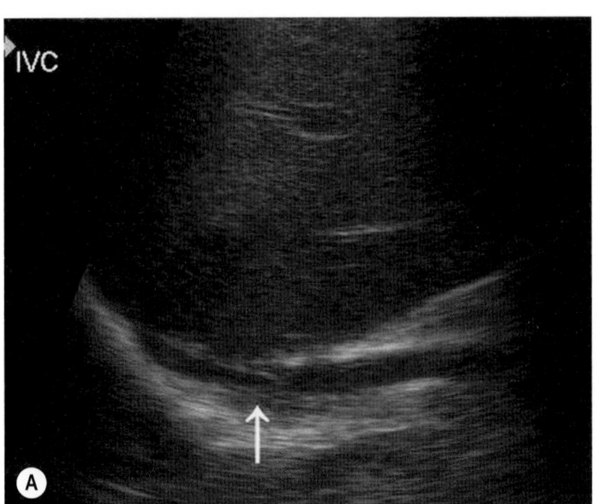

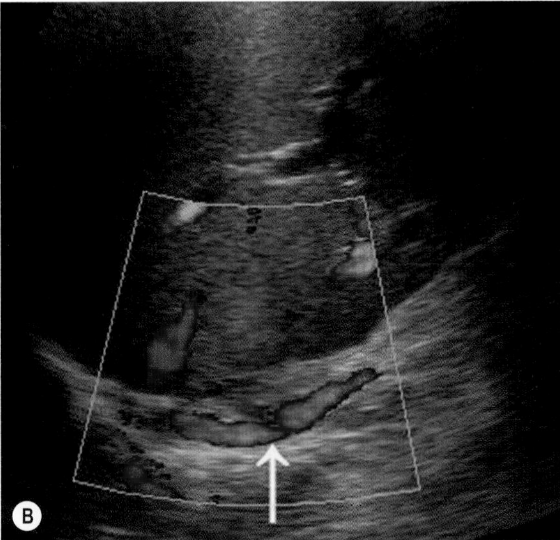

Fig. 4.33 • (A) The inferior anastomosis in the IVC post liver transplantation (arrow). (B) Power Doppler of the same case (arrow).

in the transplant recipient; cholestasis can precipitate ascending biliary infection which may subsequently form liver abscesses, a process which may be aggravated by immunosuppression.

Strictures commonly occur at the anastomosis due to scar tissue, but other, non-anastomotic strictures can result from hepatic artery insufficiency causing ischaemia. Leakage is a comparatively rare event.

Focal lesions

The most likely cause of focal lesions in the short term following transplantation is due to abscess following infection. Hepatic abscesses may be multiple and are often acoustically subtle in the early stages. Other causes of focal lesions in the early post-operative period may be due to infarction and are associated with interruption of the arterial supply or poor harvesting technique. These can be hyper- or hypoechoic, have well-defined borders and do not exert a mass effect (Fig. 4.34).

In patients with malignancy who have had a transplant, recurrence of tumour may also be a serious complication.

Post-transplantation malignancy

Patients who are immunosuppressed are at greater risk than normal for developing malignancy. PTLD (similar in appearance to non-Hodgkin's lymphoma) is a complication associated with immunocompromise, which affects up to 2% of transplant recipients (Fig. 4.34C). Ultrasound may demonstrate hypoechoic, ill-defined intrahepatic masses, lymphadenopathy and occasional involvement of the spleen and kidneys.[61]

Patients with malignant lesions pre-transplantation, such as HCC or cholangiocarcinoma, have a significant risk of recurrence after transplantation.

Fluid collections

Following liver transplantation, fluid collections are frequently demonstrated and may be monitored with ultrasound, and/or drained under ultrasound guidance. These may represent haematoma (Fig. 4.35), seroma, loculated ascites or biloma. It is not possible to differentiate different types of collection with ultrasound alone. The appearances are taken in conjunction with the clinical features and the role of ultrasound is primarily to monitor the gradual resolution of the collection or to establish if infection is present in a clinically ill patient (by aspiration) and drain the collection if appropriate.

Haematomas usually resolve if left untreated. However, a large haematoma could result from an anastomotic leak requiring surgical intervention. A

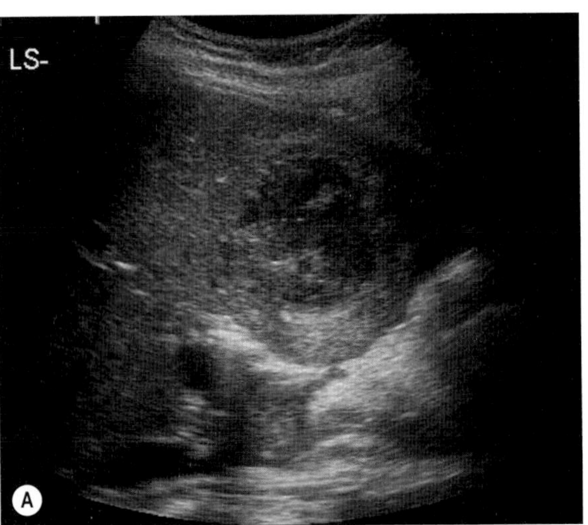

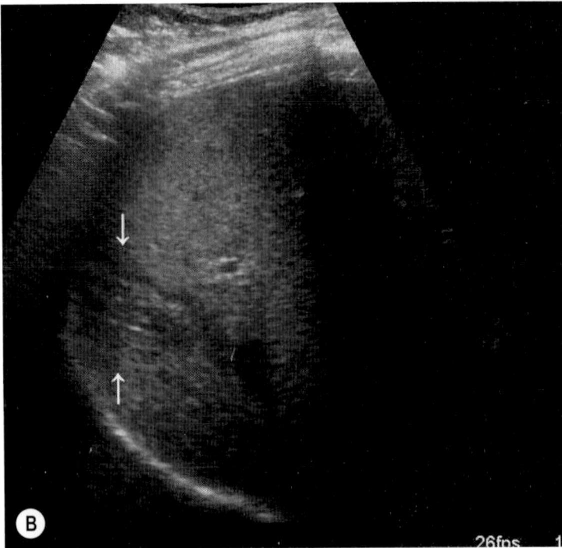

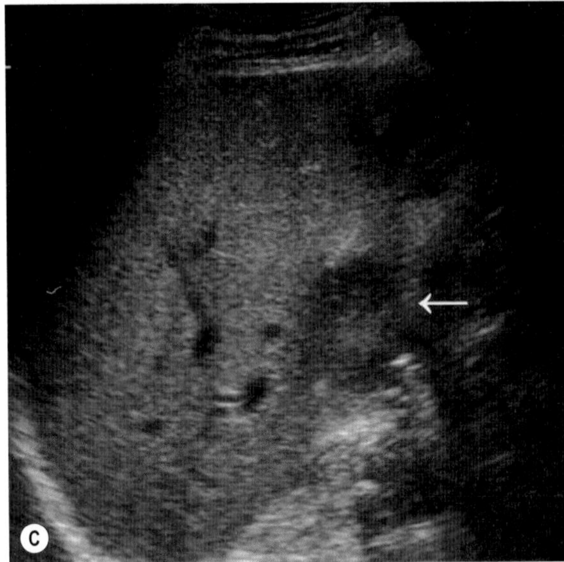

Fig. 4.34 • (A) An abscess in a liver transplant. (B) Infarct in a liver transplant (arrows) resulting from HA thrombosis. (C) PTLD, demonstrating a hypoechoic lesion near the porta hepatis in a transplant recipient.

leaking bile duct anastomosis is potentially a serious complication which could cause peritonitis. Drainage under ultrasound guidance is a temporary option but surgical repair is invariably necessary.

Recent recipients of liver transplants often have free intraperitoneal fluid and a right pleural effusion, which resolve spontaneously.

Rejection

Episodes of graft rejection are common in the first 2 weeks after transplantation. Graft rejection may be acute, in which case the immunosuppression is increased, or chronic following several acute episodes. Chronic rejection can only be treated by retransplantation.

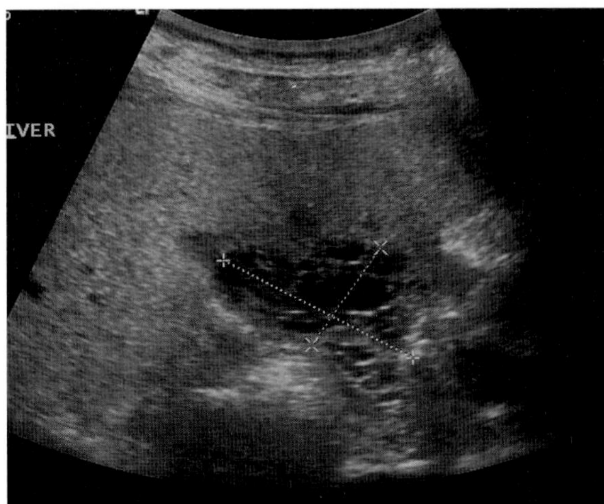

Fig. 4.35 • Subphrenic haematoma post liver transplantation. Most resolve spontaneously.

Rejection does not have any specific ultrasound features on either conventional imaging or Doppler, and the diagnosis is made from a liver biopsy following clinical suspicion.

References

1. Moorthy K, Mihssin N, Houghton PW. The management of simple hepatic cysts: sclerotherapy or laparoscopic fenestration. Ann R Coll Surg Engl 2001; 83: 409–414
2. Adam YG, Nonas CJ. Hepatobiliary cystadenoma. Southern Med J 1995; 88: 1140–1143
3. Turgut AT, Akhan O, Bhatt S, Dogra VS. Sonographic spectrum of hydatid disease. Ultrasound Q 2008; 24: 17–29
4. Voros D, Katsarelias D, Polymeneas G et al. Treatment of hydatid liver disease. Surg Infect (Larchmt) 2007; 8: 621–627
5. Huang CJ, Pitt HA, Lipsett PA et al. Pyogenic hepatic abscess: changing trends over 42 years. Ann Surg 1996; 223: 600–609
6. Doyle DJ, Hanbidge AE, O'Malley ME. Imaging of hepatic infections. Clin Radiol 2006; 61: 737–748
7. Kim TK, Jang HJ, Wilson SR. Benign liver masses: imaging with microbubble contrast agents. Ultrasound Q 2006; 22: 31–39
8. Kim TK, Jang HJ, Burns PN et al. Focal nodular hyperplasia and hepatic adenoma: differentiation with low-mechanical-index contrast-enhanced sonography. AJR Am J Roentgenol 2008; 190: 58–66
9. Morin SH, Lim AK, Cobbold JF, Taylor-Robinson SD. Use of second generation contrast-enhanced ultrasound in the assessment of focal liver lesions. World J Gastroenterol 2007; 13: 5963–5970
10. Grazioli L, Federle MP, Brancatelli G et al. Hepatic adenomas: imaging and pathologic findings. Radiographics 2001; 21: 877–892
11. Mortelé KJ, Segatto E, Ros PR. The infected liver: radiologic-pathologic correlation. Radiographics 2004; 24: 937–955
12. Lencioni R, Della Pina C, Crocetti L et al. Clinical management of focal liver lesions: the key role of real-time contrast-enhanced US. Eur Radiol 2007;17 Suppl 6: F73–F79
13. Hicks RJ, Ware RE, Lau EW. PET/CT: will it change the way that we use CT in cancer imaging? Cancer Imaging 2006; 6: S52–S62
14. Adam A. Interventional radiology in the treatment of hepatic metastases. Canc Treat Rev 2002; 28: 93–99
15. Biasco G, Derenzini E, Grazi G et al. Treatment of hepatic metastases from colorectal cancer: many doubts, some certainties. Canc Treat Rev 2006; 32: 214–228
16. Zweibel WJ. Sonographic diagnosis of diffuse liver disease. Semin Ultrasound CT MRI 1995; 16: 8–15
17. Shapiro RS, Katz R, Mendelson DS et al. Detection of hepatocellular carcinoma in cirrhotic patients: sensitivity of CT and ultrasound. J Ultrasound Med 1996; 15: 497–502
18. Forner A, Vilana R, Ayuso C et al. Diagnosis of hepatic nodules 20 mm or smaller in cirrhosis: Prospective validation of the noninvasive diagnostic criteria for hepatocellular carcinoma. Hepatology 2008; 47: 97–104
19. Llovet JM, Bruix J. Novel advancements in the management of hepatocellular carcinoma in 2008. J Hepatol 2008; 48 Suppl 1: S20–S37
20. Maruyama H, Yoshikawa M, Yokosuka O. Current role of ultrasound for the management of hepatocellular carcinoma. World J Gastroenterol 2008; 14: 1710–1719
21. Wu F, Wang ZB, Chen WZ et al. Advanced hepatocellular carcinoma: treatment with high-intensity focused ultrasound ablation combined with transcatheter arterial embolization. Radiology 2005; 235: 659–667
22. Preiss D, Sattar N. Non-alcoholic fatty liver disease: an overview of prevalence, diagnosis, pathogenesis and treatment considerations. Clin Sci (Lond) 2008; 115: 141–150
23. Chuah SK, Changchien CS, Chiu KW et al. Changes of hepatic vein waveform in chronic liver diseases. J Med Ultrasound 1995; 3: 75–80
24. Thompson Coon J, Rogers G, Hewson P et al. Surveillance of cirrhosis for hepatocellular carcinoma: a cost-utility analysis. Br J Cancer 2008; 98: 1166–1175
25. Thompson Coon J, Rogers G, Hewson P et al. Surveillance of cirrhosis for hepatocellular carcinoma: systematic review and economic analysis. Health Tech Assess 2007; 11: 1–206
26. EFSUMB study group. Guidelines for the use of contrast agents in ultrasound, 2004. Available at: www.efsumb.org/guidelines
27. Ward J, Robinson PJ. How to detect hepatocellular carcinoma in cirrhosis. Eur Radiol 2002; 12: 2258–2272

28. Kim SH, Choi BI, Lee JY et al. Diagnostic accuracy of multi-/single-detector row CT and contrast-enhanced MRI in the detection of hepatocellular carcinomas meeting the Milan criteria before liver transplantation. Intervirology 2008; 51 Suppl 1: 52–60
29. WHO. Global surveillance and control of hepatitis C. Report of a WHO Consultation organized in collaboration with the Viral Hepatitis Prevention Board, Antwerp, Belgium. J Viral Hepat 1999; 6: 35–47
30. Blonski W, Reddy KR. Hepatitis C virus infection and hepatocellular carcinoma. Clin Liver Dis 2008; 12: 661–674
31. Kumagi T, Heathcote EJ. Primary biliary cirrhosis. Orphanet J Rare Dis 2008; 3: 1
32. Dietrich C, Leuschner M, Zeuzem S et al. Perihepatic lymphadenopathy in primary biliary cirrhosis reflects progression of the disease. Eur J Gastroenterol Hepatol 1999; 11: 747–753
33. Talwalkar JA, Kurtz DM, Schoenleber SJ et al. Ultrasound-based transient elastography for the detection of hepatic fibrosis: systematic review and meta-analysis. Clin Gastroenterol Hepatol 2007; 5: 1214–1220
34. Lovet J, Fuster J, Bruix J. The barcelona approach: diagnosis, staging and treatment of hepatocellular carcinoma. Liver Transpl 2004; 10: S115–S120
35. Kok T, van der Jagt EJ, Haagsma EB et al. The value of Doppler ultrasound in cirrhosis and portal hypertension. Scand J Gastroenterol Suppl 1999; 230: 82–88
36. Gorg C, Riera-Knorrenschild J, Dietrich J. Pictorial review: colour Doppler ultrasound flow patterns in the portal venous system. Br J Radiol 2002; 75: 919–929
37. Zweibel WJ. Sonographic diagnosis of hepatic vascular disorders. Semin Ultrasound CT MRI 1995; 16: 34–48
38. Wu CC, Yeh YH, Hwang MH. Observation of portal venous flow in liver cirrhosis by Doppler ultrasound: the significance of PVH index. J Med Ultrasound 1994; 2: 180–184
39. Konno K, Ishida H, Uno A et al. Cavernous transformation of the portal vein (CTPV): role of color Doppler sonography in the diagnosis. Eur J Ultrasound 1996; 3: 231–240
40. Bach AM, Hann LE, Brown KT et al. Portal vein evaluation with US: comparison to angiography and CT arterial portography. Radiology 1996; 201: 149–154
41. Lafortune M, Patriquin H, Pomier G et al. Haemodynamic changes in portal circulation after portosystemic shunts; use of duplex sonography in 43 patients. AJR Am J Roentgenol 1987; 149: 701–706
42. Colombato L. The role of transjugular intrahepatic portosystemic shunt (TIPS) in the management of portal hypertension. J Clin Gastroenterol 2007; 41 Suppl 3: S344–S351
43. Chong WK, Malisch TW, Mazer MJ. Sonography of transjugular intrahepatic portosystemic shunts. Semin Ultrasound CT MRI 1995; 16: 69–80
44. Middleton WD, Teefey SA, Darcy MD. Doppler evaluation of transjugular intrahepatic portosystemic shunts. Ultrasound Q 2003; 19: 56–70
45. Kravetz D. Prevention of recurrent esophageal variceal hemorrhage: review and current recommendations. J Clin Gastroenterol 2007; 41 Suppl 3: S318–S322
46. Baldo V, Baldovin T, Trivello R, Floreani A. Epidemiology of HCV infection. Curr Pharm Des 2008; 14: 1646–1654
47. Gomaa A, Khan S, Toledano M et al. Hepatocellular carcinoma: Epidemiology, risk factors and pathogenesis. World J Gastroenterol 2008; 14: 4300–4308
48. Aydinli M, Bayraktar Y. Budd-chiari syndrome: etiology, pathogenesis and diagnosis. World J Gastroenterol 2007; 13: 2693–2696
49. Vogel J, Gorich J, Kramme E et al. Alveolar echinococcosis of the liver: percutaneous stent therapy of Budd–Chiari syndrome. GUT 1996; 39: 762–764
50. Mahadeva R, Webb K, Westerbeek R et al. Clinical outcome in relation to care in centres specialising in cystic fibrosis: cross sectional study. BMJ 1998; 316: 1771–1779
51. Nash KL, Allison ME, McKeon D et al. A single centre experience of liver disease in adults with cystic fibrosis 1995–2006. J Cyst Fibros 2008; 7: 252–257
52. Kawooya M, Muyinda Z, Byanyima R, Malwadde E. Abdominal ultrasound findings in HIV: a pictorial review. Ultrasound 2008; 16: 62–72
53. Geary M. The HELLP syndrome. Br J Obst Gynaecol 1997; 104: 887–891
54. O'Leary J, Lepe R, Dais G. Indications for liver transplantation. Gastroenterology 2008; 34: 1764–1776
55. Müller S, Mehrabi A, Schmied B et al. Partial liver transplantation – living donor liver transplantation and split liver transplantation. Nephrol Dial Transplant 2007; 22 Suppl 8: viii13–viii22
56. Weisner R, Edwards E, Freeman R. Model for end-stage liver disease (MELD) and allocation of donor livers. Gastroenterology 2003; 124: 91–96
57. Bruix J, Sherman M, Llovet JM et al. Clinical management of hepatocellular carcinoma. Conclusions of the Barcelona-2000 EASL conference. J Hepatol 2001; 35: 421–430
58. Tamsel S, Demirpolat G, Killi R et al. Vascular complications after liver transplantation: evaluation with Doppler US. Abdom Imaging 2007; 32: 339–347
59. Dodd GD 3rd, Memel DS, Zajko AB et al. Hepatic artery stenosis and thrombosis in transplant recipients: Doppler diagnosis with resistive index and systolic acceleration time. Radiology 1994; 192: 657–661
60. Holbert BL, Campbell WL, Skolnick ML. Evaluation of the transplanted liver and postoperative complications. Radiol Clin North Am 1995; 33: 521–540
61. Shaw AS, Ryan SM, Beese RC, Sidhu PS. Ultrasound of non-vascular complications in the post Liver Transplant Patient. Clin Radiol 2003; 58: 672–680

The pancreas

5

CHAPTER CONTENTS

THE NORMAL PANCREAS

Ultrasound techniques

The pancreas lies posterior to the stomach and duodenum, and therefore a variety of techniques must usually be employed to examine it fully. Ultrasound may still be considered the first line of investigation, but CT, MRI, EUS and/or ERCP may be required to augment and refine the diagnosis.

The operator must make the best use of acoustic windows, different patient positions and various techniques to fully investigate the pancreas. Start by scanning the epigastrium in transverse plane, using the left lobe of the liver as an acoustic window. Using the splenic vein as an anatomical marker, the body of the pancreas can be identified anterior to this. The tail of pancreas is slightly cephalic to the head, so the transducer plane should be accordingly oblique to display the whole organ (Fig. 5.1). Different transducer angulations display different sections of the pancreas to best effect.

Identify the echo-free splenic vein and the superior mesenteric artery (SMA) posterior to it. The latter is surrounded by an easily visible, hyperechoic fibrous sheath. The pancreas is 'draped' over the splenic vein (Fig. 5.1).

Where possible, use the left lobe of the liver as an acoustic window to the pancreas, angling slightly caudally. The tail, which is often quite bulky, may require the transducer to be angled towards the patient's left. The spleen also makes a good window to the tail in coronal section (Fig. 5.1E). If you can't see the pancreatic head properly, turn the patient left side raised, which moves the duodenal gas up towards the tail of the pancreas. Right side raised may demonstrate the tail better. If these manoeuvres still fail to demonstrate the organ fully, try:

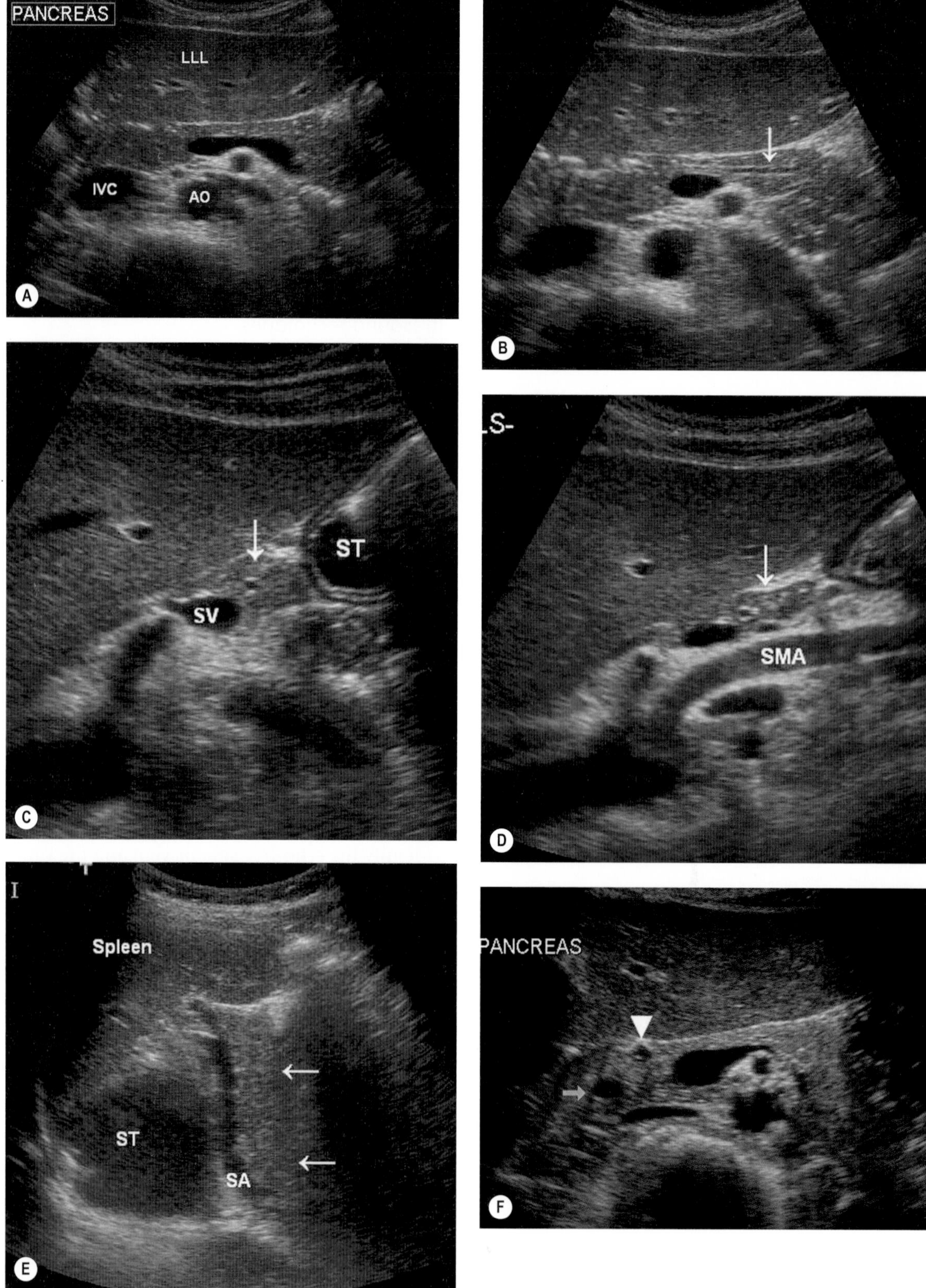
PANCREAS
LLL
IVC
AO
A
B
ST
SV
C
LS-
SMA
D
I
Spleen
ST
SA
E
PANCREAS
F

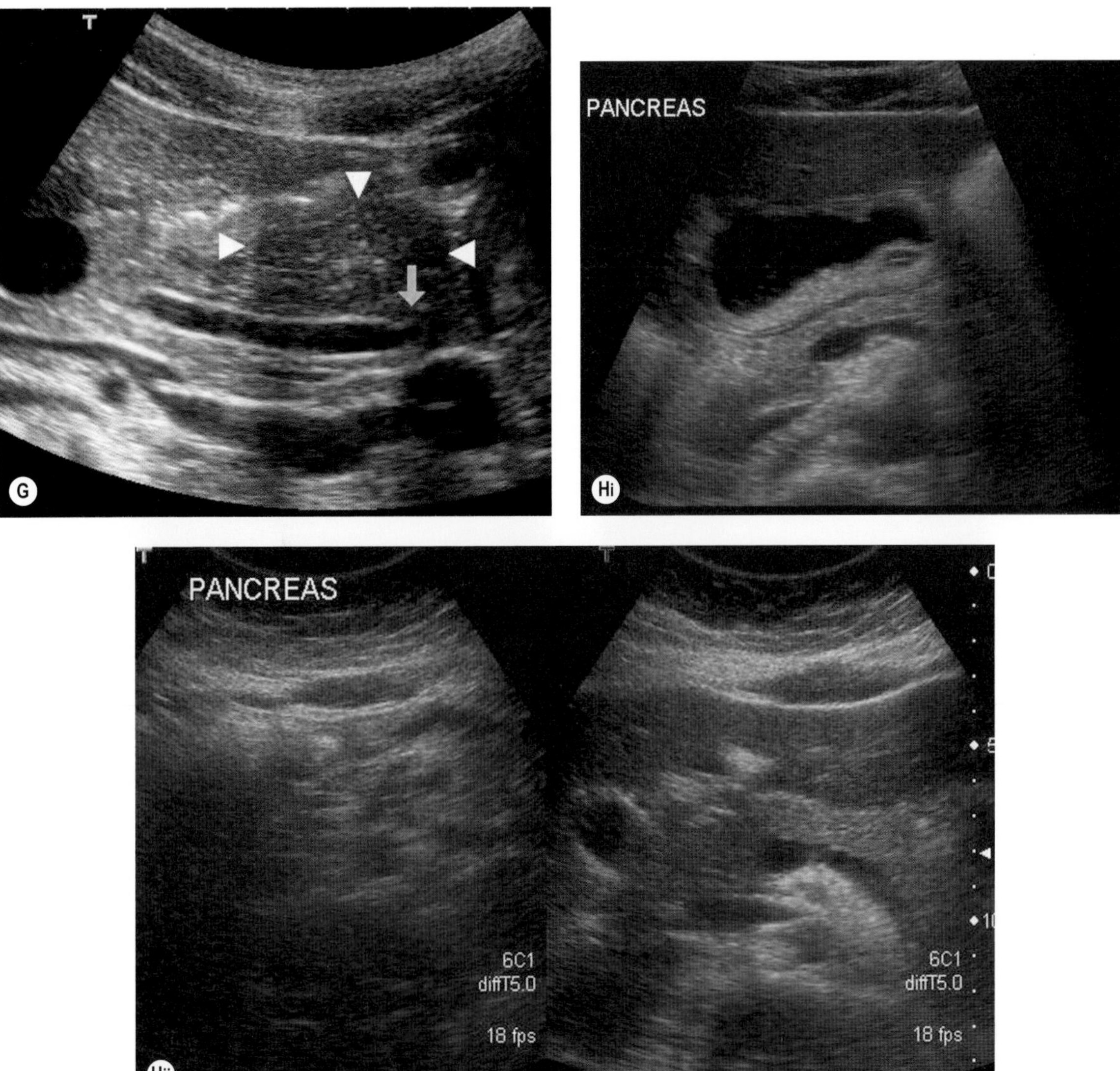

Fig. 5.1 • (A) TS showing through the epigastrium showing the normal pancreas. The left lobe of liver (LLL) makes a good acoustic window. (B) The normal pancreatic duct (arrow) is seen in the body of the pancreas. (C) LS in the epigastric midline, demonstrating the body of pancreas (arrow) with a cross-section through its normal duct. ST = stomach, SV = splenic vein. (D) The body of the pancreas (arrow) lies anterior to the SMA. (E) LS through the left upper quadrant (LUQ), using the spleen as a window to the tail of pancreas (arrows). The splenic artery (SA) lies against the tail of pancreas (TOP). (F) The normal CBD (arrow) can be seen in the head of pancreas (HOP) in TS. Gastroduodenal artery (arrowhead). (G) The lower end of the CBD (arrow) as it goes through the HOP (arrowheads). (Hi) A pancreas obscured by overlying bowel gas can be seen through the acoustic window of a water-filled stomach. (Hii) Abdominal protrusion can be a useful technique for visualizing the pancreas in a gassy abdomen; the right image displays the pancreas when the patient is asked to push the abdomen out.

- Asking the patient to perform the Valsalva manoeuvre with abdominal protrusion (Fig. 5.1Hii).
- Scanning the patient erect.
- Filling the stomach with a water load to create an acoustic window through which the pancreas can be seen (Fig. 5.1Hi).

Ultrasound appearances

The texture of the pancreas is rather coarser than that of the liver.

The echogenicity of the normal pancreas alters according to age. In a child or young person it may be quite bulky and relatively hypoechoic when compared with the liver. In adulthood, the pancreas is hyperechoic compared with normal liver, becoming increasingly so in the elderly, and tending to atrophy (Fig. 5.2).

The pancreas does not have a capsule and its margins can appear rather ill-defined, becoming infiltrated with fat in later life. These age-related changes are highly significant to the sonographer; what may be considered normal in an elderly

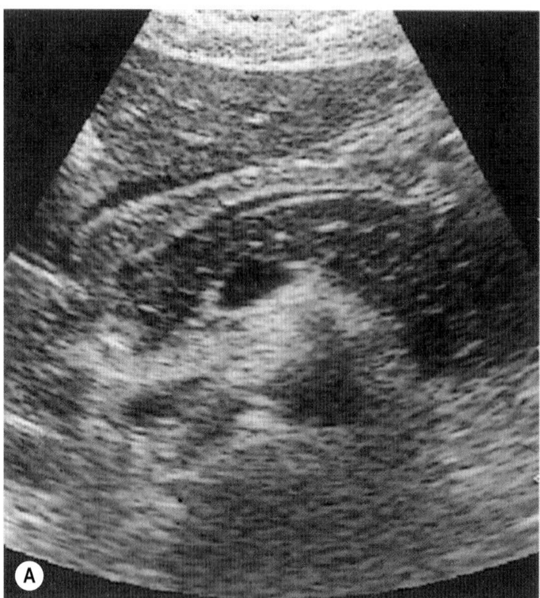

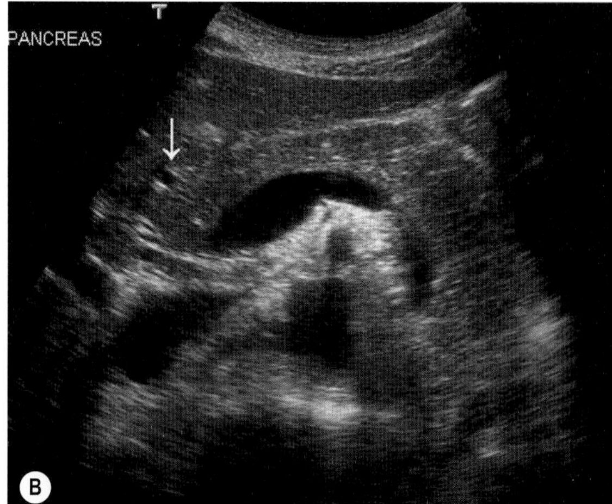

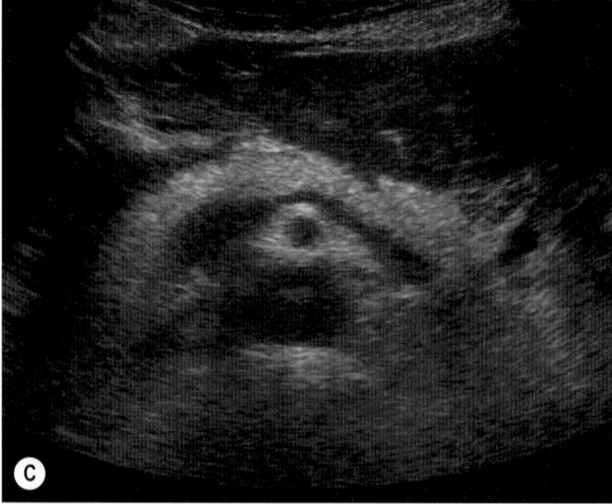

Fig. 5.2 • Age-related acoustic appearances: (A) Pancreas in a young person, demonstrating normal hypoechogenicity. (B) The normal adult pancreas is slightly more echogenic than the liver. Note the gastroduodenal artery near the HOP (arrow). (C) The pancreas becomes hyperechoic and infiltrated with fat in an older patient.

person would be abnormally hyperechoic in a younger one, and may represent a chronic inflammatory state. Conversely a hypoechoic pancreas in an older patient may represent acute inflammation, whereas the appearances would be normal in a young person.

The main pancreatic duct is most easily visualized in the body of pancreas, where its walls are perpendicular to the beam. The normal diameter is 2 mm or less. The CBD can be seen in the lateral portion of the head, and the gastroduodenal artery lies anterolaterally (Fig. 5.1F). The size of the uncinate process varies.

Pitfalls in scanning the pancreas

The normal stomach or duodenum can mimic pancreatic pathology especially if the patient is insufficiently fasted. A fluid-filled stomach can be particularly confusing when looking for pancreatic pseudocysts in patients with acute pancreatitis. Giving the patient a drink of water usually differentiates the gastrointestinal tract from a collection.

Epigastric or portal lymphadenopathy may also mimic a pancreatic mass. If careful scanning and appropriate patient positioning are unable to elucidate, CT is usually the next step.

Biochemical analysis

In many pancreatic diseases, the production of the digestive pancreatic enzymes is compromised, either by obstruction of the duct draining the pancreas or by destruction of the pancreatic cells that produce the enzymes. This can result in malabsorption of food and/or diarrhoea.

The pancreas produces the digestive enzymes amylase, lipase and peptidase, which occur in trace amounts in the blood. If the pancreas is damaged or inflamed, the resulting release of enzymes into the blood stream causes an increase in serum amylase and lipase levels. The enzymes also pass from the blood stream into the urine and therefore urinalysis can also contribute to the diagnosis.

Congenital anomalies of the pancreas

The normal pancreas is the result of the fusion of two embryonic buds – the ventral bud arises from the CBD, forming the uncinate process and part of the head, and the dorsal arises from the posterior wall of the duodenum. Developmental anomalies of the pancreas occur as a result of a failure of the dorsal and ventral pancreatic ducts to fuse – *pancreas divisum* – which is present in up to 10% of the Western population. This arrangement may cause inadequate drainage of the pancreatic duct, leading to pancreatitis. A rare developmental anomaly of the ventral bud may occur – *pancreas anulare* – in which pancreatic tissue encircles the bowel. In this latter case, patients can present with proximal small bowel obstruction in infancy, but this may also be an incidental finding at autopsy. These relatively uncommon anomalies are rarely diagnosed on ultrasound. Agenesis of the pancreas is very rare, usually in association with other defects, and children usually die soon after birth.

Other imaging

MRCP is increasingly used to examine the pancreatic duct[1] due to its relative non-invasive nature and low risk compared with ERCP.[2,3] ERCP is invasive and carries a small risk of post-procedure pancreatitis or, rarely, perforation, and so is reserved for therapeutic procedures such as the placement of a stent.

EUS is an increasingly useful modality for imaging the pancreas in detail, without the problems of intervening stomach or duodenal gas. This technique is helpful for imaging the pancreas in pancreatitis and has also been shown to be superior to CT in detecting occult neoplasms.[4] The proximity of the endoscope to the pancreas and ducts improves sensitivity and specificity for tiny stones and lesions. It also has the facility to take a biopsy if required (Fig. 5.4D), which can be accurately directed towards the area of interest, improving histological yield.

CT is most commonly used as a second-line investigation, following initial transabdominal ultrasound, especially in the presence of dilated biliary ducts. In addition to identifying pancreatic masses, it is also used to stage patients with pancreatic carcinoma. CT is generally the imaging of choice in severe acute pancreatitis, and is able to detect pancreatic necrosis, although the use of contrast ultrasound may also have a useful role in assessing vascularity,[5] diagnosing necrosis and even in identifying tumours, allowing further imaging to be directed more appropriately.

PANCREATITIS

Inflammation of the pancreas may be acute or chronic, and is usually a response to the destruction of pancreatic tissue by its own digestive enzymes (*autodigestion*) that have been released from damaged pancreatic cells.

ACUTE PANCREATITIS

Clinical features

Acute inflammation of the pancreas has a number of possible causes (Table 5.1), but is most commonly associated with gallstones or alcoholism.

Clinically it presents with severe epigastric pain, abdominal distention and nausea or vomiting. In milder cases, the patient may recover spontaneously. If allowed to progress untreated, peritonitis and other complications may occur.

Biochemically, levels of amylase and lipase (the pancreatic enzymes responsible for the digestion of starch and lipids) in the blood and urine are raised. Acute inflammation causes the pancreatic tissue to become necrosed, releasing pancreatic enzymes, which can further destroy the pancreatic tissue and also the capillary walls after entering the blood stream.

Ultrasound appearances

Mild acute pancreatitis may have no demonstrable features on ultrasound, especially if the scan is performed after the acute episode has settled. Although ultrasound is used to assess the pancreas in cases of suspected acute pancreatitis, its main role is in demonstrating the *cause* of the pancreatitis, for example biliary calculi, in order to plan further management. The ultrasound finding of microlithiasis or sludge in the gallbladder is highly significant in cases of suspected pancreatitis[7] (see Chapter 3) and is often implicated in the cause of recurrent pancreatitis.

Acute idiopathic pancreatitis (AIP) is a term used when the cause of pancreatitis has not been demonstrated, although the majority of these do turn out to have microlithiasis or biliary sludge. Improved ultrasound imaging is more readily able to detect microlithiasis, and EUS is particularly useful in such cases, as it is more sensitive in detecting tiny stones in the CBD. In more severe cases the pancreas becomes enlarged and hypoechoic due to oedema. The main duct may be dilated or prominent (Fig. 5.3).

As the condition progresses, digestive enzymes leak out forming collections, or *pseudocysts*. These are most frequently found in the lesser sac, near

Biliary calculi	Most common cause. Obstructs the main pancreatic duct/papilla of Vater and may cause reflux of bile into the pancreatic duct
Alcoholism	Alcohol overstimulates pancreatic secretions causing overproduction of enzymes
Trauma/iatrogenic	Damage/disruption of the pancreatic tissue, e.g. in a road traffic accident, or by surgery, biopsy or ESWL[6]
Drug induced	A relatively uncommon cause. Some anti-cancer drugs can cause chemical injury
Infection	E.g. mumps. A rare cause of pancreatitis
Congenital anomaly	Duodenal diverticulum, duodenal duplication, sphincter of Oddi stenosis or choledochal cyst may obstruct the pancreatic duct, giving rise to pancreatitis
Hereditary	A rare, autosomal dominant condition presenting with recurrent attacks in childhood or early adulthood

ESWL, extracorporeal shock wave lithotripsy.

Table 5.1 Causes of acute pancreatitis

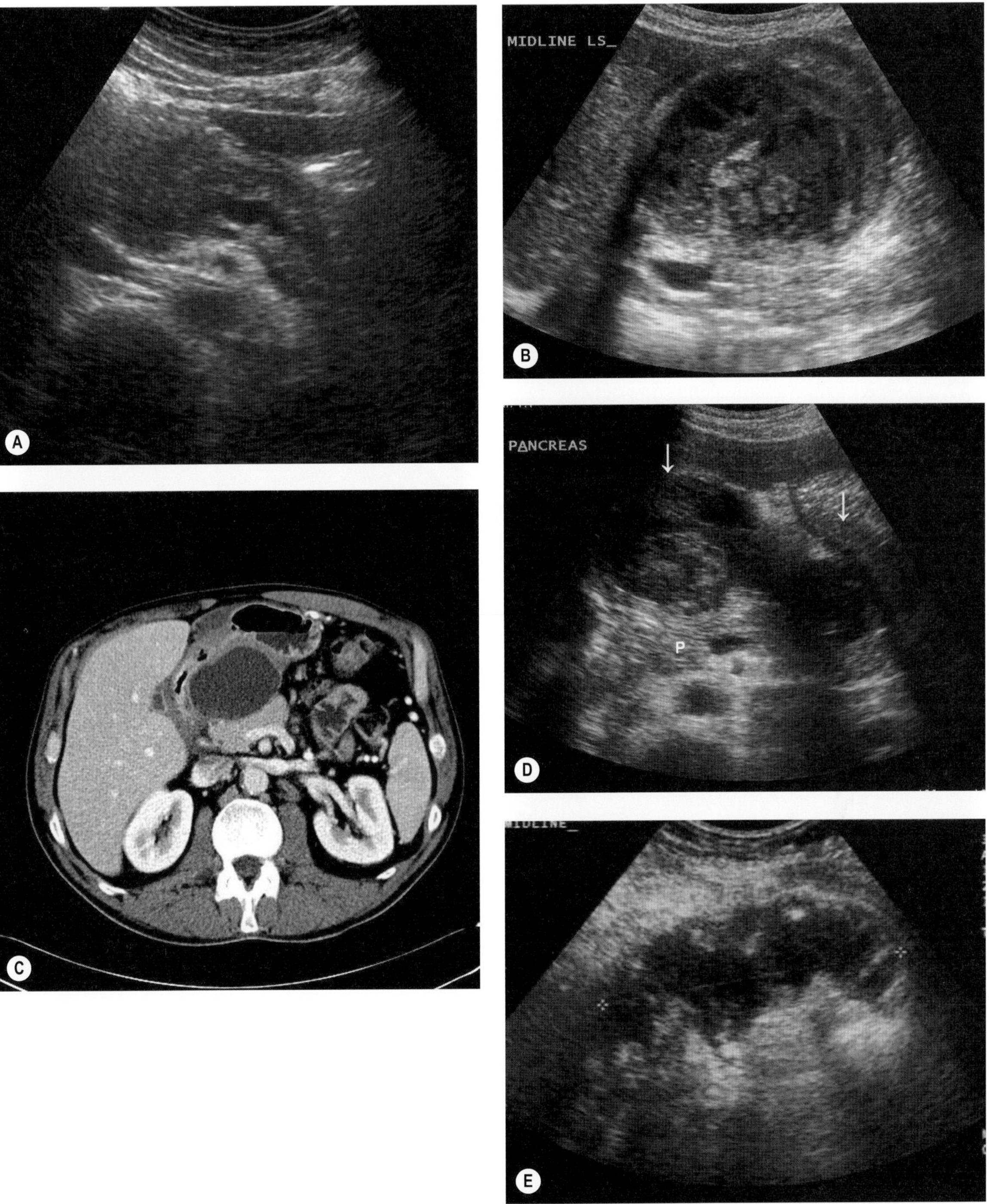

Fig. 5.3 • Acute pancreatitis: (A) Acute pancreatitis in autoimmune pancreatitis. a patient with alcoholic liver disease. The pancreas is hypoechoic and bulky with a lobulated outline and dilated main duct. (B) Large pseudocyst near the body of pancreas in acute pancreatitis. (C) CT of the case in (A), showing pseudocyst anterior to the pancreas. (D) Exudate (arrows) anterior to the body and tail of pancreas. P = head of pancreas. (E) The pancreas (calipers) has become necrotic after repeated attacks of pancreatitis.

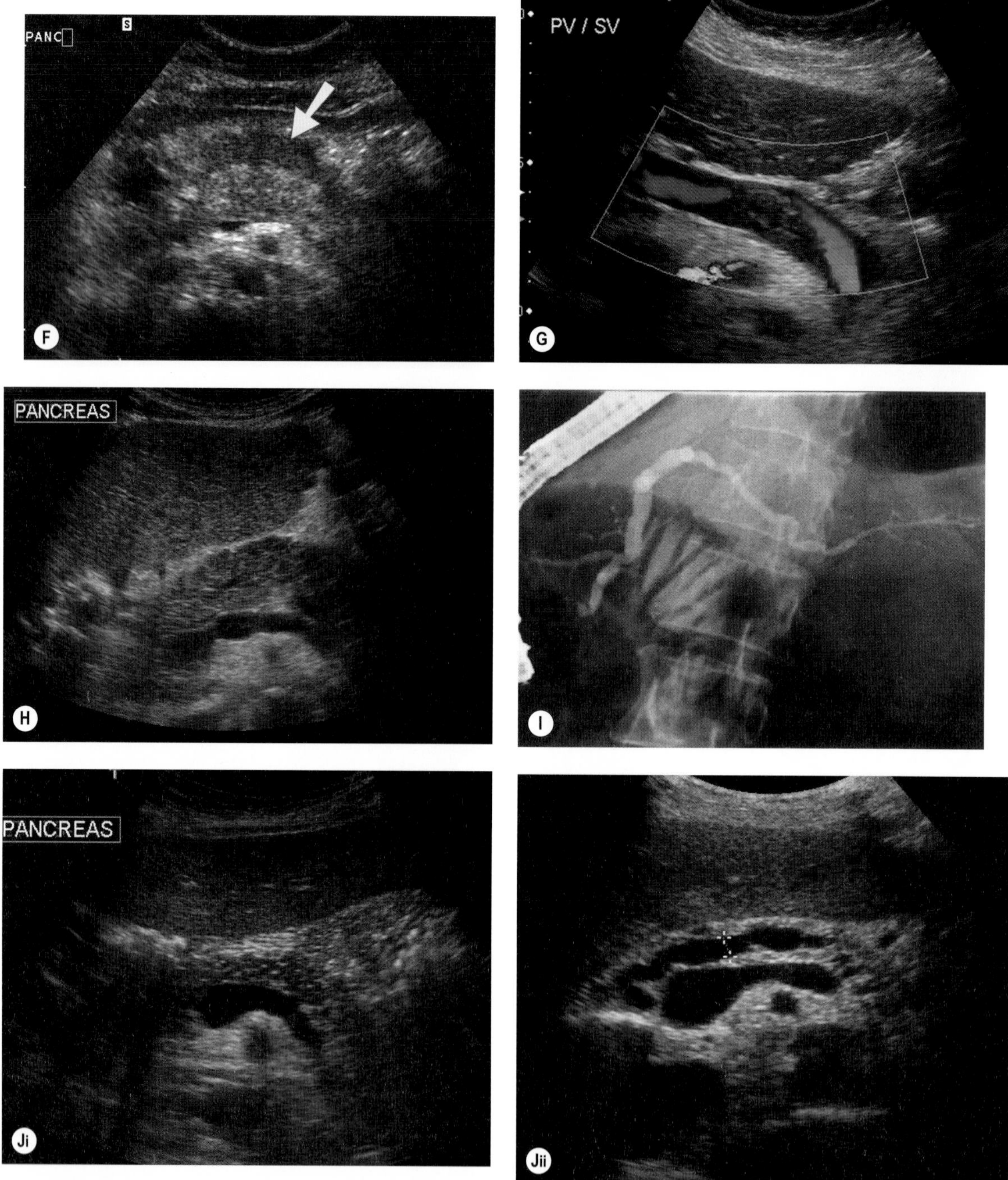

Fig. 5.3, cont'd • (F) Inflammatory exudate (arrow) is seen around the right kidney in acute pancreatitis. (G) Splenic and portal vein thrombosis is a complication of pancreatitis. (H) Acute inflammation demonstrating an enlarged, tender oedematous pancreas, which is relatively hypoechoic. (I) ERCP. A patient with pancreatitis has a dilated proximal pancreatic duct. (J) HIV with associated pancreatitis. The pancreas is relatively hypoechoic (Ji), and in another case, pancreatic duct dilatation is present (Jii).

the tail of the pancreas, but can occur anywhere in the abdomen – within the pancreatic tissue itself, anywhere in the peritoneal or retroperitoneal space or even tracking up the fissures into the liver – so a full abdominal ultrasound survey is essential on each attendance (Fig. 5.3). CT is particularly useful in demonstrating the complications of acute pancreatitis, including retroperitoneal changes, which may be obscured on transabdominal ultrasound.[8]

Pseudocysts are so-called because they do not have a capsule of epithelium like most cysts, but are merely collections of fluid surrounded by adjacent tissues. A pseudocyst may appear to have a capsule on ultrasound if it lies within a fold of peritoneum. Pseudocysts may be echo-free, but generally contain echoes from tissue debris and may be loculated. In a small percentage of cases, a pseudocyst or necrotic area of pancreatic tissue may become infected, forming a pancreatic abscess.

Although acute pancreatitis usually affects the entire organ, it may occur focally. This presents a diagnostic dilemma for ultrasound, as the appearances are indistinguishable from tumour. The clinical history may help to differentiate; suspicion of focal pancreatitis should be raised in patients with previous history of chronic pancreatitis, a history of alcoholism and normal CA 19-9 (a tumour marker for pancreatic carcinoma) levels.[9] The enlargement of the pancreas in acute pancreatitis may have other consequences, for example the enlarged pancreatic head may obstruct the CBD, causing biliary dilatation.

Doppler ultrasound is useful in assessing associated vascular complications. Prolonged and repeated attacks of acute pancreatitis may cause the splenic vein to become encased and compressed, causing splenic and/or portal vein thrombosis, with all its attendant sequelae (see Chapter 4).

Management of acute pancreatitis

While ultrasound is useful in demonstrating associated gallstones, biliary sludge and fluid collections, CT or MRI demonstrates the complications of acute pancreatitis with greater sensitivity and specificity. Localized areas of necrotic pancreatic tissue can be demonstrated on contrast-enhanced CT, together with vascular complications, such as thrombosis.

MRCP or CT is used to demonstrate the main pancreatic duct and its point of insertion into the CBD. Anomalous insertions are associated with pancreatitis, due to the reflux of bile into the pancreatic duct. ERCP, which is more invasive and subject to potential complications, is generally reserved for circumstances which require the removal of stones, alleviating the need for surgery, and in the placement of stents in the case of strictures.[10]

Pancreatitis can be difficult to treat, and management consists of alleviating the symptoms and removing the cause where possible. Patients with gallstone pancreatitis do well after cholecystectomy, but if the gallbladder is not removed, recurrent attacks of increasingly severe inflammation occur in up to a third of patients.

Pseudocysts that do not resolve spontaneously may be drained percutaneously under ultrasound or CT guidance, or, depending on the site of the collection, a drain may be positioned endoscopically from the cyst into the stomach.[11] Pseudocyst formation may cause thrombosis of the splenic vein, spreading to the portal and mesenteric veins in some cases. Other vascular complications include splenic artery aneurysm, which may form as a result of damage to the artery by the pseudocyst.

Surgery to remove necrotized or haemorrhagic areas of pancreatic tissue may be undertaken in severe cases.

CHRONIC PANCREATITIS

Patients with acute pancreatitis are at risk of repeated inflammatory episodes that eventually develop into chronic inflammation. The most common cause is alcohol abuse. In other cases, chronic pancreatitis has a gradual onset, which does not seem to be associated with previous acute attacks.

The normal pancreatic tissue is progressively replaced by fibrosis, which may encase the nerves in the coeliac plexus, causing abdominal pain, particularly post prandial. The patient has fatty stools (steatorrhoea) due to malabsorption, as there is a decreased capacity to produce the digestive enzymes.

Diagnosis of chronic pancreatitis can be difficult, especially in the early stages.[12] Serum enzyme levels are less elevated than in acute disease (if at

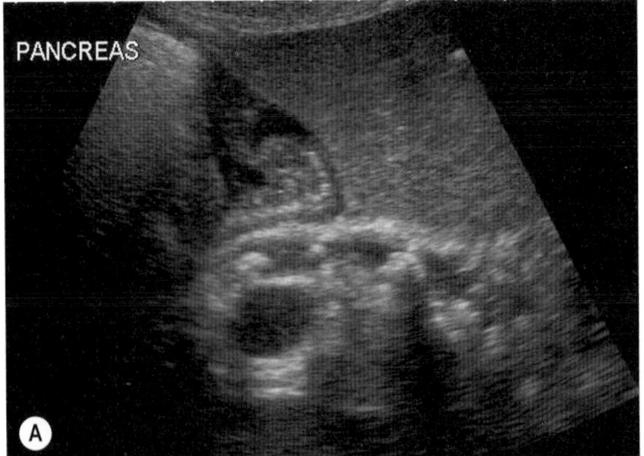

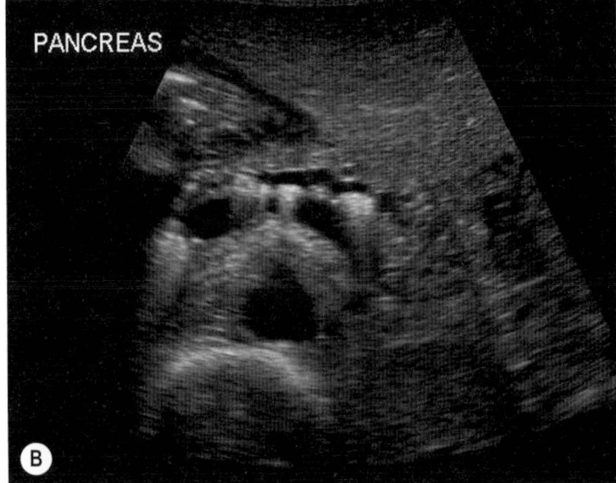

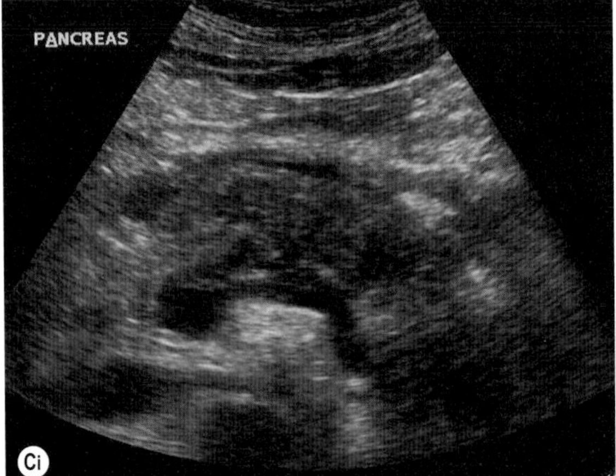

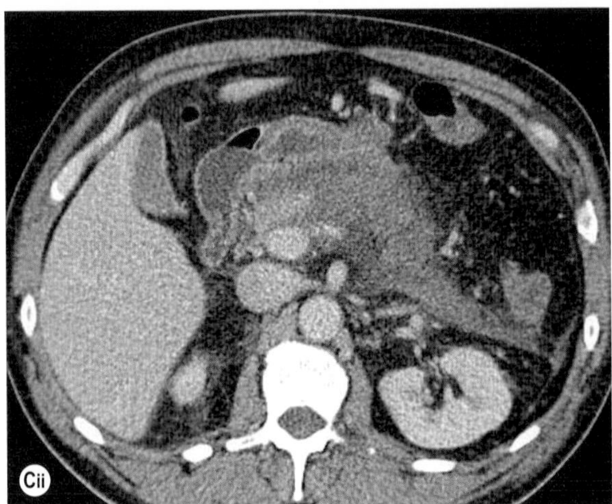

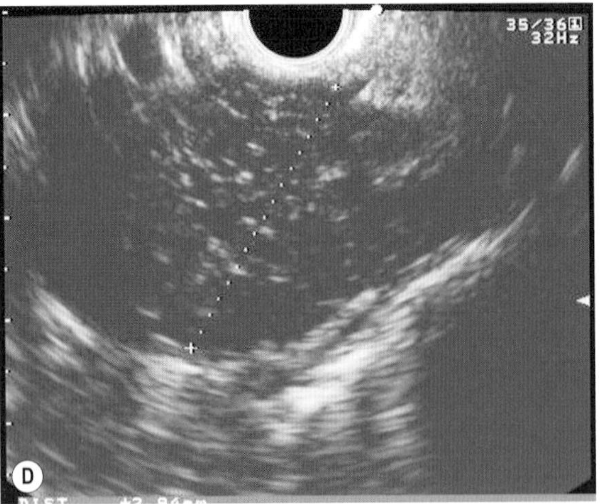

Fig. 5.4 • Chronic pancreatitis. (A) Chronic pancreatitis in a patient with hereditary pancreatitis; the pancreas is hyperechoic with stones in the dilated duct. (B) Calcification of the pancreas in alcoholic pancreatitis, with a prominent main duct. (Ci) An acute phase in a patient with a history of repeated acute on chronic pancreatitis. The pancreas is now necrotic and the SV contains thrombus. (Cii) CT demonstrates a lack of contrast in the necrotic pancreatic tissue. (D) EUS of a patient with autoimmune pancreatitis. The pancreas is swollen and hypoechoic; the operator is lined up to do an ultrasound-guided biopsy.

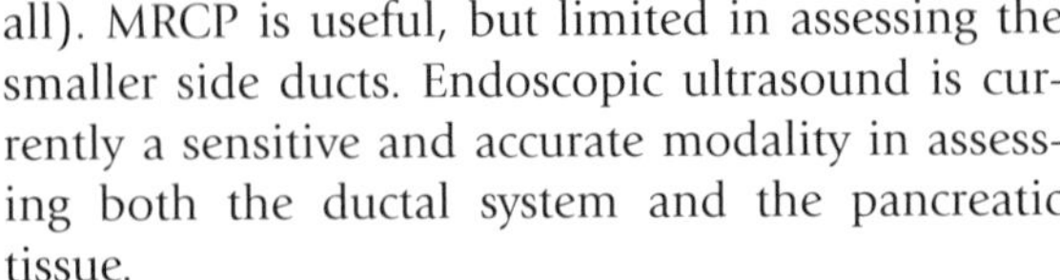

all). MRCP is useful, but limited in assessing the smaller side ducts. Endoscopic ultrasound is currently a sensitive and accurate modality in assessing both the ductal system and the pancreatic tissue.

Ultrasound appearances

The pancreas becomes abnormally hyperechoic (Fig. 5.4A). This should not be confused with the normal increase in echogenicity with age. The gland may be atrophied and lobulated and the main pancreatic duct is frequently dilated and ectatic,[13] with a beaded appearance.

Calcification may be identified in the pancreatic tissue, both on ultrasound and on a plain X-ray, and there may be stones in the duct. Generally speaking, strong shadows are cast from the calcific foci, but small flecks may be too small to shadow (Fig. 5.4B, C). As with acute inflammation, CT is the method of choice for demonstrating the complications of chronic pancreatitis.

Obstruction of the duct can cause pseudocyst formation, and other complications include biliary obstruction and portal/splenic vein thrombosis.

MALIGNANT PANCREATIC DISEASE

PANCREATIC CARCINOMA

Clinical features and management

Carcinoma of the pancreas is usually an aggressive cancer, and is currently the fourth most common cause of cancer-related death. It carries a very poor prognosis – 5-year survival is less than 5%.[14,15] Metastatic deposits from primary pancreatic adenocarcinoma occur early in the course of the disease, and 80% of patients already have nodal disease or distant metastases in the lungs, liver or bone by the time the diagnosis is made, which accounts for the poor prognosis.

The presenting symptoms depend on the size of the lesion, its position within the pancreas and the extent of metastatic deposits. Most pancreatic carcinomas (60%) are found in the head of the pancreas,[16] and patients present with the associated symptoms of jaundice due to obstruction of the CBD (Fig. 5.5). Carcinomas located in the body or tail of pancreas do not cause obstructive jaundice and are therefore more likely to present late, when treatment options become even more limited.

The majority (80%) of pancreatic cancers are ductal adenocarcinomas, most of which are located in the head of pancreas. The rest comprise a mixed bag of less common neoplasms and endocrine tumours. Endocrine tumours, which originate in the islet cells of the pancreas, tend to be either insulinomas (generally benign) or gastrinomas (malignant). These present with hormonal abnormalities while the tumour is still small and are more amenable to detection by EUS than by conventional sonography.

Cystic neoplasms of the pancreas have become increasingly recognized due to better imaging techniques,[17] and usually represent serous or mucinous tumours (Fig. 5.5E). They pose a diagnostic dilemma, appearing predominantly cystic on ultrasound, and tend to be located in the body or tail of pancreas. They follow a much less aggressive course than adenocarcinomas, metastasizing late and have a much higher curative rate with surgery.[18] The presence of calcification may be a pointer to malignancy in a cystic lesion, but is still difficult to differentiate from an inflammatory mass.

Surgical removal of the carcinoma by partial pancreaticoduodenectomy – the Whipple procedure – may be curative but only 20% of patients have a tumour that is potentially resectable, and the 5-year survival rate following resection is less than 5%.[19] Over 70% of patients die from hepatic metastases within 3 years post-operatively.[20]

Differential diagnoses of pancreatic masses must always be considered (Table 5.2); focal lesions in the pancreas may represent inflammatory rather than malignant masses. Ultrasound guided biopsy of pancreatic masses suffers from low sensitivity[21] due to the inflammatory element surrounding many carcinomas, so a negative biopsy is unhelpful.

Endosonography-guided aspiration or biopsy, however, has high sensitivity and specificity for diagnosing pancreatic cancer, and is also useful in patients with a previous negative biopsy in whom malignancy is suspected.[22] ERCP may also be used to insert a palliative stent in the CBD, to relieve biliary obstruction.

The detection of a pancreatic carcinoma by ultrasound is usefully followed by a CT scan for staging purposes as this will demonstrate invasion of peripancreatic fat, vascular involvement and lymphadenopathy.

Ultrasound appearances of pancreatic carcinoma

Adenocarcinoma, which comprises 80% of pancreatic neoplasms, is a solid tumour, usually hypoechoic or of mixed echogenicity, with an irregular border (Fig. 5.5). Because the mass is most frequently located in the head of the pancreas, which lies behind the duodenum, it may be difficult to identify at first. The major clue is in dilatation of the CBD, which must be carefully traced to its point of obstruction. Adenocarcinoma is a vascular tumour, and Doppler may demonstrate high velocity arterial flow within it in many cases. CEUS may assist in demonstrating the extent of the tumour[23] although CT is still widely considered the imaging of choice for staging purposes.[24] The pancreatic

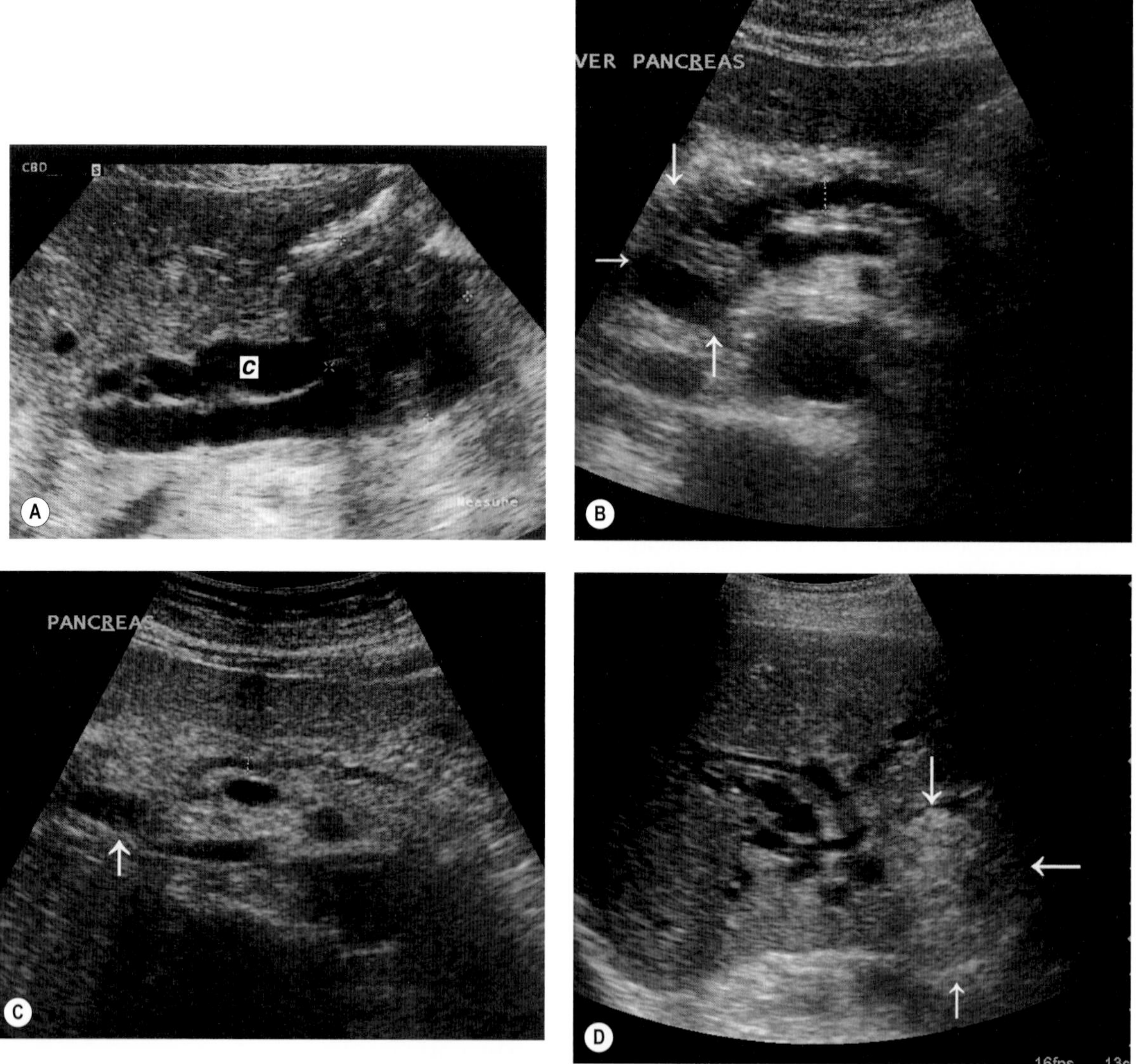

Fig. 5.5 • Pancreatic carcinoma: (A) The common bile duct, c, is obstructed by a large hypoechoic solid mass at its lower end (calipers), which is a carcinoma in the head of pancreas. (B) TS through the pancreas, demonstrating a complex mucinous cystadenocarcinoma in the head (arrows) causing dilatation of the main pancreatic duct (calipers). (C) A small, hypoechoic adenocarcinoma (arrow) in the HOP causing mild pancreatic duct dilatation. (D) Intrahepatic duct dilatation caused by a large tumour in the head of pancreas (arrows), confirmed by CT.

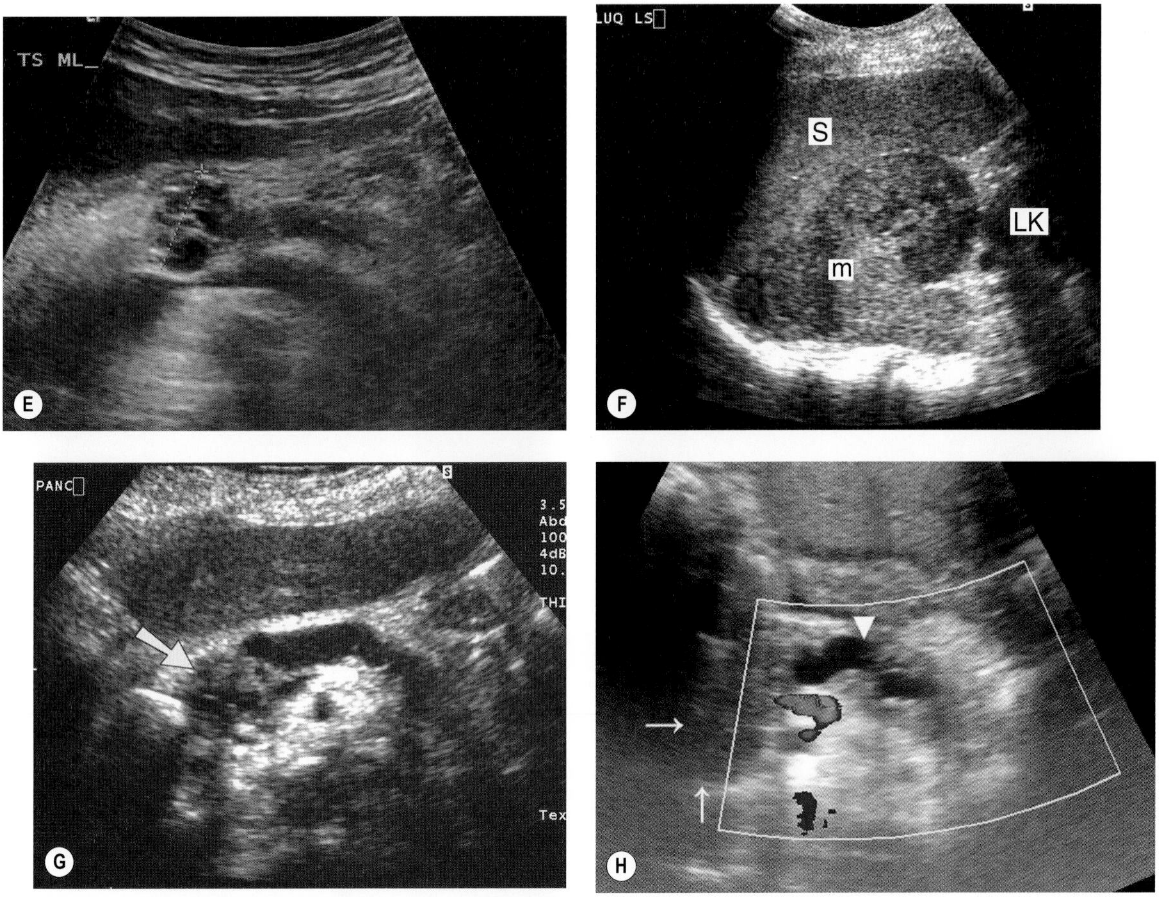

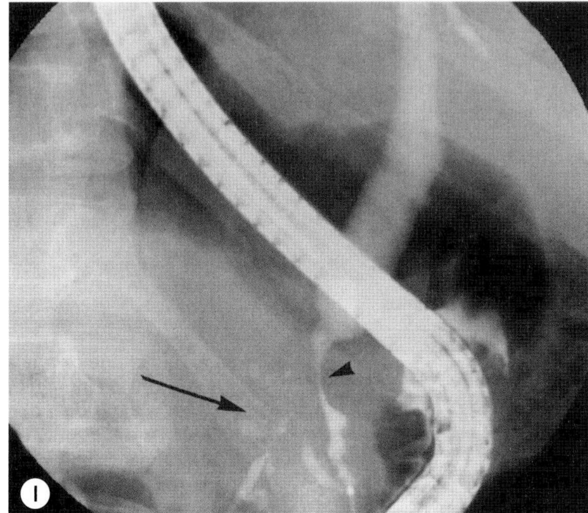

Fig. 5.5, cont'd • (E) Complex cystic mass in the head of pancreas, confirmed as a cystadenocarcinoma. (F) A complex mass (m) between the spleen (S) and the left kidney is a large carcinoma of the tail of pancreas. (G) Dilated pancreatic duct due to a carcinoma in the head (arrow). (H) Colour Doppler helps to differentiate the dilated pancreatic duct (arrowhead), which does not contain flow. The dilatation is caused by a carcinoma in the HOP (arrows). (I) ERCP demonstrating a long stricture of the pancreatic duct (arrow) involving the side branches, in a large pancreatic carcinoma. The CBD is compressed (arrowhead) by nodes, causing biliary dilatation. A palliative stent was inserted.

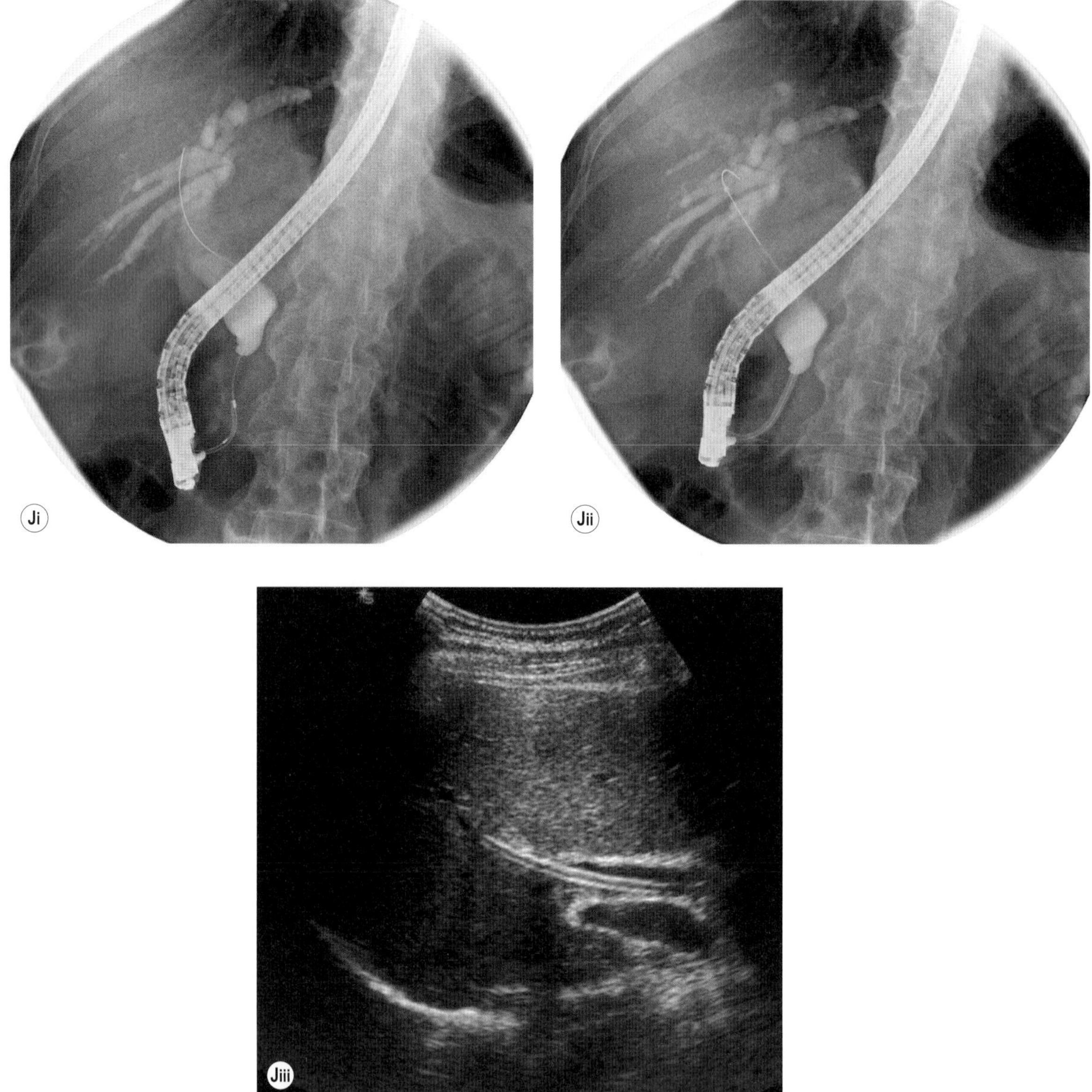

Fig. 5.5, cont'd • (Ji, ii) ERCP is used to place a stent in the CBD to decompress the ducts, later demonstrated on ultrasound (Jiii).

duct distal to the mass may be dilated. It may, in fact, be so dilated that it can be initially mistaken for the splenic vein. The walls of the duct, however, are usually more irregular than the smooth, continuous walls of the splenic vein. Colour Doppler is useful in confirming the lack of flow in the duct and in identifying the vein behind it (Fig. 5.5G, H).

Endocrine tumours, which arise from the islet cells in the pancreas, include insulinomas, which are benign, and gastrinomas, which are more often malignant. They are usually hypoechoic, well defined and exhibit a mass effect, often with a distally dilated main pancreatic duct. They are generally smaller at presentation than adenocarcinomas, and tend to arise in the body or tail of pancreas. Up to 40% of these tumours go undetected by both transabdominal ultrasound and CT, with endoscopic ultrasound and laparoscopic

SOLID	
Adenocarcinoma	Hypoechoic, usually in the HOP
Focal acute pancreatitis	Hypoechoic. Clinical history of pancreatitis
Focal chronic pancreatitis	Hyperechoic, sometimes with calcification. History of pancreatitis
Endocrine tumour	Less common. Small, hypoechoic, well-defined
Metastases	Late manifestation, widespread disease
CYSTIC[17]	
Pseudocyst	History of pancreatitis
Mucinous tumour, serous cystadenoma, intraductal papillary mucinous neoplasm (IPNM)	Less common than adenocarcinoma – tend to form in the body or tail of pancreas. More favourable prognosis following resection
Necrotic or haemorrhagic tumour	
Simple cyst	Rare. Exclude polycystic disease by scanning the liver and kidneys

Table 5.2 Differential diagnoses of focal pancreatic masses

ultrasound having the highest detection rates for insulinomas. Gastrinomas tend to be multiple and may also be extra-pancreatic.

A small proportion of pancreatic cancers contain an obvious fluid content (see above) and are similar in acoustic appearance to a pseudocyst, but unlike a pseudocyst, a mucinous neoplasm is not usually associated with a history of pancreatitis. However, some low-grade malignancies can cause pancreatitis if the duct is obstructed[25] and aspiration of fluid by EUS is useful, especially in the presence of elevated CEA.

It is also possible to see areas of haemorrhage or necrosis within a lesion, which look complex or fluid-filled. Calcification is also seen occasionally within pancreatic carcinomas.[26]

Secondary ultrasound findings in pancreatic adenocarcinoma

The most obvious secondary feature of carcinoma of the head of pancreas is the dilated biliary system (see section on obstructive jaundice in Chapter 2). In a recent series of 62 pancreatic cancers, biliary dilatation occurred in 69%, pancreatic duct dilatation in 37% and the *double duct sign* (pancreatic and biliary duct dilatation) in 34% of patients.[26]

Although the gallbladder is frequently dilated with no visible stones this is not always the case; incidental gallstones may be present, causing chronic inflammation which prevents the gallbladder from dilating. For this reason it is imperative that the CBD is carefully traced down to the head of pancreas to identify the cause of obstruction.

A thorough search for lymphadenopathy and liver metastases should always be made. If the mass is large, it is not possible to differentiate whether it arises from the ampulla of Vater (see Chapter 3) or the head of pancreas. This differentiation, however, is usually academic at this stage. Colour Doppler can demonstrate considerable vascularity within the mass, and may also identify vascular invasion of the coeliac axis, SMA, hepatic, splenic and/or gastroduodenal arteries and of the portal and splenic veins – a factor that is particularly important in assessing the suitability of the tumour for curative resection.

The recognition of involvement of peripancreatic vessels by carcinoma with colour Doppler, together with the ultrasound assessment of compression or encasement of these vessels, has been found to be highly sensitive and specific (79% and 89%) for diagnosing unresectability,[27] thus the need for further investigative procedures such as CT may be avoided, particularly in cases of large tumours.[28] Palliative care using stent insertion with ERCP (Fig. 5.5J) alleviates the biliary obstruction.

PANCREATIC METASTASES

Pancreatic metastases may occur from breast, lung and gastrointestinal tract primary tumours. They are relatively uncommon on ultrasound (Fig. 5.6), simply because they are a late manifestation in patients who already have known widespread disease and in whom investigations are generally considered unnecessary.

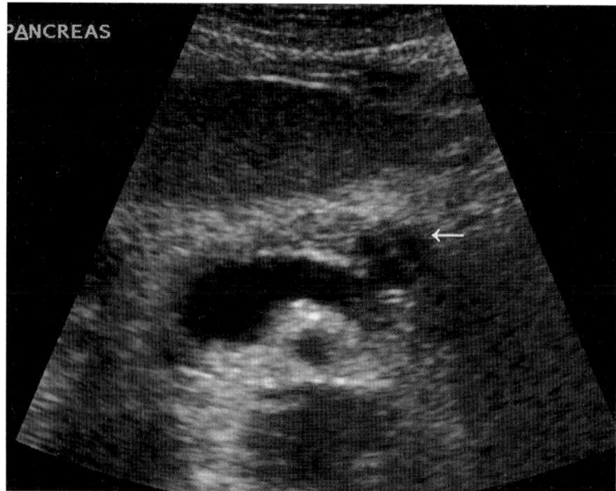

Fig. 5.6 • Metastatic deposit (arrow) from primary breast carcinoma in the body of pancreas.

Box 5.1

Pathology of the pancreas, both benign and malignant, can affect the adjacent vasculature by compression, encasement or thrombosis.

Doppler of the splenic, portal and superior mesenteric veins is useful in demonstrating the extent of vascular complication when pancreatic abnormalities are suspected.

Widespread metastatic disease can be demonstrated on ultrasound, particularly in the liver, and there is often considerable epigastric lymphadenopathy, which can be confused with the appearances of pancreatic metastases on the scan. See also Box 5.1.

BENIGN FOCAL PANCREATIC LESIONS

FOCAL FATTY SPARING OF THE PANCREAS

The uncinate process and ventral portion of the head of pancreas may sometimes appear hypoechoic in comparison with the rest of the gland (Fig. 5.7). This is due to a relative lack of fatty deposition and is often more noticeable in older patients, in whom the pancreas is normally hyperechoic. Its significance lies in not confusing it with a focal pancreatic mass. The area of fatty sparing is well defined, with no enlargement or mass effect and is regarded as a normal variation in the ultrasound appearances. If doubt exists, CT will differentiate fatty sparing from true neoplasm.[29]

FOCAL PANCREATITIS

Inflammation can affect the whole, or just part of the gland. Occasionally, areas of hypoechoic, focal acute or chronic pancreatitis are present (see Pancreatitis, above). These are invariably a diagnostic dilemma, as they are indistinguishable on ultrasound from focal malignant lesions (Fig. 5.8). Factors that point towards inflammation include a previous history of pancreatitis, and a normal CA 19-9 tumour marker level.

Because malignant lesions are frequently surrounded by an inflammatory reaction, biopsy is also of questionable help in differentiation of focal benign and malignant lesions.

OTHER BENIGN LESIONS

Benign cysts in the pancreas are rare (Fig. 5.9A) and tend to be associated with other conditions such as polycystic disease, cystic fibrosis or von Hippel–Lindau disease (an autosomal dominant disease characterized by pancreatic and renal cysts, renal carcinoma, phaeochromocytoma and/or

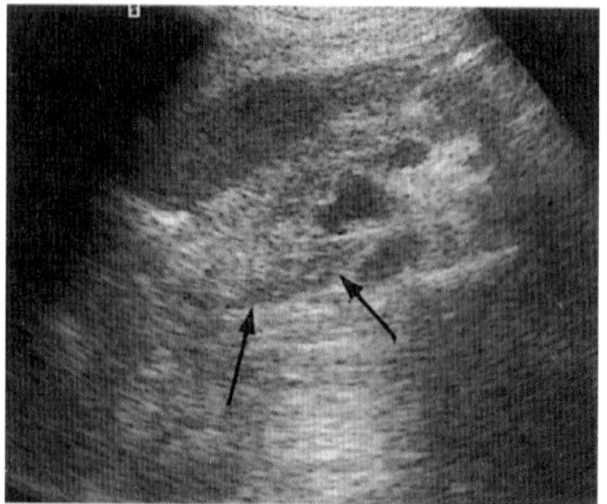

Fig. 5.7 • The uncinate process is relatively hypoechoic (arrows) due to fatty sparing.

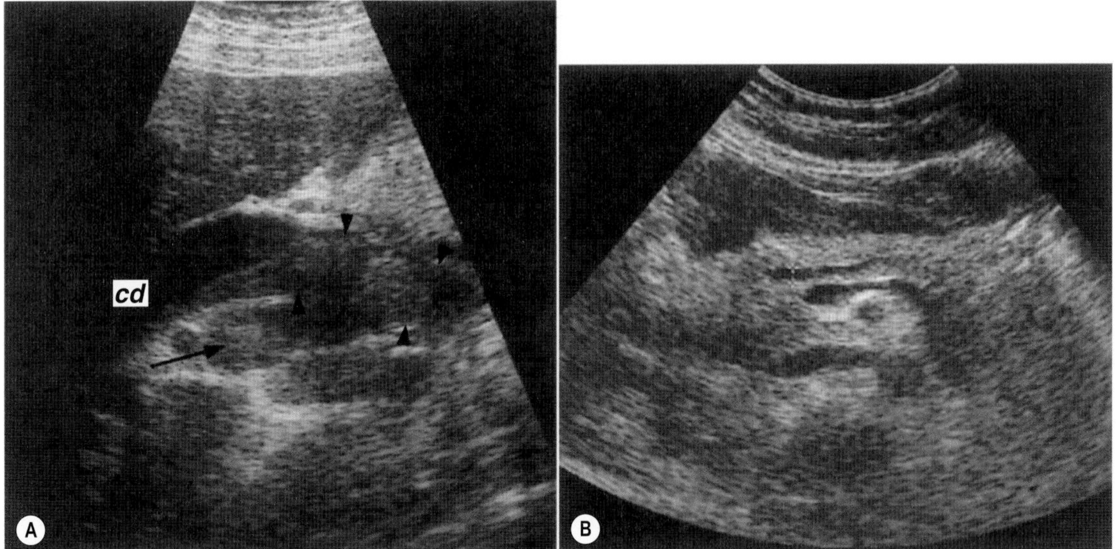

Fig. 5.8 • (A) Focal acute pancreatitis in the head of pancreas. The CBD is obstructed by a hypoechoic mass in the head, with blood clots and debris within the duct. The differential diagnosis is malignancy. (B) The same patient 8 months later. The acute inflammation has resolved, the obstruction is relieved and the pancreas now appears hyperechoic with a mildly dilated duct, consistent with chronic pancreatitis.

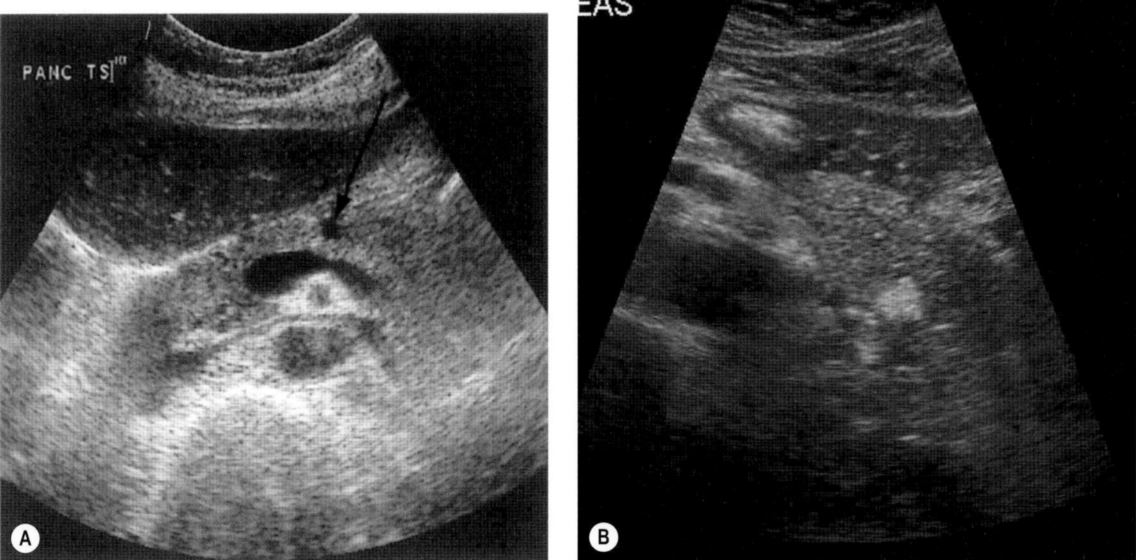

Fig. 5.9 • (A) Tiny cyst in the body of pancreas. This was confirmed on CT and remained stable over a period of 2 years. (B) Small, well-defined, hyperechoic lesion in the TOP which remained stable over a number of years. Assumed to be a rare, benign haemangioma (no histology available), although any solid mass in the pancreas is usually suspected to be malignant until proven otherwise.

haemangioblastomas in the cerebellum and spine). The presence of a cystic mass in the absence of these conditions should raise the suspicion of one of the rarer types of cystic carcinoma, or a pseudocyst associated with acute pancreatitis.

Pancreatic haemangiomas, unlike those in the liver, are extremely rare (Fig. 5.9B). Any complex cystic or solid lesion in the pancreas is usually considered suspicious for malignancy until proved otherwise.

TRAUMA OF THE PANCREAS

The pancreas is particularly vulnerable to 'blunt' trauma in road traffic accidents, in which the upper abdomen is thrown against the seat belt, resulting in laceration – often at the neck of the pancreas. The duct may be ruptured, with consequent leakage of pancreatic juice into the abdominal cavity and severe cases result in complete pancreatic transection with pancreatic ascites. The release of pancreatic enzymes triggers pancreatitis and/or peritonitis, with the gland appearing enlarged and hypoechoic.

Ultrasound may be helpful in identifying haemoperitoneum or localizing a collection, but it will not differentiate pancreatic secretions from haematoma. CT is the method of choice in cases of suspected pancreatic trauma, although even here the signs of injury can be surprisingly subtle considering the damage.[30]

PANCREATIC TRANSPLANTATION

In patients with insulin-dependent diabetes mellitus with end-stage renal disease, simultaneous pancreatic and kidney transplantation is a successful treatment that improves the quality of life and the survival of the patients.[31] Typically such patients also have severe complications, such as retinopathy and vascular disease, which may be stabilized, or even reversed, by transplantation. Simultaneous pancreas and kidney transplantation now has a 1-year graft survival of almost 90% due to improved organ preservation techniques, surgical techniques and immunosuppression.[32]

The transplanted kidney is placed in the iliac fossa with the pancreas on the contralateral side. The donor kidney is plumbed in as usual, with anastomoses to the recipient iliac artery and vein. The pancreatic vessels are anastamosed to the contralateral iliac vessels.

The pancreatic secretions are primarily by enteric drainage, as the previous method of bladder drainage was associated with an increased incidence of urological complications such as urinary tract infection, haematuria and reflux pancreatitis.[33]

Postoperative complications include rejection, sepsis, inflammation, anastomotic leak or vascular thrombosis. Localized post-operative bleeding usually resolves spontaneously. Ultrasound is useful in locating fluid collections, but CT is most often used to assess pancreatitis or anastomotic leaks.[34]

Ultrasound appearances

Ultrasound, while useful for evaluating renal transplant perfusion is less useful for the transplanted pancreas, which is frequently obscured by overlying bowel. The donor pancreas is usually situated in the iliac fossa but can be placed more centrally, particularly if a renal transplant has also been performed.

Ultrasound is limited in its ability to assess the transplanted pancreas, even if it can be located amongst the bowel loops. The lack of an adjacent reference organ, such as the liver, makes assessment of its echogenicity subjective, and therefore subtle degrees of inflammation are difficult to detect. Fluid collections are frequently concealed beneath bowel and, when identified, their appearance is non-specific. Contrast CT is more successful in detecting anastomotic leaks and collections, and is usually used for guided aspiration.

Colour Doppler can display perfusion throughout the pancreas and the main vessels may be

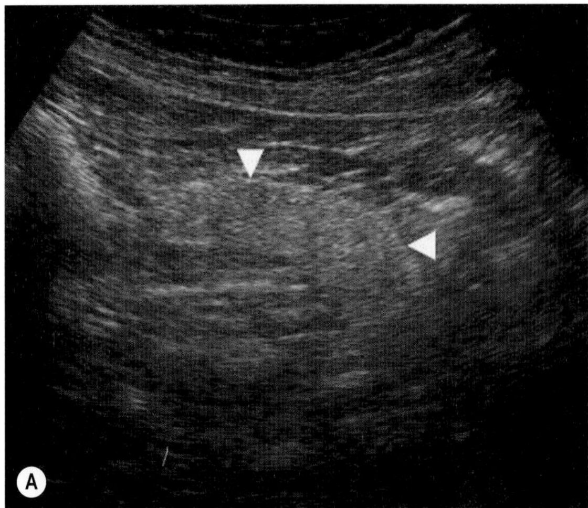

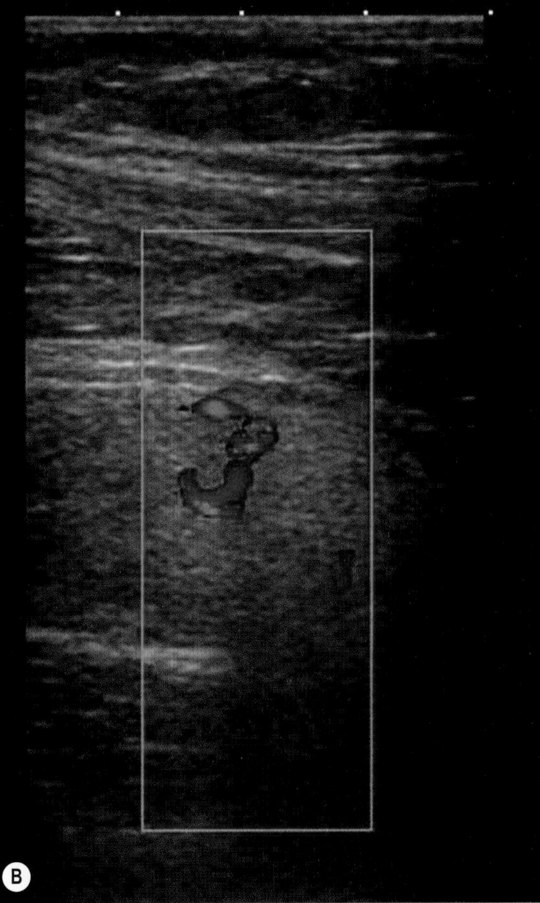

Fig. 5.10 • (A) The transplanted pancreas (arrowheads) is difficult to identify in the iliac fossa due to adjacent bowel and lack of the usual anatomical markers. (B) A high frequency helps to identify perfusion in the body of the pancreatic transplant.

traced to their anastomoses, depending on overlying bowel (Fig. 5.10).

Neither CT nor ultrasound are particularly helpful in evaluating rejection, and it is difficult to differentiate transplant pancreatitis from true rejection. The Doppler resistance index does not correlate with a rejection process and has not been found useful. MRI is able to detect vascular occlusion and both arterial and venous thrombosis, and is particularly useful in patients in whom the pancreas is obscured by overlying bowel.

References

1. Hallal AH, Amortegui JD, Jeroukhimov IM et al. Magnetic resonance cholangiopancreatography accurately detects common bile duct stones in resolving gallstone pancreatitis. J Am Coll Surg 2005; 200: 869–875
2. Brambs HJ. Developmental anomalies and congenital disorders of the pancreas. Radiologe 1996; 36: 381–388
3. Calvo MM, Bujanda L, Calderson A et al. Comparison between magnetic resonance cholangiopancreatography and ERCP for evaluation of the pancreatic duct. Am J Gastroenterol 2002; 97: 347–353
4. Rizk M, Gerke H. Utility of endoscopic ultrasound in pancreatitis: A review. World J Gastroenterol 2007; 13: 6321–6326
5. Rickes S, Mönkemüller K, Malfertheiner P. Acute severe pancreatitis: contrast-enhanced sonography. Abdom Imaging 2007; 32: 362–364
6. Siech M, Boker M, Beger HG. Extracorporeal shock wave lithotripsy as a cause of acute pancreatitis. Dig Surg 1996; 13: 210–221
7. Pezzilli R, Billi P, Barakat B et al. Ultrasonic evaluation of the common bile duct in biliary acute pancreatitis patients: comparison with endoscopic retrograde cholangiopancreatography. J Ultrasound Med 1999; 18: 391–394

8. Morgan DE. Imaging of acute pancreatitis and its complications. Clin Gastroenterol Hepatol 2008; 6: 1077–1085
9. Yamaguchi K, Chijiiwa K, Saiki S et al. 'Mass-forming' pancreatitis masquerades as pancreatic carcinoma. Int J Pancreatol 1996; 20: 27–35
10. Madhotra R, Lombard M. Endoscopic retrograde cholangiopancreatography should no longer be used as a diagnostic test: the case against. Dig Liver Dis 2002; 34: 375–380
11. Gumaste VV, Pitchumoni CS. Pancreatic pseudocyst. Gastroenterologist 1996; 4: 33–43
12. Glasbrenner B, Kahl S, Malfertheiner P. Modern diagnostics of chronic pancreatitis. Eur J Gastroenterol Hepatol 2002; 14: 935–941
13. Bolondi L, LiBassi S, Gaiani S, Barbara L. Sonography of chronic pancreatitis. Radiol Clin North Am 1989; 27: 815–833
14. Garcea G, Dennison AR, Pattenden CJ et al. Survival following curative resection for pancreatic ductal adenocarcinoma. A systematic review of the literature. Pancreas 2008; 9: 99–132
15. Iott MJ, Corsini MM, Miller RC. Evidence-based guidelines for adjuvant therapy for resected adenocarcinoma of the pancreas. Clin J Oncol Nurs 2008; 12: 599–605
16. Damjanov I. Pancreatic neoplasms. In: Pathology for health related professionals. Saunders, Philadelphia, 1996, pp 324–326
17. Mulkeen A, Yoo P, Cha C. Less common neoplasms of the pancreas. World J Gastroenterol 2006; 12: 3180–3185
18. Lichtenstein DR, Carr-Locke DL. Mucin-secreting tumours of the pancreas. Gastrointest Endosc Clin N Am 1995; 5: 237–258
19. Cooperman AM, Kini S, Snady H et al. Current surgical therapy for carcinoma of the pancreas. J Clin Gastroenterol 2000; 31: 107–113
20. Ishikawa O, Ohigashi H, Imaoka S et al. Is the long-term survival rate improved by preoperative irradiation prior to Whipple's procedure for adenocarcinoma of the pancreatic head? Arch Surg 1994; 129: 1075–1080
21. Di Stasi M, Lencioni R, Solmi L et al. Ultrasound-guided fine needle biopsy of pancreatic masses: results of a multicenter study. Am J Gastroenterol 1998; 93: 1329–1333
22. Rafique A, Freeman S, Carroll N. A clinical algorithm for the assessment of pancreatic lesions: utilization of 16- and 64-section multidetector CT and endoscopic ultrasound. Clin Radiol 2007; 62: 1142–1153
23. D'Onofrio M, Zamboni G, Faccioli N et al. Ultrasonography of the pancreas. 4. Contrast-enhanced imaging. Abdom Imaging 2007; 32: 171–181
24. Furukawa H, Uesaka K, Boku N. Treatment decision making in pancreatic adenocarcinoma: multidisciplinary team discussion with multidetector-row computed tomography. Arch Surg 2008; 143: 275–280
25. Brugge WR. Diagnosis and management of relapsing pancreatitis associated with cystic neoplasms of the pancreas. World J Gastroenterol 2008; 14: 1038–1043
26. Yassa N, Yang J, Stein S et al. Gray-scale and colour flow sonography of pancreatic ductal adenocarcinoma. J Clin Ultrasound 1997; 25: 473–480
27. Angeli E, Venturini M, Vanzulli A et al. Color Doppler imaging in the assessment of vascular involvement by pancreatic carcinoma. AJR Am J Roentgenol 1997; 168: 193–197
28. Tomiyama T, Ueno N, Tano S et al. Assessment of arterial invasion in pancreatic cancer using colour Doppler ultrasonography. Am J Gastroenterol 1996; 91: 1410–1416
29. Jacobs JE, Coleman BG, Arger PH, Langer JE. Pancreatic sparing of focal fatty inflitration. Radiology 1994; 190: 437–439
30. Craig MH, Talton DS, Hauser CJ, Poole GV. Pancreatic injuries from blunt trauma. Am Surg 1995; 61: 125–128
31. Dean PG, Kudva YC, Stegall MD. Long-term benefits of pancreas transplantation. Curr Opin Organ Transplant 2008; 13: 85–90
32. Krishnamurthi V, Philosophe B, Bartlett ST. Pancreas transplantation: contemporary surgical techniques. Urol Clin North Am 2001; 28: 833–838
33. Sutherland DE, Gruessner RW, Dunn DL et al. Lessons learned from more than 1000 pancreas transplants at a single institution. Ann Surg 2001; 233: 463–501
34. Green SJ, Sidhu PS, Deane CR. Imaging of simultaneous kidney pancreatic transplants. Imaging 2002; 14: 299–307

Ultrasound of the spleen and lymphatic system

6

CHAPTER CONTENTS

THE SPLEEN – NORMAL APPEARANCES AND TECHNIQUE

The spleen normally lies in the LUQ, posterior to the splenic flexure and stomach, making an anterior approach almost invariably unsuccessful due to overlying bowel gas. It is best approached via a left lateral intercostal aspect with the patient supine. In this way, gas-filled bowel is usually anterior to the spleen. Gentle respiration is frequently more successful than deep inspiration, as the latter brings the lung bases downwards, and may obscure a small spleen altogether.

Lying the patient decubitus, left side raised, may also be successful but sometimes has the effect of causing the gas-filled bowel loops to rise to the left flank, once again obscuring the spleen. A posterior approach may overcome this.

Ultrasound appearances

The normal spleen has a fine, homogeneous texture, with smooth margins and a pointed inferior edge. It has similar echogenicity to the liver (but may be slightly hypo- or hyperechoic in some subjects) but the echoes tend to be finer and more closely packed than the liver.

Sound attenuation through the spleen is less than that through the liver, requiring the operator to 'flatten' the TGC controls to maintain an even level of echoes throughout the organ.

The main splenic artery and vein and their branches may be demonstrated at the splenic hilum (Fig. 6.1). The spleen provides an excellent acoustic window to the upper pole of the left kidney, the left adrenal gland and the tail of the pancreas.

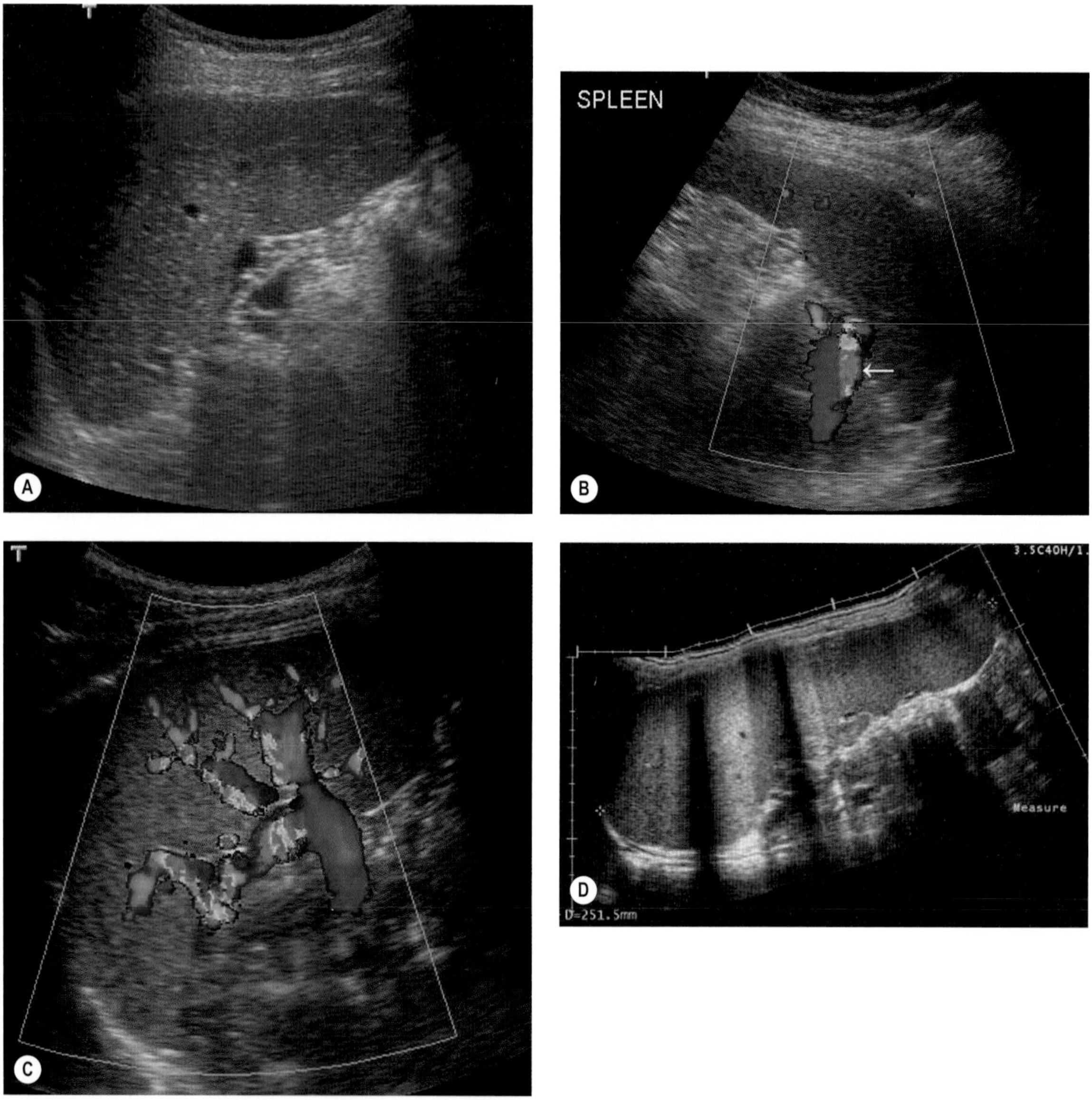

Fig. 6.1 • (A) Left coronal view of the normal spleen demonstrating vessels at the hilum. (B) Left coronal view of the normal spleen at the hilum. The splenic artery (arrow) lies alongside the vein. The PRF is set for the lower, venous velocity so the artery demonstrates 'aliasing'. (C) By increasing the Doppler sensitivity, (decreasing the PRF) the perfusion within the spleen is demonstrated. (D) An enlarged spleen can be displayed more fully using an extended field of view, allowing measurement of the length (25 cm). Shadowing from the ribs is evident.

SPLENIC VARIANTS

Spleen size and shape are both highly variable, with a gradual age-related decrease in volume. A splenic length – inferior (lateral) edge to superior medial (subdiaphragmatic) aspect – of below 12 cm is generally considered normal, although this is subject to variation in shape and the plane of measurement used.

Rarely, the diaphragmatic surface of the spleen may be lobulated, or even completely septated. This appearance may give rise to diagnostic uncertainty, and Doppler may be helpful in establishing the vascular supply, and differentiating this from other masses in the LUQ, or from scarring or infarction in the spleen.

The spleen may lie in an ectopic position, in the left flank or pelvis, or posterior to the left kidney. The ectopic (or wandering) spleen is situated on a long pedicle, allowing it to migrate within the abdomen.

The significance of this rare condition is that the pedicle may twist, causing the patient to present acutely with pain from splenic torsion. Ultrasound demonstrates the enlarged, hypoechoic organ in the abdomen, with the absence of the spleen in its normal position.

Splenomegaly

Enlargement of the spleen is a highly non-specific sign associated with numerous conditions, the most common being infection, portal hypertension, haematological disorders and neoplastic conditions (Box 6.1).

As with the liver, measurement of splenic volume is unreliable and not reproducible, due to variation in shape and subdiaphragmatic access. However, the length of the spleen is an adequate indicator of size for most purposes and provides a useful baseline for monitoring changes in disease status. The length (infero-superior) of the normal adult spleen is less than 12 cm.

The spleen enlarges downwards and medially. Its inferior margin becomes rounded (Figs 6.1D, 6.2A) and it may extend below the left kidney and into the pelvis.

Although the etiology of splenomegaly may not be obvious on ultrasound, the causes can be narrowed down by considering the clinical picture and by identifying other relevant appearances in the abdomen. Splenomegaly due to portal hypertension, for example, is frequently accompanied by other associated pathology such as cirrhotic liver changes, varices (Fig. 6.2A, B) or ascites (see Chapter 4).

BOX 6.1 Examples of causes of splenomegaly

- Portal hypertension
- Acute or chronic systemic infection – e.g. hepatitis, AIDS, infectious mononucleosis, sepsis
- Haemolytic anaemia, sickle cell disease, thalassaemia, pernicious anaemia, spherocytosis
- Malignancy – leukaemia, Hodgkin's and non-Hodgkin's lymphoma, myeloproliferative disorders
- Storage disorders
- Immunological diseases

Splenunculi

In around 10% of the population, a small accessory spleen, or splenunculus, may be located at the splenic hilum. These small, well-defined ectopic nodules of splenic tissue (Fig. 6.2C) rarely exceed 2 cm in diameter. Splenunculi enlarge under the same circumstances as those which cause splenomegaly, and may also hypertrophy in post-splenectomy patients.

The importance of recognizing these lies in differentiating them from lymph nodes, left adrenal nodules or masses in the tail of pancreas. Colour Doppler may identify the vascular supply as being common to the main spleen (Fig. 6.2D).[1]

Pitfalls in scanning the spleen

- In hepatomegaly, the left lobe of liver may extend across the abdomen to the LUQ, displacing the spleen. This can give the appearance of a homogeneous, intrasplenic 'mass' when the spleen is viewed coronally (Fig. 6.2E). A transverse scan at the epigastrium should demonstrate the extent of

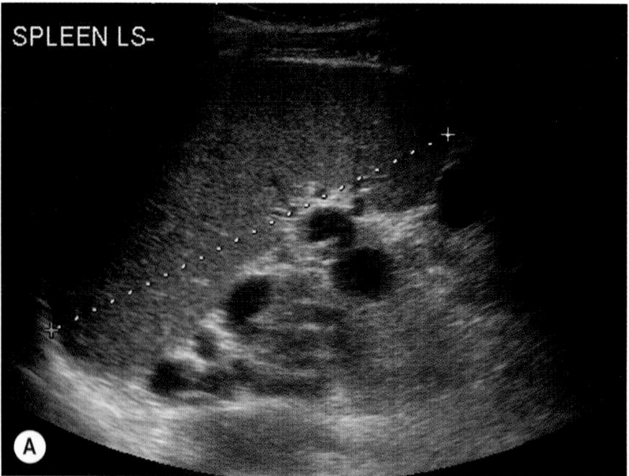

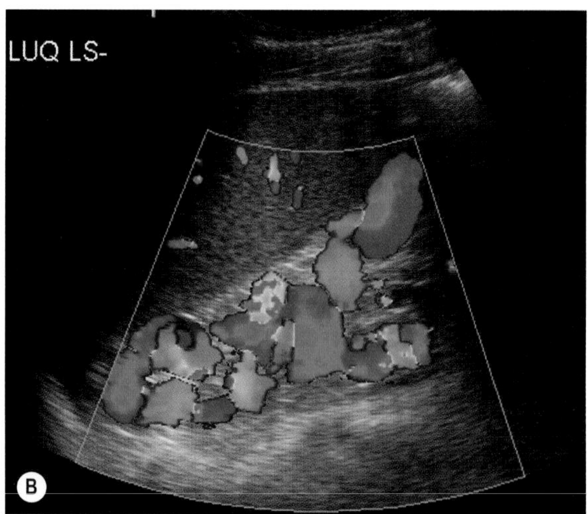

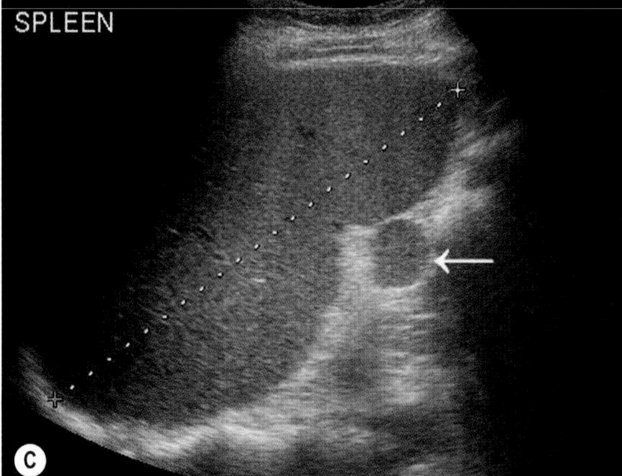

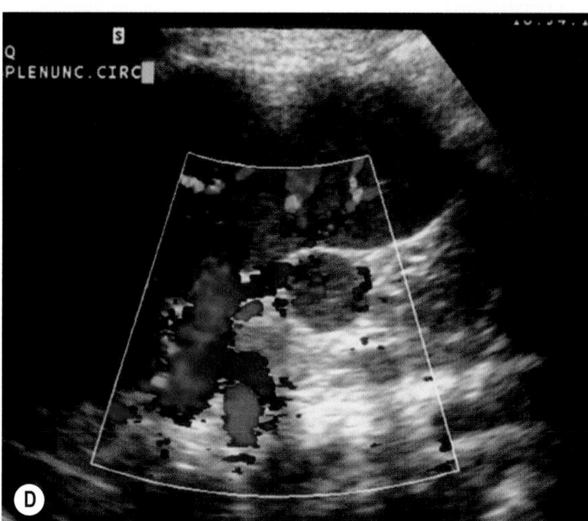

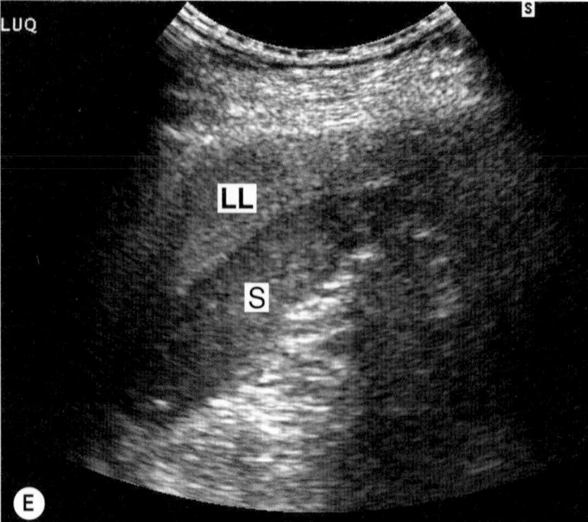

Fig. 6.2 • (A) Splenomegaly in portal hypertension. The inferior splenic margin is blunted, descending below and medial to the left kidney. Varices are present around the hilum. (B) Varices, in the form of a spleno-renal shunt, in portal hypertension. (C) A splenunculus (arrow) at the hilum of a mildly enlarged spleen. (D) The circulation of the splenunculus derives from the main splenic artery and drains into the main splenic vein. (E) The left lobe of the liver, LL, extends across the abdomen and above the spleen, S, in hepatomegaly, giving the appearance of a well-defined splenic 'mass'.

left hepatic enlargement and confirm its relationship to the spleen.

- Splenunculi may be mistaken for enlarged lymph nodes at the splenic hilum. Colour Doppler can confirm the vascular drainage and supply are shared by the spleen.
- The normal tail of pancreas may mimic a perisplenic mass.
- A left adrenal mass, or upper pole renal mass, may indent the spleen making it difficult to establish the origin of the mass.

MALIGNANT SPLENIC DISEASE

Lymphoproliferative disorders

These are malignant haematologic conditions, comprising Hodgkin's and non-Hodgkin's lymphoma, leukaemias and myeloma.

Lymphoma is the most common malignant disease affecting the spleen (Fig. 6.3). Malignant cells can infiltrate the spleen, lymph nodes, bone marrow and thymus and can also involve the liver, gastrointestinal tract, kidney and other organs. Approximately 3% of malignant diseases are lymphomas.

Splenic involvement may be found in up to 60% of lymphomas as a result of dissemination of the disease. Primary splenic lymphoma, limited to the spleen, is very rare, and accounts for less than 1% of lymphomas.

Lymphoma is also associated with AIDS and infection with HIV has given rise to a broad spectrum of lymphomatous conditions which may be demonstrated on ultrasound and CT.[2] These include masses in the liver, spleen, kidneys, adrenal gland, bowel and other retroperitoneal and nodal masses. In addition, the increased use of immunosuppression in transplant patients, and the increased survival in this group, has also been the cause of an increased incidence of immunodeficiency-related lymphoma known as PTLD (Fig. 6.3D) (see also Chapter 4).

Clinical features and management

Patients may present with a range of non-specific symptoms which include lymph node enlargement, anaemia, general fatigue, weight loss, fever, sweating and infections associated with decreased immunity. If the disease has spread to other organs, these may produce symptoms related to the organs in question. Prognosis depends upon the type of the disease, which must be determined histologically, and its stage.

Diagnosis is usually by biopsy of the lymph node or mass, and ultrasound is useful in guiding this procedure. CT is most frequently used for staging purposes, and is superior to ultrasound in demonstrating lymphadenopathy, although ultrasound can be useful in helping to characterize focal lesions and detecting renal obstruction.[3] FDG-PET is increasingly useful in staging[4] with a high diagnostic accuracy for identifying residual or recurrent tumour, and it can also help to predict the patient's response to therapy.

Depending on the type of lymphoma, chemotherapy regimens may be successful and, if not curative, can cause remission for lengthy periods. High-grade types of lymphoma are particularly aggressive with a poor survival rate.

Ultrasound appearances

Patients may present with a varied and broad spectrum of appearances in lymphoma (Fig. 6.3). In many cases the spleen is not enlarged and shows no acoustic abnormality.[5] Lymphoma may produce a diffuse splenic enlargement with normal, hypo- or hyperechogenicity.

Focal lesions may be present in up to 16% of lymphomas.[6,7] They tend to be hypoechoic and hypovascular, and may be single or multiple. In larger lesions the margins may be ill-defined and the echo contents vary from almost anechoic to heterogeneous, often with increased through transmission. In such cases, they may be similar in appearance to cysts, however, the well-defined capsule is absent in lymphoma, which has a more indistinct margin.[8] Smaller lesions may be hyperechoic or mixed. Tiny lymphomatous foci may affect the entire spleen, making it appear coarse in texture.

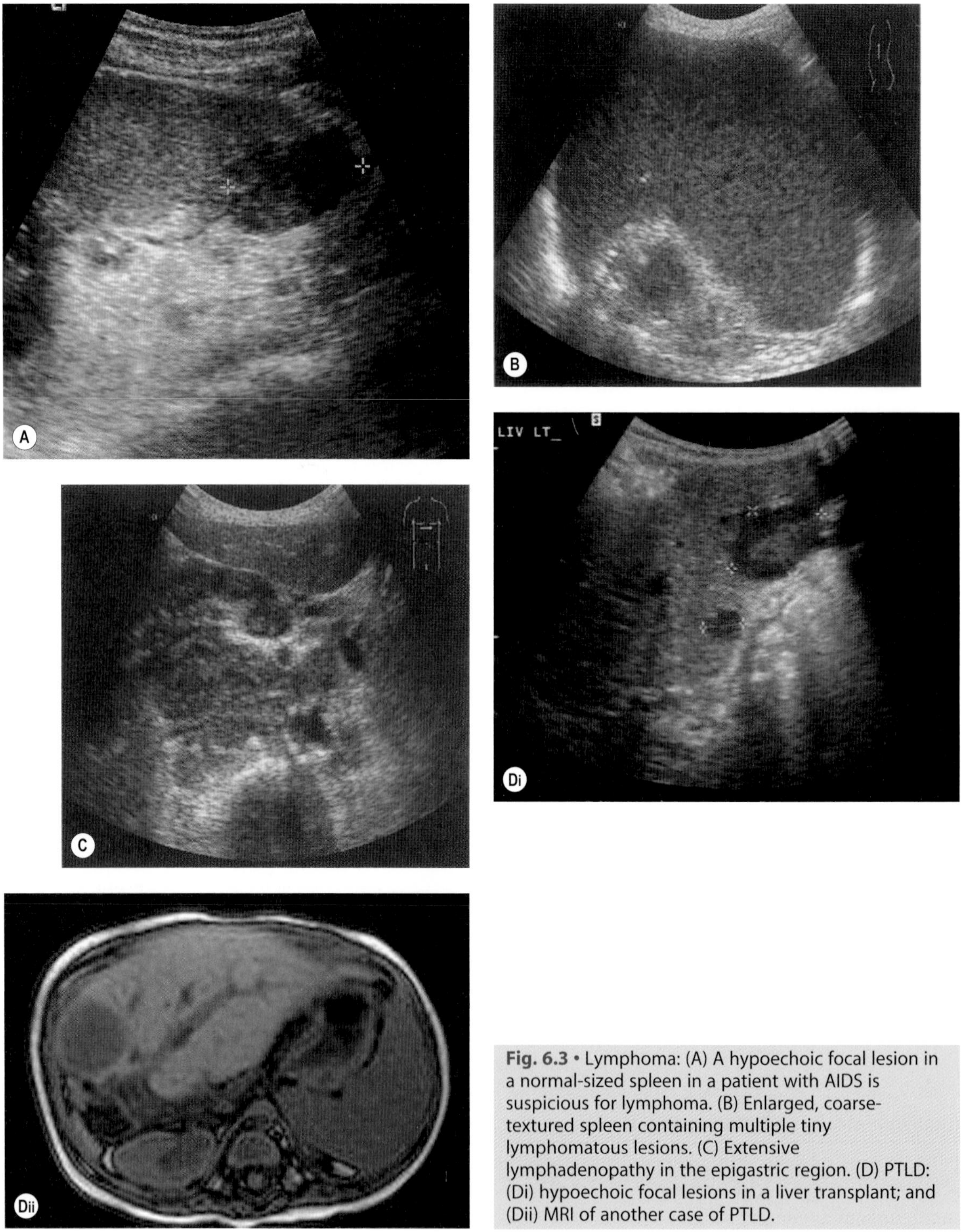

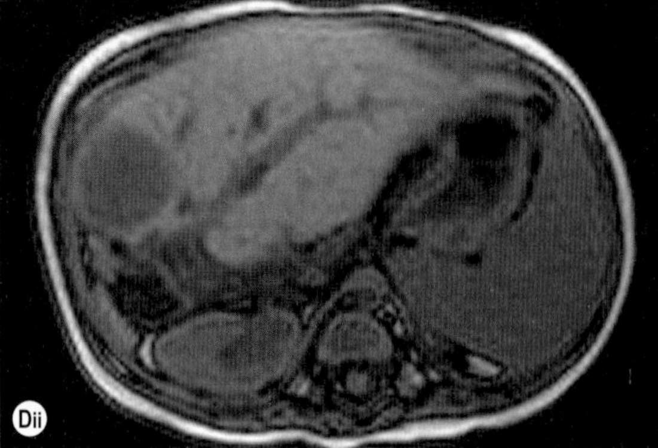

Fig. 6.3 • Lymphoma: (A) A hypoechoic focal lesion in a normal-sized spleen in a patient with AIDS is suspicious for lymphoma. (B) Enlarged, coarse-textured spleen containing multiple tiny lymphomatous lesions. (C) Extensive lymphadenopathy in the epigastric region. (D) PTLD: (Di) hypoechoic focal lesions in a liver transplant; and (Dii) MRI of another case of PTLD.

Lymphadenopathy may be present elsewhere in the abdomen. If other organs, such as the kidney or liver are affected, the appearances of mass lesions vary but are commonly hypoechoic or of mixed echo pattern.

A differential diagnosis of metastases should be considered in the presence of multiple solid hypoechoic splenic lesions, but most cases are due to lymphoma.[9] In patients who are immunocompromised, and who are at risk from PTLD, the main differential diagnosis with multiple hepatic or splenic lesions would be abscesses, as both PTLD and abscess may have similar acoustic characteristics.

Leukaemia

Leukaemia (literally meaning 'white blood,' from the Greek) is characterized by an increased number of malignant white blood cells. Unlike lymphoma, which affects the lymphatic system, leukaemia affects the circulation. There are two main types: myeloid and lymphoid, both of which can be either acute or chronic. The bone marrow becomes infiltrated with malignant cells which cause the blood to have increasing levels of immature blood cells.

Patients present with fatigue, anaemia, recurrent infections and a tendency to bleed internally. The patient's inability to overcome infections may eventually lead to death.

Chemotherapy is successful in curing acute lymphoblastic leukaemia in approximately half the patients, and may induce remission in others. The long-term prognosis is poor for other types of leukaemia, although patients may survive for 10 years or more with the slow-growing chronic lymphocytic leukaemia.

Leukaemia produces diffuse splenic enlargement, but rarely with any change in echogenicity. Abdominal lymphadenopathy may also be present.

Metastases

Metastatic deposits occur in the spleen relatively rarely in comparison with the liver.[10] Autopsy reports an incidence of around 10%, although a proportion of these are microscopic and not amenable to radiological imaging.

The most commonly found splenic metastases on ultrasound are from lymphoma, but may occur with any primary cancer. Intrasplenic deposits are more likely in later stage disease and favour melanoma, pulmonary, ovarian, colon or breast primaries.

As with liver metastases, the ultrasound appearances vary enormously, ranging from hypo- to hyperechogenic or of mixed pattern (Fig. 6.4). They may be solitary, multiple or diffusely infiltrative giving a coarse echo-pattern.[11]

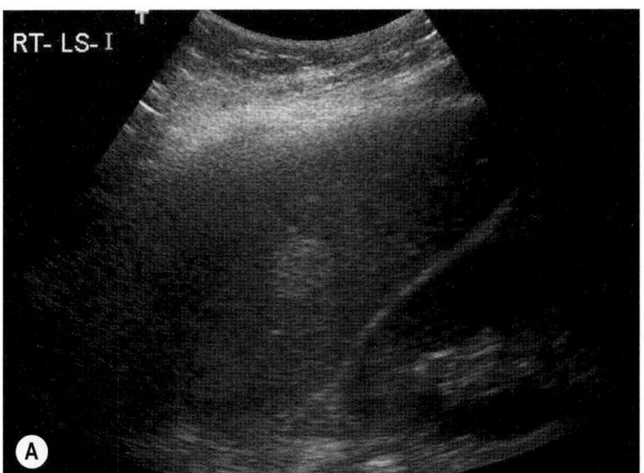

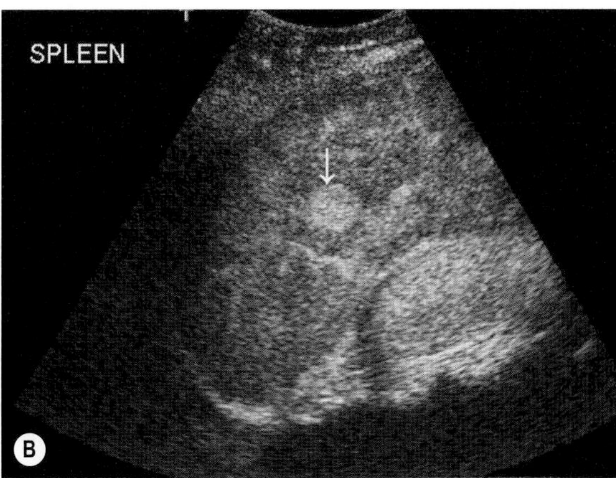

Fig. 6.4 • (A) Solitary hyperechoic splenic lesion in a patient with melanoma. This is suspicious for metastasis. (B) CEUS demonstrates the arterial vascularity in the metastasis and several other lesions (C). (D) MRI confirms splenic metastases.

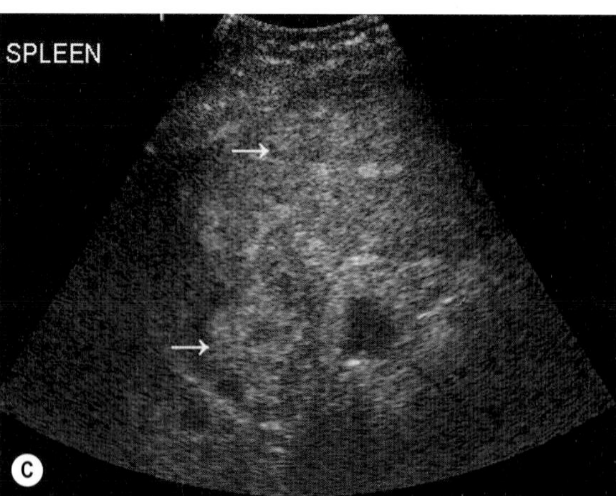

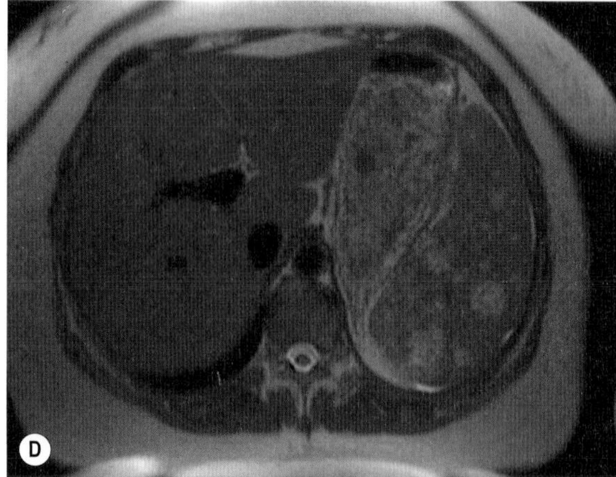

Fig. 6.4, cont'd

BENIGN SPLENIC CONDITIONS

Many benign focal lesions that occur in the spleen are of similar nature and ultrasound appearances to those in the liver. Focal lesions are less common in the spleen, however.

CYSTS

Splenic cysts have a relatively low incidence, but are nevertheless the most common benign mass found in the spleen. They demonstrate the usual acoustic characteristics of well-defined capsule, no internal echoes and posterior enhancement. Splenic cysts may occasionally be associated with autosomal dominant polycystic disease.

Other causes of cystic lesions in the spleen include post-traumatic cysts (liquefied haematoma), hydatid cysts (*Echinococcus granulosus* parasite) pseudocysts or cystic metastases (for example from primary ovarian carcinoma, which may contain mucin).[12]

As with hepatic cysts, haemorrhage may occur, causing LUQ pain. Large cysts may be resected, in order to avoid rupture.

HAEMANGIOMA

The benign haemangioma occurs rarely in the spleen. As in the liver, it is usually found as an incidental lesion of uncertain significance on ultrasound. They exhibit a spectrum of possible ultrasound appearances, from hyper- to hypoechoic, and may, rarely, contain cystic areas.

Like the hepatic haemangioma, they may pose a diagnostic dilemma as characterization is difficult with ultrasound alone. In cases with a low clinical suspicion of malignancy, such lesions may be followed up with ultrasound, and tend to remain stable in size. Contrast ultrasound is also useful in characterizing the lesions.[13] Less commonly, haemangiomas may also be multiple (Fig. 6.5B).

ABSCESS

Splenic abscesses usually result from bloodborne bacterial infection, but can also be due to amoebic infection, post-traumatic or fungal infection. Patients with splenomegaly resulting from typhoid fever, malaria and sickle cell disease are particularly predisposed to the formation of multiple pyogenic abscesses in the spleen.

Splenic abscesses are also particularly associated with immunosuppression, AIDS and high-dose chemotherapy. Such patients become susceptible

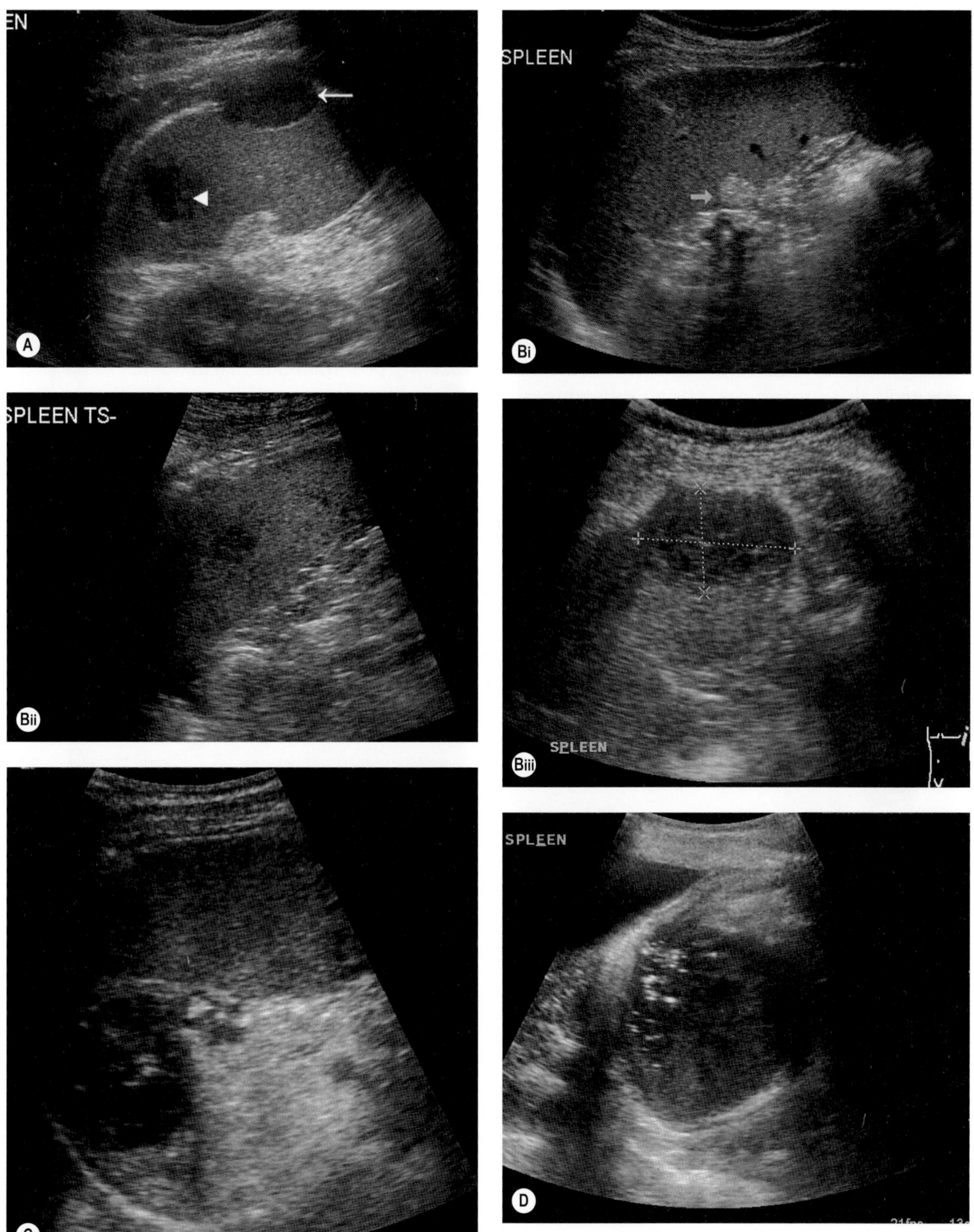

Fig. 6.5 • (A) A subcapsular haematoma in the spleen (arrow) following injury, with blood surrounding the spleen and a left pleural effusion. Another haematoma is seen superior to this (arrowhead). (B) Splenic haemangiomas: (Bi) a small well-defined hyperechoic haemangioma near the splenic hilum; (Bii) a solitary, hypoechoic splenic haemangioma; and (Biii) a large complex splenic haemangioma. (C) Large splenic abscess in an immunosuppressed patient following hepatic transplantation. (D) Large splenic abscess, resulting from an infected haematoma. Note the left pleural effusion.

to invasive fungal infections, which can cause multifocal microabscesses in the liver and spleen.[14] Patients present, as might be expected, with LUQ pain and fever.

The ultrasound appearances are similar to liver abscesses; they may be single or multiple, hyperechoic and homogeneous in the early stages, progressing to complex, fluid-filled structures with increased through transmission (Fig. 6.5C, D).

Splenic abscesses are frequently hypoechoic and it may not be possible to differentiate abscess from lymphoma or metastases on ultrasound appearances alone. This applies both in cases of large solitary abscesses and in multifocal microabscesses. They may also contain gas, posing difficulties for diagnosis as the area may be mistaken for overlying bowel.

As with liver abscesses, percutaneous drainage with antibiotic therapy is the management of choice for solitary abscesses.

CALCIFICATION

Calcification may occur in the wall of old, inactive abscess cavities, forming granulomatous deposits. Other infective processes, particularly in association with AIDS, may cause multiple small calcific foci throughout the spleen and liver (Fig. 6.6). Calcification is also associated with post-traumatic injury and may be seen around the wall of an old, resolving post-traumatic haematoma.

Conditions that predispose to the deposition of calcium in tissues, such as renal failure requiring dialysis, are also a source of splenic calcification.

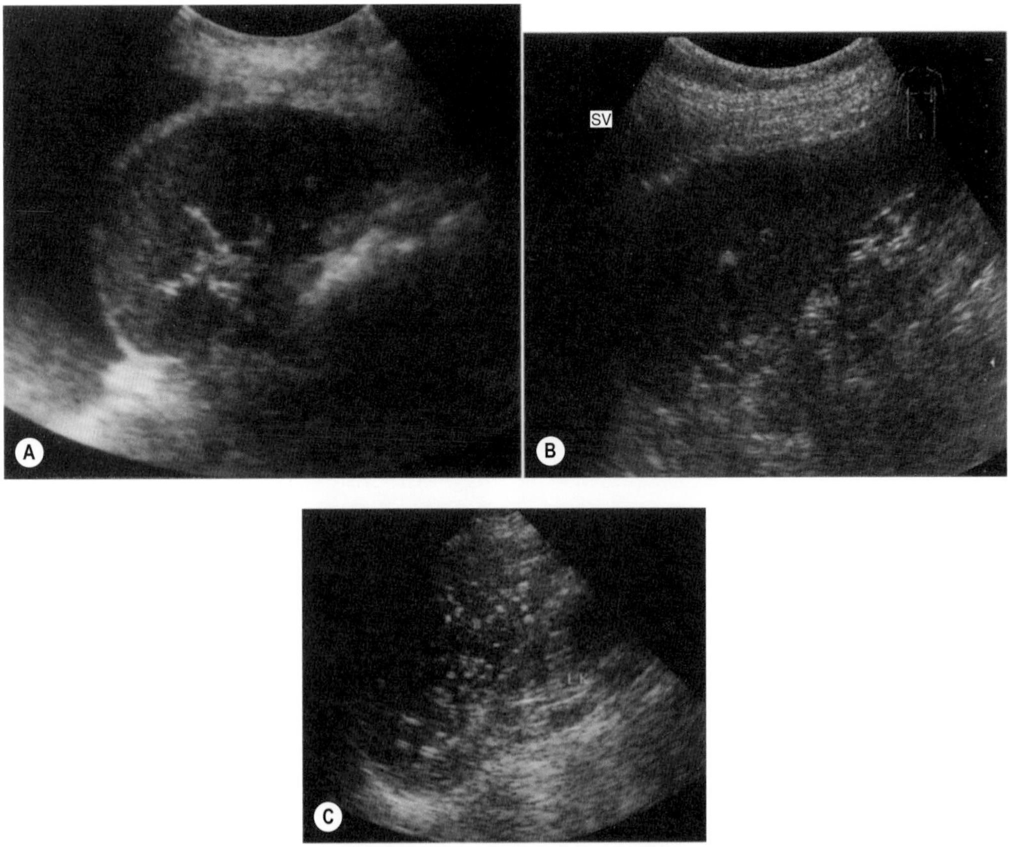

Fig. 6.6 • (A) Calcification in the spleen in a patient with nephrotic syndrome. Note the left pleural effusion. (B) Small calcified foci in the spleen of a patient with hepatitis. (C) Multiple granulomas throughout the spleen.

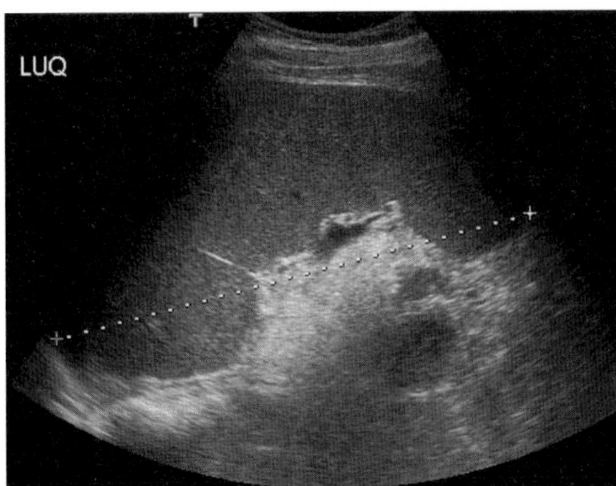

Fig. 6.7 • Splenomegaly in hereditary spherocytosis.

HAEMOLYTIC ANAEMIA

Increased red blood cell destruction, or *haemolysis*, occurs under two circumstances; when there is an abnormality of the red cells – as in sickle cell anaemia, thalassaemia or hereditary spherocytosis – or when a destructive process is at work, such as infection or autoimmune conditions. Fragile red cells are destroyed by the spleen, which becomes enlarged (Fig. 6.7).

Sickle cell anaemia is most prevalent in the black American and African populations. Progression of the disease leads to repeated infarcts in various organs, including the spleen, which may eventually become shrunken and fibrosed. Patients have (non-obstructive) jaundice because the increased destruction of red blood cells releases excessive amounts of bilirubin into the blood.

VASCULAR ABNORMALITIES OF THE SPLEEN

A range of vascular neoplasms may occur in the spleen, most of which are relatively rare.[15] These include haemangiomas (see above), hamartoma, lymphangioma and the (malignant) angiosarcoma. These may be demonstrated (but not characterized) on ultrasound, and a definitive diagnosis will usually require further imaging, such as MRI, and splenectomy may be performed in cases of a mass with atypical features.

SPLENIC INFARCT

Splenic infarction is most commonly associated with endocarditis, sickle cell disease and myeloproliferative disorders,[16] and also with lymphoma and cancers. It usually results from thrombosis of one or more of the splenic artery branches. Because the spleen is supplied by both the splenic and gastric arteries, infarction tends to be segmental rather than global. Patients may present with LUQ pain, but not invariably.

Initially the area of infarction is hypoechoic and usually wedge-shaped, solitary and extending to the periphery of the spleen (Fig. 6.8A, B). The lesion may decrease in time, and gradually fibrose, becoming hyperechoic. It demonstrates a lack of Doppler perfusion compared with the normal splenic tissue, and CEUS may be particularly helpful in outlining the area of non-perfusion, allowing a definitive diagnosis. In rare cases of total splenic infarction (Fig. 6.8D), due to occlusion of the proximal main splenic artery, grey-scale sonographic appearances may be normal in the early stages.

Occasionally infarcts may become infected or may haemorrhage. Sonography can successfully document such complications and is used to serially monitor their resolution. In patients with multiple infarcts, such as those with sickle cell disease, the spleen may become scarred, giving rise to a patchy, heterogeneous texture.

Splenic vein thrombosis

This is frequently accompanied by portal vein thrombosis and results from the same disorders. The most common of these are pancreatitis and tumour thrombus. Colour and spectral Doppler are an invaluable aid to the diagnosis, particularly when the thrombus is fresh and therefore echo-poor. Contrast agents may be administered if doubt exists over vessel patency.

Splenic vein occlusion causes splenomegaly and varices may be identified around the splenic hilum.

Splenic artery aneurysm

This is rare, although more common than hepatic artery aneurysms. It is only clinically significant if over 2 cm in diameter, when the risk of rupture and fatal haemorrhage is present.

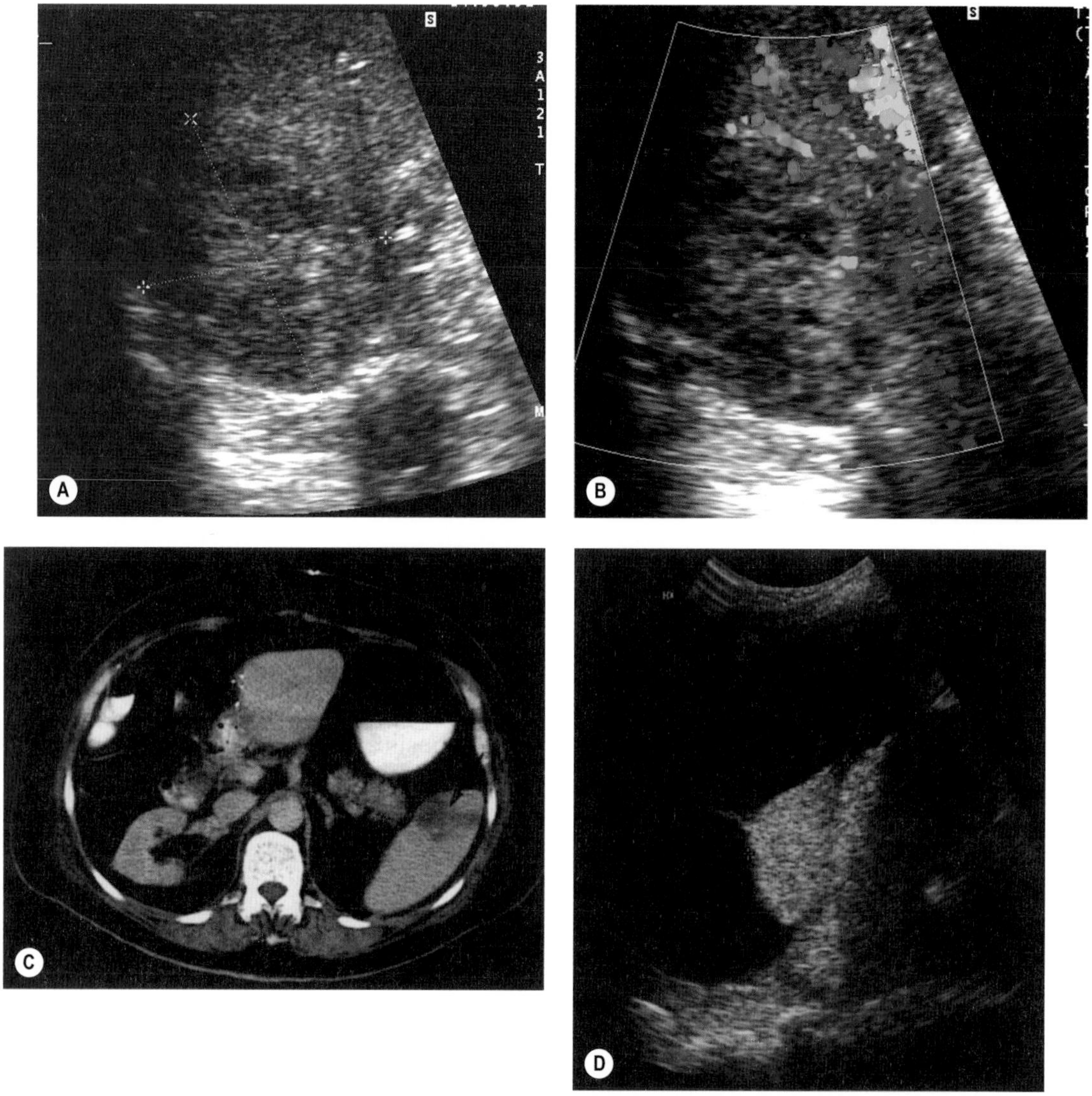

Fig. 6.8 • Splenic infarction. (A) Splenic infarct due to an embolus following recent liver resection. (B) Colour Doppler of the same patient demonstrates a lack of perfusion in the infarcted area. (C) CT scan of a splenic infarct. (D) Complete splenic infarction. The spleen is small and hyperechoic. Considerable free fluid is present.

Colour and spectral Doppler confirm arterial flow through the aneurysm and help to differentiate it from other possible cystic masses near the splenic hilum, such as pancreatic pseudocysts. Splenic artery aneurysms are usually asymptomatic and are associated with pregnancy or liver disease with portal hypertension.

Surgical resection or ligation is performed to prevent rupture, although smaller aneurysms may be safely monitored with ultrasound.[17]

Pseudoaneurysm

Pseudoaneurysm in the spleen occurs in a minority of cases following splenic trauma. An echo-free or 'cystic' area may be observed, which demonstrates flow on colour Doppler.

In rare cases, pseudoaneurysm is also a complication of splenic infarct, infiltration of the spleen by malignancy, inflammatory disease such as pancreatitis, or infection,[18] and usually occurs in association with non-traumatic splenic rupture.

SPLENIC TRAUMA

(See also Chapter 10.)

Splenic laceration may be particularly difficult to detect on ultrasound, particularly in the immediate post-trauma phase. The presence of free fluid in the abdomen of a trauma victim should alert the sonographer to the strong possibility of organ injury following blunt abdominal injury. The laceration may appear as a subtle, hyperechoic line within the spleen immediately after the injury. A frank area of haemorrhage, easily identifiable on ultrasound, may not develop until later.

CT is usually performed as the first imaging step in patients with blunt trauma, as it can also detect laceration to the gastrointestinal tract and other extra-visceral injury. However, if the patient is too unstable to be moved from the emergency department, a careful ultrasound scan can detect solid organ injury, even before a haemoperitoneum is apparent, provided the equipment is of appropriate standard. CEUS is often useful in demonstrating lacerations of the spleen and liver following blunt trauma[19] (see Chapter 10).

Iatrogenic splenic trauma has been known due to the 'blind' insertion of a drain in the case of left pleural effusion. Thankfully the guidance from the British Thoracic Society and the National Patient Safety Agency to perform such procedures under ultrasound guidance, following proper training, has reduced such incidents.

Intrasplenic pseudoaneurysm is a recognized, but rare complication of splenic trauma, which can be demonstrated on colour Doppler. In rare cases, spontaneous splenic rupture may be encountered, most usually associated with massive splenomegaly of the sort seen in infectious mononucleosis.

LYMPHATICS

Normal lymph nodes are difficult to demonstrate on ultrasound, but in certain, acoustically accessible areas, such as the hepato-duodenal ligament at the porta hepatis, normal lymph nodes can be demonstrated using a suitable acoustic window, such as the normal liver (Fig. 6.9A), particularly in young and/or thin patients.[20]

The search for lymphadenopathy should include the para-aortic and para-caval regions, the splanchnic vessels and epigastric regions, and the renal hila (Fig. 6.9). Ultrasound has a low sensitivity for

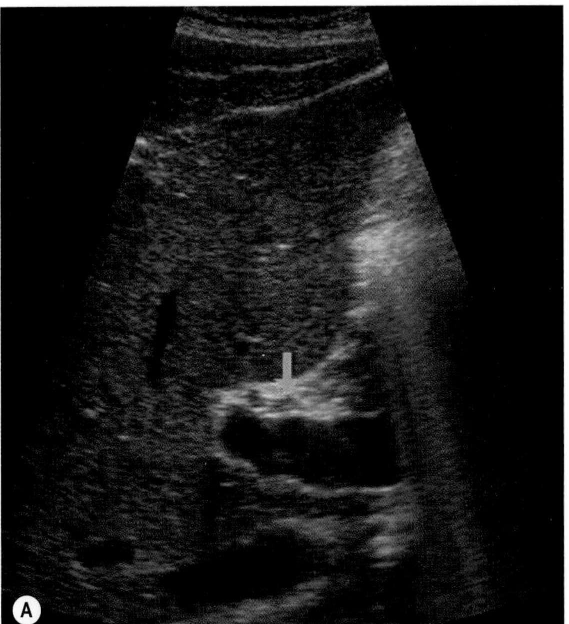

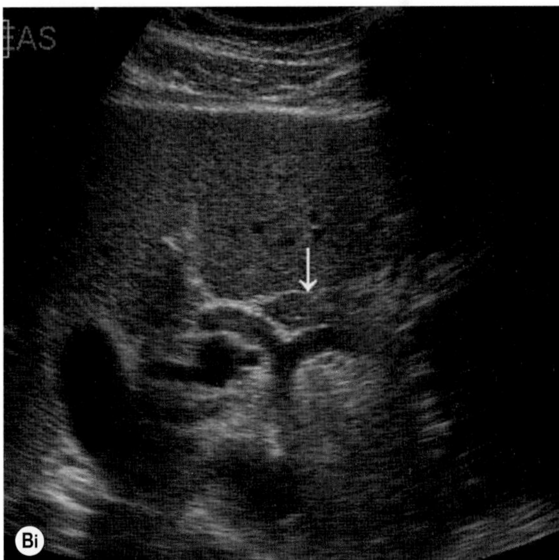

Fig. 6.9 • (A) Normal lymph nodes can be demonstrated at the porta in slim patients. (Bi) Small lymph node (arrow) at the coeliac axis, typical of the findings in hepatitis C.

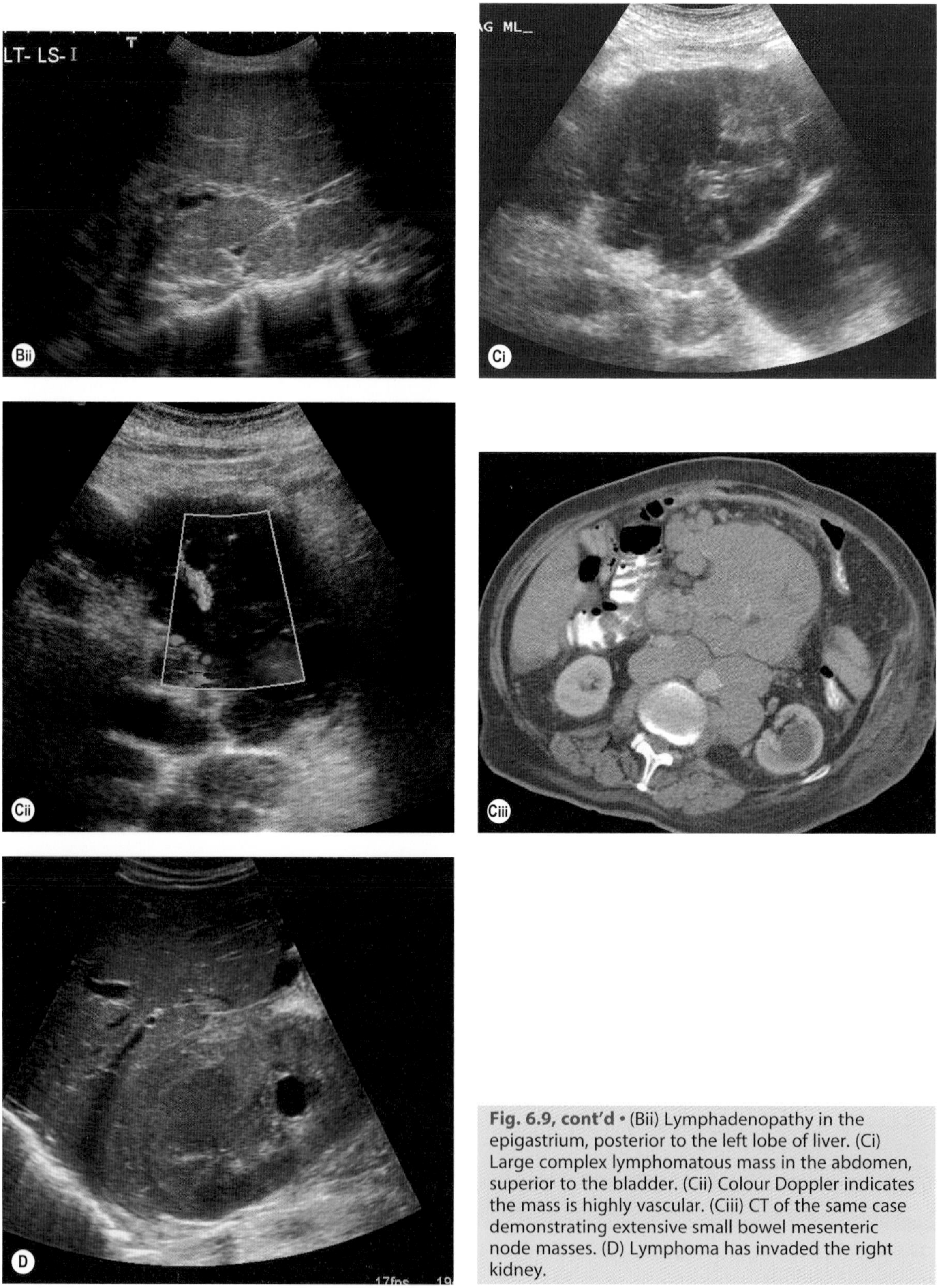

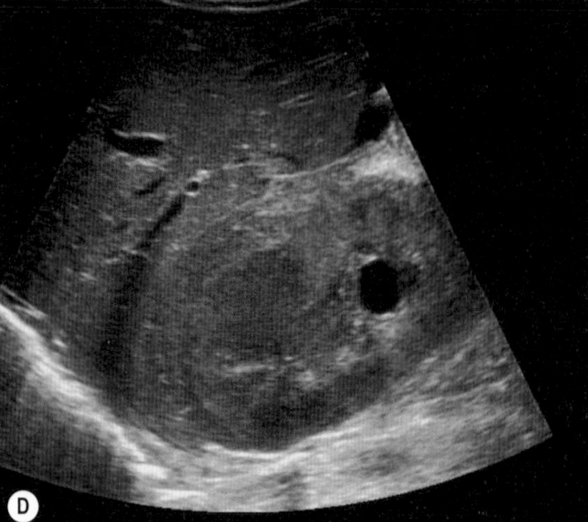

Fig. 6.9, cont'd • (Bii) Lymphadenopathy in the epigastrium, posterior to the left lobe of liver. (Ci) Large complex lymphomatous mass in the abdomen, superior to the bladder. (Cii) Colour Doppler indicates the mass is highly vascular. (Ciii) CT of the same case demonstrating extensive small bowel mesenteric node masses. (D) Lymphoma has invaded the right kidney.

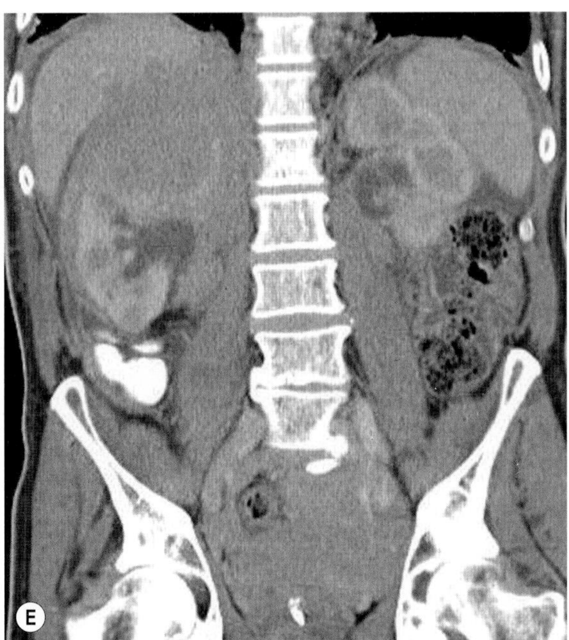

Fig. 6.9, cont'd • (E) CT of case in (D) confirms the right kidney invasion and obstructive retroperitoneal lymphadenopathy.

demonstrating lymphadenopathy in the retroperitoneum, as bowel contents frequently obscure the relevant areas. CT or MRI are better able to define the extent of lymphadenopathy, particularly in the pelvis.

The presence of lymphadenopathy is highly non-specific, being associated with a wide range of conditions including malignancy, infections and inflammatory disorders. Benign lymphadenopathy is commonly seen in conjunction with hepatitis and other inflammatory disorders such as pancreatitis, cholangitis and colitis.[21] Ultrasound may be used to guide fine needle biopsy of a nodal mass for diagnosis.

Nodes of 1.5 cm or over are generally considered pathological. Enlarged nodes are most often hypoechoic, rounded or oval in shape and well defined. Less frequently nodes are hyperechoic, or may combine to form large, lobulated masses. Nodes must be differentiated from other masses (such as gastrointestinal tract or other inflammatory masses) and Doppler is helpful here. Larger nodes display colour or power Doppler radiating from a central hilum.

There is some evidence that colour Doppler may assist in differentiating benign from malignant

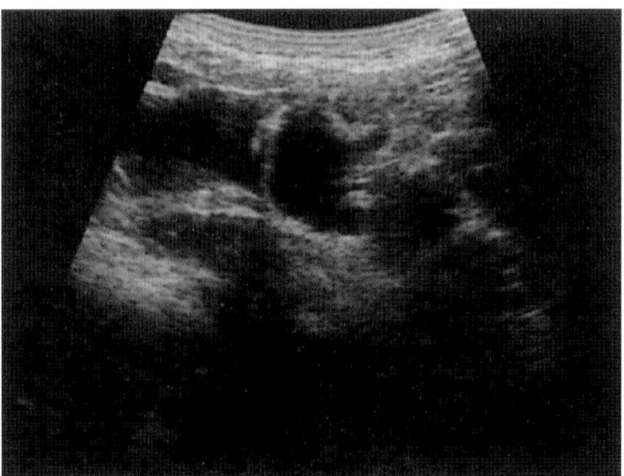

Fig. 6.10 • Lymphangioma. This large, septated cystic mass was present in the chest wall of this 2-year-old girl.

superficial nodes, the latter displaying a significantly higher resistance on spectral analysis.[22,23] Other suspicious lymph node features include increasing size, lobulated shape, absence of a hilum on grey-scale appearances, presence of microcalcification and cystic changes, but these are all relatively non-specific changes.

Lymphadenopathy occasionally causes obstructive jaundice due to compression of the CBD near the porta hepatis, or venous thrombosis due to compression of the adjacent vein.

LYMPHANGIOMA

These are benign tumours of the lymphatic vessels, usually diagnosed in the neonatal period or on prenatal sonography. They are predominantly cystic, frequently septated, and may be large (Fig. 6.10). They can compress adjacent organs and vessels and their severity depends to a large extent upon their location. They are most common in the neck (cystic hygroma) but can be found in various locations, including the abdomen,[24] and are occasionally found in adults after a long asymptomatic period.

References

1. Bertolotto M, Gioulis E, Ricci C et al. Ultrasound and Doppler features of accessory spleens and splenic grafts. Br J Radiol 1998; 71: 595–600
2. Townsend R, Laing F, Jeffrey B, Bottles K. Abdominal lymphoma in AIDS. Evaluation with ultrasound. Radiology 1989; 171: 719–724

3. Leite N, Kased N, Hanna R et al. Cross-sectional imaging of extranodal involvement in abdominpelvic lymphoproliferative malignancies. Radiographics 2007; 27: 1613–1634
4. Jhanwar Y, Straus D. The role of PET in lymphoma. J Nucl Med 2006; 47: 1326–1334
5. Siniluoto T, Paivansalo M, Alavaikko M. Ultrasonography of spleen and liver in staging Hodgkin's disease. Eur J Radiol 1991; 13: 181–186
6. Di-Stasi M, Cavanna L, Fornari F et al. Splenic lesions in Hodgkin's and non-Hodgkin's lymphomas. An ultrasonographic study. Eur J Ultrasound 1995; 2: 117–124
7. Gorg C, Weide R, Schwerk WB. Malignant splenic lymphoma: sonographic patterns, diagnosis and follow-up. Clin Radiol 1997; 52: 535–540
8. Ishida H, Konno K, Naganuma H et al. Splenic lymphoma: differentiation from splenic cysts with ultrasonography. Abdomin Imag 2001; 26: 529–532
9. Goerg C, Schwerk WB, Goerg K. Sonography of focal lesions of the spleen. AJR Am J Roentgenol 1990; 157: 965–966
10. Kamaya A, Weinstein S, Desser TS. Multiple lesions of the spleen: differential diagnosis of cystic and solid lesions. Semin Ultrasound CT MR 2006; 27: 389–403
11. Siniluoto T Paivansalo M, Lahde S. Ultrasonography of splenic metastases. Acta Radiol 1989; 30: 463
12. Warshauer DM, Hall HL. Solitary splenic lesions. Semin Ultrasound CT MR 2006; 27: 370–388
13. von Herbay A, Barreiros AP, Ignee A et al. Contrast-enhanced ultrasonography with SonoVue: differentiation between benign and malignant lesions of the spleen. J Ultrasound Med 2009;28:421-434
14. Gorg C, Weide R, Schwerk WB et al. Ultrasound evaluation of hepatic and splenic microabscesses in the immunocompromised patient: sonographic patterns, differential diagnosis and follow-up. J Clin Ultrasound 1994; 22: 525–529
15. Abbott RM, Levy AD, Aguilera NS et al. From the archives of the AFIP: primary vascular neoplasms of the spleen: radiologic-pathologic correlation. Radiographics 2004; 24: 1137–1163
16. Georg C, Schwerk WB. Splenic infarction; sonographic pattern, diagnosis, follow-up and complications. Radiology 1990; 174: 803–807
17. Mattar SG, Lumsden AB. The management of splenic artery aneurysms: experience with 23 cases. Am J Surg 1995; 169: 580–584
18. Görg C, Cölle J, Wied M et al. Spontaneous nontraumatic intrasplenic pseudoaneurysm: causes, sonographic diagnosis and prognosis. J Clin Ultrasound 2003; 31: 129–134
19. Görg C. The forgotten organ: contrast enhanced sonography of the spleen. Eur J Radiol 2007; 64: 189–201
20. Metreweli C, Ward S. Ultrasound demonstration of lymph nodes in the hepatoduodenal ligament ('daisy chain nodes') in normal subjects. Clin Radiol 1995; 50: 99–101
21. Gimondo P, Mirk P, Messina G, Pizzi C. Abdominal lymphadenopathy in benign diseases: sonographic detection and clinical significance. J Ultrasound Med 1996; 15: 353–359
22. Dong GN, Hyo KL, Hong SB et al. Differential diagnosis of cervical lymphadenopathy: usefulness of colour Doppler sonography. AJR Am J Roentgenol 1997; 168: 1311–1316
23. Min YC, Jun WL, Kyung JJ. Distinction between benign and malignant causes of cervical, axillary and inguinal lymphadenopathy: value of Doppler spectral waveform analysis. AJR Am J Roentgenol 1995; 165: 981–984
24. Schmidt M. Intra-abdominal lymphangioma. Kans Med 1995; 93: 149–150

7 Ultrasound of the renal tract

CHAPTER CONTENTS

THE NORMAL RENAL TRACT

Ultrasound technique

The kidneys are best evaluated with ultrasound by first obtaining an LS of the kidney, including the upper and lower poles, with the kidney roughly perpendicular to the beam. This may necessitate using various angles and patient positions, and it may be necessary to scan from the posterior aspect. Finding the maximum length at the start of the procedure, by twisting the probe to include both poles, enables the operator to establish the lie of the kidney and provides a good starting point from which to fully and carefully evaluate the organ. In this way the operator is less likely to miss pathology or underestimate renal length.

The right kidney is readily demonstrated through the right lobe of the liver. Generally a subcostal approach displays the (more anterior) lower pole to best effect, while an intercostal approach is best for demonstrating the upper pole (Fig. 7.1). The left kidney (LK) is not usually demonstrable in a true sagittal plane because it lies posterior to the stomach and splenic flexure. The spleen can be used as an acoustic window to the upper pole by scanning coronally, from the patient's left side, with the patient supine or decubitus (left side raised) but, unless the spleen is enlarged, the lower pole must usually be imaged from the left side posteriorly. Coronal sections of both kidneys are particularly useful as they display the renal pelvicalyceal system and its relationship to the renal

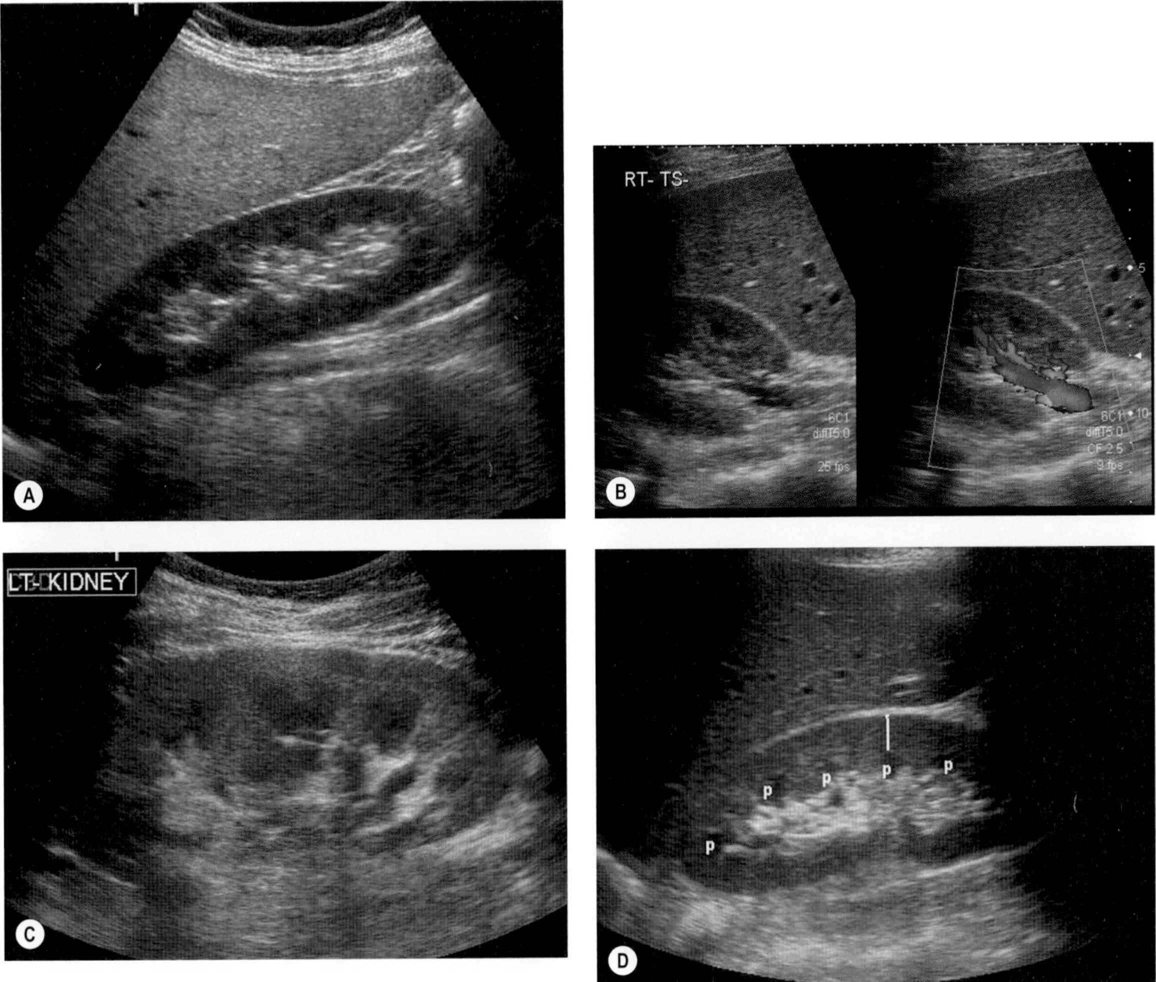

Fig. 7.1 • (A) Sagittal section through the normal RK, using the liver as an acoustic window. The central echoes from the renal sinus are hyperechoic due to the fat content. The hypoechoic, triangular, medullary pyramids are demonstrated in a regular arrangement around the sinus. The cortex is of similar echogenicity to the liver. (B) Transverse section through the hilum of the RK. Colour Doppler shows flow in the main renal vein and artery. (C) LK in coronal section. The renal hilum is seen furthest from the transducer. (Compare this with the sagittal section of the RK in which cortex is seen all the way around the PCS.) (D) Pyramids (p) are arranged regularly around the pelvicalyceal system. The renal cortical thickness is represented by the white line.

hilum (Fig. 7.1C). This section demonstrates the main blood vessels and ureter (if dilated). As with any other organ, the kidneys must be examined in both longitudinal and transverse (axial) planes and the operator must be flexible in his/her approach to obtain the necessary results.

The bladder should be filled and examined to complete the renal tract scan. An excessively full bladder may cause mild dilatation of the pelvicalyceal system, which will return to normal following micturition.

Normal ultrasound appearances of the kidneys

The cortex of the normal kidney is slightly hypoechoic when compared to the adjacent liver parenchyma, although this is age dependent. In young people it may be of similar echogenicity and in the elderly it is not unusual for it to be comparatively hyperechoic and thinner. The medullary pyramids are seen as regularly spaced, hypoechoic (not echo-free) triangular structures between the cortex and the renal sinus (Fig. 7.1). The tiny reflective structures often seen at the margins of the pyramids are echoes from the arcuate arteries which branch around the pyramids.

The renal sinus containing the pelvicalyceal system is hyperechoic due to sinus fat which surrounds the vessels. The main artery and vein can be readily demonstrated at the renal hilum and should not be confused with a mild degree of pelvicalyceal dilatation. Colour Doppler can help differentiate.

The kidney develops in the fetus from a number of lobes that fuse together. Occasionally the traces of these lobes can be seen on the surface of the kidney, forming *fetal lobulations* (Fig. 7.2A); these may persist into adulthood. The issue for the sonographer is being able to recognise these as normal variations, as distinct from a renal mass, or renal scarring.

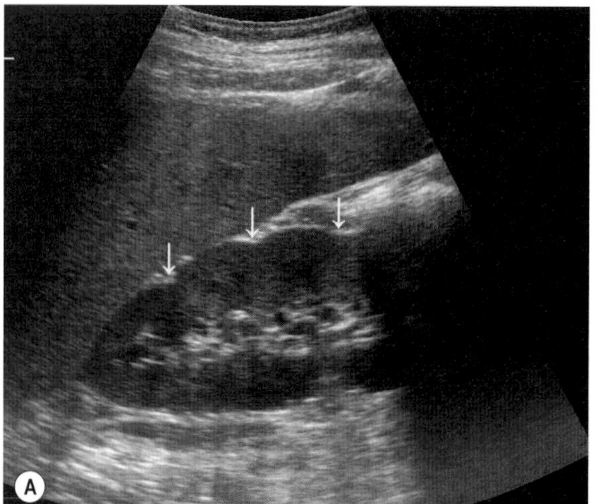

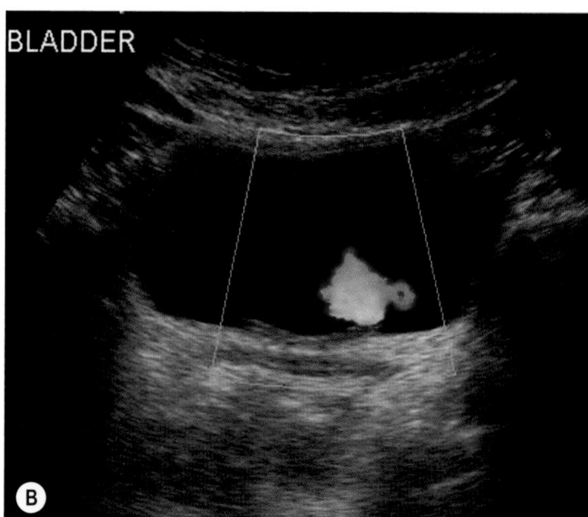

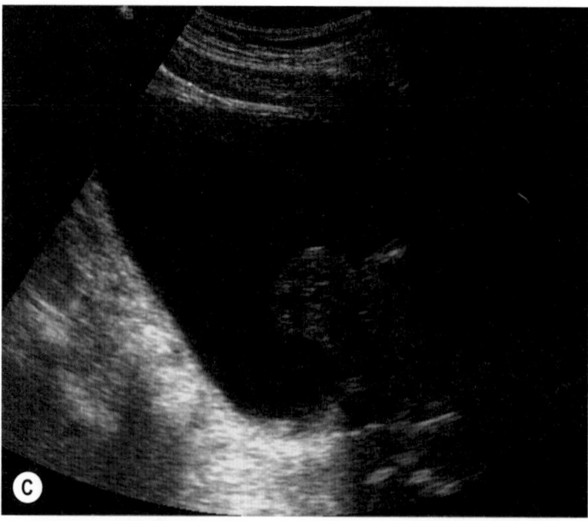

Fig. 7.2 • (A) RK demonstrating fetal lobulations (arrows). (B) TS through the base of the bladder demonstrating a left ureteric jet. (C) An enlarged prostate indents the bladder. This may be associated with incomplete emptying and/or retention. A post-micturition scan is useful in estimating residual volume.

Normal ultrasound appearances of the lower renal tract

When the bladder is distended with urine, the walls are thin, regular and hyperechoic. The walls may appear thickened or trabeculated if the bladder is insufficiently distended, making it difficult to exclude a bladder lesion. The ureteric orifices can be demonstrated in a transverse section at the bladder base. Ureteric jets can easily be demonstrated with colour Doppler at this point and normally occur between 1.5 and 12.4 times per minute (a mean of 5.4 jets per minute) from each side (Fig. 7.2B).[1]

It is useful to examine the pelvis for other masses, e.g. related to the uterus or ovaries, which could exert pressure on the ureters causing proximal dilatation. The prostate is demonstrated transabdominally by angling caudally through the full bladder (Fig 7.2C). The investigation of choice for the prostate is transrectal ultrasound, however, an approximate idea of its size can be gained from transabdominal scanning.

When prostatic hypertrophy is suspected, it is useful to perform a post-micturition bladder volume measurement to determine the residual volume of urine (see next section).

Measurements

The normal adult kidney measures between 9 cm and 12 cm in length. A renal length outside the normal range may be an indication of a pathological process and measurements should therefore form part of the protocol of renal scanning. Technique is extremely important if the renal length is not to be underestimated (see above.) Obtaining the maximum renal length may involve an intercostal scan with rib shadowing over the central portion of the kidney, or may necessitate scanning from the posterior of the patient. A subcostal section, which foreshortens the kidney, often underestimates the length and it is more accurate to measure a coronal or posterior longitudinal section with the beam perpendicular to the renal axis.

The cortical thickness of the kidney is generally taken as the distance between the capsule and the margin of the medullary pyramid (Fig. 7.1D). This varies between individuals and within individual kidneys, and tends to decrease with age.

The bladder volume can be estimated for most purposes by taking the product of three perpendicular measurements and multiplying by 0.56:

$$\text{Bladder volume (mL)} = \text{Length} \times \text{width} \times \text{AP diameter (cm)} \times 0.56$$

Haemodynamics

The vascular tree of the kidney can be effectively demonstrated with colour Doppler (Fig. 7.3). By manipulating the system sensitivity and using a low PRF, small vessels can be demonstrated at the periphery of the kidney.

Demonstration of the extrarenal main artery and vein with colour Doppler is most successful in the coronal or axial section by identifying the renal hilum and tracing the artery back to the aorta or the vein to the IVC. The best Doppler signals – i.e. the highest Doppler shift frequencies – are obtained when the direction of the vessel is parallel to the beam, and taken on suspended respiration. The LRV is readily demonstrated between the SMA and aorta by scanning just below the body of the pancreas in transverse section. The origins of the renal arteries may be seen arising from the aorta in a coronal section (Fig. 7.3D).

The normal adult renal vasculature is of low resistance with a fast, almost vertical systolic upstroke and continuous forward end diastolic flow. Resistance generally increases with age.[2] The more peripheral arteries are of lower velocity with weaker Doppler signals, and are less pulsatile than the main vessel.

ASSESSMENT OF RENAL FUNCTION

Blood and urine tests can be useful indicators of pathology. Frequently, the request to perform ultrasound is triggered by biochemical results outwith the normal range.

Raised serum levels of urea and creatinine are associated with a reduction in renal function. However, any damage is usually quite severe before this becomes apparent. The creatinine clearance rate estimates the amount of creatinine excreted over 24 hours, and is a guide to the GFR (normal

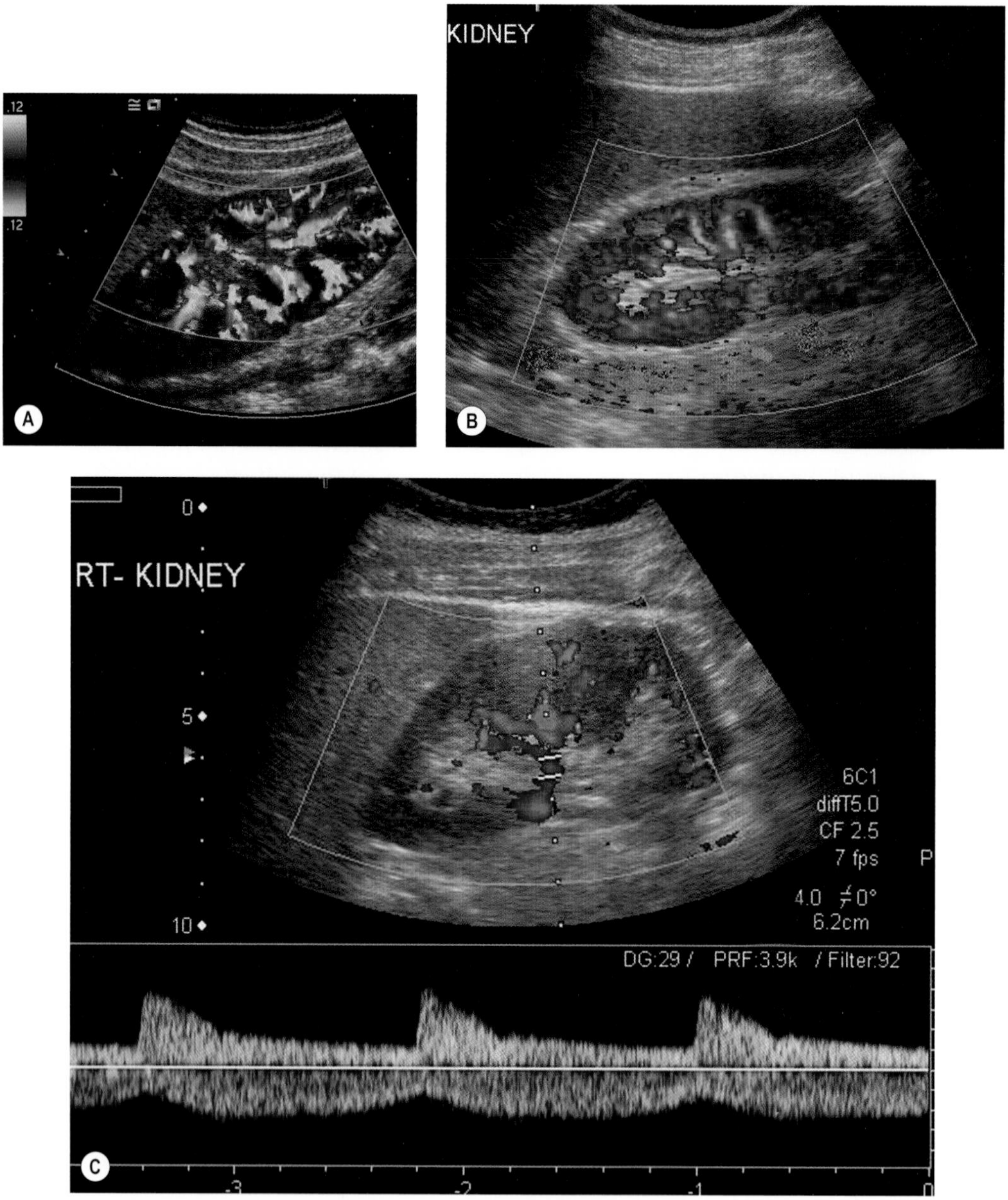

Fig. 7.3 • (A) Colour Doppler of the RK demonstrating normal intrarenal perfusion throughout the kidney. (B) Power Doppler demonstrating renal perfusion. (C) The waveform from the main renal artery at the hilum of the kidney is of low resistance with good EDF. The spectrum from the adjacent vein can be seen below the baseline.

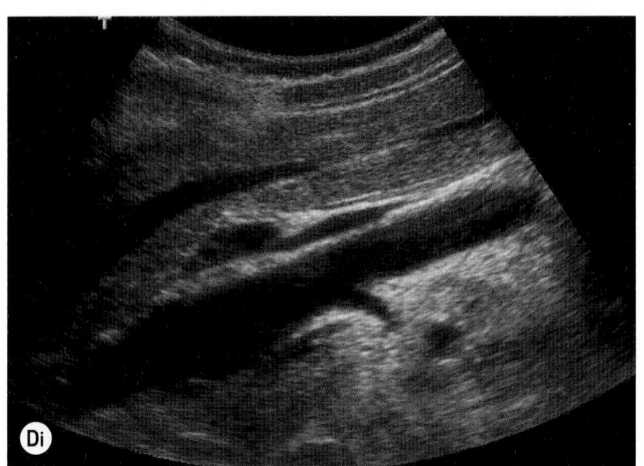

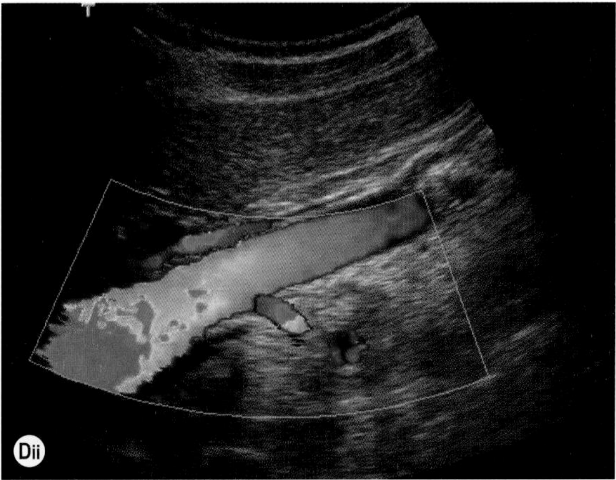

Fig. 7.3, cont'd • (Di) Coronal section through the aorta taken from the patient's right side showing the origin of the left renal artery (LRA). (Dii) The LRA appears in blue as it is flowing away from the transducer.

GFR 100–120 mL/min). A poor rate of clearance (mL/min) is indicative of renal failure.

Blood in the urine is a potentially serious sign that should prompt investigation with ultrasound. Frank haematuria may be a sign of renal tract malignancy. Microscopic haematuria may reflect inflammation, infection, calculi or malignancy. The urine can be easily examined for protein, glucose, acetone and pH using chemically impregnated strips.

Radioisotope scans

Although the ultrasound scan is invaluable in assessing the morphology of the kidneys, it is not able to assess function. The administration of a radioactive tracer, however, reveals valuable information regarding renal function and an isotope scan may often be performed in addition to ultrasound.

A DTPA (diethylene triaminepenta-acetic acid) scan, in which the isotope is intravenously injected as a bolus, can assess renal perfusion, with further data reflecting renal uptake, excretion and drainage during later images. A DMSA (dimercaptosuccinic acid) scan shows uptake of isotope which is proportional to functioning renal tissue. Relative renal function can be determined between kidneys and localized areas of poor or absent function, such as scars, are clearly demonstrated.

RENAL ANATOMICAL VARIANTS

Duplex kidney

This term is used to describe a spectrum of possible appearances, from two separate kidneys with separate collecting systems and duplex ureters, to a more simple division of the pelvicalyceal system at the renal hilum (Fig. 7.4A). The latter is more difficult to recognize on ultrasound, but the two moieties of the pelvicalyceal system are separated by a zone of normal renal cortex which invaginates the kidney – a *hypertrophied column of Bertin* (see below).

Duplex kidney is the most common congenital renal abnormality. It may be associated with other anomalies such as reflux, ectopic ureteric orifice or ureterocele, and may predispose the patient to infection or obstruction of the upper moiety or, rarely, the lower moiety.[3] The main issue for the sonographer here is that one moiety may be mistaken on ultrasound for the entire kidney, especially if bowel gas overlies part of the kidney, and the operator must ensure that both renal poles are properly demonstrated. A chronically obstructed moiety in an adult patient may masquerade as a renal cyst or as fluid-filled bowel.

The main renal artery and vein may also be duplicated, which can occasionally be identified using colour or power Doppler.

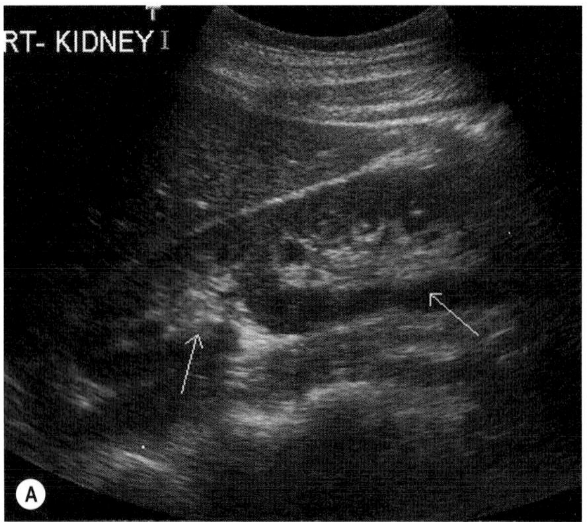

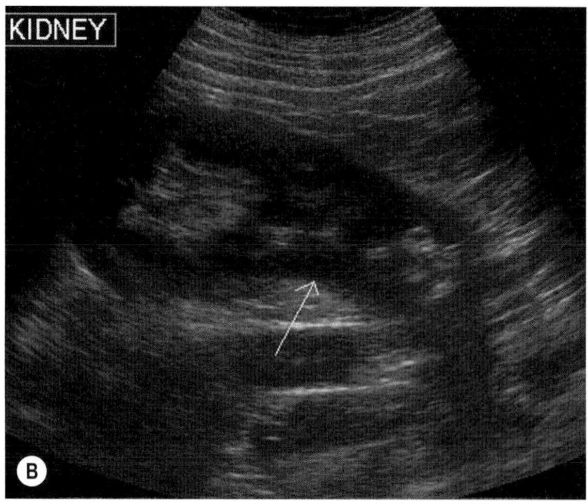

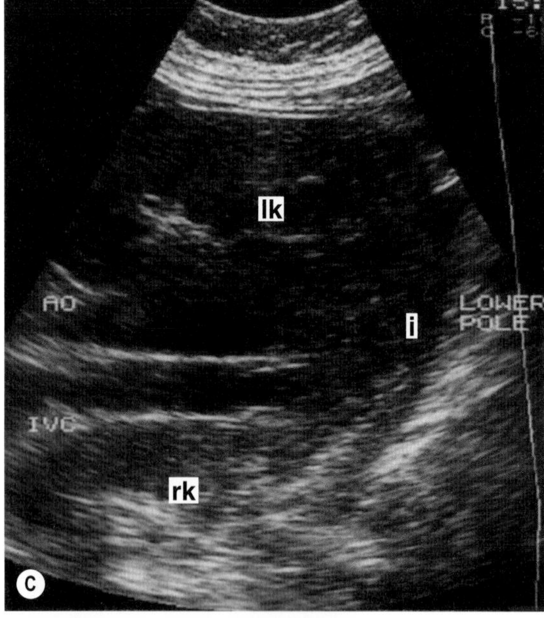

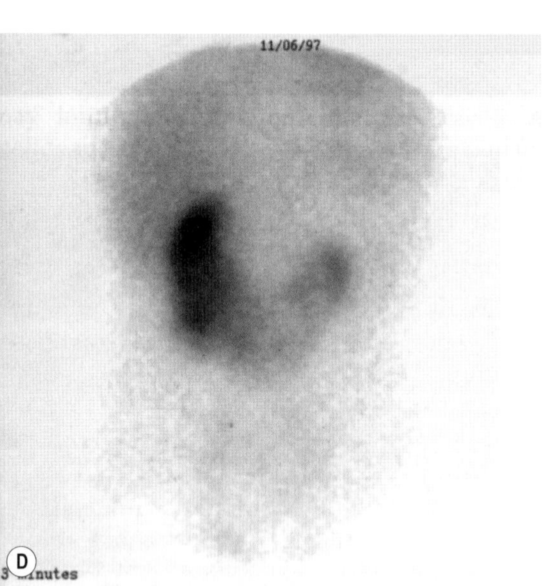

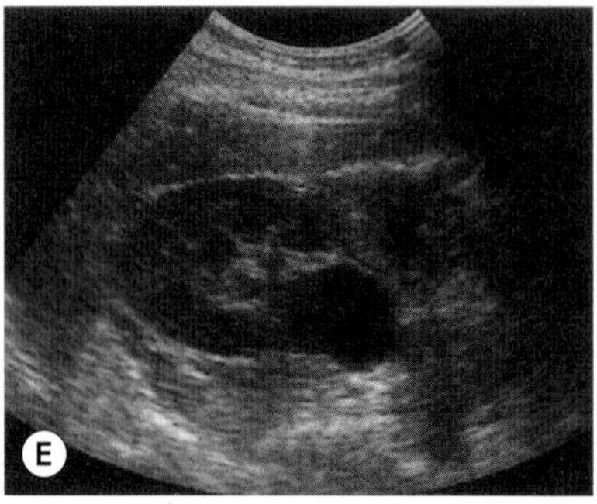

Fig. 7.4 • (A) Duplex kidney showing two separate intrarenal collecting systems (arrows). These drained into a single ureter on intravenous urethrogram (IVU). (B) TS through the abdomen demonstrating the fused lower poles of the horseshoe kidney (arrow) anterior to the spine. (C) Coronal section through a horseshoe kidney with the isthmus of the kidney (i) anterior to the aorta and IVC. (D) MAG3 scan demonstrating a horseshoe kidney with a poorly functioning LK and isthmus. Differential function is 86% on the right and 14% on the left. (E) TS through the RK demonstrating a baggy extrarenal pelvis. The pelvicalyceal system remains undilated and this should not be confused with hydronephrosis.

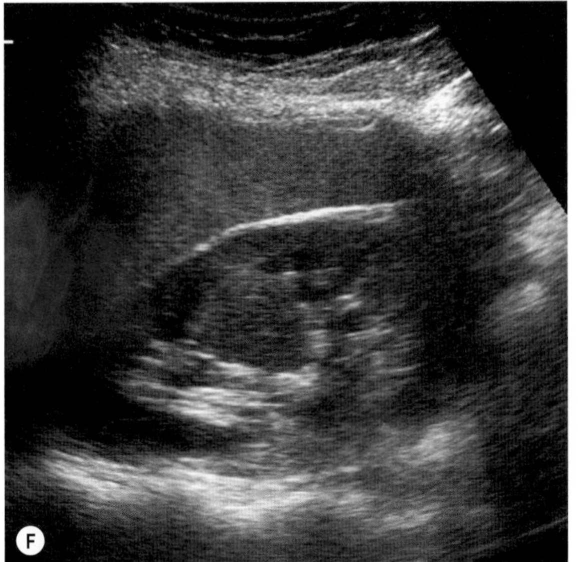

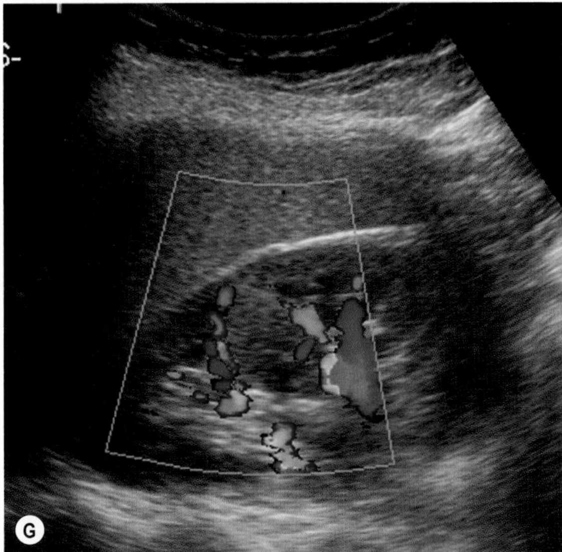

Fig. 7.4, cont'd • (F) Hypertrophied column of Bertin. (G) Colour Doppler of the hypertrophied column reveals regular, normal interlobar vessels (as opposed to the irregularly distributed, increased flow through a renal cell carcinoma [RCC]).

Ectopic kidneys

The kidney normally ascends from the pelvis into the renal fossa during its course of development. During this 'migration' it rotates inwards so that the renal hilum faces medially. A failure of this mechanism causes the kidney to fall short of its normal position, remaining in the pelvis, i.e. a pelvic kidney. Usually it lies on the correct side, however ,occasionally it can cross to the other side, lying inferior to its normally placed partner – *crossed renal ectopia*. Frequently it may fuse with the lower pole of the other kidney – *crossed fused renal ectopia* – resulting in what appears to be a very long, unilateral organ.

Horseshoe kidneys

In the horseshoe kidney, the kidneys lie one on each side of the abdomen but their lower poles are fused by a connecting band of renal tissue, or *isthmus*, which lies anterior to the aorta and IVC (Fig. 7.4B–D). The kidneys tend to be rotated and lie with their lower poles medially.

It may be difficult to visualize the isthmus due to bowel gas anterior to it, but a horseshoe kidney should always be suspected when the operator is unable to confidently identify the lower poles of the kidneys, or when the lower pole seems unusually anterior and medial.

When the isthmus can be seen, it is important not to confuse it with other abdominal masses, such as lymphadenopathy. CT is occasionally performed because of this and normally clarifies the findings.

Extrarenal pelvis

Not infrequently, the renal pelvis projects outside the kidney, medial to the renal sinus. This is best seen in a transverse section through the renal hilum. It is frequently 'baggy' containing anechoic urine, which is prominently demonstrated on the ultrasound scan (Fig. 7.4E). The importance of recognizing the extra-renal pelvis lies in not confusing it with dilatation of the PCS, or with a para-pelvic cyst or collection.

Hypertrophied column of Bertin

The septum of Bertin is an invagination of renal cortex down to the renal sinus. It occurs at the junctions of original fetal lobulations and is present in Duplex systems, (see above) dividing the two moieties. Particularly prominent, hypertrophied columns of Bertin may mimic a renal tumour. It is usually possible to distinguish between the two as the column of Bertin does not affect the renal outline and has the same acoustic characteristics as the adjacent cortex (Fig. 7.4F, G).

Colour or power Doppler are helpful in revealing the normal, regular vascular pattern (as opposed to the chaotic and increased blood flow pattern of malignant renal tumours). If doubt persists, particularly in a symptomatic patient, CEUS reliably differentiates a prominent column of Bertin from tumour.[4] An isotope scan can also be helpful demonstrating normally functioning renal tissue.

Renal humps

These are areas of renal cortex, which form a bulge in the renal outline. Like the hypertrophied column of Bertin, a hump may mimic a renal mass. Careful scanning can usually solve the dilemma as the cortex remains constant in thickness. The most usual manifestation is the *splenic hump* on the left kidney, which is a flattening of the upper pole with a lateral prominence just below the margin of the spleen.

Humps are basically a variation in the shape of the kidney rather than an area of hypertrophied tissue.

RENAL CYSTS AND CYSTIC DISEASE

CYSTS

The most common renal mass is a simple cyst which can be found in up to 50% of the population, the incidence increasing with age. Most cysts are asymptomatic and may be solitary or multiple. Generally they are peripheral but may occur within the kidney adjacent to the renal pelvis. A parapelvic cyst may be difficult to distinguish from pelvicalyceal dilatation, a calyceal diverticulum or an extrarenal pelvis and careful scanning is required to differentiate. A parapelvic cyst may be the cause of a filling defect on IVU and CT can differentiate a cyst from a diverticulum if necessary, as the latter will fill with contrast.

Occasionally cysts can haemorrhage causing pain. Large cysts, particularly of the lower pole, may be palpable, prompting a request for an ultrasound scan.

Ultrasound appearances

Like cysts in any other organ, they must display three basic characteristics – anechoic, a thin, well-defined capsule and exhibit posterior enhancement – if they are to be legitimately called 'simple'. It can be difficult to appreciate the posterior enhancement if the hyperechoic perirenal fat lies distal to the cyst; scanning from a different angle (Fig. 7.5) is helpful.

Haemorrhage or infection can give rise to low-level echoes within a cyst and in some cases the capsule may display calcification.

Whilst a solitary, simple cyst can almost certainly be ignored, cysts with more complex acoustic characteristics may require further investigation, e.g. CT. A calcified wall may be associated with malignancy. Increasingly small renal cysts are incidentally discovered on ultrasound due to improved technology and they are by no means always simple. In 1989 Bosniak[5] proposed a classification of cysts to be used with CT to differentiate benign from malignant lesions (Fig. 7.5B, C; Table 7.1). This has been used over the years in conjunction with ultrasound findings in order to highlight possible malignancy. Whilst it broadly works, it is by no means a definitive test[6] and complex renal cysts should normally be monitored or undergo CT to evaluate further.

These lesions can now be successfully characterized into the Bosniak classification using CEUS[7] (see also Fig. 7.10.) CEUS is able to differentiate the vascularized solid components of complex renal masses at least as well as CT, and can also be used to monitor lesions, thereby reducing the radiation dose from CT.

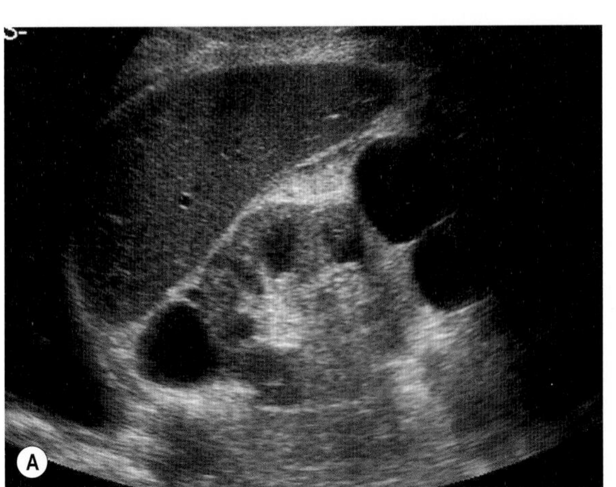

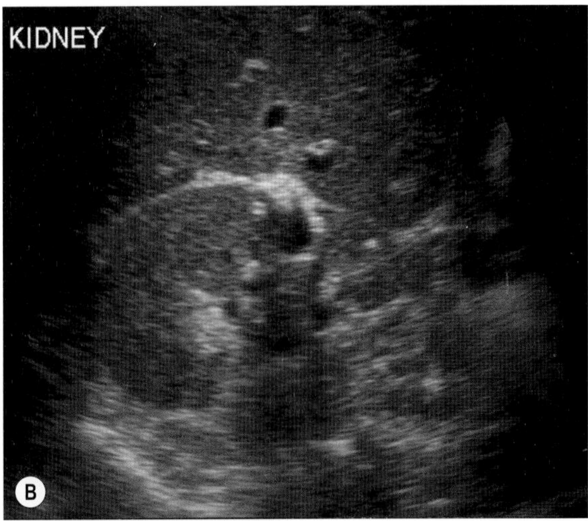

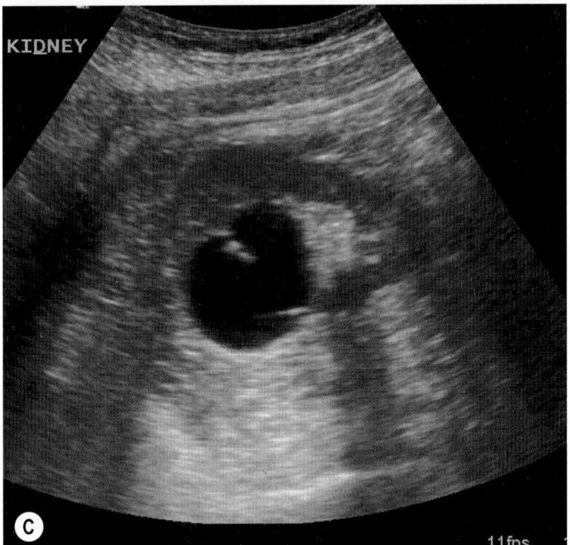

Fig. 7.5 • (A) 3 Simple renal cysts with posterior enhancement. (B) Small renal cyst, Bosniak 2, containing calcification following episodes of infection. This remained stable on follow-up. (C) Example of a Bosniak 2F cyst with a thin septum and nodule of calcification on the wall. No contrast enhancement was demonstrated and the cyst remained stable.

AUTOSOMAL DOMINANT POLYCYSTIC KIDNEY DISEASE

Autosomal dominant polycystic kidney disease (ADPKD) is the most common genetically linked renal disorder and it is associated with progressive renal failure. Renal transplant offers a successful 'cure' for many patients. APKD demonstrates a spectrum of severity, with some patients having renal failure in early life, and others achieving a normal life span with no appreciable symptoms. In about 50% of cases, cysts are also present in the liver; they are also found in the spleen and pancreas in a small proportion of patients.

Ultrasound screening for APKD is performed in families with a positive history, as patients may then be monitored and treated for hypertension. A negative scan does not entirely exclude disease

CATEGORY	FEATURES
I	Benign simple cyst, thin walled, no septae, calcification or solid components. No contrast enhancement with CT
II	May contain hairline septae, possible fine calcification in the wall. Sharp margins. Benign
IIF	More hairline septae. Minimal thickening of septa or wall. May contain nodular calcification. No contrast enhancement of any soft tissue elements. Well marginated. Usually benign
III	Indeterminate cystic mass with thickened irregular wall or septa in which enhancement can be seen
1V	Clearly malignant, containing enhancing soft tissue components

Table 7.1 Bosniak renal cyst classification for CT[5]

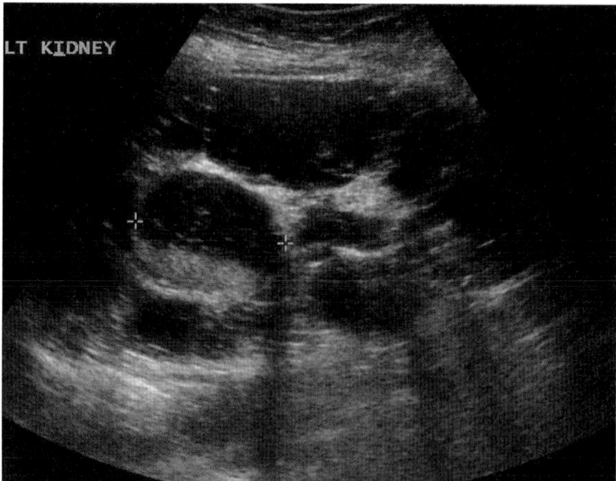

Fig. 7.6 • Autosomal dominant ('adult') polycystic disease. Numerous cysts of varying size are seen within in the renal bed. No discernable renal architecture is apparent. A cyst containing debris i.e. haemorrhage (calipers) is present.

especially in the paediatric group and multiple examinations over years may need to be performed.

Ultrasound appearances

The disease is always bilateral, causing progressively enlarging kidneys with multiple cysts of various sizes, many having irregular margins (Fig. 7.6). There may be little or no demonstrable normal renal tissue and the kidneys may become so large that they visibly distend the abdomen.

APKD predisposes the patient to urinary tract infections, stones and cyst haemorrhage. The liver, spleen and pancreas should also be examined on ultrasound for associated cysts. Although there have been reports of an increased incidence of RCC in APKD, there is no substantial evidence for this and it is generally considered that the risk of RCC is the same as the general population.[8,9]

VON HIPPEL–LINDAU DISEASE

Von Hippel–Lindau disease (VHL) is an inherited autosomal dominant disease that affects the central nervous system and retina with haemangioblastomas. Renal disease may present later, with cysts occurring in approximately 60–70% of sufferers. Because there is a recognized association with renal adenocarcinoma in up to 45% of patients, ultrasound is useful in screening patients with the disease.

TUBEROSE SCLEROSIS

Tuberose sclerosis is a rare, multisystem disorder with a wide spectrum of possible presentation. Up to 75% of patients may develop multiple renal cysts and/or multiple angiomyolipomas (AMLs).[10] Rarely, renal cell carcinoma may occur, although it is thought that the occurrence is similar to that of the general population. However, RCC tends to occur at a younger age in patients with TS (see Fig. 7.8B).

AUTOSOMAL RECESSIVE ('INFANTILE') PCKD

This autosomal recessive condition is part of a spectrum of congenital fibrocystic hepatorenal diseases, and may often be diagnosed prenatally on ultrasound. The disease carries a high mortality rate in early childhood, and is rarely seen on ultrasound in children.

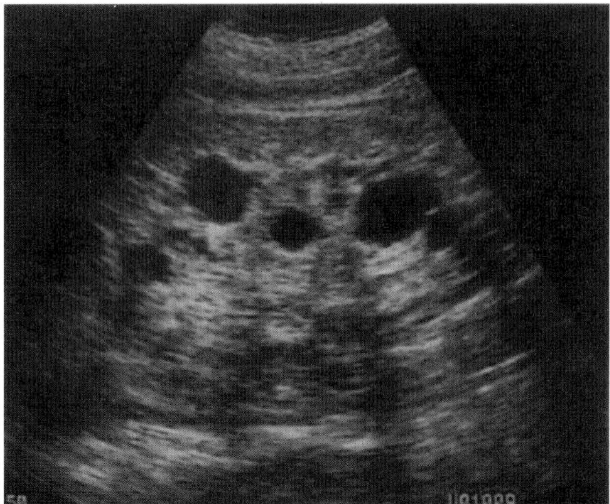

Fig. 7.7 • Acquired cystic disease in a patient with chronic renal failure who has been on long-term dialysis.

Tiny cysts replace both kidneys, giving them a hyperechoic appearance due to the multiple reflections from the cyst walls and the overall increased through-transmission.

ACQUIRED CYSTIC DISEASE

This condition tends to affect patients on long-term dialysis who may already have shrunken, end-stage kidneys. Its frequency increases with the duration of dialysis.

Multiple cysts form in the kidneys, which may, like autosomal dominant PCKD, haemorrhage or become infected. The disease tends to be more severe the longer the patient has been on dialysis. The proliferative changes which cause acquired cystic disease also give rise to small adenomata and the ultrasound appearances maybe a combination of cysts and solid, hypoechoic nodules. In particular, acquired cystic disease has the potential for malignancy[11,12] and it is therefore prudent to screen native kidneys, even after renal transplantation has been performed (Fig. 7.7).

MULTICYSTIC DYSPLASTIC KIDNEY

Multicystic dysplastic kidney (MCDK) is a congenital malformation of the kidney, in which the renal tissue is completely replaced by cysts. It is frequently diagnosed prenatally (although it is naturally a lethal condition if bilateral). Most MCDKs shrink with age, although a minority (around 10%) are stable or increase in size. By adulthood, the MCDK be so small that it is difficult to detect and may be mistaken for an absent kidney. Contralateral renal hypertrophy is often present.

MCDK can be associated with contralateral pelviureteric junction obstruction, which is also frequently diagnosed in utero. It is thought that MCDK occurs as a result of severe, early renal obstruction during development in utero. Obstructed calyces become blocked off, forming numerous cysts which do not connect.

BENIGN FOCAL RENAL TUMOURS

Angiomyolipoma

These are usually solitary, asymptomatic lesions, found incidentally on the scan. They tend to be well-defined and highly reflective, often rounded lesions containing blood vessels, muscle tissue and fat as the name suggests. They are usually asymptomatic, although the larger lesions can haemorrhage, causing haematuria and pain. AMLs are also associated with tuberose sclerosis, when they are often multiple and bilateral (Fig. 7.8). Because the contrast between the hypoechoic renal parenchyma and the hyperechoic AML is so great, very small lesions in the order of a few millimetres can be recognized on ultrasound.

An AML may cause a diagnostic dilemma, particularly in patients presenting with haematuria. They tend to be smaller and more echogenic than RCCs, and sometimes demonstrate shadowing, which is not normally seen in small carcinomas.[13] When doubt persists, CT is usually able to differentiate in these cases by identifying the fat content of the lesion. However this is not infallible as a small number of AMLs (<5%) do not contain fat

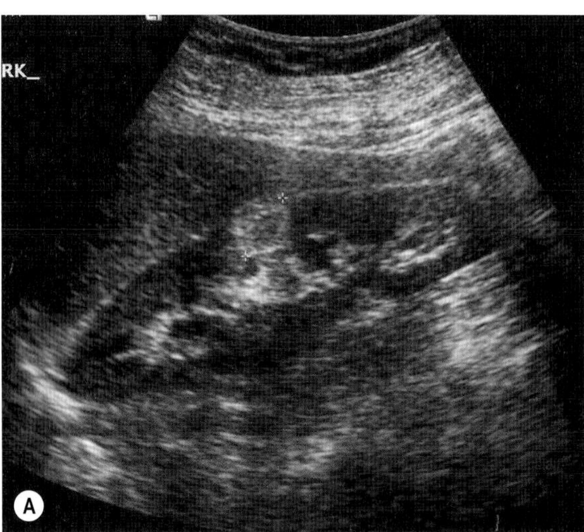

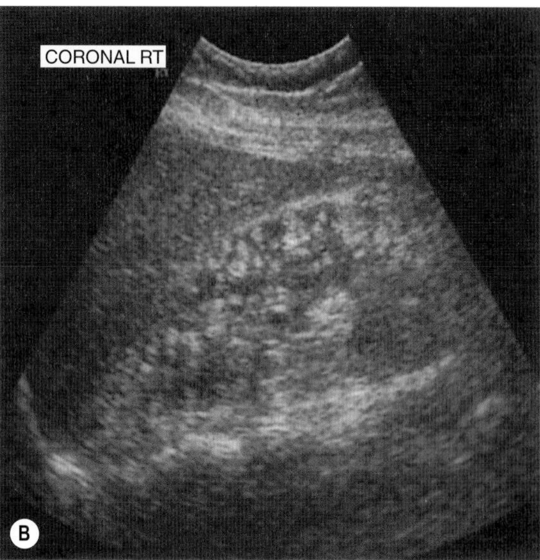

Fig. 7.8 • (A) AML in the RK (calipers). (B) Multiple, small AMLs in a patient with tuberose sclerosis.

and a number of other tumours, such as lipoma, liposarcoma and some RCCs, also may contain fat.[14]

Adenoma

The renal adenoma is usually a small, well-defined hyperechoic lesion, similar in appearance to the AML. It is felt that adenomas are frequently early manifestations of renal carcinoma as distinct from a benign lesion[14,15] and the two may be histologically indistinguishable.

Renal adenomas are often found in association with an RCC in the same or contralateral kidney,[16] although these are radiologically indistinguishable from metastases. Because of the controversy surrounding the distinction between adenomas and small RCCs, the management of patients with these masses is uncertain. Most incidentally discovered, small (less than 3 cm) parenchymal renal masses are slow growing and may safely be monitored with CT or ultrasound, particularly in the elderly.[17]

There are a number of other benign renal tumours including leiomyoma, haemangioma, fibroma, oncocytoma and lymphangioma. Ultrasound is usually unable to characterize these, and CT may be helpful in evaluating the kidney further.[14]

MALIGNANT RENAL TRACT MASSES

IMAGING AND MANAGEMENT OF MALIGNANT RENAL MASSES

Ultrasound is the first line of investigation in patients with haematuria. It is highly sensitive in detecting renal masses over 2.5 cm in diameter, and readily differentiates them from renal cysts. Smaller masses maybe missed with ultrasound however, as they are frequently isoechoic (in 86% of cases); CT is more sensitive in small lesion detection. MRI also detects small renal masses more frequently than ultrasound but is generally reserved for patients with equivocal CT scans. If imaging is not able to characterize a renal lesion, then biopsy will provide a histological diagnosis.

Renal malignancy is not infrequently detected incidentally on ultrasound. Such lesions tend to be small (<4 cm) and isolated, with a good prognosis. Surveillance with ultrasound is an option in older patients or those with comorbidities, as many small lesions in older patients are stable in size. Any increase in size triggers more aggressive treatment.[18]

There is now a range of treatment options for renal malignancy; in addition to nephrectomy – still the treatment of choice in most centres – it is possible to offer minimally invasive techniques such as laparoscopic removal, nephron-preserving partial nephrectomy or percutaneous ablation (CT or ultrasound-guided.) CEUS may be used to guide percutaneous ablation for small renal tumours, and is useful in demonstrating tumour devascularization post ablation, or to monitor ablated tumours for signs of recurrence[19] (see below and also Fig. 7.10).

Staging of renal cancers is usually performed with CT.

RENAL CELL CARCINOMA

Adenocarcinoma is the most common type of renal malignancy (referred to as RCC) occurring less commonly in the bladder and ureter. RCCs are frequently large at clinical presentation, but are increasingly identified as an incidental finding in asymptomatic patients, due to increasing use and quality of imaging techniques, particularly ultrasound.

Ultrasound appearances

The RCC is a heterogeneous mass that often enlarges and deforms the shape of the kidney (Fig. 7.9). The mass may contain areas of cystic degeneration and/or calcification. It has a predilection to spread into the ipsilateral renal vein and IVC (see also Chapter 8). The increasing use of ultrasound, and its improved quality has led to an increase in the detection of small tumours, often in asymptomatic patients. Around 50% of all RCCs diagnosed fall into this category.[20]

Colour Doppler reveals a disorganized and increased blood flow pattern in larger masses with high velocities from the arteriovenous (AV) shunts within the carcinoma. CEUS may demonstrate a variety of contrast uptake patterns, with heterogeneous uptake, or hyper-enhancement in the sinusoidal phase.[4–7,21] CEUS is also helpful in identifying residual tissue after tumours have been ablated (Fig. 7.10).

Smaller renal cell carcinomas can be hyperechoic and may be confused with benign angiomyolipoma. The latter has well-defined borders whilst a renal cell carcinoma is ill-defined: differentiation may not be possible on all occasions – biopsy or interval scan may be required.

Clearly smaller masses have a better prognosis and are likely to be early in stage with no metastases.[20] With larger masses, liver, adrenal and lymph node metastases may be demonstrated on ultrasound. CT is used to stage the disease and will also demonstrate if metastases are present in the lungs.

TRANSITIONAL CELL CARCINOMA

Transitional cell carcinoma (TCC) is the most common bladder tumour, occurring less frequently in the collecting system of the kidney and the ureter. It usually presents with haematuria whilst still small. It is best diagnosed with cystoscopy. Small tumours in the renal collecting system are difficult to detect on ultrasound unless there is proximal dilatation. Depending on its location it may cause hydronephrosis, particularly if it is situated in the ureter (rare) or at the vesicoureteric junction (VUJ). The exact position and extent of the tumour is best demonstrated with CT urography.

TCCs in the renal pelvis account for approximately 10% of renal tumours. Spread to the contralateral collecting system is a recognized risk,[22] and patients are regularly monitored following treatment.

Ultrasound appearances

The TCC is typically a relatively hyperechoic, solid mass distending the renal sinus (Fig. 7.11A). Some pelvicalyceal dilatation is not unusual. The TCC is less likely to distort the renal outline (compared with RCC) and so is more easily missed by the unwary operator. A TCC can mimic a hypertrophied column of Bertin (see above); CT may differentiate in cases of doubt.

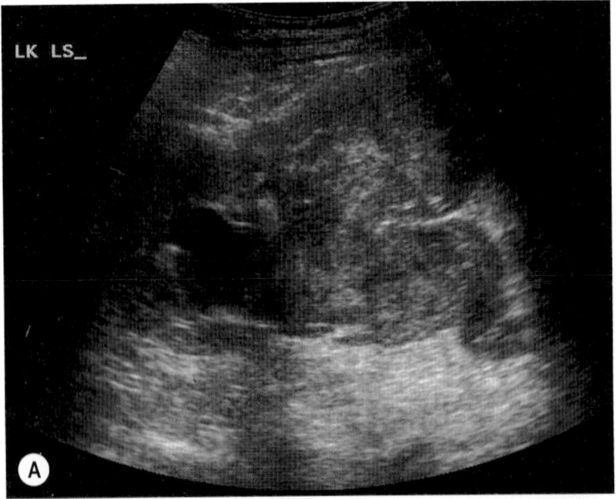

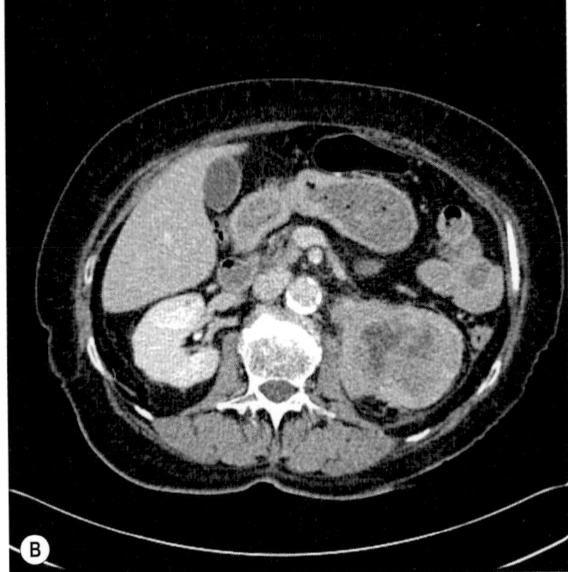

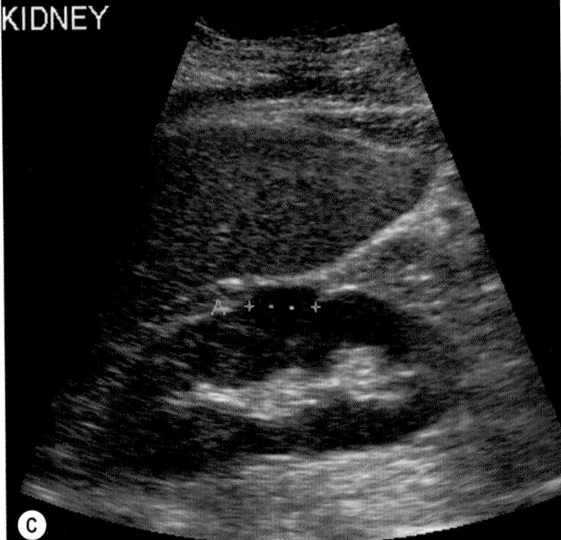

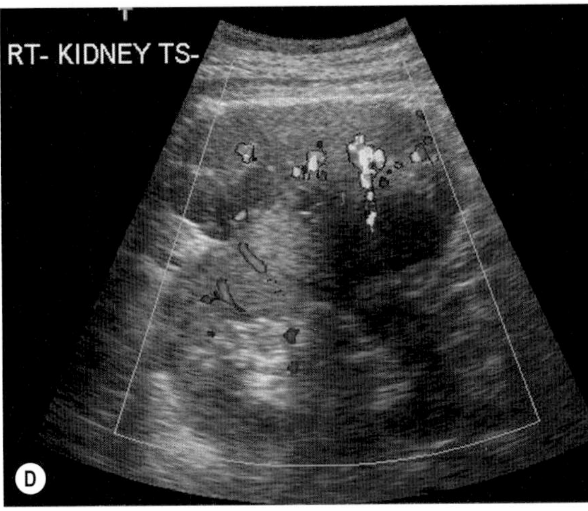

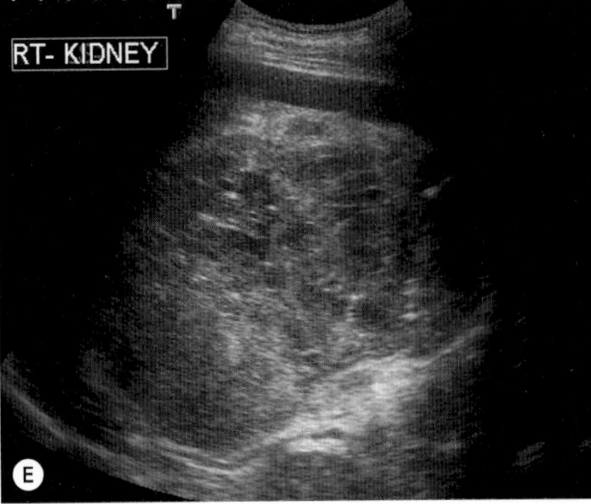

Fig. 7.9 • (A) The LK is almost completely replaced by a large renal carcinoma. The ureter also contains tumour thrombus. (B) CT of the case in (A). (C) A small RCC (calipers) discovered incidentally during abdominal US. (D) Colour Doppler of an exophytic RCC reveals disorganized, multidirectional blood flow. (E) Large RCC completely replacing the right kidney.

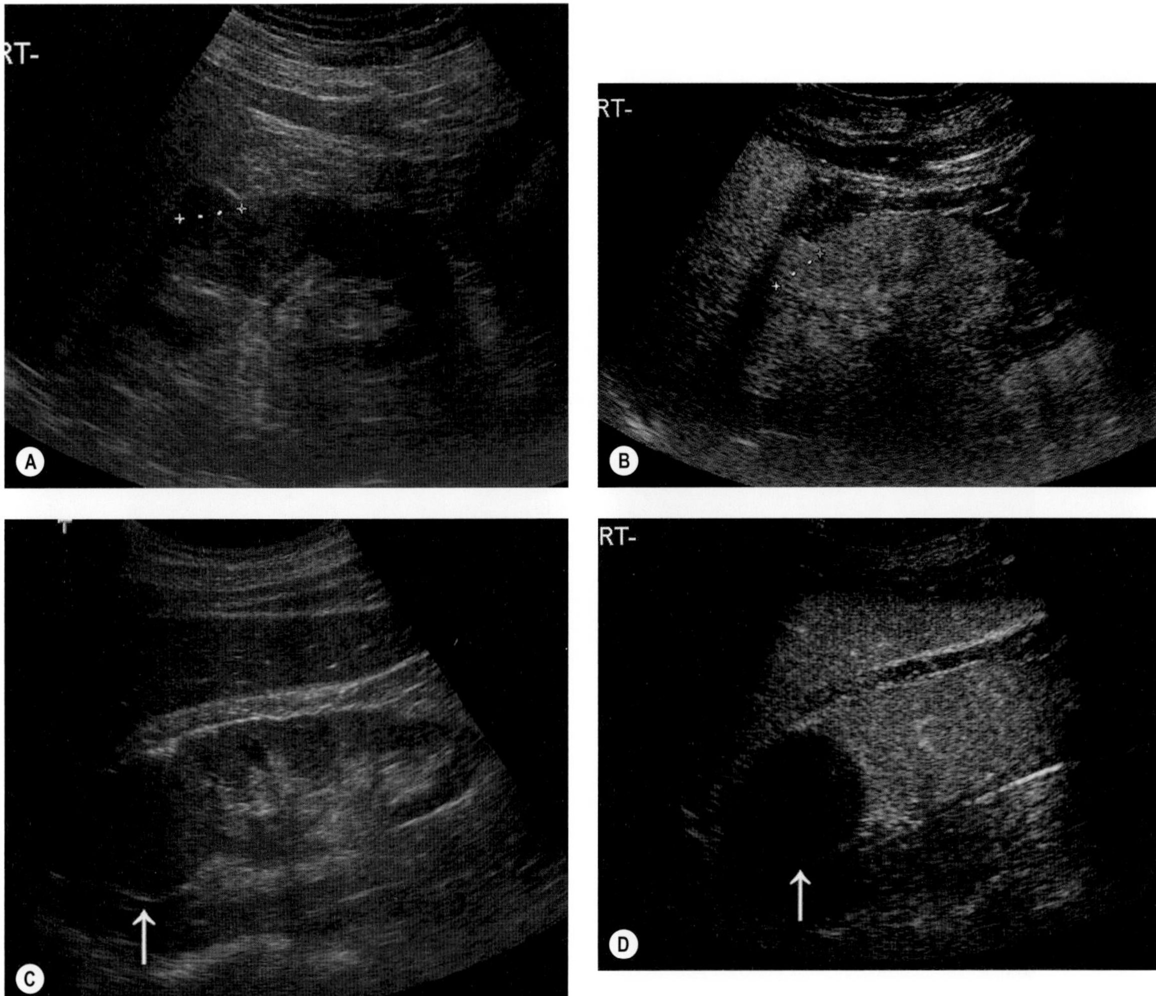

Fig. 7.10 • CEUS: (A) Small RCC (calipers) pre-contrast. (B) The lesion in (A) is hypervascular and takes up contrast throughout. (C) Another small RCC post-ablation (arrow) before contrast. (D) The lesion in (C) is avascular following successful ablation – note the normal contrast uptake in the background kidney.

Once large, they invade the surrounding renal parenchyma and become indistinguishable from renal cell carcinoma on ultrasound. They frequently spread to the bladder and the entire renal tract must be carefully examined.

The role of ultrasound here is usually limited to that of a first line investigation in haematuria, particularly as the ureters are not well demonstrated. CT urography has higher sensitivity especially in demonstrating ureteric lesions.

In the bladder, TCCs are potentially easier to see as they are surrounded by urine (Fig. 7.11B). Invasion of the bladder wall can be identified on ultrasound in the larger ones but biopsy is necessary to formally determine the level of invasion.

LYMPHOMA

Renal involvement of non-Hodgkin's or Hodgkin's lymphoma is not uncommon and depends

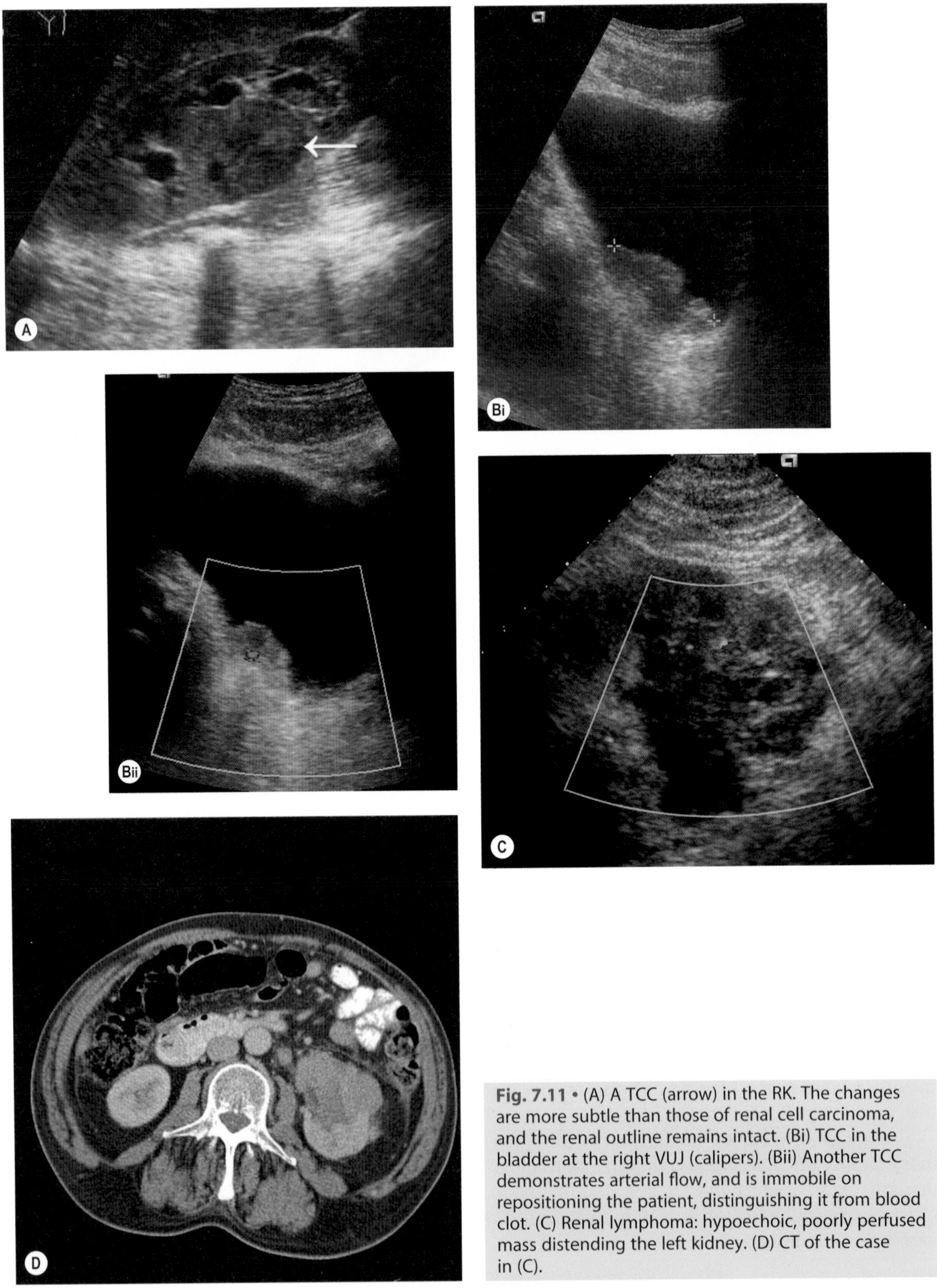

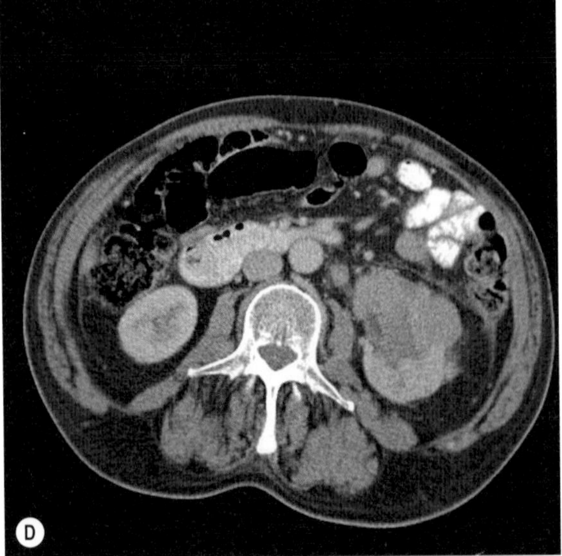

Fig. 7.11 • (A) A TCC (arrow) in the RK. The changes are more subtle than those of renal cell carcinoma, and the renal outline remains intact. (Bi) TCC in the bladder at the right VUJ (calipers). (Bii) Another TCC demonstrates arterial flow, and is immobile on repositioning the patient, distinguishing it from blood clot. (C) Renal lymphoma: hypoechoic, poorly perfused mass distending the left kidney. (D) CT of the case in (C).

upon the stage of the disease. The ultrasound appearances are highly variable and range from solitary to multiple masses, usually hypoechoic but sometimes anechoic, hyperechoic or mixed (Fig. 7.11C, D).

The masses may have increased through transmission of sound and may mimic complex fluid lesions such as haematoma or abscess. The clinical history should help to differentiate these cases. Occasionally diffuse enlargement may occur secondary to diffuse infiltration.

METASTASES

Renal metastases from a distant primary are usually only found in cases of widespread metastatic disease and are frequently multiple. In such cases, the primary diagnosis is usually already known and other abdominal metastases, such as liver deposits and/or lymphadenopathy are commonly seen on ultrasound.

Rarely, a single metastasis is seen in the kidney without other evidence of metastatic spread making the diagnosis difficult, (as the question arises of whether this could be a primary or secondary lesion.) CT may identify the primary and frequently picks up other, smaller metastases not identified on ultrasound.[23]

VON HIPPEL–LINDAU DISEASE

VHL is a comparatively rare autosomal dominant multisystem disorder which is associated with the development of tumours, both benign and malignant. Retinal and CNS haemangioblastomas, pancreatic cysts and tumours and pheochromocytomas are among the varied possible spectrum of disease. RCC is one of the most common causes of death in these patients,[24] and screening with ultrasound is advocated in some centres. Where early detection of RCC occurs, timely treatment options are available and patient morbidity and mortality is reduced.

PELVICALYCEAL SYSTEM DILATATION AND OBSTRUCTIVE UROPATHY

Not all pelvicalyceal system dilatation is pathological, or indeed obstructive; there can be dilatation without physiological obstruction. Conversely not all obstructive uropathy necessarily results in pelvicalyceal system dilatation.

PHYSIOLOGICAL DILATATION

Mild dilatation of the renal collecting system is a common finding, most commonly being secondary to an overdistended bladder. Following micturition, the collecting system decompresses and returns to normal. An external renal pelvis (see above) is a non-obstructive 'baggy' dilatation of the pelvis and can be regarded as a normal variant. The intrarenal collecting system is normal in this situation (Fig. 7.4D).

Pregnancy is another common cause of mild pelvicalyceal dilatation, more frequently on the right, particularly in the second and third trimester. This is thought to be due partly to pressure on the ureters from the advancing pregnancy and partly hormonal. It is, however, wrong to assume that the kidney is not obstructed just because the patient is pregnant. If symptomatic, the suspicion of obstruction in a dilated system is increased, particularly if echoes are present in the pelvicalyceal system.

OBSTRUCTIVE UROPATHY

Causes of renal obstruction vary (Table 7.2) but the most common is due to stone obstruction, either in the pelviureteric junction (PUJ), ureter or VUJ. Renal obstruction, particularly if longstanding, can irreversibly damage the kidney or kidneys, leading eventually to renal failure. If diagnosed early enough, renal function can be preserved and therefore ultrasound plays an important role as one of the first-line investigations in

INTRINSIC FACTORS	
Stones	Accompanied by renal colic. May be situated anywhere along the renal tract
Tumour	In the bladder, pelvicalyceal system or ureter
Blood clot	From infection or trauma
Papillary necrosis	Sloughed papillae can travel down the ureter, causing obstruction
INFECTIVE PROCESSES	
Stricture	Caused by chronic, repeated infection
Fungal balls	Rare
Tuberculosis	
CONGENITAL	
Idiopathic PUJ obstruction	Usually unilateral; pelvicalyceal system dilatation only
Posterior urethral valves	Entire renal tract dilatation. Frequently diagnosed antenatally.
Ureterocoele	Unilateral hydronephrosis with hydroureter
OUTFLOW OBSTRUCTION	
Prostate enlargement	Benign or malignant
Urethral stricture	May be iatrogenic, congenital or as a result of infection. Accompanied by disturbed micturition
EXTRINSIC PELVIC MASS	
Cervical carcinoma	Proximity to the ureters causes obstruction
Endometriosis	Endometriotic lesions adhere to the peritoneal and/or ureteric surfaces, causing compression
Others: lymphadenopathy, inflammatory bowel masses, gynaecological masses	Always scan the kidneys to exclude obstruction when a pelvic mass is present
IATROGENIC	
Post-surgical procedure	Ligation of ureters in gynaecological procedures
Trauma	Can cause a stricture of the ureter or can cause the renal tract to be blocked by blood clot from damage to the kidney

Table 7.2 Causes of renal tract obstruction

patients with loin pain, renal colic or micturition disorders. CT urography is the imaging modality of choice when acute obstruction is suspected, as the ureters are clearly demonstrated, unlike ultrasound, and tiny stones are confidently demonstrated (Fig. 7.12B).

In the vast majority of cases, urinary tract obstruction causes dilatation of the collecting system proximal to the site of obstruction (Fig. 7.12). Whether the hydronephrosis is bilateral or unilateral and whether or not it involves the ureter(s) depends on the cause and site of the obstructing lesion.

Dilatation of the collecting system may be localized. Sometimes only one moiety of the kidney may be obstructed by a stone or tumour, while the rest of the kidney remains normal. In a duplex kidney, dilatation of the upper pole moiety is a common occurrence due to a ureterocele at the VUJ.

If the obstruction is long-standing, the renal cortex may atrophy and become thin. Normal thickness of cortex is a good prognostic indicator. Function may be assessed with a nuclear medicine (DTPA) scan prior to further management.

FURTHER MANAGEMENT OF RENAL OBSTRUCTION

CT urography has been recognized as the most suitable investigation in patients with suspected renal stones or obstruction.[25,26] Ultrasound is useful in pregnant or paediatric patients, when it is particularly necessary to minimize radiation dose. It is important to assess the *function* of the obstructed side, as a chronic, long-standing obstruction with no residual function cannot be treated, but a kidney that still has function is worth saving. A DTPA scan can assess the relative functions of the obstructed and non-obstructed side.

Most stones pass without intervention and are conservatively managed. If conservative treatment fails, then surgical or radiological removal is necessary.

Percutaneous nephrostomy (the placing of a tube into the PCS to drain the urine) in the case of unilateral obstruction is performed to relieve the obstruction, minimizing damage to the kidney and maintaining renal function and drainage. This may be done under either ultrasound or fluoroscopic guidance or a combination of both (Fig. 7.12G).

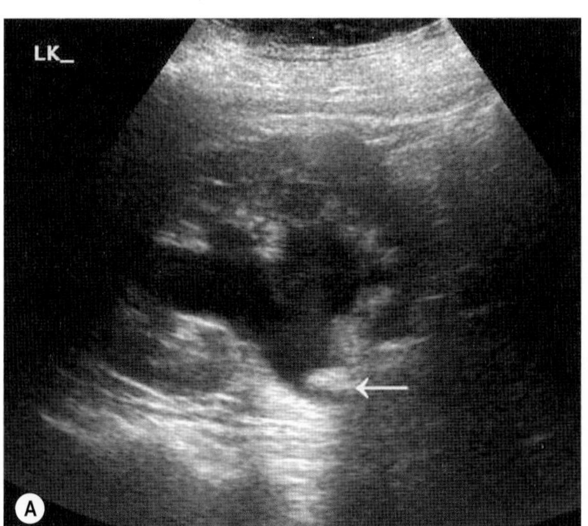

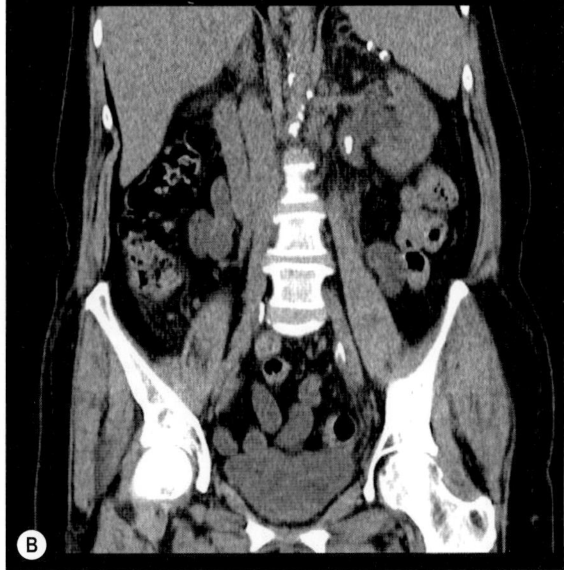

Fig. 7.12 • (A) Hydronephrosis of the left kidney, secondary to a stone in the PUJ (arrow). (B) CT urography of the same case demonstrating left VUJ stone.

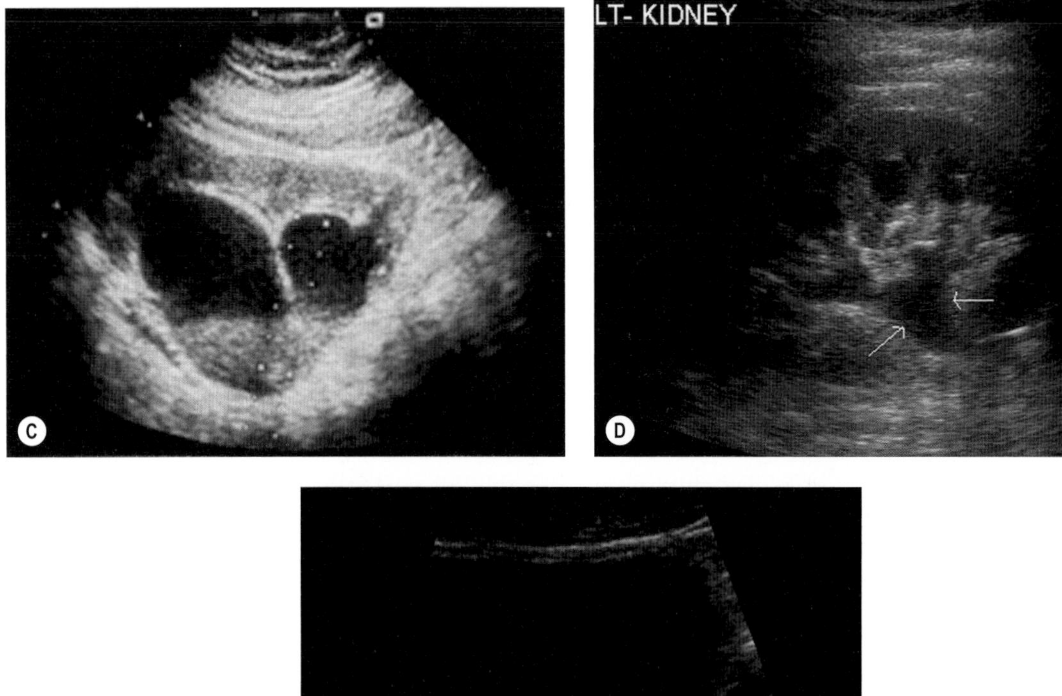

Fig. 7.12, cont'd • (C) Hydronephrosis of the lower moiety of a duplex kidney containing debris within the dilated pelvicalyceal system, prior to percutaneous nephrostomy. (D) Mild dilatation of the left pelvicalyceal system (arrows) heralds obstruction. (E) A stone in the left VUJ, with acoustic shadowing, is the cause of the obstruction in case (D).

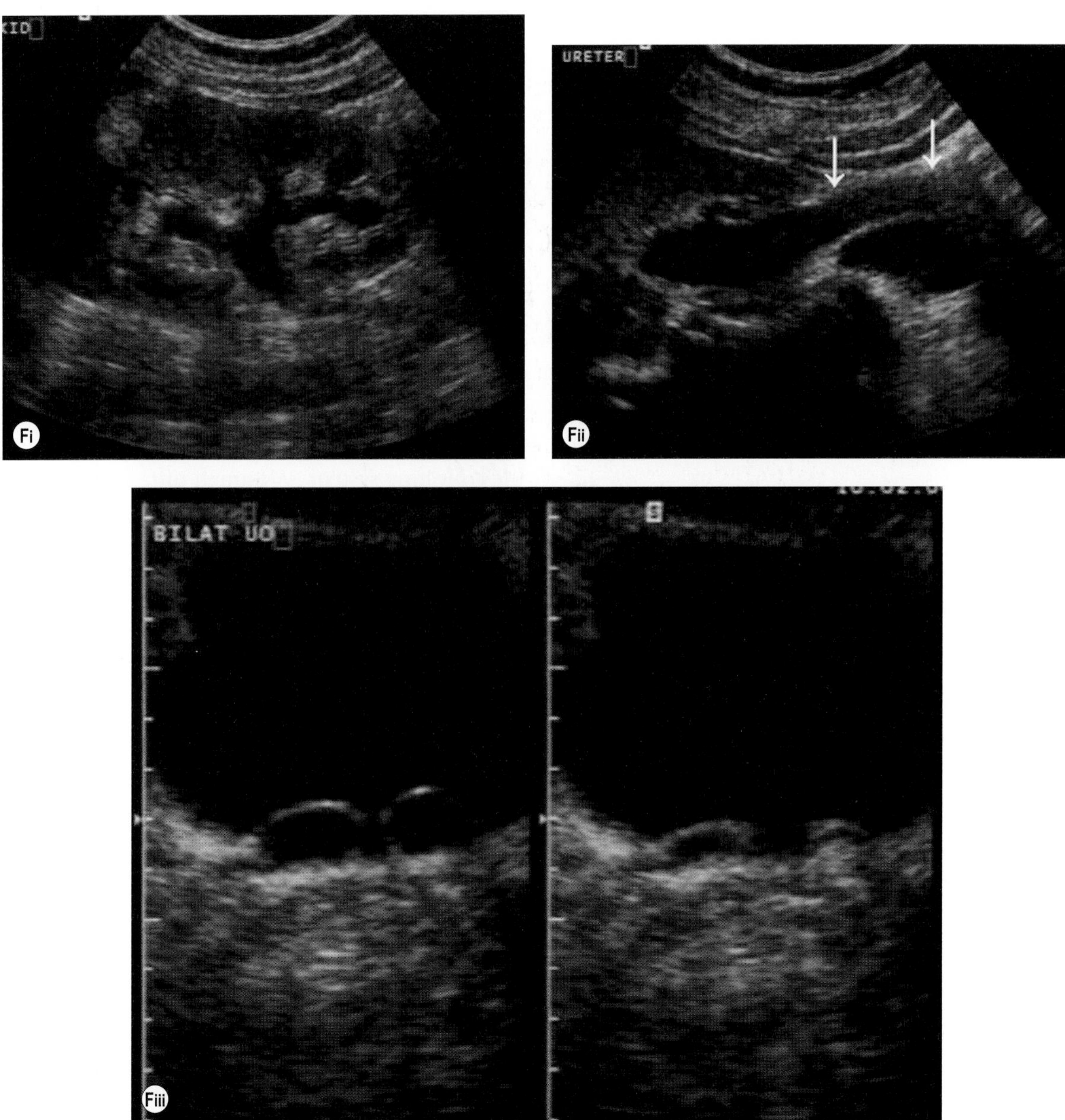

Fig. 7.12, cont'd • (Fi) Hydronephrosis and (Fii) hydroureter (arrows) are bilateral and caused by bilateral ureteroceles, (Fiii), seen at the VUJ.

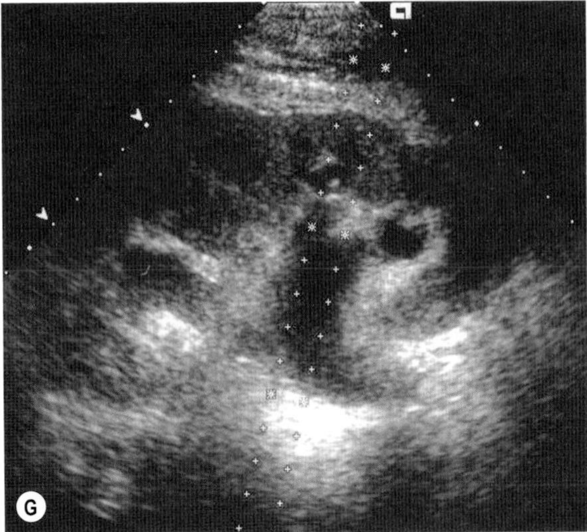

Fig. 7.12, cont'd • (G) A dilated kidney is about to undergo percutaneous nephrostomy under ultrasound guidance; the needle guide is lined up to enter the dilated collecting system.

Pyonephrosis

Pyonephrosis is a urological emergency. An obstructed kidney is prone to become infected. High fever and loin pain can suggest obstructive pyonephrosis. Pus or pus cells may also be detected in the urine.

Low level echoes can be seen within the dilated PCS on ultrasound, which may represent pus. Sometimes, however, the urine may appear anechoic, despite being infected. The clinical history should help differentiate pyo- from simple hydronephrosis (Fig. 7.13). Percutaneous drainage by ultrasound or fluoroscopically guided nephrostomy is usually necessary, partly as diagnostic confirmation and partly as a therapeutic procedure.

Haemo-hydronephrosis

Blood within the dilated PCS may be due to trauma or other local or semi local pathological processes such as infection or tumour. It is not usually possible to determine whether obstruction is caused by a blood clot or whether the blood is the result of an obstructing lesion which is also causing bleeding.

Renal colic as a result of obstruction by a blood clot in the absence of trauma or blood dyscrasia, must naturally be thoroughly investigated to exclude an underlying lesion. Like pyonephrosis, low level echoes may be seen on ultrasound within the collecting system . Although ultrasonically it is not possible to differentiate pyo- from haemo-hydronephrosis, the clinical picture can be suggestive of one or the other.

Non-dilated renal obstruction

The finding of a non-dilated PCS on ultrasound does not exclude obstruction in a patient with symptoms of renal colic. Obstruction may occasionally be present in the acute stages before renal dilatation is apparent. Spectral Doppler is useful in diagnosing acute, early renal obstruction, before pelvicalyceal dilatation develops, because of the associated increase in blood flow resistance in the affected kidney (Fig. 7.14). This causes an increase in the resistance and pulsatility indices (RI and PI) on the obstructed side, due to a reduction in diastolic flow.

A raised RI in itself is a non-specific finding, not necessarily indicating obstruction; it is known to be age related or can be associated with extrinsic compression of the kidney (for example by a fluid collection or mass [Table 7.3]) or with some chronic renal diseases or vascular disorders. This can be overcome by analysing Doppler spectra from both kidneys and evaluating any difference between the two sides. A marked *difference* in RI between the kidneys in a patient with renal colic points towards obstruction of the kidney with the higher

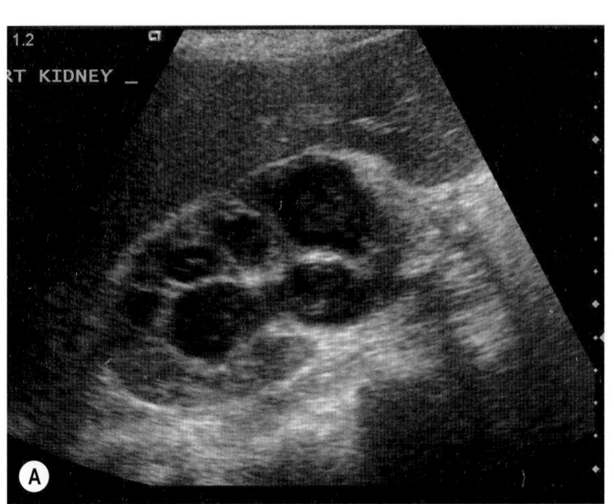

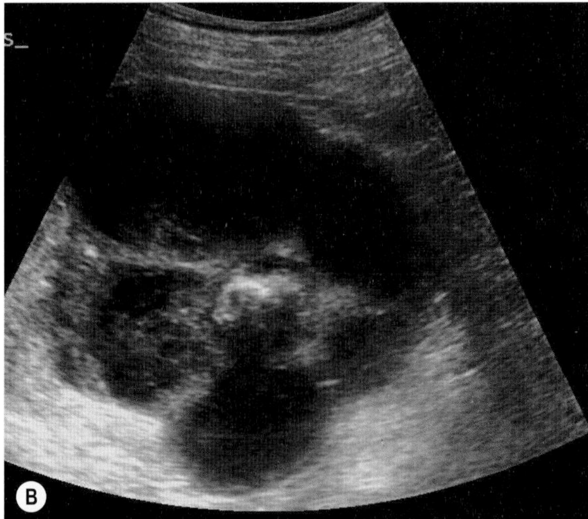

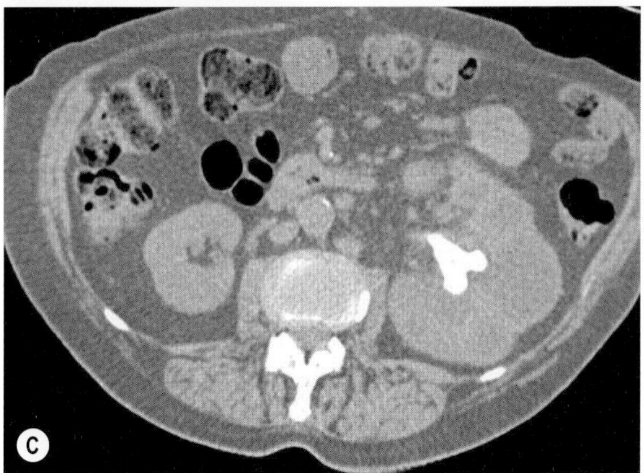

Fig. 7.13 • Pyonephrosis: (A) Low-level echoes from pus can be seen in the dilated pelvicalyceal system. (Note that absence of echoes does not exclude pyonephrosis). (B) This obstructed kidney contains a large central staghorn calculus. The echoes within the pelvicalyceal system represent pus. (C) CT of the case in (B), demonstrating the staghorn calculus and pyonephrosis.

resistance.[27,28] A difference in RIs of greater than 6 is highly suspicious of obstruction in a patient with renal colic; a reduction in the RI on the affected side can be observed when the obstruction has been relieved or after the renal PCS has become dilated.

This effect often does not persist once the kidney dilates, presumably because the intrarenal pressure is relieved, which emphasizes the use of Doppler in acute cases, before dilatation has become established.[29] Because of the vagaries of the stage of obstruction, renal pressure, etc. the interpretation of RI should be made cautiously.

Vesicoureteric junction

The normal ureters may be identified on ultrasound as they enter the bladder. Jets of urine emerge into the bladder at these points and can be demonstrated with colour Doppler (Fig. 7.2B). An absent or reduced number of jets may indicate obstruction on that side. This finding again should be interpreted cautiously; ureteric jet analysis is not a useful test of renal obstruction. Careful scanning at the VUJs can identify significant anomalies (Fig. 7.12):

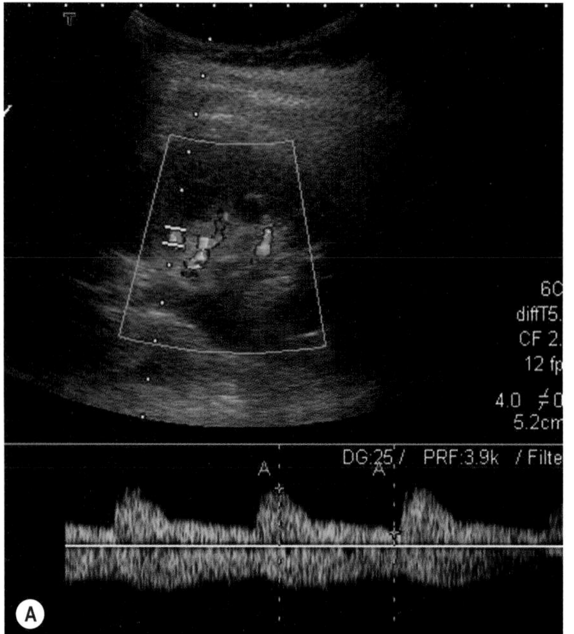

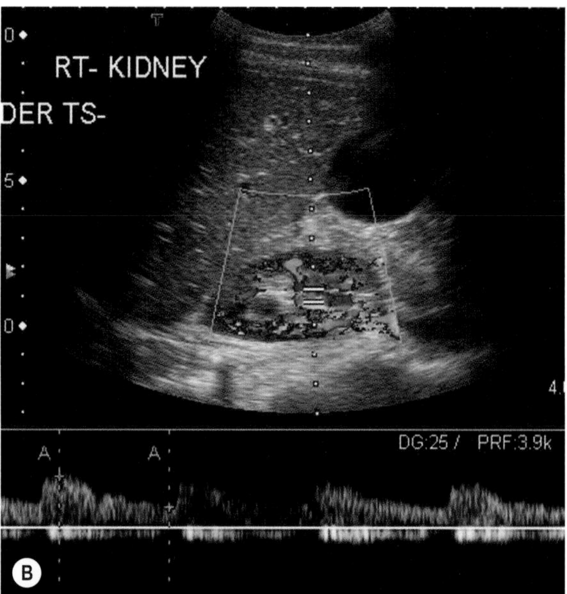

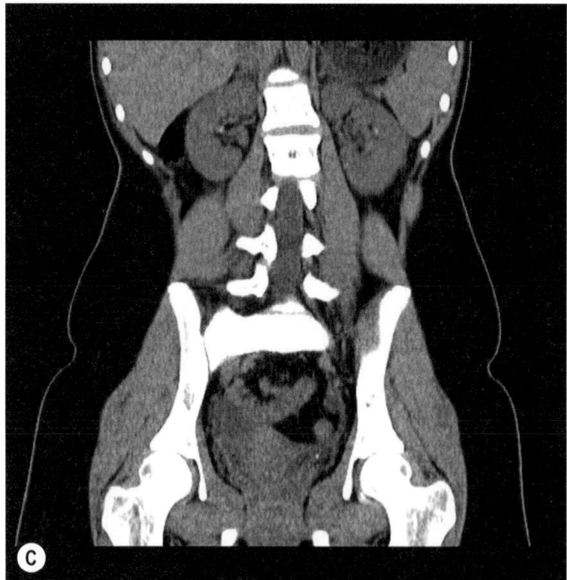

Fig. 7.14 • Doppler in obstruction: (A) A patient with acute left-sided renal colic has a non-dilated LK with a raised resistance index of 75.8. (B) In the same patient, the contralateral, normal kidney has a much lower resistance index of 61. (C) CT confirms a tiny stone in the left VUJ, causing the obstruction, before dilatation becomes apparent.

Solitary lesions	Simple cyst Infected or haemorrhagic cyst Hydatid cyst (rare)
Complex fluid lesions	Haematoma Abscess Lymphoma Necrotic primary or secondary tumour Tuberculosis
Pelvicalyceal system dilatation	Obstructive or non-obstructive causes Xanthogranulomatous pyelonephritis
Multiple cystic lesions	Polycystic or acquired cystic disease Multiple abscesses

Table 7.3 Differential diagnoses for fluid-filled renal masses

- Reflux can be seen to dilate the ureter intermittently (see below)
- A ureterocele may be diagnosed as it dilates with the passage of urine – it may not be obvious until the operator has watched carefully for a few minutes
- Stones may become lodged at the VUJ, causing proximal dilatation.

NON-OBSTRUCTIVE HYDRONEPHROSIS

Not all renal dilatation is the result of an obstructive process, and the kidney may frequently be dilated for other reasons.

Reflux

This is the most common cause of non-obstructive renal dilatation, and is usually diagnosed in children. Reflux is associated with recurrent urinary tract infections (UTIs) and can result in reflux nephropathy, in which the renal parenchyma is irretrievably damaged.

Reflux can be distinguished from other causes of renal dilatation by observing the dilatation of the ureters at the bladder base, due to the retrograde passage of urine. For a more detailed consideration of the diagnosis of reflux see Chapter 9.

Post-obstructive dilatation

Dilatation of a once severely obstructed kidney may persist. The pelvicalyceal system remains baggy and dilated despite the obstruction having been relieved.

Papillary necrosis

The renal papillae, which are situated in the medulla adjacent to the calyces, are susceptible to ischaemia due to relatively low oxygenation in the region of the medullary junction. This is particularly associated with diabetic patients and those on long-term anti-inflammatory or analgesic medication. The condition is also associated with sickle cell disease, pyelonephritis and tuberculosis.

The papillae tend to necrose and slough off, causing blunting of calyces on IVU. Sloughed off papillae may lodge in the entrance to the calyces, causing obstruction.

Papillary necrosis is difficult to detect on ultrasound unless advanced. It appears as prominent calyces with increased cortico-medullary differentiation. IVU is the traditional imaging method of choice, although CT is now able to demonstrate early ischaemic change around the medullae[30] (Fig. 7.15).

Congenital megacalyces

A congenital condition in which the pelvicalyceal system is dilated due to poor development of the papillae. The calyces are usually markedly enlarged but the cortex is normal; the ureters are of normal calibre and not dilated.[31] Occasionally this is associated with *congenital megaureter*, in which the muscular layer of the ureter is atonic.

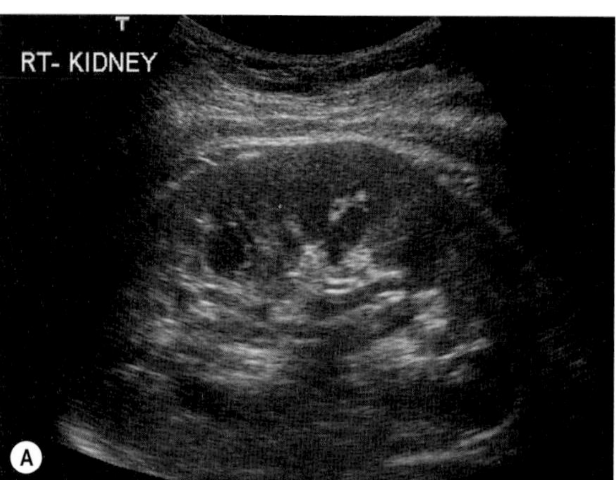

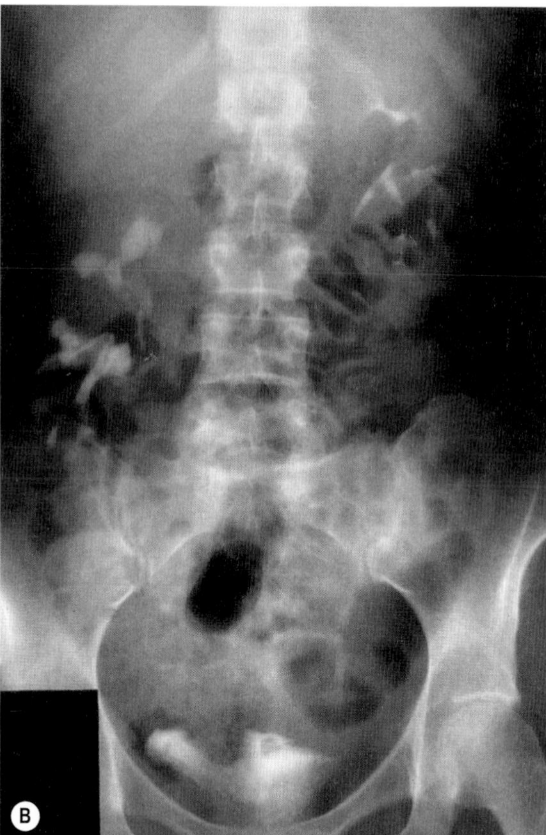

Fig. 7.15 • (A) Papillary necrosis. The calyces are mildly dilated with blunted, irregular margins and contain low-level echoes from sloughed papillae. (B) IVU of another patient demonstrating the blunted calyces.

RENAL TRACT CALCIFICATON

Calcification within the kidney usually occurs in the form of stones. Smaller foci of calcium, which do not shadow on ultrasound, are associated with conditions such as tuberculosis, xanthogranulomatous pyelonephritis, nephrocalcinosis or some neoplastic tumours.

RENAL TRACT STONES

Renal calculi are a common finding on ultrasound. They may be an incidental discovery in an asymptomatic patient; alternatively they maybe present in patients with acute renal colic and complete or partial obstruction of the ipsilateral renal tract. They may cause haematuria and can also be associated with urinary tract infections. The composition of calculi can vary. The common types include:

- *Calcium stones* – these are the most common type and are frequently associated with patients who have abnormal calcium metabolism.
- *Struvite (triple phosphate) stones* – these have a different composition of salts and are associated with urinary tract infections. They may form large, staghorn calculi (see below).

- *Uric acid stones* – these are rare, and tend to be associated with gout.
- *Cystine stones* – these are the rarest of all and result from a disorder of amino acid metabolism – cystinuria.

Ultrasound appearances

Most renal calculi are calcified foci located in the collecting system of the kidney. Careful scanning with modern equipment can identify over 90% of these.[32] Most stones are highly reflective structures which display distal shadowing (Figs 7.13B, C, 7.16). The shadowing may, however, be difficult to demonstrate due to the proximity of hyperechoic sinus echoes distal to the stone, or due to the relatively small size of the stone compared to the beamwidth.

Differentiation of stones from sinus fat and reflective vessel walls is dependent on careful technique and optimal use of the equipment. Tiny stones must be within the focal zone of the beam

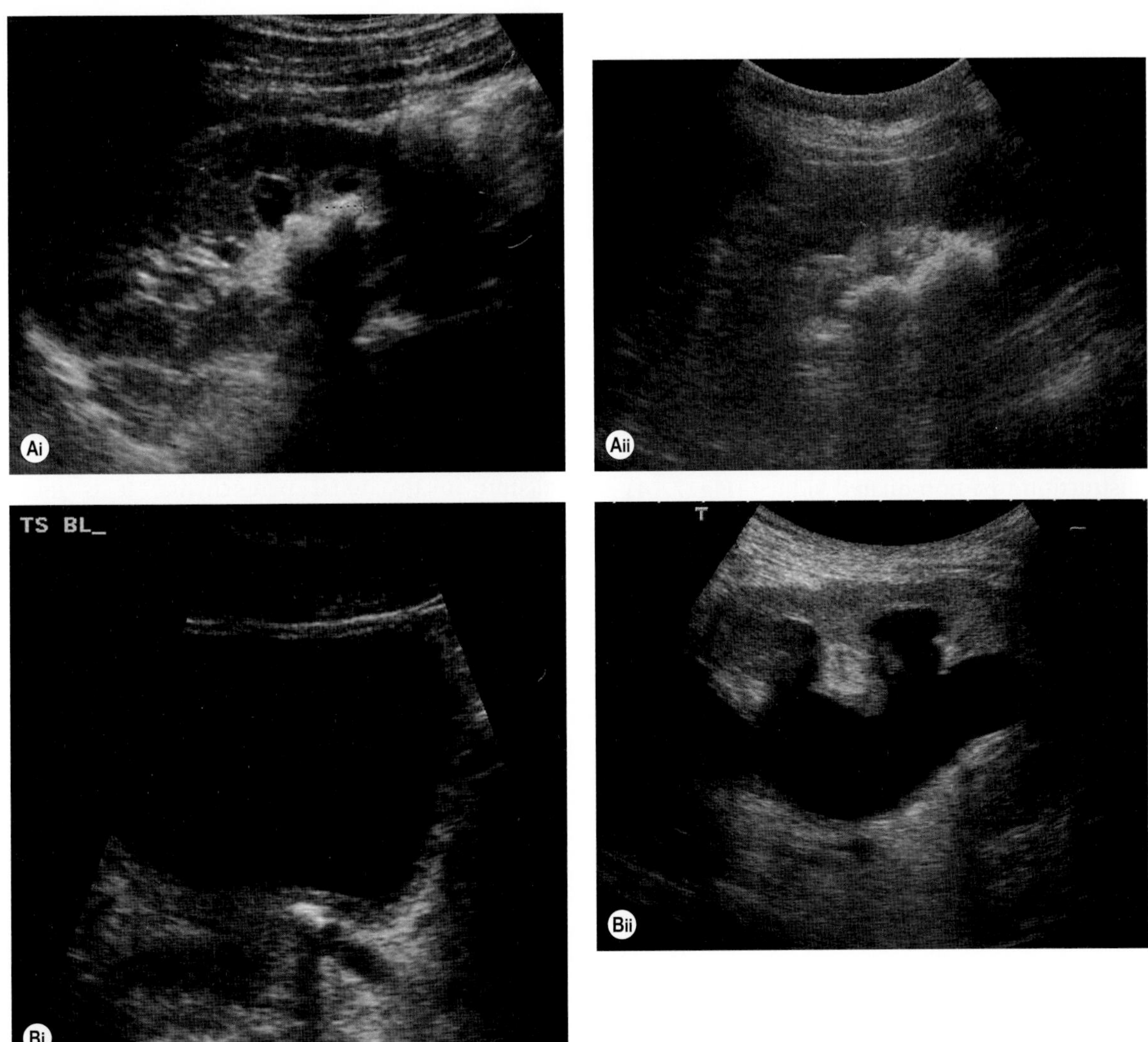

Fig. 7.16 • (Ai) Two calculi within the pelvicalyceal system of the RK cast distal acoustic shadows. (Aii) A staghorn calculus fills the collecting system of the kidney. (Bi) A stone in the left VUJ with posterior shadowing, causing left hydronephrosis (Bii).

to be demonstrated clearly. A high frequency is also necessary to maximize the chances of seeing small stones. Clearly, the identification of large calculi is usually straightforward, however, for many of the reasons above, identification of small calculi can be difficult especially in a patient with pain. Both false positive and false negative studies are well recognized. Patients with acute pain suspicious for renal stones may have CT urography as the first investigation, unless there is some contraindication[33] (Figs 7.12B, 7.14C).

Ultrasound still has a major role, however, not just in calculus detection but in identifying the secondary effects, i.e. hydronephrosis and where necessary guiding renal drainage. The pelvicalyceal system may be obstructed proximal to the stone. Obvious hydronephrosis may be present and a dilated ureter may be apparent when the stone has travelled distally. The stone can sometimes be identified in the dilated ureter, but this is unusual as the retroperitoneum is frequently obscured by overlying bowel.

Early obstruction occurs *before* the pelvicalyceal system can become dilated, making the diagnosis more difficult on ultrasound. Occasionally there will be mild separation of the pelvicalyceal system to give a clue, but sometimes the kidney appears normal. Doppler ultrasound can help to diagnose obstruction in a non-dilated kidney (Fig. 7.14) as discussed previously, however this may not always be definitive.

Staghorn calculi

These large calculi are so-called because they occupy a significant proportion of the collecting system (Fig. 7.16), giving the appearance of a staghorn on X-ray. On ultrasound they cast a dense shadow from the pelvicalyceal system, which may obscure any associated dilatation and can, in small, atrophied kidneys, be misinterpreted as shadowing from bowel gas. Because of the lobulated shape of the calculus it may appear as several separate calculi on ultrasound. A coronal section may therefore be more successful in confirming a staghorn calculus than a sagittal section.

Cystinuria

This rare metabolic disease causes crystals of cystine to precipitate in the kidneys and be excreted in the urine (Fig. 7.17). Cystine stones form in the kidneys and may result in obstruction.

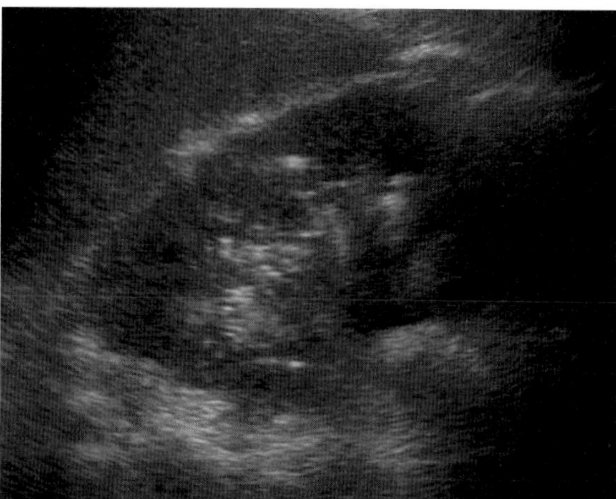

Fig. 7.17 • Cystinuria. The left kidney demonstrates small, highly reflective crystals of cystine with some reverberative artefact posterior to the crystals.

NEPHROCALCINOSIS

This term is used to describe the deposition of calcium in the renal parenchyma. It is most often related to the medullary pyramids, but may also affect the cortex, sparing the pyramids. It is frequently associated with medullary sponge kidney (see below.) It may also be seen in papillary necrosis, in patients with disorders of calcium metabolism, e.g. hyperparathyroidism and in renal tubular acidosis, sarcoidosis and metastatic disease.

Ultrasound appearances

Nephrocalcinosis is usually bilateral, but may affect one kidney and can be present in some or all of the pyramids. A regular arrangement of hyperechoic pyramids are seen which may shadow if large calcific foci are present, but not if the foci are numerous and tiny, as they are smaller than the beamwidth (Fig. 7.18).

Cortical nephrocalcinosis is less common and may occur with acute cortical necrosis, chronic conditions such as glomerulonephritis and hyper-

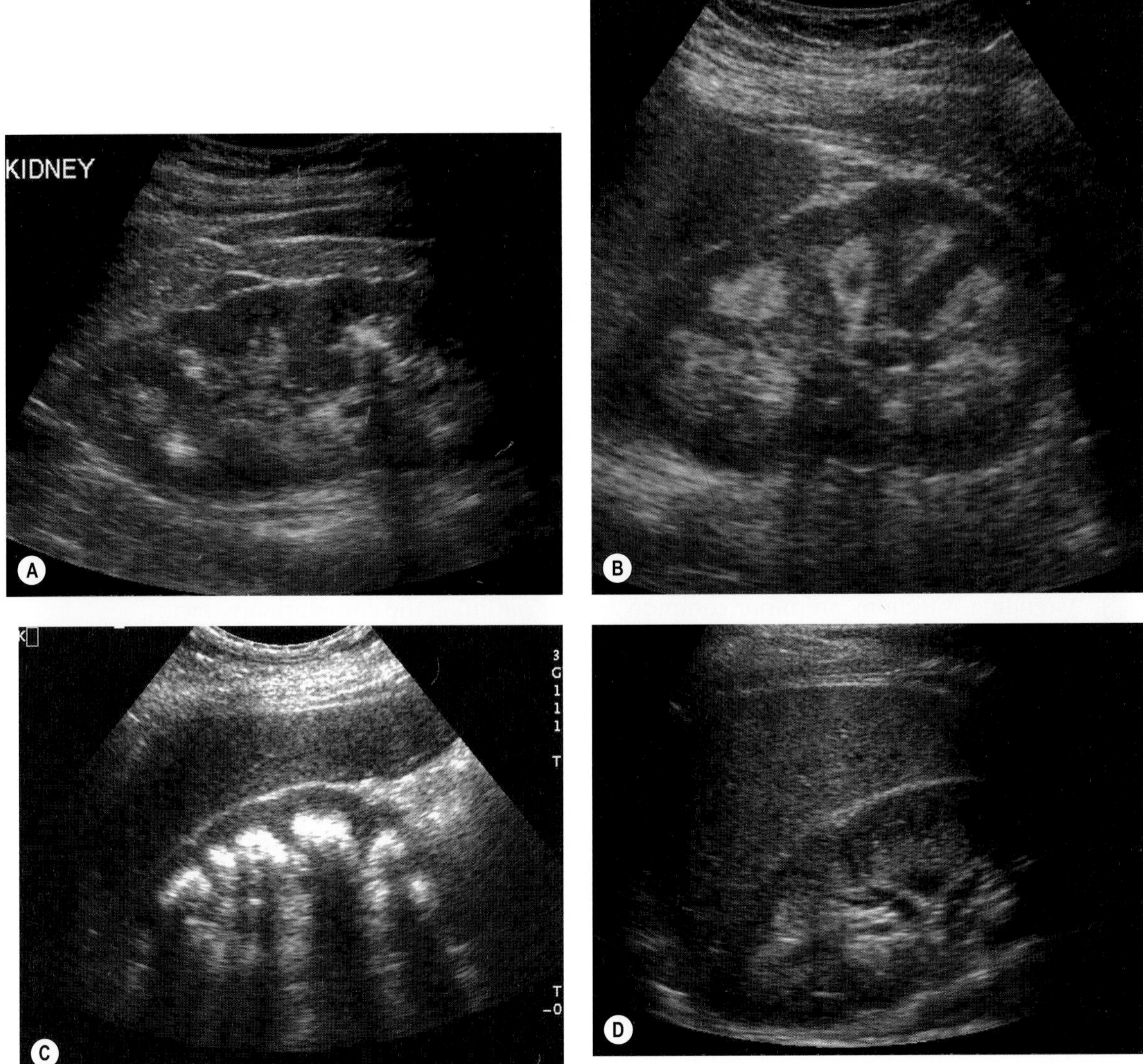

Fig. 7.18 • Nephrocalcinosis: (A) Deposits of calcium within the renal pyramids are too small to cast an acoustic shadow. A larger, frank stone at the lower pole, however, casts a shadow. (B) Hyperechoic, non-shadowing renal pyramids in nephrocalcinosis. (C) Calcification in the renal pyramids with strong acoustic shadowing. (D) Medullary sponge kidney, with hyperechoic renal pyramids.

calcaemia and sickle cell disease, and in AIDS-related infection.

HYPERPARATHYROIDISM

The (normally) four parathyroid glands in the neck regulate calcium metabolism in the body. Patients with *primary hyperparathyroidism* (due to an adenoma or hyperplasia of one or more of the parathyroid glands) have hypercalcaemia, which makes them prone to nephrocalcinosis or stones in the kidneys.

Secondary hyperparathyroidism is associated with chronic renal failure. Hypocalcaemia, which results from the chronic renal failure, induces compensatory hyperplasia of the parathyroid glands. There is a high incidence of hyperparathyroidism secondary to chronic renal failure in patients on dialysis; scintigraphy may demonstrate the region of increased activity and ultrasound is particularly suitable for demonstrating the enlarged parathyroid, guiding diagnostic aspiration and, if necessary, ablating the gland with ethanol to control symptoms in non-surgical patients.

RENAL TRACT INFLAMMATION AND INFECTION

The most common UTIs are bacterial in origin, with viral and fungal infections being comparatively rare. The diagnosis is made by urine analysis after the patient presents with symptoms of dysuria, haematuria and/or suprapubic or renal angle pain. The origin of the infection may be via the blood stream (haematogenous) or the urethra (ascending). Ascending infections are more common in women due to the short urethra.

Ultrasound is often requested, particularly in children, to identify any unsuspected renal pathology which may be associated with the infection, e.g. a duplex collecting system, pelvic kidney, etc.

Common conditions which may be identified on ultrasound include renal cystic diseases, calculi, obstructive uropathy, reflux and anatomical variants. Infection may be either acute or chronic. Ultrasound signs of acute renal infection may be absent altogether, and this is the commonest scenario as the subtler signs of interstitial nephritis are not usually demonstrable on ultrasound. The infection may be confined to the bladder – *cystitis* – in which case low-level echoes and/or hyperechoic debris may be identified, or may have progressed to the kidneys. Scarring and/or cortical thinning may be present in cases of repeated infections (see 'Chronic pyelonephritis' below).

PYELONEPHRITIS

Acute pyelonephritis

Acute inflammation of the kidney rarely results in any ultrasound abnormality. Occasionally the kidney may be enlarged and hypoechoic – the contrast between the kidney and the hepatic or splenic parenchyma is increased due to oedema – but the ultrasound changes are generally subtle. Other possible ultrasound findings include congenital anomalies, hydronephrosis, stones and a loss of the hyperechoic sinus fat echoes, due to oedema, and loss of corticomedullary differentiation.[31]

CT is useful for detecting subtle, inflammatory changes within the kidney and has the advantage of outlining the entire urinary tract.

Chronic pyelonephritis

This chronic inflammatory state is usually the result of frequent previous inflammatory/infective episodes. The kidney may be small and often has focal scarring present. Scar tissue has the appearance of a hyperechoic, linear lesion which affects the smooth renal outline and crosses the renal cortex. The cortex can appear focally thinner (Fig. 7.19A). (Do not confuse focal scarring with fetal lobulation, the latter being smooth, thin, continuous with the capsule and forming an indentation between the pyramids.)

The renal cortex is frequently thin and scarred in chronic pyelonephritis and may appear abnormally hyperechoic. Overall the kidneys may be reduced in length.

Bladder diverticula

Repeated infections can cause the bladder wall to thicken and become trabeculated. In such cases, a bladder diverticulum may form, making treatment of subsequent infections particularly difficult. The diverticulum may harbour debris or stones and may fail to empty properly, often enlarging as the urine refluxes into it when the patient micturates (Fig. 7.19B).

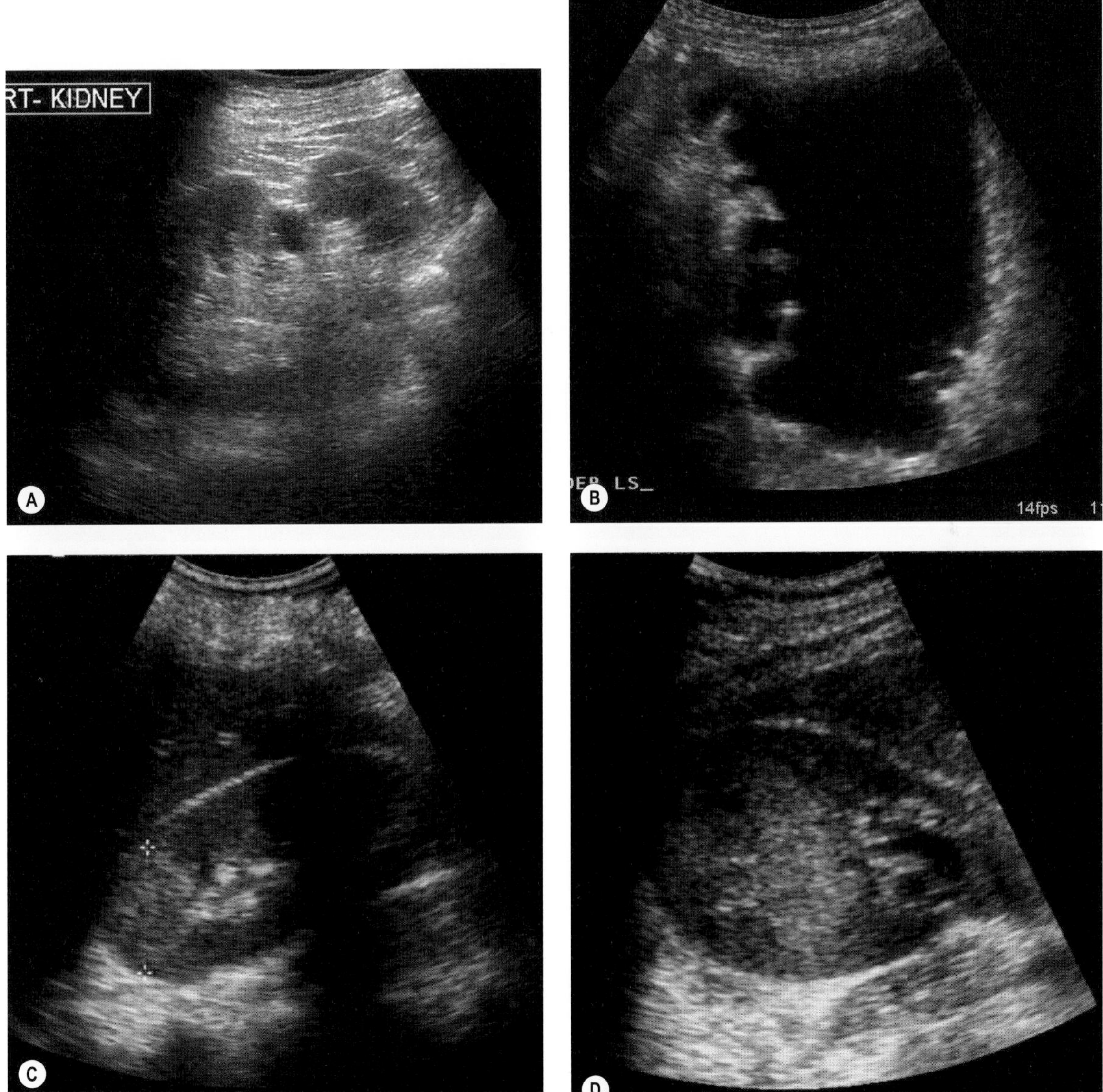

Fig. 7.19 • (A) Cortical scar tissue, demonstrating a focal area of cortical thinning, following repeated episodes of UTI. (B) Numerous bladder diverticulae in chronic infection. (C) Focal pyelonephritis (calipers). This subtle area of altered echogenicity in the kidney corresponds to the patient's pain. (D) Another case of focal inflammation in an enlarged RK with an area of increased echogenicity.

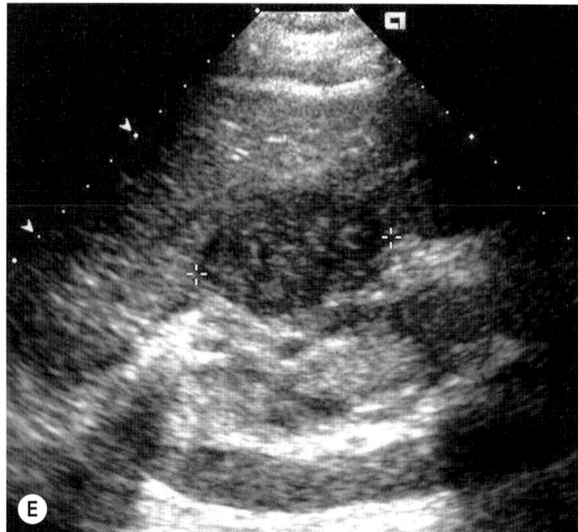

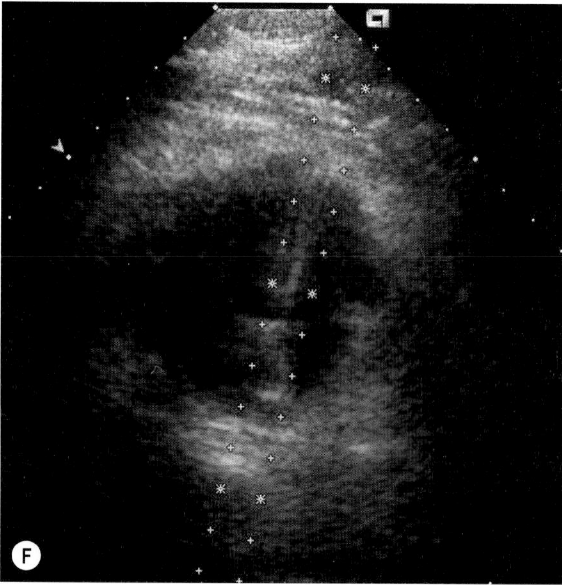

Fig. 7.19, cont'd • (E) Focal renal infection (calipers) is developing into a renal abscess. Note the posterior acoustic enhancement. (F) The abscess in (E) undergoes ultrasound-guided drainage before antibiotic therapy.

Focal pyelonephritis

The presence of acute infection within the kidney may progress in focal regions of the renal parenchyma. This phenomenon is particularly associated with diabetes. The ultrasonic changes are subtle, as in diffuse pyelonephritis, but it is possible to detect a slight change in echogenicity when it is surrounded by normal-looking parenchyma.

Focal pyelonephritis (sometimes called focal or lobar nephronia) may be either hypo- or hyperechoic compared with normal renal tissue. Depending on the size of the lesion, it may cause a mass effect, mimicking a renal tumour. The outline of the kidney is preserved, however (Fig. 7.19C).

The patient presents with fever and tenderness on the affected side and frequently has a history of UTI. A focal renal mass under these circumstances is highly suggestive of focal pyelonephritis and is also well demonstrated on CT.[34] It usually responds to antibiotic therapy and resolution of the lesion can be monitored with ultrasound scans. Focal pyelonephritis can progress to form an abscess in the kidney, which can be usually treated with antibiotics and ultrasound-guided percutaneous drainage if it is large (Fig. 7.19D–F).

Pyonephrosis

Pyonephrosis describes a dilated and obstructed renal collecting system which has become infected. It is important to recognise the condition as early as possible, as permanent damage will occur to the kidney if left untreated. Presentation is usually associated with UTI, fever and pain.[31] The obstruction may be from a variety of causes – usually stone – and ultrasound demonstrates low-level echoes and debris in the dilated system (Fig. 7.13).

Renal abscess

A renal abscess is generally a progression of focal inflammation within the kidney (see above). The area liquefies and may enlarge to form a complex mass with distal acoustic enhancement. Low-level echoes from pus may fill the abscess cavity, giving it the appearance of increased echogenicity but it may also be hypoechoic. The margins of the abscess may be ill-defined at first, but may develop a more obvious capsule as the lesion becomes established (Fig. 7.19D–F); the capsule often has an easily identifiable thick rim. Flow may be seen in the inflammatory capsule with colour Doppler, but not in the liquefied centre.

A renal abscess may mimic a lymphoma as both may be hypoechoic on ultrasound, and both may have either single or multiple foci. The abscess may be intrarenal, subcapsular or perirenal. Frequently, drainage under ultrasound guidance is the preferred treatment; gradual resolution of the abscess can also be monitored with ultrasound.

HIV and AIDS

The kidneys may be involved in a range of processes in patients affected with HIV or AIDS.[35] These can include infections, for example fungal infection or tuberculosis, malignancy such as lymphoma or Kaposi's sarcoma and other HIV-associated nephropathy. Renal disease may also arise due to the burden of antiretroviral therapy as treatments are frequently nephrotoxic. Stone formation is common with some medical treatments.

Ultrasound findings may include renal enlargement, cortical hyperechogenicity, pelvicalyceal thickening and loss of sinus fat.

Tuberculosis

Renal tuberculosis is an uncommon finding, although its incidence is rising due to HIV infection. The renal tract is the most common site for tuberculosis outside the lungs. It is a difficult diagnosis to make on ultrasound. The subtle inflammatory changes which affect the calyces in the early stages are best demonstrated with CT. In the later stages ultrasound may show calcific foci and obstructed calyces as a result of thickened inflammatory calyceal walls and papillary necrosis. Calcification and debris may be present. Tuberculosis may spread to other adjacent sites in the abdomen, including the psoas muscle and gastrointestinal tract.

The differential diagnosis is xanthogranulomatous pyelonephritis, which is often indistinguishable from tuberculosis on ultrasound, or a necrotic renal neoplasm.

Xanthogranulomatous pyelonephritis

This condition (which gets its name from the yellow colour of the kidney) is the result of chronic recurrent bacterial infection. It is most frequently associated with renal dilatation and obstruction by calculi in the pelvicalyceal system. Frequently, a staghorn calculus is present.

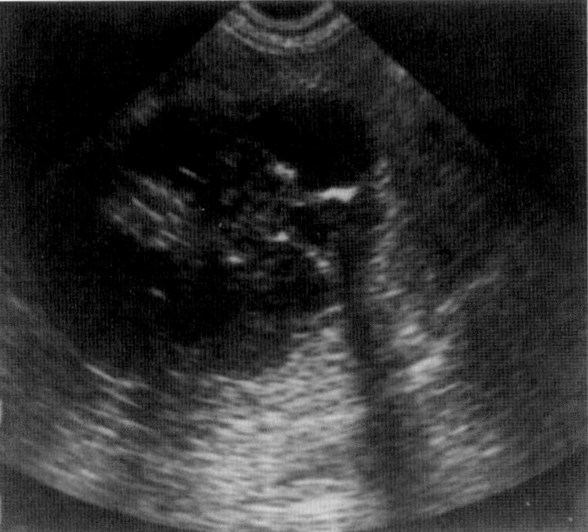

Fig. 7.20 • Xanthogranulomatous pyelonephritis. Numerous stones have obstructed the pelvicalyceal system, which contains debris. The renal cortex is thin and the architecture of the kidney is difficult to recognize.

The kidney becomes chronically infected and the calyces enlarge and become filled with infected debris. The cortex may be eroded and thin (Fig. 7.20).

On ultrasound, these appearances are similar to tuberculosis or to pyonephrosis. The latter is usually accompanied by a more severe, acute pain and fever whereas in xanthogranulomatous pyelonephritis or tuberculosis there is lower grade, chronic pain. The kidney may be enlarged with strong reflection and shadowing from a staghorn calculus. The dilated collecting system contains inflammatory debris.

CT may differentiate tuberculosis from xanthogranulomatous pyelonephritis and is also more sensitive to extrarenal spread of disease.

Hydatid cysts

The *Echinococcus* parasite spends part of its lifecycle in dogs. The larvae may be transmitted to humans through contact with dog faeces, finding its way to the lungs, liver and, less frequently, the kidneys.

The parasite forms a cyst that has a thickened wall, often with smaller, peripheral daughter cysts. Frequently the main cyst contains echoes.

The condition is rare in the UK, but may be diagnosed when small, grape-like cysts are passed in the urine.

DIFFUSE RENAL DISEASE AND RENAL FAILURE

Most diffuse medical renal conditions have non-specific appearances on ultrasound, the kidneys often appearing normal in the early stages of disease. Renal failure may be acute or chronic and its causes are numerous. If acute, an increase in overall renal size may be observed and there may be a diffuse alteration in the renal echogenicity, however, this can be either hypo- or hyperechoic compared with normal. Either increased or decreased corticomedullary differentiation may also be observed (Fig. 7.21). Although ultrasound is successful in detecting renal parenchymal disease, the acoustic changes are not specific and the cause must usually be diagnosed histologically,[36] ultrasound being invaluable in directing the biopsy procedure.

In chronic renal failure the kidneys shrink and the cortex becomes thin. The end-stage kidney can be quite tiny and hyperechoic and may be difficult to differentiate from the surrounding tissues (Fig. 7.21C). Depending on the cause, either one, but generally both, of the kidneys are affected.

ACUTE TUBULAR NECROSIS

Acute tubular necrosis is the result of ischaemia, which destroys the tubules of the kidney resulting in acute renal failure. It occurs when there is a sudden decrease in renal perfusion as a result of a severely hypotensive episode, e.g. cardiac arrest, massive haemorrhage, drug toxicity or septicaemia.

Patients are treated temporarily by dialysis. Tubular damage is capable of regeneration once the blood supply and perfusion pressure returns to normal, reversing the renal failure. If suspected, it is useful to perform a biopsy to determine the cause of renal failure, in order to plan further management.

On ultrasound the kidneys are normal in size or slightly enlarged. Occasionally, there may be increased cortical echogenicity with increased corticomedullary differentiation. However, this is a very non-specific sign and in most cases there is no detectable abnormality on grey-scale ultrasound. Spectral Doppler may be normal or demonstrate increased arterial resistance with reduced or even reversed EDF.

GLOMERULONEPHRITIS

Glomerulonephritis is an inflammatory condition which affects the glomeruli of the kidney. It may be either acute or chronic, and frequently follows prolonged infection.

Patients may present in acute renal failure, with oliguria or anuria, or with features of nephrotic syndrome – oedema, proteinuria and hypoalbuminaemia. Depending on aetiology, acute renal failure may be reversible or may progress to chronic renal failure requiring dialysis. Glomerulonephritis can be caused by numerous mechanisms:

- *Immunologic mechanisms* – e.g. in systemic lupus erythematosus (SLE) or AIDS
- *Metabolic disorders* – e.g. diabetes
- *Circulatory disturbances* – e.g. atherosclerosis or disseminated intravascular coagulation (DIC).

As with acute tubular necrosis, the ultrasound appearances are non-specific. In the acute stages the kidneys may be slightly enlarged; changes in the echogenicity of the cortex may be observed. In the chronic stages the kidneys shrink, become hyperechoic, lose cortical thickness and have increased corticomedullary differentiation.[36]

MEDULLARY SPONGE KIDNEY

In medullary sponge kidney the distal tubules, which lie in the medullary pyramids, dilate. This may be due to a developmental anomaly but this is not certain. In itself it is usually asymptomatic and therefore rarely seen on ultrasound. However,

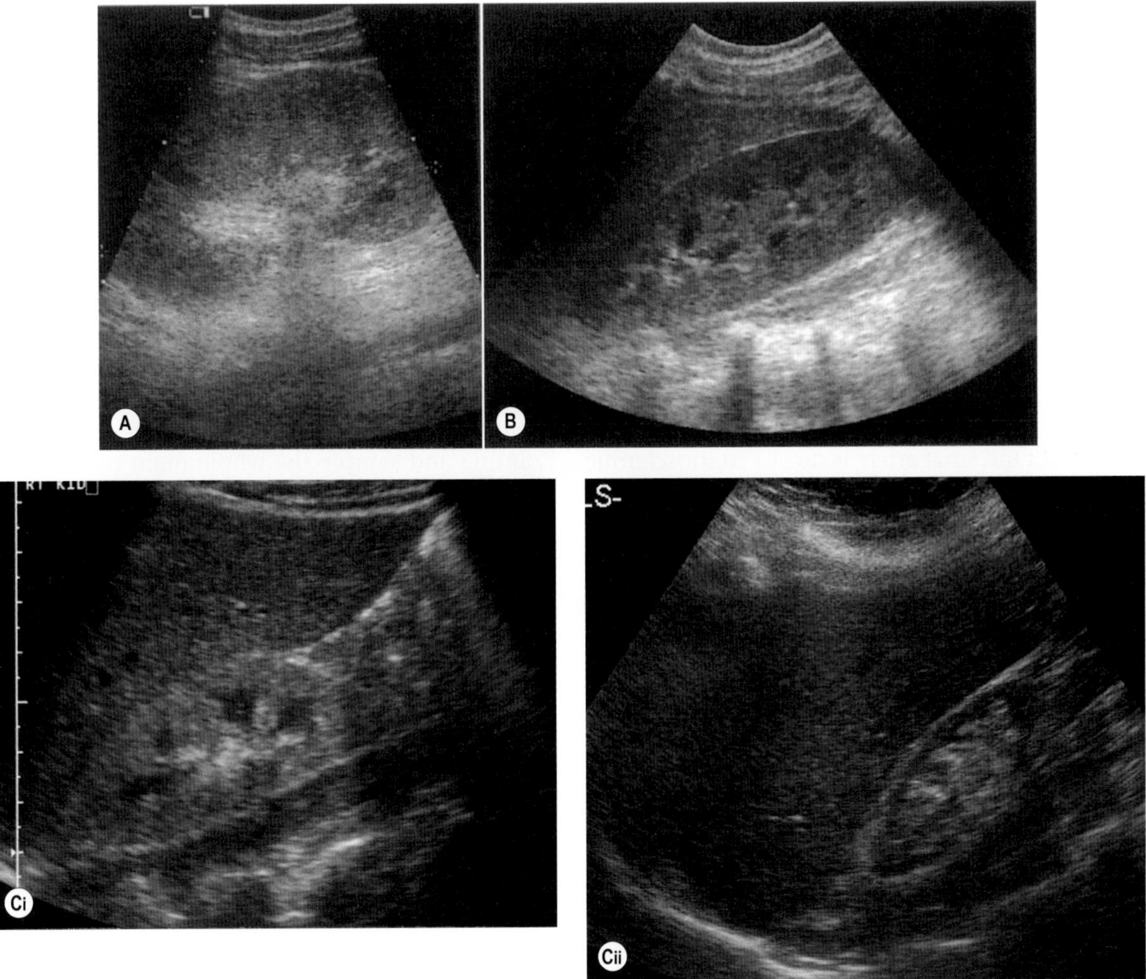

Fig. 7.21 • (A) Acute renal failure demonstrating an enlarged, diffusely hyperechoic kidney with loss of corticomedullary differentiation. (B) Acute renal failure in paracetamol overdose. The kidney is large (16 cm) and hyperechoic with increased corticomedullary differentiation. (C) Chronic renal failure. (Ci) The kidney is small and hyperechoic compared with the adjacent liver. (Cii) Another example of chronic renal failure, with a small kidney in which the cortex is of similar echogenicity to the liver, but very thin.

the condition is prone to nephrocalcinosis particularly at the outer edges of the pyramids and stone formation, (see above), which may cause pain and haematuria. Involvement is usually bilateral, but may be unilateral or segmental. On ultrasound the kidneys tend to be normal in size, and the pyramids may be hyperechoic – regardless of the presence of nephrocalcinosis. Other possible ultrasound findings include possible nephrocalcinosis (Fig. 7.18), stones and the results of stone obstruction and/or chronic infection if present.

AMYLOID

In amyloid disease, excess protein is deposited in the renal parenchyma, predominantly the cortex. This causes proteinuria and may progress to nephrotic syndrome (oedema, proteinuria and hypoalbuminaemia.) Amyloidosis can cause acute renal failure and is particularly associated with longstanding rheumatoid arthritis.

Ultrasound findings are non-specific. As with other diffuse renal diseases, the acute stage may cause renal enlargement and the parenchyma tends to be diffusely hyperechoic. By the time the chronic stage of disease has been reached, the kidneys become shrunken and hyperechoic in keeping with all end stage appearances.

RENAL VASCULAR PATHOLOGY

RENAL ARTERY STENOSIS

Stenosis of the renal artery is due to arteriosclerotic disease in the vast majority of patients, or to fibromuscular dysplasia of the arterial wall in the younger, generally female patient. Renal artery stenosis (RAS) may cause hypertension and may eventually cause renal failure. It is frequently bilateral, and is responsible for up to 15% of patients who require long-term dialysis. It is associated with aortic aneurysm, neurofibromatosis or can be traumatic in origin.

Stenosis generally affects the main vessel at its origin and involves the aorta (ostial) or occurs within 1 cm of its origin (non-ostial). It can occur in both native and transplanted organs. It is frequently bilateral.

Ultrasound appearances

If the stenosis is long-standing and/or severe, the kidney is likely to be small. Loss of renal mass is associated with a stenosis of 60% or greater.[37] However, the ultrasound appearances are often normal with milder grades of RAS.

The role of ultrasound is diagnosing RAS is limited. Digital subtraction angiography is still considered the gold standard, but is invasive and carries a small risk. MRA is now regarded as the first-line imaging modality of choice. Colour and spectral Doppler techniques can demonstrate a stenosis[38] by identifying a high velocity jet in the MRA. However, it has poor sensitivity as acoustic access to the entire artery is often limited by overlying bowel, and accessory arteries are infrequently demonstrated.

At the site of a stenosis, an increase in peak systolic velocity may be found (greater than 1.5–1.8 m/s) with post-stenotic turbulence. Although, it is often not technically possible to confidently examine and sample the whole main renal artery and thus make a definitive diagnosis it nevertheless remains the best Doppler technique for diagnosis.

A more reliable and reproducible sign of RAS is demonstrated in the intrarenal vessels, distal to the stenosis. Within the kidney, the perfusion may appear subjectively reduced in the number of vessels and velocity of flow and it may be necessary for the operator to use a low PRF value to detect blood flow. This is very subjective and variable. The spectral waveforms of arteries distal to the stenosis also reflect changes which suggest a proximal stenosis; the normally fast systolic upstroke is replaced by a delayed *parvus tardus* pattern (Fig. 7.22), making the waveform less pulsatile with a rounded envelope.[39]

This type of waveform can be appreciated subjectively, but quantitative measurements may be used to support the diagnosis. The *acceleration time* (*AT*) or *acceleration index* (*AI*) are the most common; a normal AT is <0.07 seconds, and a normal AI >3 m/s.

The actual value of these indices, however, does not reflect the severity of stenosis; unfortunately stenoses of <70–80% narrowing do not usually demonstrate the *parvus tardus* effect (although these tend to be less clinically significant) and these spectral phenomenon may be obscured altogether if the vessels are rigid and severely diseased[40] or if a good collateral circulation has developed. In such cases the Doppler result is falsely negative and the operator should bear this in mind when attempting to exclude RAS.

Renal artery occlusion may occur as a result of further progression of the same disease process

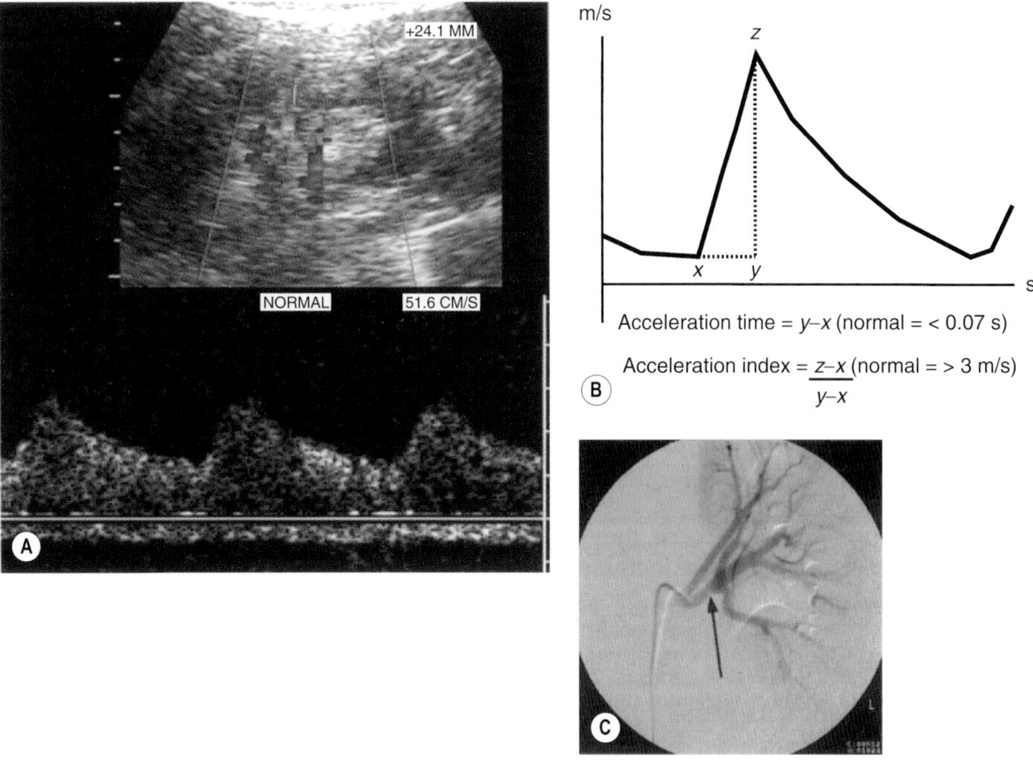

Fig. 7.22 • Renal artery stenosis. (A) The kidney is small, with subjectively reduced perfusion on colour Doppler. (B) The spectrum displays the *parvus tardus* pattern with delayed systolic upstroke. (C) The arteriogram in case A confirms a stenosis (arrow).

which causes stenosis. Doppler will confirm the lack of renal perfusion. The kidney shrinks in response to deteriorating arterial perfusion.

Management

Stenosis of the main renal artery is amenable to percutaneous angioplasty and/or stenting, which can effect a cure or more realistically stabilize or slow disease progression. A post-angioplasty ultrasound scan can confirm vessel patency, and may play a role in monitoring the patient for disease recurrence. For those with deteriorating function, for whom percutaneous techniques have failed, renal failure will ultimately necessitate dialysis. Renal transplant is a viable option, particularly for those who have been treated in the long term.

RENAL VEIN THROMBOSIS

This can occur when chronic renal disease is already present or in cases of a coagulation disorder with increased tendency to thrombose e.g. polycythaemia. It is frequently associated with nephrotic syndrome. Other associated factors include the contraceptive pill and the use of steroids.[41]

Tumour thrombus from renal cell carcinoma is also prone to invade the ipsilateral renal vein, and sometimes may extend into the IVC and even into the right atrium. Thrombus in the renal vein, whether secondary to a malignancy or thrombocythaemia can travel up the IVC forming a source of emboli. If non-malignant, the thrombus may be successfully treated medically and the renal function can be preserved even if the vein is totally occluded.

Ultrasound appearances

It is often possible to see echo-poor thrombus within a dilated renal vein. Colour Doppler confirms absent venous flow. Perfusion within the kidney itself is reduced and there may be a highly pulsatile arterial waveform with reversed diastolic flow, although this is not commonly seen in the native kidney.

If the thrombus produces a total and sudden occlusion, the kidney becomes oedematous and swollen within the first 24 hours (Fig. 7.23). Eventually it will shrink and become hyperechoic. Partially occluding thrombus is more difficult to diagnose as the changes in the kidney may not be apparent. However, a non-dilated renal vein with good colour Doppler displayed throughout has a high negative predictive value.

Incomplete thrombosis may still demonstrate venous flow within the kidney, although the arterial waveforms are of lower velocity than normal, with a marked reduction in the systolic peak.[42] Forward diastolic flow may be preserved at this stage.

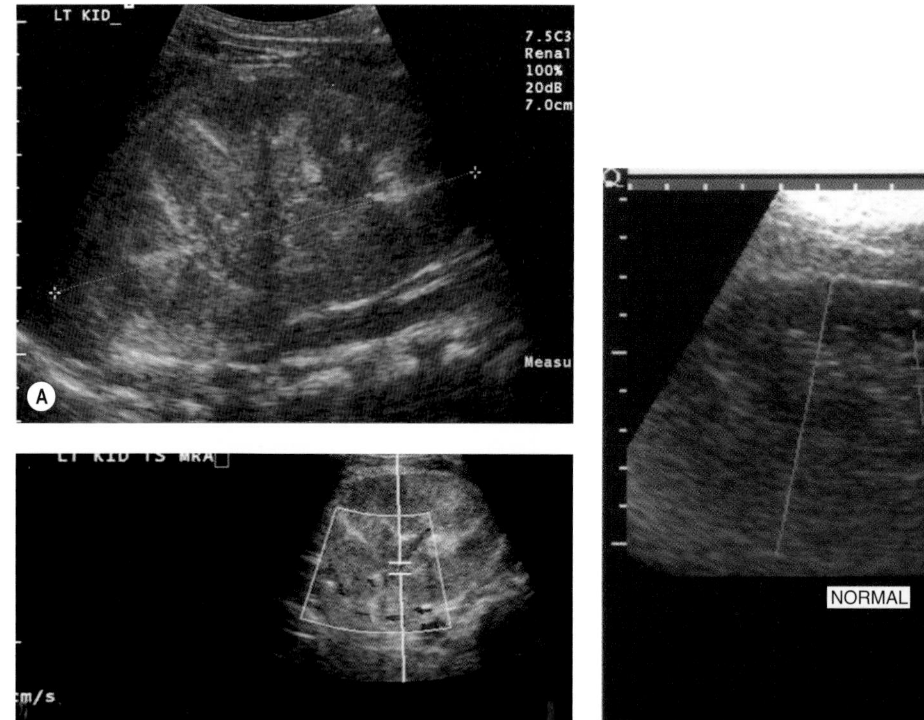

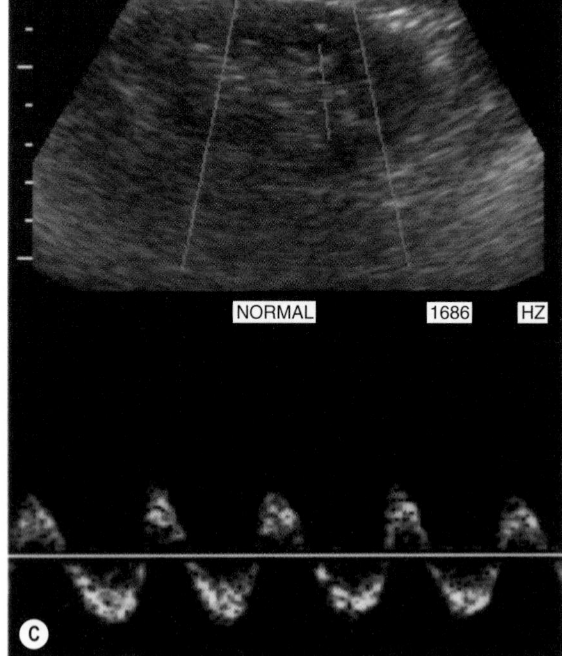

Fig. 7.23 • Renal vein thrombosis. (A) Acute renal vein thrombosis demonstrating an enlarged, diffusely hyperechoic kidney. (B) Doppler demonstrates high resistance bi-directional arterial flow with no venous flow. (C) Small shrunken kidney (6 cm) demonstrating hardly any perfusion, apart from a tiny interlobar artery with bidirectional flow.

ARTERIOVENOUS FISTULA

AV fistulas most usually occur as a result of biopsy and are recognized on colour and spectral Doppler by localized vessel enlargement with turbulent, sometimes high velocity flow. A 'pool' of colour flow is often present. The vein may show a regular, pulsatile pattern and be dilated. These iatrogenic fistulae usually resolve spontaneously and are clinically insignificant. If bleeding is a clinical problem and is ongoing, recurrent and/or severe then embolisation may be necessary.

ULTRASOUND IN DIALYSIS

Patients with chronic renal failure may undergo either haemodialysis, (in which a subcutaneous arteriovenous shunt is created, usually in the arm) or continuous ambulatory peritoneal dialysis (CAPD), (in which a catheter is inserted through the abdominal wall). Ultrasound may be used to assess the patency of the shunt or catheter, and may identify localized areas of infection along the CAPD tract, which can be drained under ultrasound guidance if necessary.

Ultrasound may also be used to diagnose acquired cystic kidney disease in long-term dialysis patients (see above) (Box 7.1).

BOX 7.1 Causes of haematuria

- Urinary tract infection
- Stones
- Neoplasm (renal cell or transitional cell carcinoma in the kidney, ureter or bladder)
- Prostatic pathology (benign hypertrophy or carcinoma)
- Renal cyst haemorrhage
- Papillary necrosis
- Glomerulonephritis
- Trauma
- Tuberculosis
- Renal infarct

RENAL TRAUMA

A direct injury can rupture the kidney. This will result in blood and/or urine leaking out into the perinephric space to form a urinoma or haematoma. The main renal vessels may also be damaged, causing lack of perfusion. Trauma resulting in haematuria and suspected renal damage is usually imaged with CT as a first line. This has the advantage of demonstrating a range of possible injuries to all the abdominal viscera.

The role of ultrasound in such cases is more usually reserved for guiding drainage of subsequent fluid collections such as urinoma or infected haematoma. The insertion of a drain carries a risk of infection and is therefore limited to infected collections in symptomatic patients. Patients who are unable to attend a CT department (for example unstable patients in intensive care) may benefit from a careful bedside ultrasound scan to identify free fluid and organ damage. Occasionally contrast ultrasound is useful in demonstrating a rupture of the kidney (see Chapter 10). The causes of haematuria are listed in Box 7.1.

RENAL TRANSPLANTS

Although there are a number of treatment choices for patients with renal failure including peritoneal and haemodialysis, undoubtedly the treatment of choice is renal transplantation. From the very early days of Carrel's experimental attempts at transplantation in the 1900s resulting in the Nobel Prize of 1912,[43] to the non-immunosuppressed allografting of the 1950s, the more successful and encouraging outcome of twin-to-twin transplants,[44] a better understanding of tissue rejection and the introduction of azathioprine and steroid in 1963,[45] and more specifically ciclosporin A by Calne in the 1970s,[46] have all contributed immensely to slow but positive progress in this field. Improvements in surgical technique, newer, more effective and less toxic anti-rejection therapy, the routine use of ultrasound in the 1970s and then Doppler a decade later, and the development of interventional radiology have all combined to make this the successful operation and clinical outcomes we now take so much for granted.

Although many different imaging modalities are available, ultrasound is still the single most useful investigation in the post-operative monitoring of the transplant. Among its many roles, it is sensitive to early pelvicalyceal dilatation, can be used to guide biopsy procedures and to guide the drainage of fluid collections and placement of nephrostomy tubes.

Normal anatomy

Most renal transplants are *heterotopic* – i.e. they are placed in addition to the diseased, native kidneys, which remain in situ. The transplanted organ is usually positioned in the iliac fossa anterior to the psoas and iliacus muscles. It lies outside the peritoneal cavity.

Within the UK, the majority of transplanted kidneys are cadaveric, and are harvested with their main vessels intact, which are then anastomosed to the recipient iliac artery and vein. Increasingly, live donors are supplementing the transplant programme, and ultrasound is useful in both donor (in confirming normality prior to donation) and recipient.

Normal ultrasound appearances

The transplanted kidney is particularly amenable to ultrasonic investigation; its position relatively near to the skin surface allows a high frequency transducer – 5–6 MHz – to be used for better detail.

The ultrasonic appearances of the transplant kidney are the same as would be expected for a native kidney, allowing for the higher resolution (Fig. 7.24). The transplant kidney should be assessed in the same way as the native organ, i.e. in two planes. Features to be observed include:

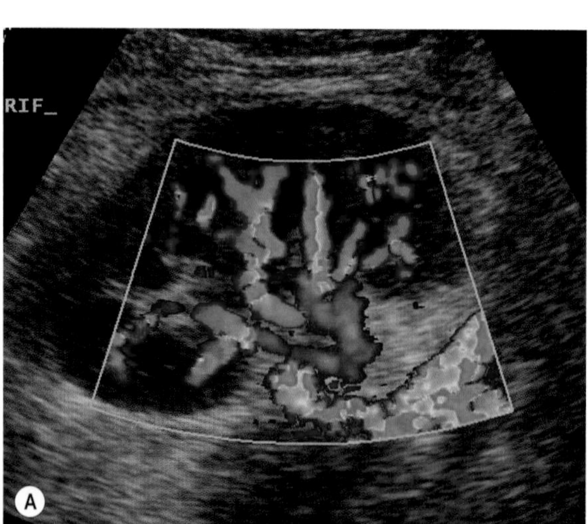

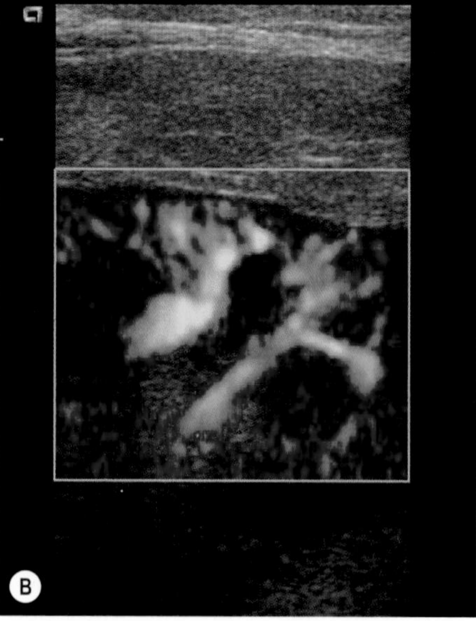

Fig. 7.24 • (A) Perfusion within the transplanted kidney is easily displayed. A higher frequency may be used as the kidney is usually superficially situated in the iliac fossa. (B) By using an even higher frequency, and power Doppler, tiny vessels can be displayed in the periphery of the transplant kidney.

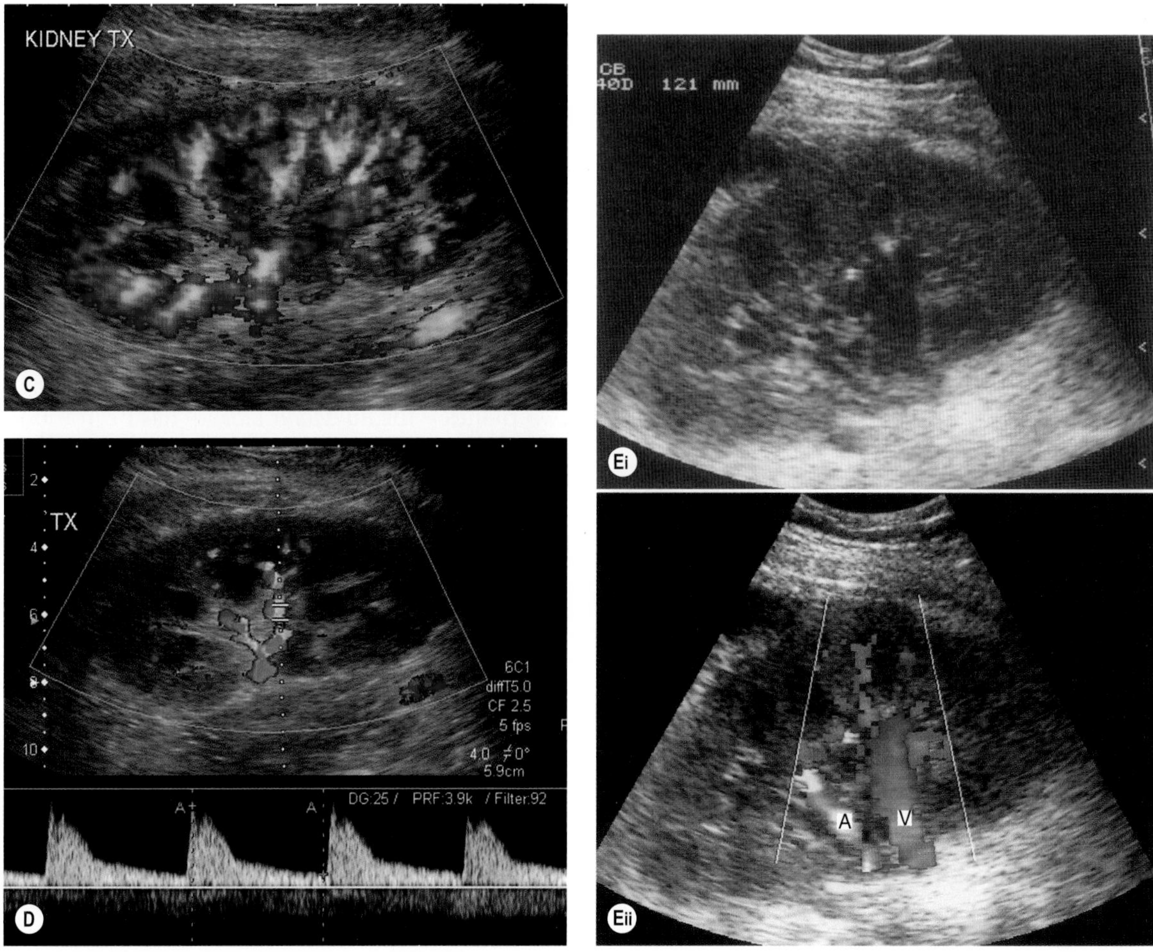

Fig. 7.24, cont'd • (C) The increased sensitivity of power Doppler is valuable in demonstrating perfusion in the transplanted kidney. (D) Normal spectrum from the interlobar renal artery, demonstrating good EDF (low resistance) with a vertical systolic upstroke. (E) (Ei) Large vessels at the hilum may mimic dilatation; (Eii) Colour Doppler demonstrates this is the main renal vein.

- *Morphological appearances*: this should include an assessment of the relative echogenicity of the cortex, medulla and renal sinus and cortico-medullary differentiation. Focal or diffuse changes in echogenicity may be observed, but are non-specific findings associated with inflammation, infection or infarction.
- *Pelvicalyceal system dilatation*: even mild pelvicalyceal dilatation may be significant, as it may represent an early obstructive process. The bladder should be empty before assessing the pelvicalyceal system, to eliminate physiological dilatation. Any degree of hydronephrosis should be correlated with the clinical findings and biochemistry – hydronephrosis in isolation is not a reason for nephrostomy.
- *Vascular anatomy*: the main transplant artery and vein are anastomosed to the recipient's external iliac artery and vein respectively and can usually be visualized throughout their length. Overall global perfusion can be assessed with colour or power Doppler and

the smaller vessels at the periphery of the kidney (Fig. 7.24) should be discernable. The normal spectral Doppler waveform is a low-resistance waveform with continuous forward end diastolic flow.

- *Perirenal fluid*: A small amount of free fluid is not unusual post-operatively. This usually resolves spontaneously.

Fluid collections around the kidney are a common complication. They may resolve on further scanning; drainage is only performed for good clinical reasons. (See below.)

POST-OPERATIVE COMPLICATIONS

Ultrasound has an essential role in assessing the transplant and makes a significant contribution towards graft survival through the early recognition of post-operative complications.[46,47] Complications are varied and include acute rejection, ureteric obstruction, vascular occlusions, perirenal fluid collections, renal dysfunction (of various aetiologies) and infection. Drug toxicity from the immunosuppressive therapy can also compromise graft function. Finally, in the long term, the original disease, for which transplantation was performed, may recur.

Complications can be divided into three main categories; immediate post-operative complications and primary and secondary renal dysfunction.

- Immediate:
  - Non-perfusion. This is usually the result of an occluded or twisted renal artery; correction is usually surgical
  - Haematoma.
- Primary dysfunction:
  - Non-perfusion (arterial occlusion) – total or lobar
  - Acute tubular necrosis
  - Renal vein thrombosis
  - Obstruction
  - Acute or accelerated acute rejection.
- Secondary dysfunction:
  - Acute rejection
  - Ciclosporin nephrotoxicity
  - Acute tubular necrosis
  - Obstruction
  - RAS
  - Post-biopsy fistula
  - Infection
  - Chronic rejection.

RENAL TRANSPLANT DILATATION

A mild degree of pelvicalyceal system dilatation is normal post-operatively, due to oedema, at the site of the vesicoureteric anastomosis. This phenomenon is usually transient, and serial scans in conjunction with biochemistry (urea, creatinine) is usually all that is required.

More severe dilatation may be indicative of obstruction, especially if the individual calyces are also dilated. A trend of increasing dilatation is a poor prognostic indicator. A ratio between the area of the pelvicalyceal system and the renal outline in two planes – the *dilatation index* – has been found to predict obstruction and differentiate obstructive from non-obstructive dilatation[48] (Fig. 7.25). The degree of dilatation of the pelvicalyceal system correlates well with the severity of obstruction.

Obstruction of the transplant kidney may be due to an ischaemic related stricture at the vesicoureteric anastomosis, or may be the result of a blood clot or infected debris in the ureter. Haematoma or debris within the pelvicalyceal system may appear echogenic but require to be differentiated from fungal balls. Percutaneous nephrostomy (X-ray and/or ultrasound guided) is the method of choice to relieve obstruction.

REJECTION

This can be acute or chronic. Acute rejection may be responsible for delayed graft function whereas chronic rejection is a gradual deterioration in renal function that may begin any time after 3 months of transplantation. Ongoing episodes of acute rejection should raise the possibility of non-compliance with therapy. Acute rejection cannot be differentiated on ultrasound from other causes of delayed function, particularly, acute tubular necrosis and therefore biopsy is invariably necessary.

Pathologically, rejection can be either cellular (98%) or vascular (now accounting for only 2% of cases). Improved immunosuppressive therapy has greatly reduced the problems of rejection.

Ultrasound appearances

These are varied and non-specific. In the majority of cases the kidney appears normal, however, greyscale findings can include enlargement due to

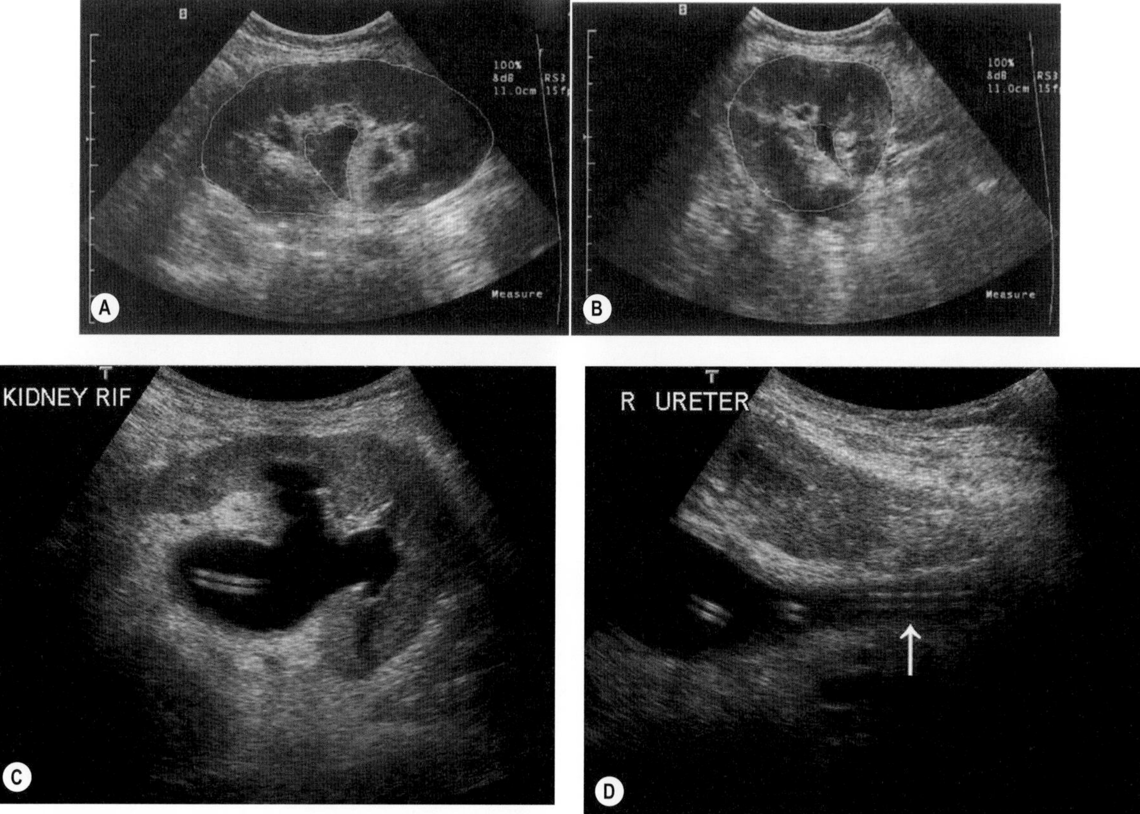

Fig. 7.25 • (A) LS and (B) TS of a dilated transplant kidney showing the measurements used to calculate the ratio between the dilated pelvicalyceal system and the kidney. This kidney was dilated but not obstructed. (C) Ureteric stenosis: A dilated transplant kidney with a stent seen in the pelvicalyceal system. (D) The stent is seen in the ureter shortly following its insertion through the stenosis (arrow). The collecting system subsequently returned to normal.

oedema (this change is subtle in the early stages and not a reliable ultrasonic indicator), increased corticomedullary differentiation with prominent pyramids, infundibular thickening (thickening of the Acute tubular necrosis walls) and decreased fat in the renal sinus[49] (Fig. 7.26). These findings are subjective, non-specific and limited in the diagnosis of rejection.

In chronic rejection there may be an overall increase in the echogenicity of the kidney with reduced corticomedullary differentiation. Eventually the kidney will shrink. The Doppler RI are increased in rejection but, again, this finding is non-specific[50] (see Table 7.4 below) (Fig. 7.26B). In general the higher the RI the more likely is the diagnosis of acute rejection.

The cause of renal dysfunction is established by ultrasound-guided biopsy.

Fluid collections associated with transplantation

Up to 50% of renal transplants will demonstrate perirenal fluid.[51] The size of the collection should be monitored with ultrasound, as significant growth may require intervention. While it is not possible to classify the collection on the ultrasound appearances alone, the clinical picture, including the time interval following transplantation, can often give a clue.

- *Lymphocoele*: the commonest perirenal fluid collection, lymphocoeles usually occur several

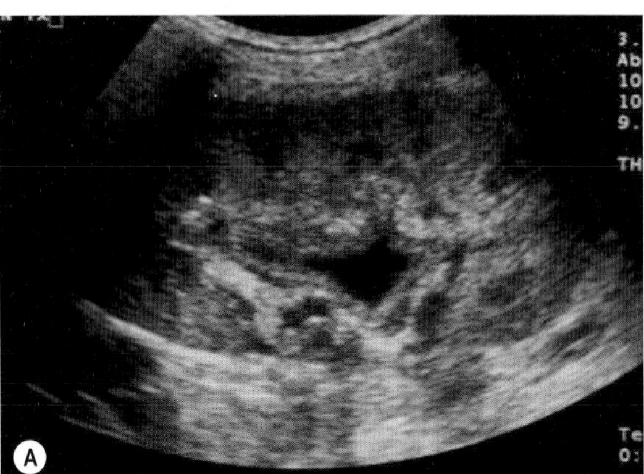

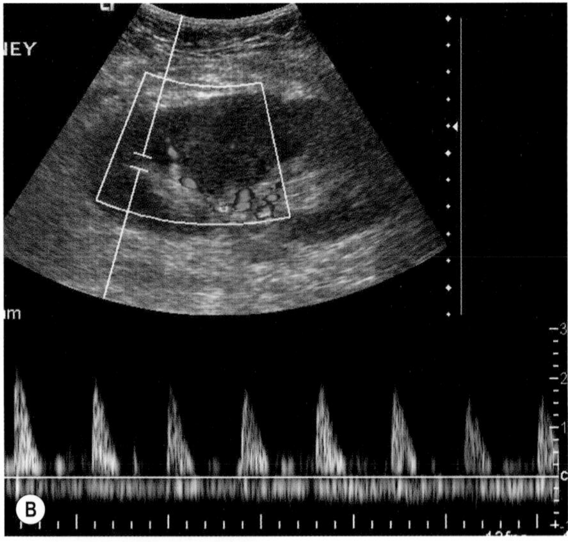

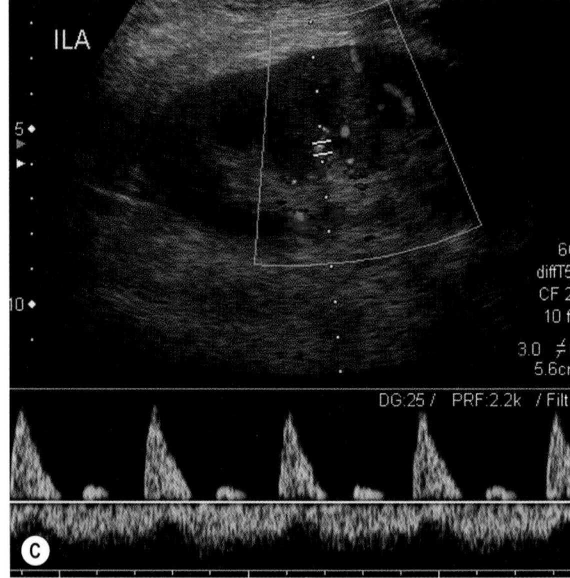

Fig. 7.26 • Transplant rejection. (A) Peri-infundibular or mural thickening is present in the pelvicalyceal system. (B) Perfusion is reduced throughout the kidney, and the high resistance vasculature demonstrates a high Doppler RI, with no EDF. (C) Another example of high resistance vasculature in transplant rejection with a pulsatile arterial waveform with no EDF.

weeks or months after the transplant. They may resolve spontaneously but occasionally require percutaneous drainage if large. They may compress the kidney, causing an increase in vascular resistance on spectral Doppler (Fig. 7.27). The collection is anechoic but may contain loculations or septa. If treated, then surgical laparoscopic marsupialization is the treatment of choice.

- *Haematoma*: an immediate post-operative phenomenon, which usually resolves spontaneously. If the haematoma is due to an anastomotic leak at the main artery or vein, it can compress the renal vein, causing

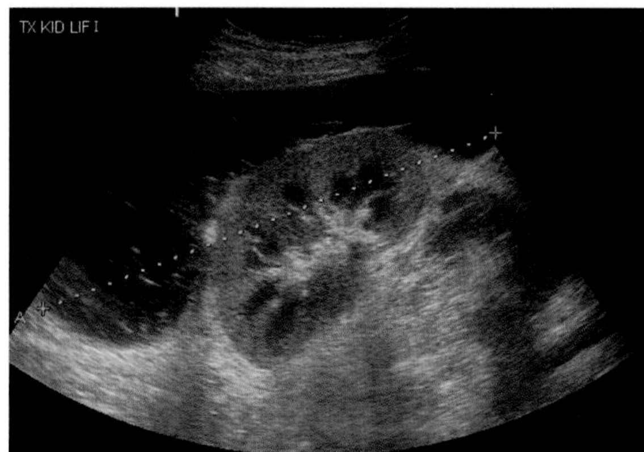

Fig. 7.27 • A large seroma around the transplanted kidney. This was drained under ultrasound guidance.

Acute rejection	does not occur in the first 48 hours
ATN	occurs in the first 48 hours
Obstruction	has a relatively *slight* increase in RI and is accompanied by pelvicalyceal system dilatation
Cyclosporin nephrotoxicity	has to be prolonged and severe to affect the EDF and blood levels.
	A late complication of renal transplants.
Renal vein thrombosis	has a characteristic reversed EDF pattern. The artery has a low velocity systolic peak in the early stages. No venous flow identified.
Peri-renal fluid collections	Compression of the kidney causes an increase in intra-renal pressure.

Table 7.4 Causes of high resistance Doppler (low EDF) in renal transplants

thrombosis in rare cases. On ultrasound, the haematoma can appear hyperechoic and ill-defined in the early stages. As it resolves and liquefies, the margins become more defined and the centre becomes anechoic. Hyperechoic blood clots and strands of fibrin may be seen within the haematoma.

- *Urinoma*: this occurs as a result of an anastomotic leak in the ureter. Urinomas are uncommon, but may progress to urinary ascites. They occur early following the surgical procedure, unlike lymphocoeles.
- *Abscess*: if any of the above fluid collections becomes infected, this leads to an abscess. Hyperechoic debris can be seen in the collection and this may be treated with ultrasound-guided percutaneous drainage.

VASCULAR COMPLICATIONS

Vascular occlusion

Colour and spectral Doppler are essential for the diagnosis of post-operative vascular complications. Non-perfusion may be total or lobar (Fig. 7.28). Focal areas of hypoperfusion may be due to oedema in focal infection, AV fistula or severing of an accessory artery during harvesting of the transplant or at the time of implantation causing infarction. Total vascular occlusion is rare, but occurs early. Patients may be asymptomatic and non-perfusion of the transplant may be inadvertently seen on either a routine scan or isotope study. Graft nephrectomy is the most likely outcome. Conversely, the appearance of good renal perfusion throughout the kidney on colour or power Doppler does not necessarily indicate normal vascularity and severe vascular rejection or acute tubular necrosis can be present under such circumstances.[52] Vascular complications may include arterial stenosis or thrombosis, venous stenosis or thrombosis, pseudoaneurysms and AV fistulae.[50]

RAS

This is one of the most common post-transplant vascular complications, affecting up to 10% of transplants. It generally occurs at the site of the anastomosis close to the iliac artery but also along the length of the artery or even affecting the intra renal branches. The patient may present with severe, difficult to control hypertension, graft dysfunction, or both. Alternatively the patient's renal function may deteriorate following angiotensin-converting enzyme (ACE) inhibitor therapy and

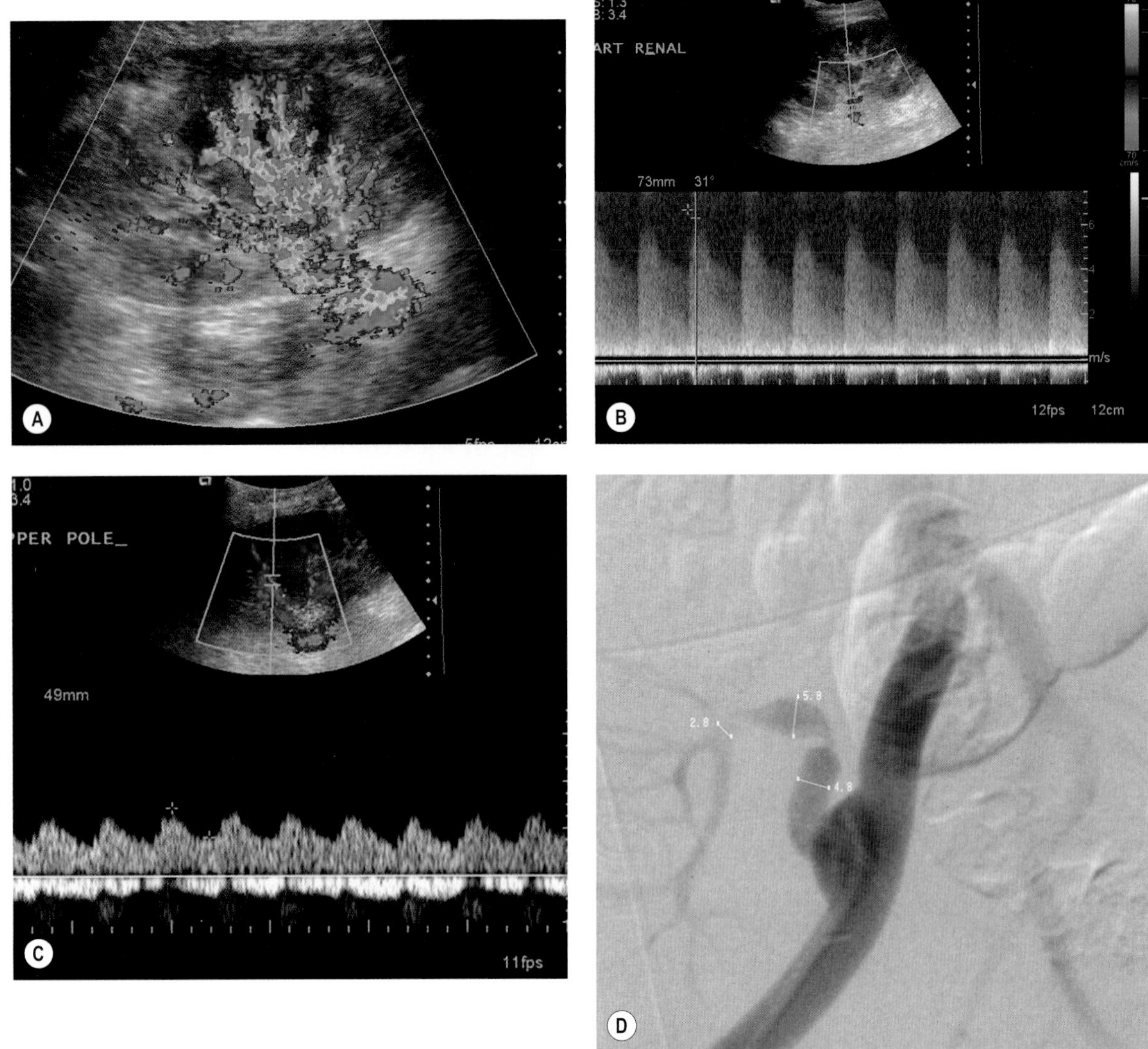

Fig. 7.28 • (A) The upper pole of this transplant kidney lacks perfusion, (despite reducing the PRF setting) due to infarction. (B) High-velocity jet at the site of an MRA stenosis in a transplant kidney. The patient had increasing, badly controlled hypertension since transplantation. (C) Downstream from an arterial stenosis Doppler displays a tardus parvus pattern of delayed systolic upstroke. (D) Arteriography of the case in (C) demonstrates two stenoses.

this is also an indication of a possible underlying RAS.

Careful Doppler examination is now the accepted first-line investigation in the diagnosis of RAS. It most cases it is possible to trace the artery back to its anastomosis with the iliac artery, using colour Doppler. If the site of the stenosis is identified, spectral Doppler will demonstrate an increase in peak systolic velocity at the lesion, followed by post-stenotic turbulence (Fig. 7.28B, C). The point of stenosis can be difficult to pinpoint in the main renal artery, especially if bowel is overlying the vessel.

A delayed systolic rise (the *parvus tardus* waveform) can be identified in the intrarenal spectral Doppler waveforms, as for the native kidney (see above). The diagnosis, however, is primarily made on the peak systolic velocity within the renal artery. A value of <2.5 m/s is normal whereas >2.5 m/s constitutes RAS. If the stenosis is severe, it may be difficult to identify colour flow in the kidney and the waveform may be reduced in velocity with a tiny, damped trace in the main vessel.

A stenosis affecting an interlobar artery may result in focal, segmental non-perfusion or ischaemia on Doppler ultrasound. In general, contrast angiography is only used to grade and treat stenoses after a positive ultrasound scan, or when a high index of clinical suspicion persists, despite a negative ultrasound.[51]

Renal vein thrombosis

This is uncommon, and usually the result of surgical technique or vein compression. The occlusion may be partial or complete and the venous Doppler spectrum may therefore be absent (Fig. 7.29). If venous thrombosis is partial, the arterial spectral

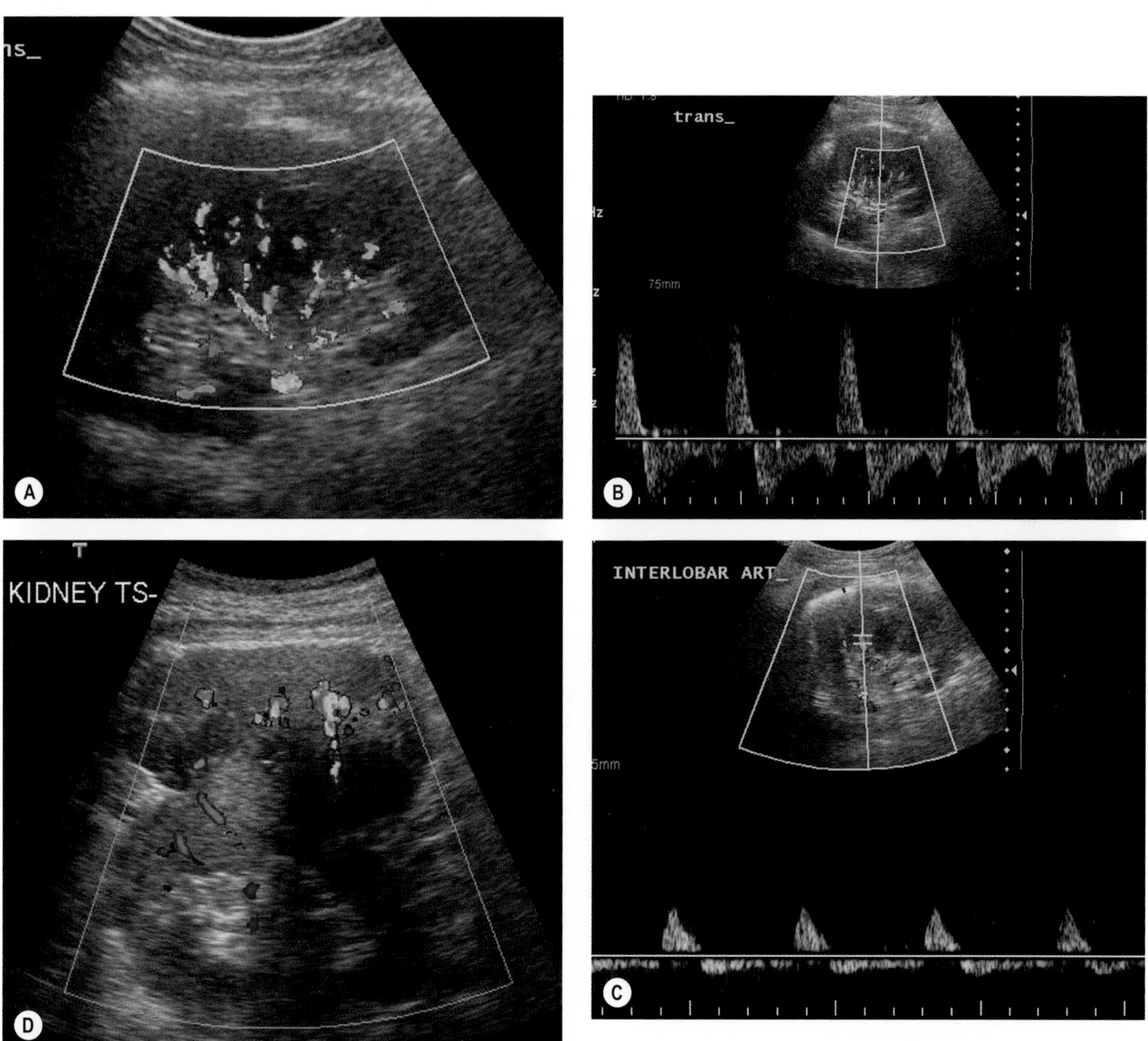

Fig. 7.29 • Renal vein thrombosis. (A) Only the arteries are demonstrated in this transplant kidney, flashing alternately red and blue. (B) Doppler of case (A) demonstrates reversed flow in the arteries with an absence of venous flow. (C) Another example of transplant renal vein thrombosis (D).

waveform becomes very pulsatile, with reverse EDF, which in the clinical setting of an oliguric patient with a tender graft in the early post operative period is highly suspicious for RVT.

During the early stages, when thrombosis is incomplete, venous flow may be seen in the kidney, but the artery is of reduced velocity.[41] The ultrasound findings of RVT may be indistinguishable from severe rejection, however, venous flow is generally unaffected in the latter.

Thrombosis is rare, occurring typically in the immediate post-operative period.[51] It may be associated with a faulty venous anastomosis, secondary to compression of the vein, for example by a large, peri-venous collection or the patient may have an increased thrombotic tendency for a number of reasons.

Pseudoaneurysms and AV fistulae

These may sometimes form as a result of vascular damage during biopsy procedures. They are usually not significant and tend to resolve spontaneously (Fig. 7.30A). An AV fistula follows damage to an artery and vein, showing an irregular knot of vessels on colour or power Doppler with a pulsatile venous waveform and high peak and end diastolic velocity in the feeding artery. A large draining vein may also be seen.

A pseudoaneurysm is the result of arterial damage and may appear cystic on the grey-scale image, but will demonstrate filling on colour Doppler with a pulsatile flow velocity waveform (Fig. 7.30B, C). Careful, ultrasound-guided biopsy technique helps to avoid such lesions (see Chapter 11).

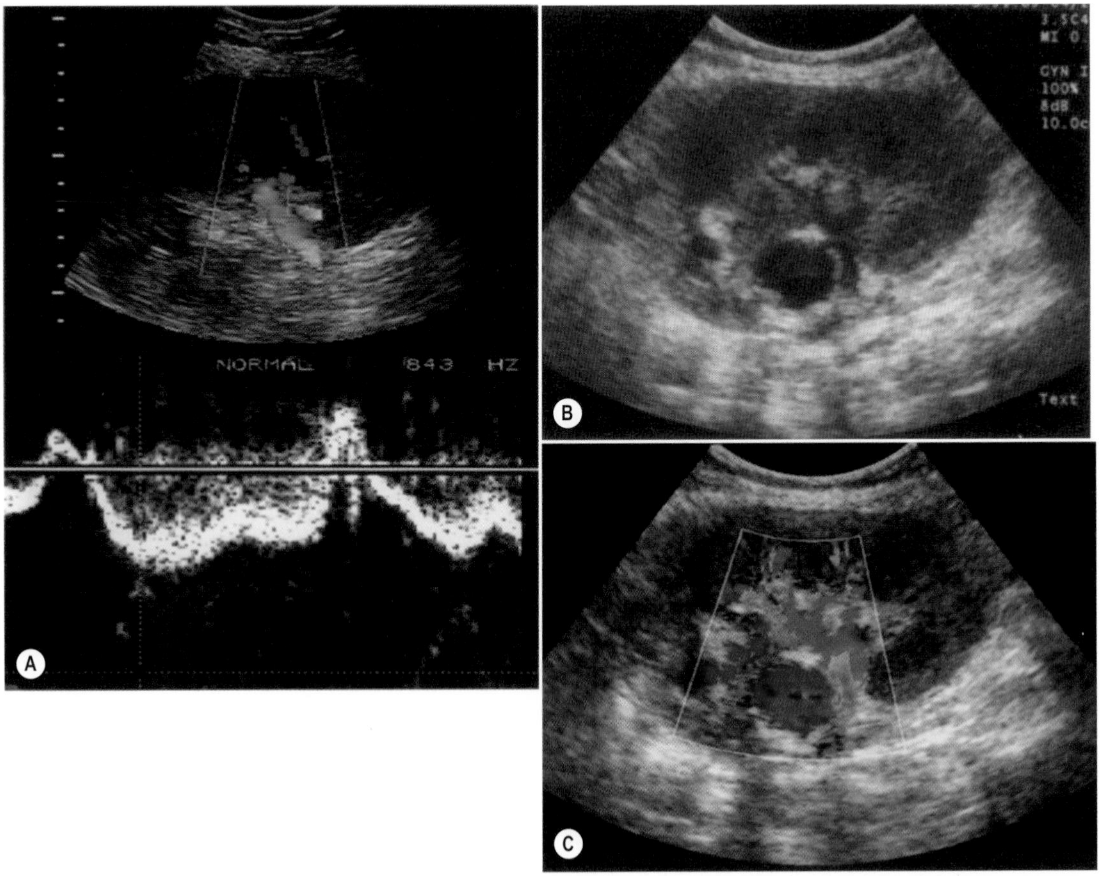

Fig. 7.30 • (A) Pulsatile venous waveform is seen as a result of a small AV fistula following biopsy procedure. (B) This renal artery aneurysm appears cystic on grey-scale. (C) Colour Doppler demonstrates arterial flow.

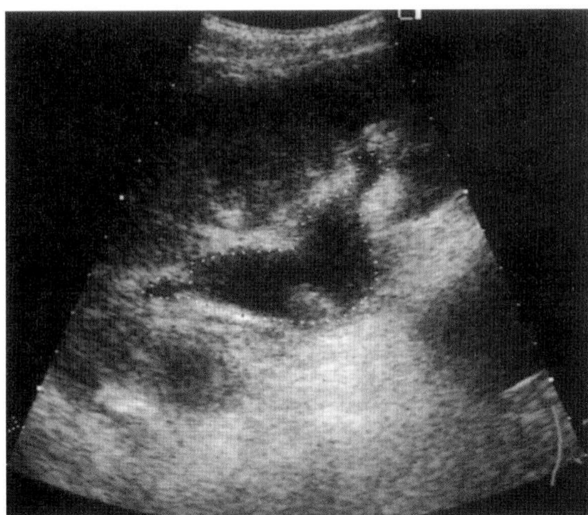

Fig. 7.31 • Fungal ball in the dilated pelvicalyceal system.

INFECTION

This is characterized by swelling of the uroepithelium, especially with fungal infections. Fungal balls may be visible as relatively hyperechoic structures within the pelvicalyceal system (Fig. 7.31).

ACUTE TUBULAR NECROSIS

Acute tubular necrosis is the most common form of delayed graft function immediately following transplant. It is associated with ischaemia after removal from the donor, and reperfusion injury. Mild acute tubular necrosis may resolve spontaneously. On ultrasound, it may demonstrate prominent medullary pyramids, with Doppler demonstrating low EDF. Reverse EDF is uncommon but recognized. A biopsy is required for confirmation.

CYCLOSPORIN NEPHROTOXICITY

The toxic nature of the immunosuppressive regimen requires the dose to be very carefully adjusted. Drug toxicity is a recognized cause of poor renal function and decreased perfusion. There may be increased Doppler resistance, as for acute tubular necrosis, but normally indices remain unaffected. Histology is required to confirm the diagnosis, or a clinical improvement following reduction or withdrawal of the immunosuppressive agent.

RENAL TRANSPLANT DYSFUNCTION AND DOPPLER CORRELATION

Doppler correlation with the different types of renal graft dysfunction is not possible. However, by taking the *clinical picture* into account it *is* possible to differentiate these situations (Table 7.4).

References

1. Burge HJ, Middleton WD, McClennan BL et al. Ureteral jets in healthy subjects and in patients with unilateral ureteral calculi: comparison with color Doppler US. Radiology 1991; 180: 437–442
2. Brkljacic B, Drinkovic I, Delic-Brkljacic D, Hebrang A. Age-related changes of renal vascular resistance in normal native kidneys: colour duplex Doppler ultrasound assessment. Radiol Oncol 1995; 29: 102–106
3. Wah T, Weston M, Irving H. Lower moiety pelvic-ureteric junction obstruction (PUJO) of the duplex kidney presenting with pyonephrosis in adults. Br J Radiol 2003; 76: 909–912
4. Fan L, Lianfang D, Jinfang X et al. Diagnostic efficacy of contrast-enhanced ultrasonography in solid renal parenchymal lesions with maximum diameters of 5 cm. J Ultrasound Med 2008; 27: 875–885, 4278–4297
5. Bosniak M. The current radiological approach to renal cysts. Radiology 1986; 158: 1–10
6. Warren K, McFarlane J. The Bosniak classification of renal cystic masses. BJU Int 2008; 95: 939–942
7. Ascenti G, Mazziotti S, Zimbaro G et al. Complex cystic renal masses: characterisation with Contrast-enhanced US. Radiology 2007; 243: 158–165
8. Glassberg KI. Renal dysgenesis and cystic disease of the kidney. In: Walsh PC, Retik AB, Vaughan ED, Wein AJ, eds. Campbell's urology, 8th edn. Elsevier Science, Philadelphia, 2002, p 1925
9. Badani K, Hemal AK, Menon M. Autosomal dominant polycystic kidney disease and pain – A review of the disease from aetiology, evaluation, past surgical treatment options to current practice. JPGM 2004; 50: 3, 222–226
10. Umeoka S, Koyama T, Miki Y et al. Pictorial review of tuberous sclerosis in various organs. Radiographics 2008; 28: e32
11. Heinz-Peer G, Schoder M, Rand T et al. Prevalence of acquired cystic kidney disease and tumours in native kidneys of renal transplant recipients: a prospective study. Radiology 1995; 195: 667–671
12. Levine E. Acquired cystic kidney disease. Radiol Clin North Am 1996; 34: 947–964
13. Siegel CL, Middleton WD, Teefey SA, McClennan BL. Angiomyolipoma and renal cell carcinoma: US differentiation. Radiology 1996; 198: 789–793

14. Prasad SR, Surabhi VR, Menias CO et al. Benign renal neoplasms in adults: cross-sectional imaging findings. AJR Am J Roentgenol 2008; 190: 158–164
15. Curry NS, Schabel SI, Betsill WL. Small renal neoplasms: diagnostic imaging, pathologic features and clinical course. Radiology 1986; 158: 113–117
16. Licht MR. Renal adenoma and oncocytoma. Semin Urol Oncol 1995; 13: 262–266
17. Bosniak MA, Birnbaum BA, Krinsky GA, Waisman J. Small renal parencymal neoplasms: further observations on growth. Radiology 1996; 197: 589–597
18. Mattar K, Jewett MA. Watchful waiting for small renal masses. Curr Urol Rep 2008; 9: 22–25
19. Correas J, Tranquart F, Claudon M. Guidelines for contrast enhanced ultrasound (CEUS). J Radiol 2009; 90: 123–140
20. Sánchez-Martín FM, Millán-Rodríguez F, Urdaneta-Pignalosa G et al. Small renal masses: incidental diagnosis, clinical symptoms, and prognostic factors. Adv Urol 2008; 310694.
21. Haendl T, Strobel D, Legal W et al. Renal cell cancer does not show a typical perfusion pattern in contrast-enhanced ultrasound. Ultraschall Med 2009; 30: 58–63
22. Browne RF, Meehan CP, Colville J et al. Transitional cell carcinoma of the upper urinary tract: spectrum of imaging findings. Radiographics 2005; 25: 1609–1627
23. Jamis-Dow CA, Choyke PL, Jennings SB et al. Small (<3 cm) renal masses: Detection with CT versus US and pathologic correlation. Radiology 1996; 198: 785–788
24. Leung RS, Biswas SV, Duncan M, Rankin S. Imaging features of von Hippel-Lindau disease. Radiographics 2008; 28: 65–79
25. Dhar M, Denstedt JD. Imaging in diagnosis, treatment, and follow-up of stone patients. Adv Chronic Kidney Dis 2009; 16: 39–47
26. Shine S. Urinary calculus: IVU vs. CT renal stone? A critically appraised topic. Abdom Imaging 2008; 33: 41–43
27. Rodgers PM, Bates JA, Irving HC. Intrarenal Doppler ultrasound studies in normal and acutely obstructed kidneys. Br J Radiol 1992; 65: 207–212
28. Miletic D, Fuckar Z, Sustic A et al. Resistance and pulsatility indices in acute renal obstruction. J Clin Ultrasound 1998; 26: 79–84
29. Hak-JL, Seung HK, Yoong KJ, Kyung MY. Doppler sonographic resistive index in obstructed kidneys. J Ultrasound Med 1996; 15/9: 613–618
30. Jung DC, Kim SH, Jung SI et al. Renal papillary necrosis: review and comparison of findings at multi-detector row CT and intravenous urography. Radiographics 2006; 26: 1827–1836
31. Craig WD, Wagner BJ, Travis MD. Pyelonephritis: radiologic-pathologic review. Radiographics 2008; 28: 255–277
32. Haddad MC, Sharif HS, Shahed MS et al. Renal colic: diagnosis and outcome. Radiology 1992; 184: 83–88
33. Abdominal radiography after CT reveals urinary calculi: a method to predict usefulness of abdominal radiography on the basis of size and CT attenuation of calculi. AJR Am J Roentgenol 2001; 176: 1117–1122
34. Li Y, Zhang Y. Diagnosis and treatment of acute focal bacterial nephritis. Chinese Med J 1996; 109: 168–172
35. Symeonidou C, Standish R, Sahdev A et al. Imaging and histopathologic features of HIV-related renal disease. Radiographics 2008; 28: 1339–1354
36. Page JE, Morgan SH, Eastwood JB et al. Ultrasound findings in renal parenchymal disease: comparison with histological appearances. Clin Radiol 1994; 49: 867–870
37. Strandness DE. Natural history of renal artery stenosis. Am J Kidney Dis 1994; 24: 630–635
38. Olin JW, Piedmonte MR, Young JR et al. The utility of duplex ultrasound scanning of the renal arteries for diagnosing significant renal artery stenosis. Ann Intern Med 1995; 122: 833–838
39. Baxter GM, Aitchison F, Sheppard D et al. Colour Doppler ultrasound in renal artery stenosis: intrarenal waveform analysis. Br J Radiol 1996: 69/825: 810–815
40. Bude RO, Rubin JM, Platt JF et al. Pulsus Tardus: Its cause and potential limitations in detection of arterial stenosis. Radiology 1994; 190: 779–784
41. Witz M, Kantarovsky A, Morag B, Shifin EG. Renal vein occlusion: a review. J Urol 1996; 155: 1173–1179
42. MacLennan AC, Baxter GM, Harden P, Rowe PA. Renal transplant vein occlusion: an early diagnostic sign? Clin Radiol 1995; 50/4: 251–253
43. Hamilton D. Alexis Carrel and the early days of tissue transplantation. Transplant Rev 1987; 2: 1–15
44. Murray JE, Merrill JP, Harrison JH. Kidney transplantation between seven pairs of identical twins. Ann Surg 1958; 148: 343–359
45. Starzl TE. Experience in renal transplantation. Saunders, Philadelphia, 1964
46. Calne RY, White DJG, Thiru S et al. Cyclosporin A in patients receiving renal allografts from cadaveric donors. Lancet 1978; ii: 1323–1327
47. Cosgrove DO, Chan KE. Renal transplants: what ultrasound can and cannot do. Ultrasound Q 2008; 24: 77–87
48. Kashi SH, Irving HC. Improving the evaluation of renal transplant collecting system dilatation by computerised ultrasound imaging digitisation. Br J Radiol 1993; 66: 1002–1008
49. Townsend RR, Tomlanovich SJ, Goldstein RB et al. Combined Doppler and morphologic sonographic evaluation of renal transplant rejection. J Ultrasound Med 1990; 9: 199–206
50. Perella RR, Duerincky AJ, Tessler FN et al. Evaluation of renal transplant dysfunction by duplex Doppler sonography; a prospective study and review of the literature. Am J Kidney Dis 1990; 15: 544–550
51. Tublin ME, Dodd GD. Sonography of renal tranplantation. Radiol Clin North Am 1995; 33: 447–459
52. Hilborn MD, Bude RO, Murphy KJ et al. Renal transplant evaluation with power Doppler sonography. Br J Radiol 1997; 70: 39–42

Ultrasound of the retroperitoneum and gastrointestinal tract

8

CHAPTER CONTENTS

NORMAL ANATOMY

The peritoneum is the large sheet of serous membrane that lines the abdominal cavity and surrounds the organs. The peritoneum has several 'extensions', which bind the organs together: the mesentery, which loosely anchors the small bowel, ensuring it does not twist; the transverse mesocolon, which attaches the transverse colon to the posterior abdominal wall and the greater and lesser omentum. These projections coat the viscera and form pouches, or sacs, within the peritoneal cavity in which dependent fluid can collect.

The retroperitoneal space contains the kidneys and ureters, adrenal glands, pancreas and duodenal loop, great vessels and the ascending and descending portions of the large bowel, including the caecum (Fig. 8.1).

THE ABDOMINAL AORTA

The proximal abdominal aorta can usually be visualized in the midline, inferior to the xiphisternum, by using the left lobe of liver as an acoustic window. The coeliac axis and SMA are easily demonstrated in LS, arising from its anterior aspect (Fig. 8.2); the coeliac axis branches – the main hepatic and splenic arteries – are better appreciated in a transverse section. Just below this level, the origin of the SMA is seen with the renal arteries inferior to this.

The distal abdominal aorta runs more anteriorly, towards the bifurcation. Here, bowel gas may obscure the structures in sagittal section. A coronal approach overcomes this problem: from the patient's left side the aorta can be demonstrated using the left kidney as an acoustic window, and from the patient's right side, the right lobe of liver affords good access (Fig. 8.2D, E). A coronal view

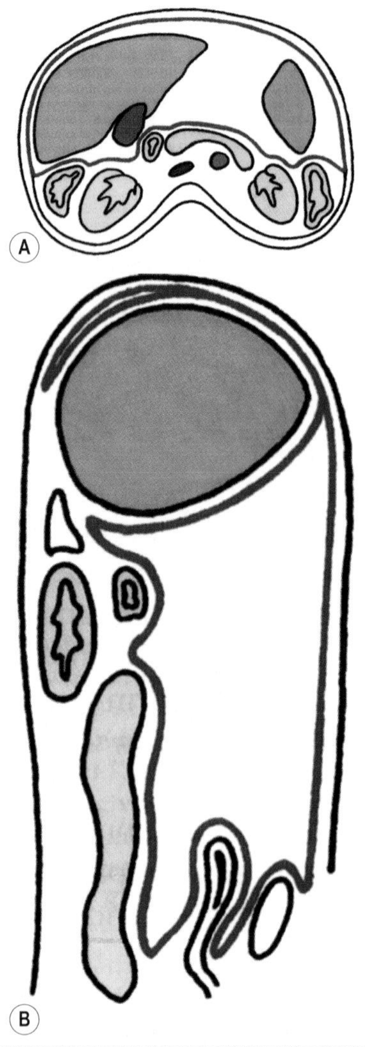

Fig. 8.1 • (A) Axial and (B) sagittal sections through the abdomen showing the relationship of the abdominal viscera to the peritoneum (red).

is also useful in displaying the origin of the renal arteries.

The aorta often becomes ectatic and tortuous with age, and it is not unusual to detect considerable calcification of the walls (Fig. 8.2G).

Aortic aneurysm

Abdominal aortic aneurysm (AAA) is a common and potentially deadly condition. The risk factors for AAA include male gender, age over 65, smoking and a family history. AAA is found in up to 10% of men aged 65 and over. The risk of aneurysm rupture increases with diameter, increasing dramatically when it reaches 6 cm, with a 1-year mortality of 50%.[1]

Screening of the high-risk population with ultrasound is increasingly being adopted. Small aneurysms may then be monitored to allow timely treatment (open or endovascular repair) with a subsequent fall in mortality.[2,3] It is generally accepted that repair is indicated in any aneurysm of over 5.5 cm diameter due to the imminent risk of rupture.[4]

Post-operative complications of grafts, such as infection or pseudoaneurysm, are usually monitored with CT or MRI.

Ultrasound appearances and measurements

Most aneurysms are associated with atherosclerosis, which weakens the media of the wall, causing the vessel to dilate and eventually rupture. The aneurysm may be fusiform or saccular (Fig. 8.3). Blood flow within it is turbulent, and the slow flowing blood at the edges of the vessel tends to thrombose.

Surgery is always complicated by the involvement of the renal arteries. Fortunately, the vast majority of aneurysms are infrarenal, but it may be difficult to determine the relationship of the aneurysm to the renal artery origins on ultrasound, and CT is helpful in such cases. Occasionally the aneurysm affects the bifurcation and common iliac arteries, which should also be examined during the scan as far as possible.

The true maximum diameter of the aneurysm should be ascertained in LS, where the calipers can be placed perpendicular to the walls for an accurate diameter at the widest part of the aneurysm. This is a reliable and reproducible measurement in trained hands. CT measurements and ultrasound measurements done in a transverse plane tend to overestimate the diameter, as the aorta often runs obliquely (Fig. 8.2F). When the aorta is scanned in TS, care must be taken to keep the transducer perpendicular to the (often tortuous) axis of the vessel to avoid inaccurate measurements. The ability of ultrasound to locate the correct plane for measurement, regardless of vessel tortuosity, is an advantage over CT, which may overestimate the size of the aneurysm in an axial plane.

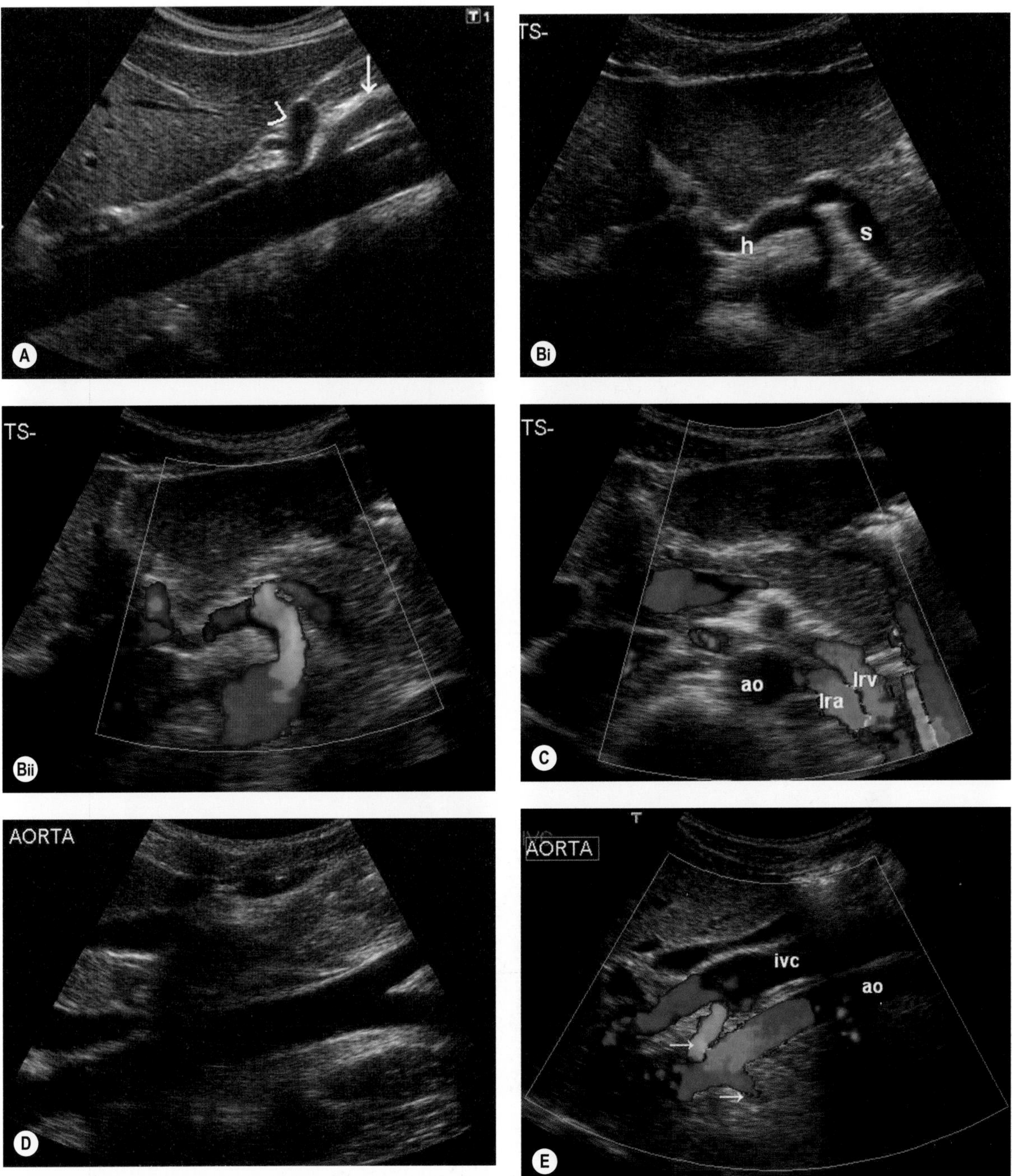

Fig. 8.2 • (A) LS through the abdominal aorta demonstrating the coeliac axis (arrowhead) and the SMA (arrow). The SV is seen anterior to the SMA. (Bi) TS through the proximal abdominal aorta. The coeliac axis divides into the hepatic (h) and splenic (s) arteries. (Bii) Colour Doppler demonstrates the direction of flow with respect to the transducer. (C) TS, distal to the coeliac axis, demonstrating the origin of the renal arteries. The left renal vein (lrv, red) passes anterior to the left renal artery (lra, blue) and aorta (ao) to drain into the IVC. (D) A coronal plane, from the patient's right side, demonstrates the aortic bifurcation. (E) Coronal section, from the patient's right side, demonstrating the IVC and aorta at the level of the renal arteries (arrows).

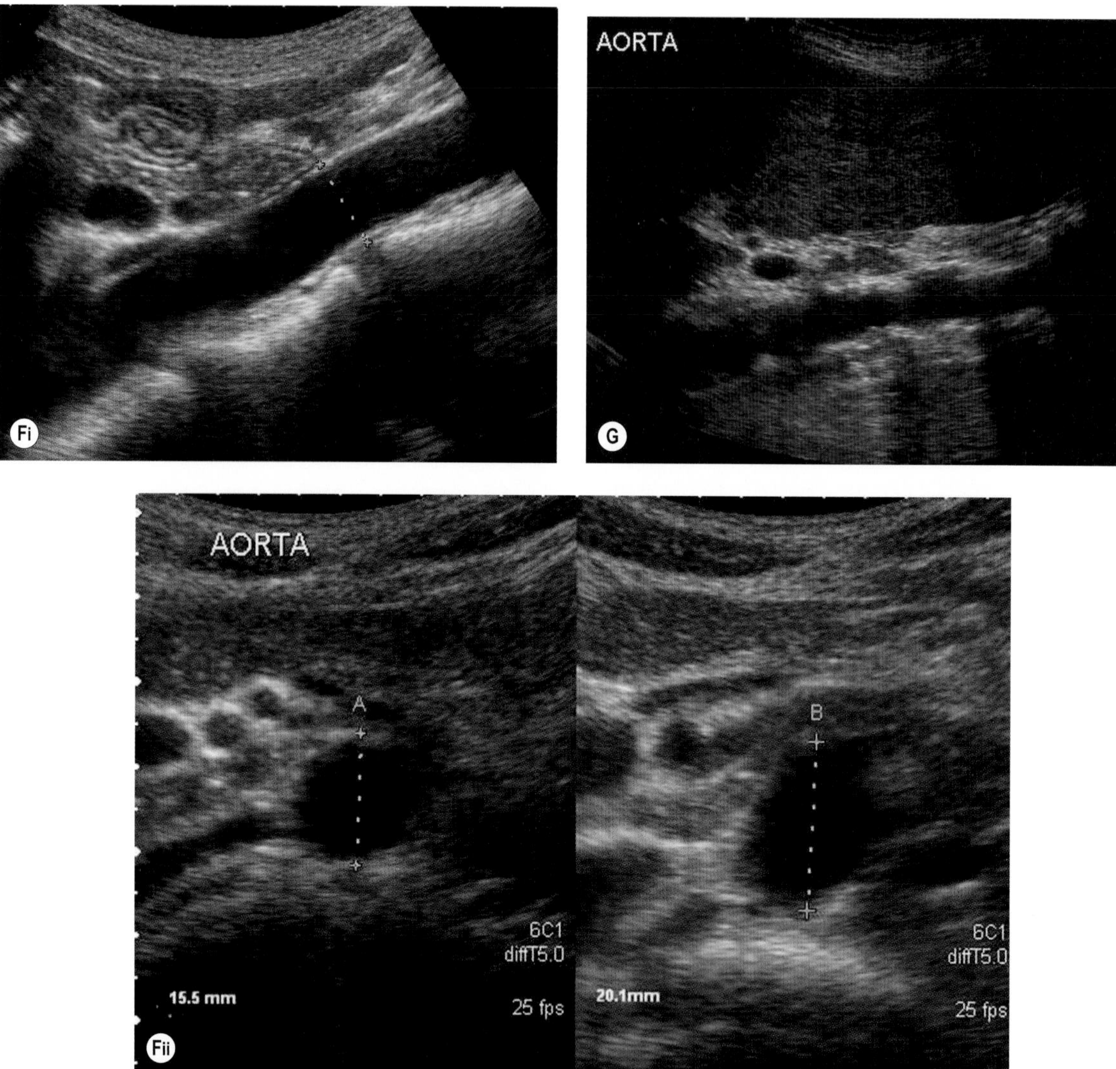

Fig. 8.2, cont'd • (Fi) Sagittal LS through the aorta demonstrating the correct measurement technique – calipers perpendicular to the walls. (Fii) Incorrect technique in TS: in the left image the probe is angled caudally and is probably perpendicular to the vessel but the right image has the probe perpendicular to the abdominal wall (similar to CT), overestimating the aortic diameter by almost 20%. (G) The aorta of an elderly patient containing calcification in the walls, causing acoustic shadowing.

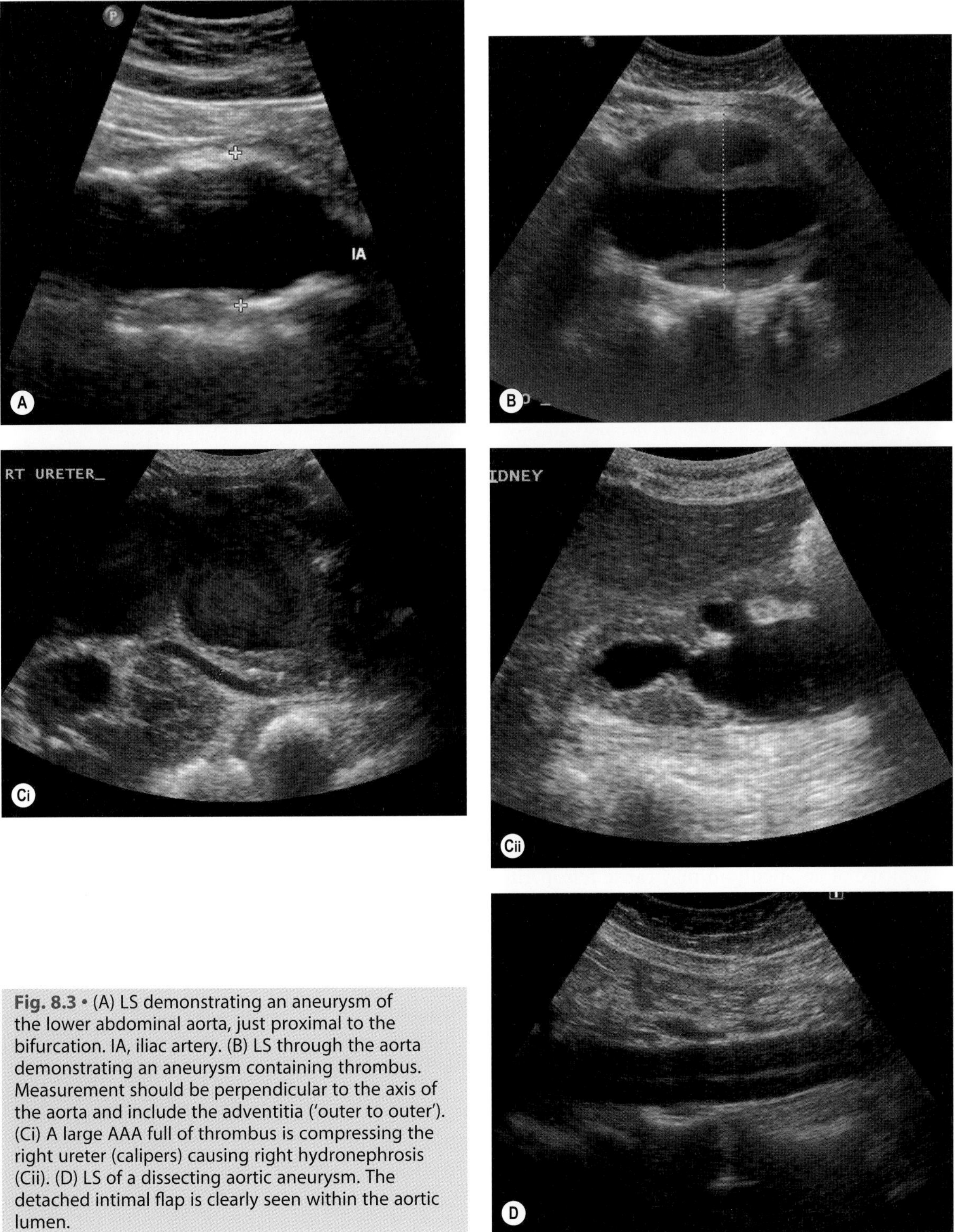

Fig. 8.3 • (A) LS demonstrating an aneurysm of the lower abdominal aorta, just proximal to the bifurcation. IA, iliac artery. (B) LS through the aorta demonstrating an aneurysm containing thrombus. Measurement should be perpendicular to the axis of the aorta and include the adventitia ('outer to outer'). (Ci) A large AAA full of thrombus is compressing the right ureter (calipers) causing right hydronephrosis (Cii). (D) LS of a dissecting aortic aneurysm. The detached intimal flap is clearly seen within the aortic lumen.

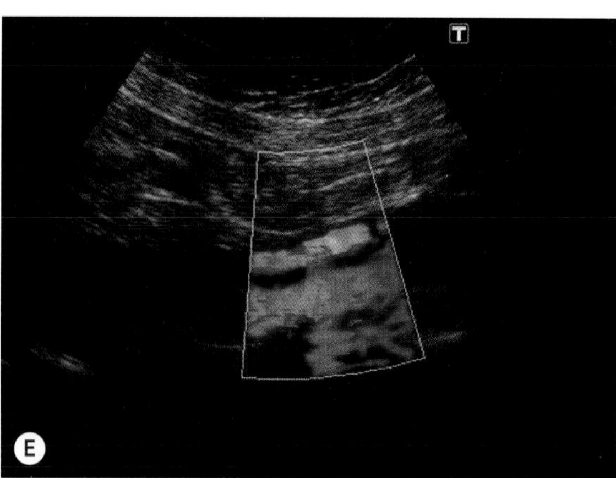

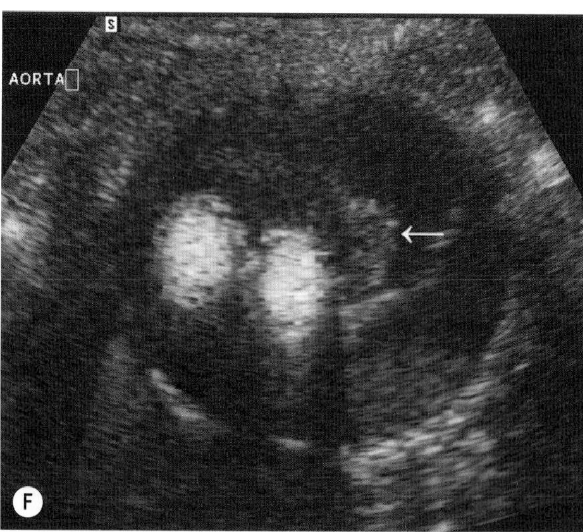

Fig. 8.3, cont'd • (E) Colour Doppler demonstrates flow on both sides of the intima. (F) CEUS of the aorta post Y graft demonstrates enhancement of the lumens of the iliac arteries with slight leakage (arrow) in the region of the bifurcation.

Complications of aortic aneurysm

Dissection of the aneurysm, in which the intima becomes detached, is uncommon in the abdomen. Ultrasound may visualize the intimal flap and the false lumen created between the media and intima often contains slower, more turbulent or even reversed flow. Layers of thrombus may mimic a dissection, and colour flow Doppler is particularly useful in such cases.

Leakage of an aneurysm may cause retroperitoneal haematoma, but CT is usually more reliable in detecting leaks than ultrasound. CEUS has had success in identifying leaks following AAA repair, and has been reported to be more sensitive than CT in this group (Fig. 8.3F).[5,6] This has the added advantage of reducing radiation dose due to CT, especially in patients who are regularly monitored with imaging.

Rupture of an aortic aneurysm is a surgical emergency associated with high mortality. It is accompanied by abdominal pain and severe hypotension. Involvement of the renal arteries may cause renal artery thrombosis and subsequently small kidney(s). Always check the kidneys at the time of scanning to ensure they are of normal size and appearance.

THE INFERIOR VENA CAVA

Ultrasound is highly successful in demonstrating the proximal IVC, by using the liver as an acoustic window, especially if the patient is right side raised. The distal IVC may be obscured by overlying bowel gas and, unlike the aorta, is susceptible to compression, making visualization difficult in some cases. In comparison with the aorta in LS, the course of the IVC is anterior as it passes through the diaphragm.

The normal IVC has thinner walls and a more flattened profile than the aorta, and its lumen alters with changing abdominal pressure, for example during respiration the lumen decreases on inspiration, or with the Valsalva manoeuvre (Fig. 8.4). The main renal veins may be seen in TS, entering the IVC just below the level of the pancreas.

Haemodynamically, the blood flow spectrum from the IVC alters according to the distance of the sample volume from the right atrium. The blood flow through the IVC and proximal hepatic veins is pulsatile, with reverse flow during right atrial systole. Pulsatility reduces in the distal IVC.

The most common anomaly of the IVC is that of duplication. However, this is infrequently picked up on ultrasound and is best demonstrated with

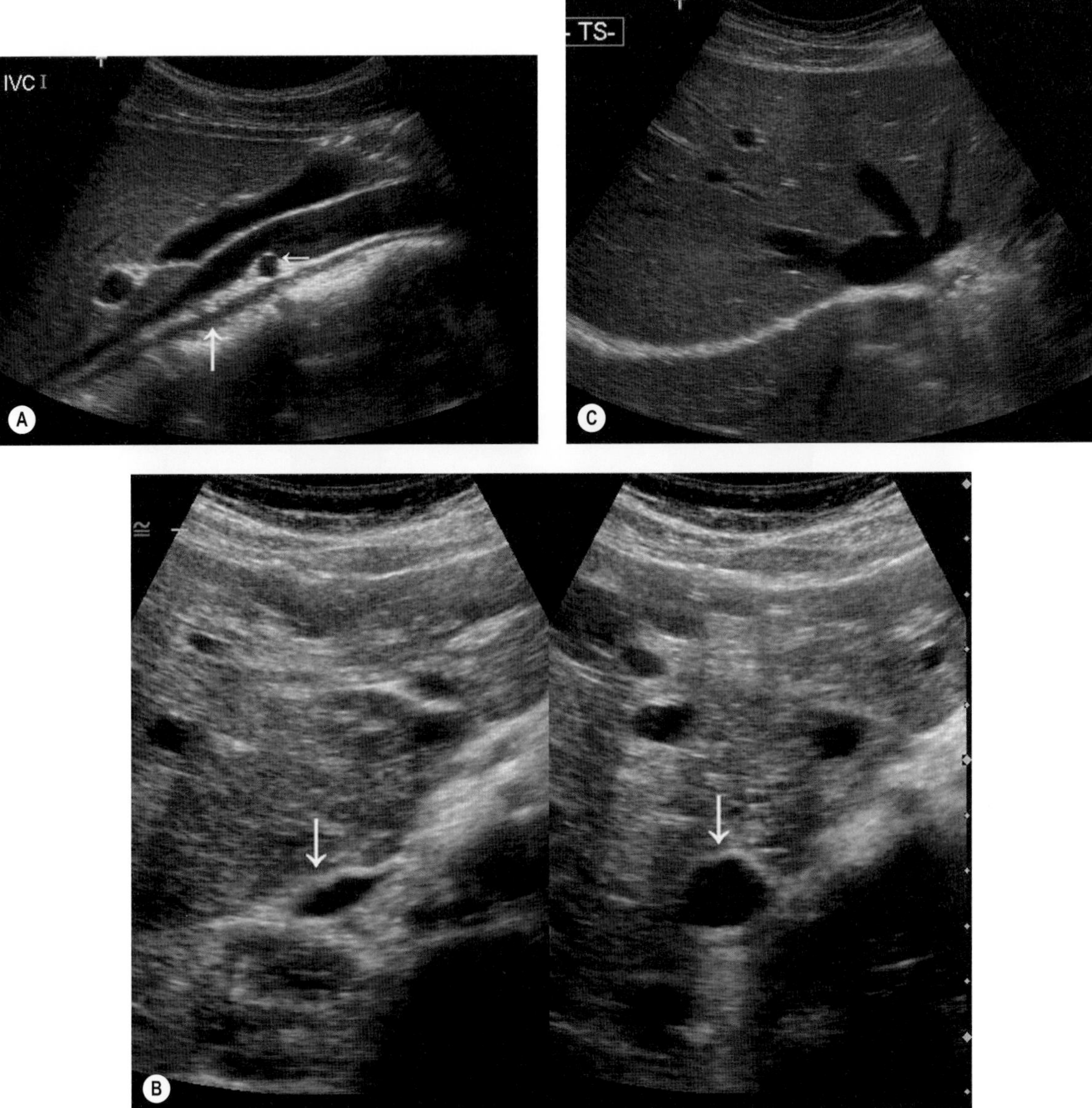

Fig. 8.4 • (A) LS through the IVC. The right renal artery (RRA, small arrow) is seen passing posterior to the IVC. The diaphragmatic crus lies posterior to this (large arrow). (B) TS through the IVC demonstrating the difference in profile during the Valsalva manoeuvre (left) compared with normal expiration (right). (Liver cysts are present.) (C) IVC at the level of the confluence of the hepatic veins, just beneath the diaphragm.

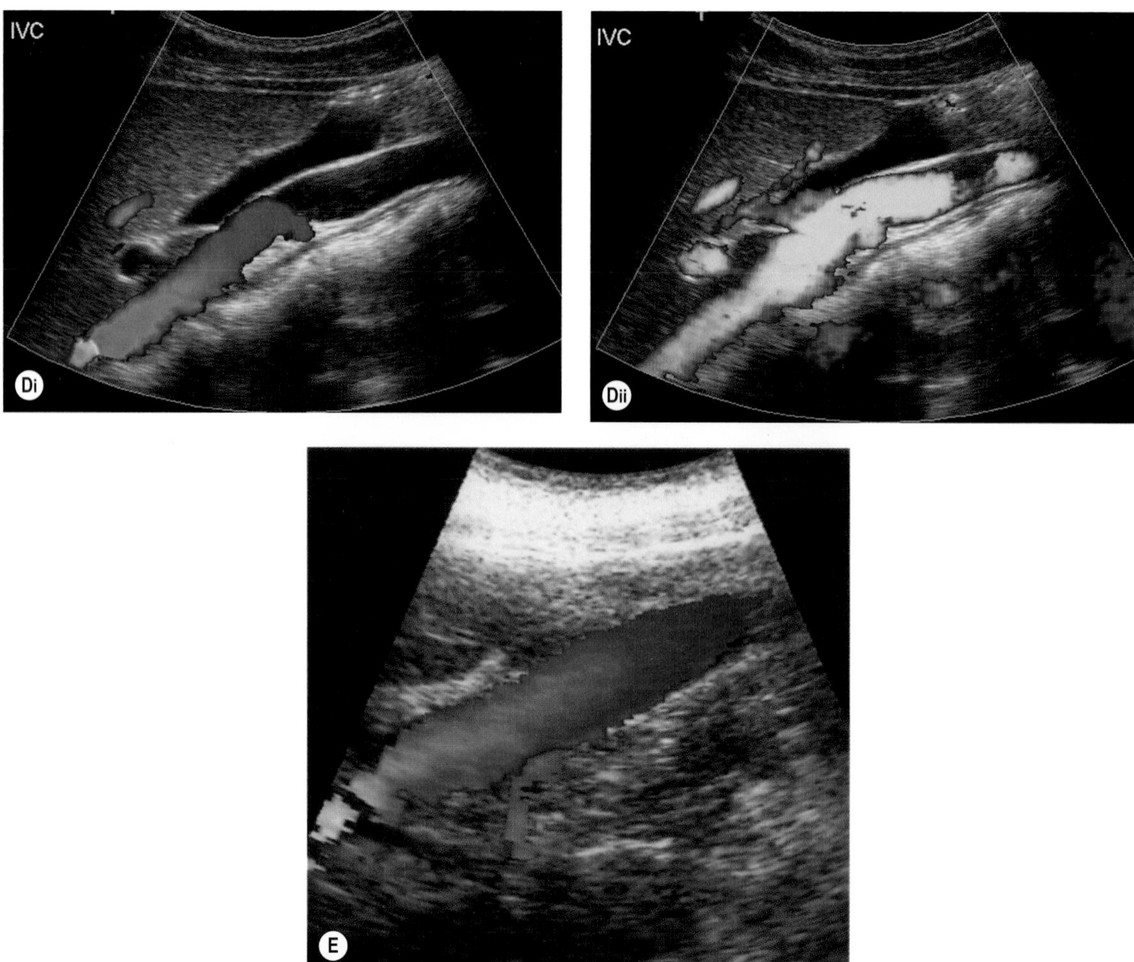

Fig. 8.4, cont'd • (Di) Colour Doppler fails to demonstrate flow when the IVC is perpendicular to the beam, (Dii) Power Doppler overcomes this, as it is less angle-dependent. (E) The RRV (in red) is seen draining into the IVC on colour Doppler.

CT or MRI. Transposition of the IVC may be seen in situs inversus.

Pathology of the IVC

Thrombus in the IVC may be due to benign causes, or the result of tumour. It is not usually possible to tell the difference on grey-scale appearances alone, but vascularity may be demonstrated on power or colour Doppler within tumour thrombus, and the clinical history is helpful. Tumour thrombus invades the renal vein and enters the IVC in around 10% of renal carcinoma cases. Tumour thrombus from hepatic or adrenal masses can also invade the IVC (Fig. 8.5).

Coagulation disorders, which cause Budd–Chiari syndrome (see Chapter 4) predominantly affect the hepatic veins, but may also involve the IVC (Fig. 8.6). Patients may require the insertion of a caval filter, which is performed under X-ray guidance, but may be monitored for patency using ultrasound with Doppler. Dilatation of the IVC is a finding commonly associated with congestive heart failure, and is frequently accompanied by hepatic vein dilatation.

Compression of the IVC by large masses is not uncommon. This may be due to retroperitoneal masses, such as lymphadenopathy, or liver masses such as tumour or caudate lobe hypertrophy. Colour or power Doppler is particularly useful in confirming patency of the vessel and differentiating extrinsic compression from invasion. Insertion of metallic stents may be performed under angiographic control to maintain the vessel patency, particularly if the compression is due to inoperable hepatic metastasis (Fig. 8.6).

Tumours of the IVC are rare. Leiomyosarcoma is a primary IVC tumour, appearing as a hyperechoic mass in the lumen of the vein.[7,8] This may cause partial or complete obstruction of the IVC resulting in Budd–Chiari syndrome. In partial

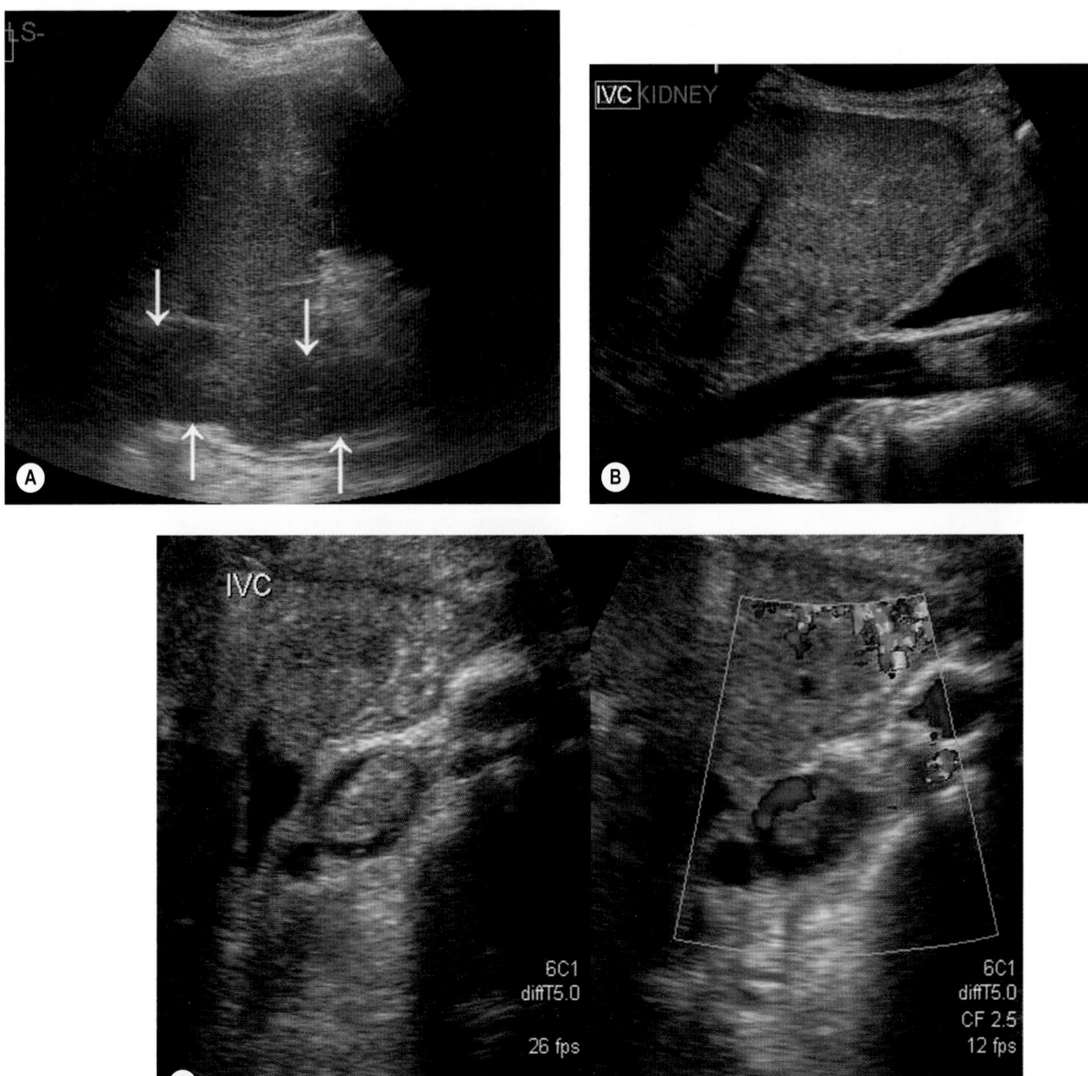

Fig. 8.5 • (A) Tumour thrombus, from a left renal carcinoma completely occludes the IVC (arrows). (B) Advanced renal carcinoma. The IVC contains tumour thrombus. (C) TS through the IVC containing non-occlusive thrombus. Flow is demonstrated around the thrombus on the right hand image.

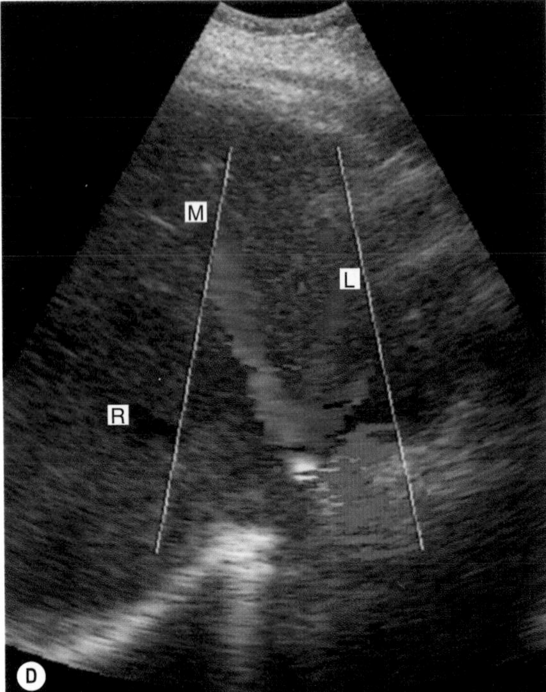

Fig. 8.5, cont'd • (D) Tumour thrombus from a renal carcinoma has spread up the IVC and invaded the RHV causing a partial Budd–Chiari effect. M, L, R: middle, left and right hepatic veins.

occlusion, the hepatic veins and proximal IVC may be considerably dilated. Resection of the tumour, with repair of the IVC, is possible provided the adjacent liver is not invaded.[7]

THE ADRENAL GLANDS

Normal appearances

The normal adrenal glands can be seen on ultrasound in the vast majority of patients,[9,10] if you know where and how to look. Each adrenal gland is constructed with a central fold or ridge, which points anteromedially, from which extend two thin 'wings' of tissue – a medial and a lateral wing (Fig. 8.7).

The ultrasound appearances are therefore of a smaller shape in longitudinal section, or a thin, linear structure as the transducer is moved medially towards the central ridge. The wings of the gland appear hypoechoic and are no more than 2 mm in thickness.

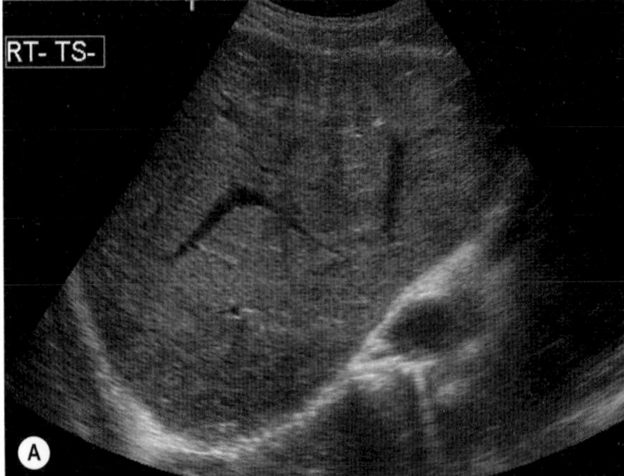

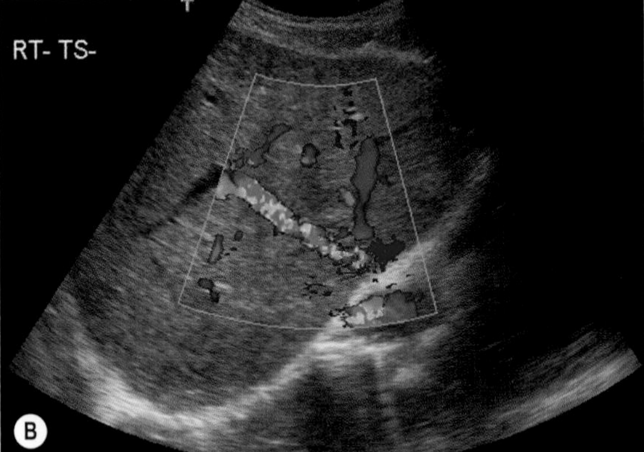

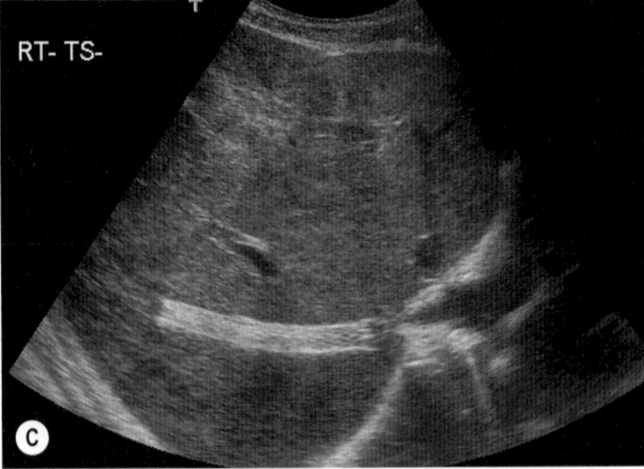

Fig. 8.6 • (A) Budd–Chiari syndrome, with an occluded RHV. (B) Confirmed with colour Doppler. (C) A stent has been inserted under angiographic guidance to restore flow in the vein.

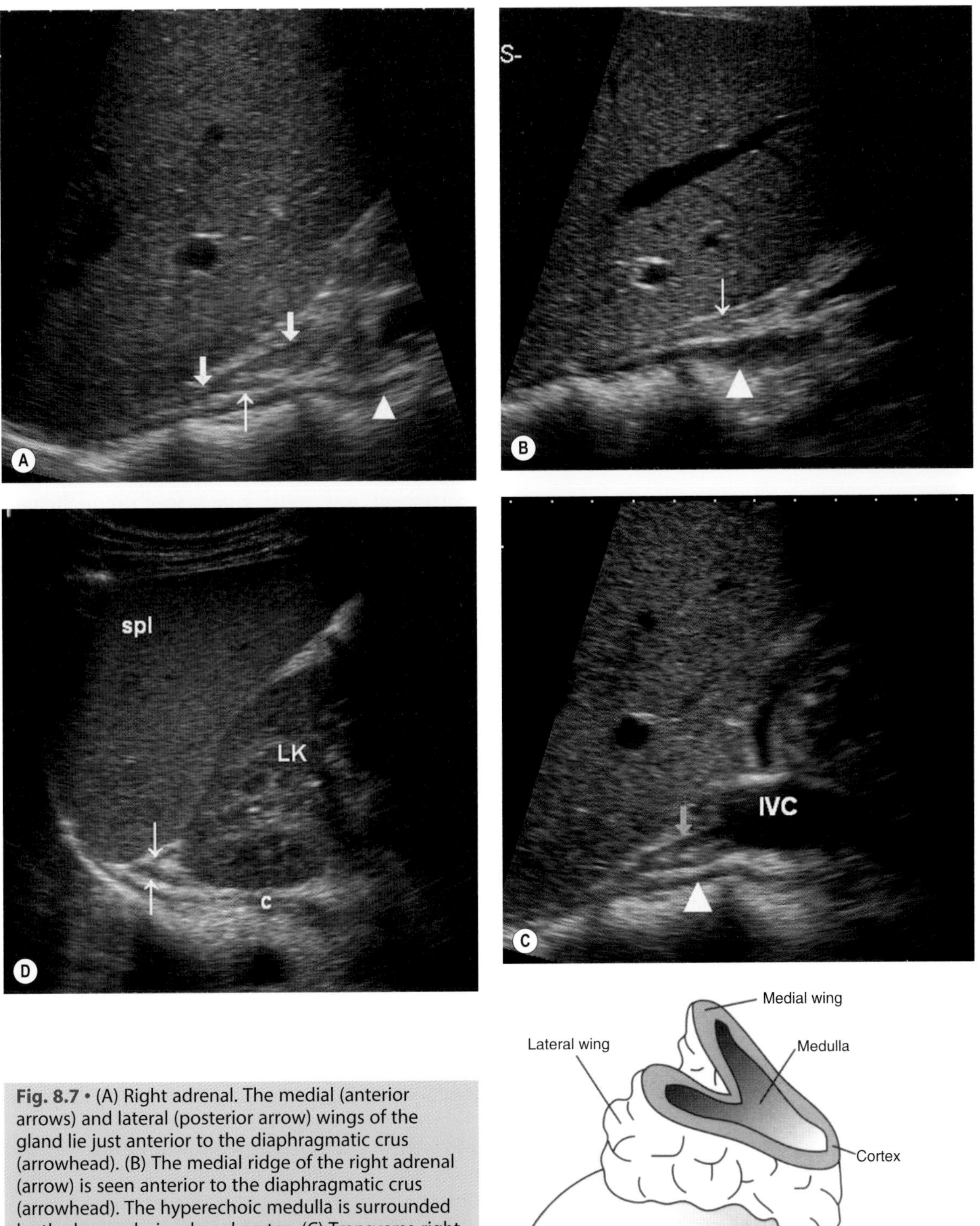

Fig. 8.7 • (A) Right adrenal. The medial (anterior arrows) and lateral (posterior arrow) wings of the gland lie just anterior to the diaphragmatic crus (arrowhead). (B) The medial ridge of the right adrenal (arrow) is seen anterior to the diaphragmatic crus (arrowhead). The hyperechoic medulla is surrounded by the hypoechoic adrenal cortex. (C) Transverse right adrenal (arrow) between the IVC and crus (arrowhead). (D) The two hypoechoic wings of the left adrenal (arrows) can be seen in the space between the spleen, LK and the crus, c. (E) Section through the right adrenal gland.

Ultrasound technique

For the right adrenal, use the liver as an acoustic window. Scan the upper pole of the kidney intercostally through the liver, and angle just medially to the kidney, where the gland can be located between the liver and the diaphragmatic crus (Fig. 8.7A). Continue angling medially towards the IVC to see the central ridge of the gland posterior to the IVC (Fig. 8.7B).

For the left gland the spleen must be used as a window. To avoid overlying bowel this is best achieved with the patient supine, using a coronal section. When the upper pole of the left kidney is located through the spleen, the left adrenal is located in the small triangular area between the spleen, kidney and diaphragmatic crus (Fig. 8.7D).[9,10]

Pathology of the adrenal glands

It is not unusual to find small incidental adrenal nodules on ultrasound. While these are usually benign non-functioning adenomas, and can be ignored if small, ultrasound is unable to characterize adrenal masses. A diagnostic dilemma occurs if patients are symptomatic or have a history of malignancy. CT is usually able to adequately characterize a non-functioning adenoma, and MRI or scintigraphy may be useful in cases in which the CT is not diagnostic.[11]

Adenoma

Small (less than 3 cm) solid adrenal nodules are a common, incidental finding in non-symptomatic patients (Fig. 8.8A). Benign, non-hyperfunctioning adenomas account for the majority of adrenal nodules, and are of no clinical significance. Their incidence increases with age and they are present in around 2% of adult autopsies. Small nodules in asymptomatic patients generally require no further action, but endocrine function may be evaluated to rule out a functioning mass. A hyperfunctioning adenoma (a determination made by evaluation of the endocrine function), although an essentially benign mass, usually requires surgical resection.

As a solitary abdominal finding in a patient with no relevant clinical history, it is generally safe to assume a small adrenal nodule requires no further action. However, because it is not possible to distinguish benign, incidental nodules from other forms of more serious pathology on ultrasound, incidental nodules of greater than 3 cm should be investigated further to confirm their benign nature.[12] Almost all incidental adrenal nodules below 3 cm are benign, with the likelihood of malignancy related to increasing size.[13] In patients with no history of malignancy and normal endocrine function, small nodules may be treated conservatively. Non-functioning adenomas remain stable in size on ultrasound follow-up.

A small study with CEUS has been found to characterize adrenal adenomas with similar sensitivity to CT and MRI,[14] and distinguish them from malignant masses. Adenomas displayed a pattern of late or slow enhancement while more rapid arterial phase enhancement with late-phase hypoenhancement was more often seen in malignant lesions. However, acoustic access to small, and particularly to left, adrenal nodules limits this technique and CT remains the next imaging step of choice.

Metastasis

The adrenal glands are a common site for metastases, particularly from lung, breast, bowel cancer, and melanoma. The adrenal glands are also commonly involved in non-Hodgkin's lymphoma. Although frequently accompanied by liver metastases, an adrenal metastasis may be present in the absence of any other obvious abdominal deposits, and therefore the adrenal glands should routinely be examined when staging malignant disease.

Like adenomas, they are often small, well-defined and hypoechoic on ultrasound (Fig. 8.8B). It is not possible to differentiate between benign adenoma and metastasis on the ultrasound appearances alone, but a small adrenal mass in the absence of a known primary carcinoma or suspicion of malignancy is highly likely to be benign, and will remain stable on follow-up. Larger metastases may be irregular in outline, and some demonstrate areas of necrosis or haemorrhage.

A solitary adrenal mass in a patient with known or suspected carcinoma requires further imaging for diagnosis. CT is usually the next step, as it is able to characterize the lesion in most cases in addition to staging the disease and demonstrating

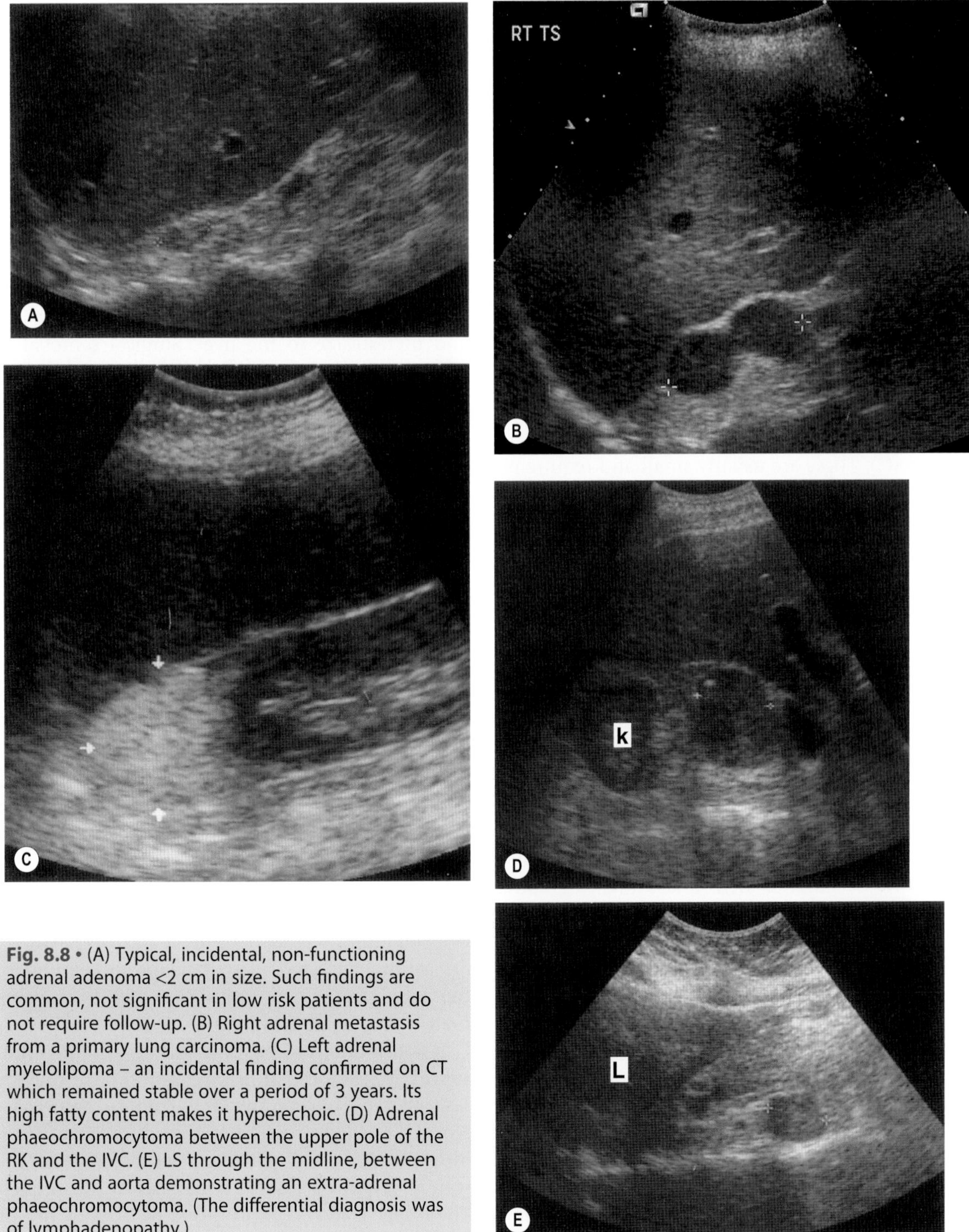

Fig. 8.8 • (A) Typical, incidental, non-functioning adrenal adenoma <2 cm in size. Such findings are common, not significant in low risk patients and do not require follow-up. (B) Right adrenal metastasis from a primary lung carcinoma. (C) Left adrenal myelolipoma – an incidental finding confirmed on CT which remained stable over a period of 3 years. Its high fatty content makes it hyperechoic. (D) Adrenal phaeochromocytoma between the upper pole of the RK and the IVC. (E) LS through the midline, between the IVC and aorta demonstrating an extra-adrenal phaeochromocytoma. (The differential diagnosis was of lymphadenopathy.)

lesions not visible on ultrasound, such as peritoneal deposits.

Adrenal cysts

Simple cysts are uncommon in the adrenal gland, but are easily differentiated from solid lesions with ultrasound. Some cysts may be the sequelae of previous haemorrhage, but most are simple, epithelial cysts. The usual acoustic characteristics of a cyst (anechoic, thin, regular capsule and posterior enhancement) apply.

Myelolipoma

The adrenal myelolipoma is a rare, benign non-functioning mass found incidentally. It is highly echogenic and well defined, due to its fatty content (Fig. 8.8C). These are usually small and require no further management.

Phaeochromocytoma

The phaeochromocytoma is uncommon, but may be found in up to 1% of patients with hypertension. It is a tumour arising in the chromaffin cells of the adrenal medulla (most commonly) or in autonomic nervous tissue. It may be bilateral and appears solid on ultrasound, although larger masses may have areas of necrosis within them. Most are benign, but 5–10% are malignant. It presents on a background of episodic, severe hypertension and secretes catecholamines, which can be found in the urine. (Although this is also a feature of adrenal neuroblastoma, the latter is predominantly a childhood tumour.) These lesions should be treated with great care – vigorous palpation may precipitate a severe hypertensive episode and biopsy should therefore be avoided.

Although most phaeochromocytomas arise in the adrenal glands, and are therefore demonstrable on ultrasound, those arising in the sympathetic chain may be obscured by bowel gas and are not possible to exclude on ultrasound (Fig. 8.8D, E). Tumours which arise from extra-adrenal chromaffin cells are termed paragangliomas. If there remains biochemical evidence of phaeochromocytoma in the presence of normal adrenal glands, a metaiodobenzylguanidine (MIBG) isotope scan may demonstrate increased activity and CT scan can then be targeted to the appropriate area. More recently, PET has been found to be superior in locating phaeochromocytomas in some at risk patient groups.[15]

Phaeochromocytomas are associated with some hereditary syndromes such as von Hippel–Lindau disease. Treatment is usually surgical removal.

Adrenal carcinoma

Primary adrenal carcinomas are rare in the adult. They are commonly endocrinologically inactive in adults, and therefore tend to present late when they are quite large. They may invade the IVC and metastasize to the liver. Surgical removal of tumours in the absence of liver metastases has a good prognosis[16] and in patients with metastases, radiofrequency (RF) ablation of the adrenal mass may have some benefit in prolonging survival.[17]

GASTROINTESTINAL TRACT

Contrast radiographic investigations, including CT and fluoroscopy, are frequently the first line of investigation for suspected gastrointestinal tract disease, in conjunction with endoscopic examination. Although ultrasound is not considered a primary tool in the investigation of bowel lesions, it is remarkably successful in diagnosing gastrointestinal tract pathology in the hands of an experienced operator,[18] and is much underestimated in its ability to evaluate the bowel. Gastrointestinal tract ultrasound can be time-consuming, but a wealth of information can be obtained in a symptomatic patient with a high-frequency linear probe. Considerable diagnostic benefit has been shown for careful, targeted, percutaneous ultrasound of the large and small gastrointestinal tract using high-frequency transducers.[19]

It is important to be aware of the variable ultrasound appearances of normal bowel, as it may be responsible for mimicking other pathology. Normal bowel is frequently difficult to examine on ultrasound as the gas-filled lumen reflects the sound, requiring careful compression techniques. The image is also compromised by obesity and by bowel contents. Abnormal bowel is particularly accessible to ultrasound, however. A fluid-filled lumen also facilitates demonstration of valvulae conniventes of the small bowel and haustra of the large colon.

Technique

A high-frequency curved or linear array (up to 12 MHz) is ideal. It is helpful for the patient to self-locate any areas of pain prior to scanning. The area may then be carefully examined by applying graded compressions to displace luminal gas and faeces and to reduce the depth of tissue being scanned.

Normal large intestine is compressible, does not undergo peristalsis and has a mural thickness of less than 4 mm; small intestine is less than 2 mm and undergoes peristalsis.

Oesophagus and stomach

The oesophagus is not usually accessible to percutaneous ultrasound, however, the lower end can be demonstrated as it passes through the diaphragm in the midline, just anterior to the aorta (Fig. 8.9A). Its normal appearances should not be confused with a mass. Occasionally, ultrasound demonstrates the thickened wall associated with an oesophageal carcinoma involving the lower oesophagus. EUS is excellent for imaging the oesophagus as it can also be used for biopsy and stent placement (Fig. 8.9B).

Although percutaneous ultrasound has had modest success in revealing stomach masses if the stomach is filled with water[20] it can never replace endoscopy. However, if such lesions are discovered, this helps to direct subsequent radiological management (Fig. 8.10).

EUS, with its high frequency and proximity to the relevant structures, is able to demonstrate the layers of the gut wall, and to demonstrate pathology and accurately stage malignant disease in both the oesophagus and stomach, and also to guide invasive procedures.[21,22] It is regarded as the gold standard for investigating the lining of the stomach and duodenum and can be combined with biopsy when necessary.

Accurate tumour staging is essential in order to plan the most appropriate management of the patient and determine prognosis. Cancers are staged using the 'TNM' classification, in which T determines the depth of invasion of the tumour, N represents the presence (or absence) of regional lymph node involvement and M indicates distant metastases. EUS is particularly good at determining the T stage of oesophageal cancers, and is also more accurate than CT in identifying regional node involvement, although it performs less well in staging gastric cancers.[23]

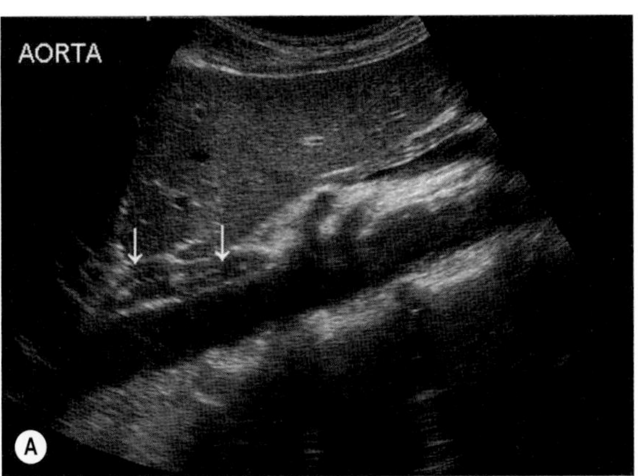

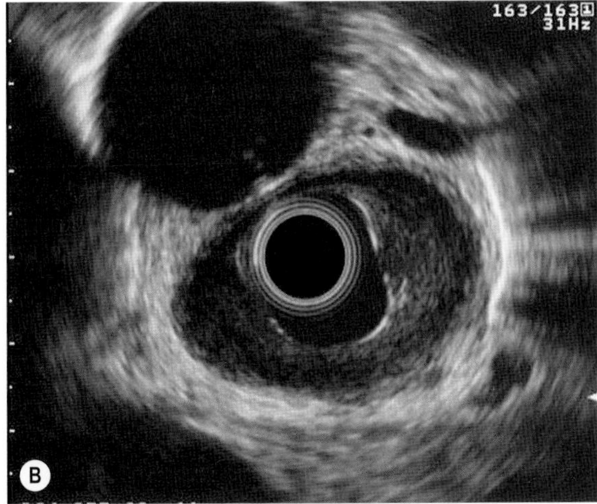

Fig. 8.9 • (A) Normal oesophagus (arrow) between the aorta and the left lobe of liver. Thin, hypoechoic walls with a hyperechoic lumen due to the presence of air. (B) EUS demonstrates the thickened wall of oesophageal carcinoma prior to stent insertion.

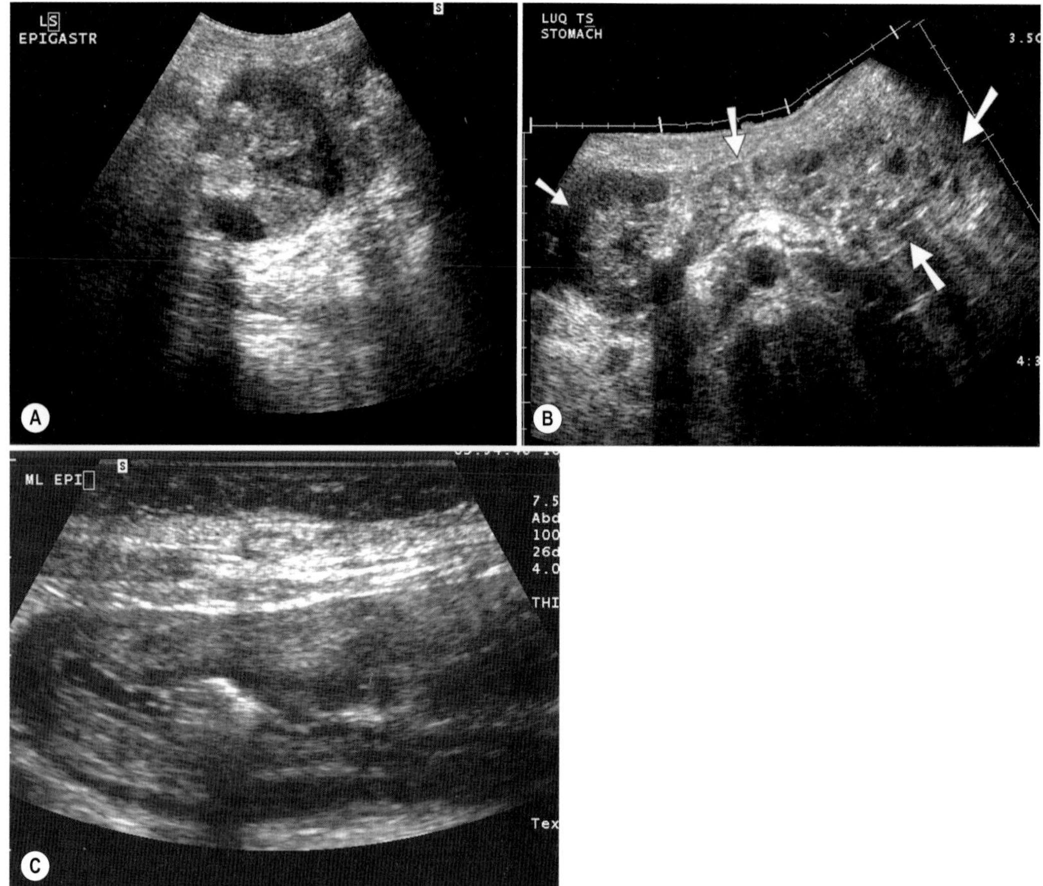

Fig. 8.10 • (A) LS through the epigastrium demonstrating a gastric carcinoma, with eccentric, grossly thickened stomach wall with fluid in the lumen. (B) TS through the epigastrium demonstrating a gastric carcinoma (arrows). (C) Gastric carcinoma, presenting with altered LFTs. The patient had multiple liver metastases.

Mesenteric ischaemia

Mesenteric ischaemia is a potentially lethal condition, associated with atherosclerosis of the mesenteric vessels, which can cause bowel necrosis and death if left untreated. It is a difficult diagnosis to make on clinical grounds because the symptoms are varied and non-specific – including acute abdominal pain following meals, diarrhoea and subsequent weight loss. Patients frequently undergo a number of comparatively invasive investigations before a diagnosis is reached, and this delay increases the mortality and morbidity of the condition.[24,25]

Treatment involves restoring the blood flow via angioplasty or surgery and, if necessary, resecting segments of necrosed bowel.

Atherosclerosis may be demonstrated in the SMA in a number of cases. Signs of occlusion or stenosis of the SMA may be identified with colour or power Doppler[26] as a filling defect within the lumen of the vessel. However, significant stenoses have been diagnosed with Doppler in a relatively high percentage (18%) of the asymptomatic, elderly population. The finding of a stenosis on ultrasound, therefore, is an indication for further imaging in symptomatic patients, rather than an absolute indicator of mesenteric ischaemia.[27]

In a normal patient, the response of the SMA to food can be demonstrated as an increase in EDF velocities (Fig. 8.11). Mesenteric compromise has also been associated with an abnormal post-prandial response; Doppler waveforms of the SMA have

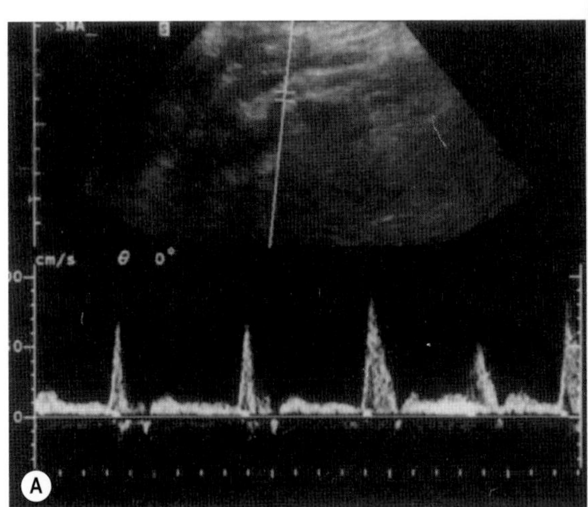

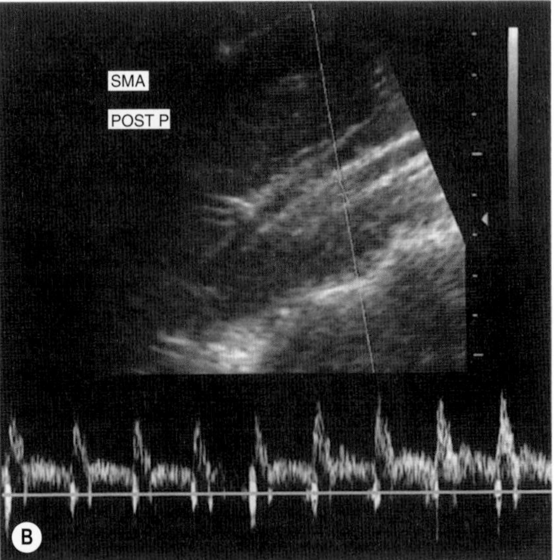

Fig. 8.11 • (A) Normal spectral waveform from the SMA in a fasting patient is highly pulsatile with little or no EDF and reverse flow in early diastole. (B) Post-prandially, the waveform becomes much less pulsatile, with low resistance and good end diastolic flow.

decreased peak systolic and EDF velocities after food.[28]

None of these ultrasound signs and appearances are specific for mesenteric ischaemia; the mesentery is supplied by three arteries, which cannot all be evaluated with ultrasound and, in addition, numerous other conditions are associated with altered SMA Doppler resistance, including inflammatory bowel conditions, haemorrhage, elevation of venous pressure and cirrhosis.

Inflammatory bowel conditions

Appendicitis

Acute appendicitis is a common diagnosis on admission to the casualty department with right lower abdominal pain. However, around 15–25% of patients who undergo laparotomy turn out to have normal appendices. The use of ultrasound in the investigation of acute abdominal pain is well-established and increases the reliability of the diagnosis of acute appendicitis when performed by an experienced operator.[29]

The normal appendix is located using a high frequency (10 MHz or more) linear or curved array probe, with gentle, graduated compression to move overlying bowel. Raising the patient's left side may encourage bowel gas to move away from the area of interest. The normal appendix is compressible by gentle transducer pressure.

The ultrasound features of acute appendicitis include an enlarged, usually hypoechoic, fluid-filled appendix greater than 6 mm in diameter. The inflamed appendix is non-compressible, and hyperechoic peri-appendiceal fat can be demonstrated (Fig. 8.12A). Attempted compression of the acutely inflamed appendix obviously requires great care from the operator. Compression must be very slow and the release of compression must be equally as gentle. These features have a high sensitivity and specificity for acute appendicitis (74% and 94%, respectively).[29] Acute appendicitis often demonstrates hypervascularity on power Doppler.

Perforation of the appendix may result in a demonstrable peri-appendiceal fluid collection, or free fluid plus or minus dilated loops of small bowel that is not undergoing peristalsis (Fig. 8.12B). The presence of an ill-defined fluid mass in the right iliac fossa of a symptomatic patient is highly suggestive of acute appendicitis with perforation. This may become infected, leading to peritonitis.

Occasionally, a hyper-reflective appendicolith may be seen in the blind end of the inflamed appendix, casting an acoustic shadow.

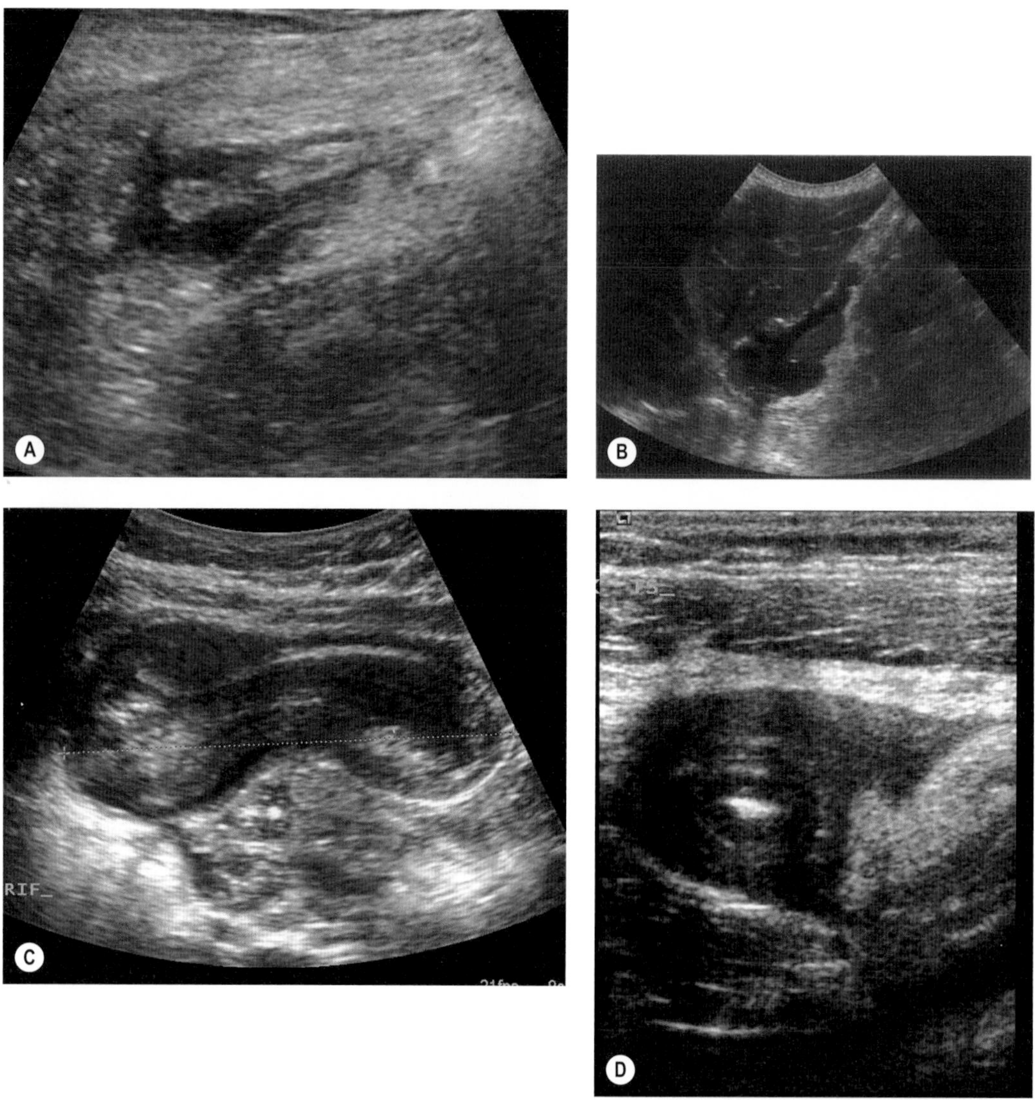

Fig. 8.12 • (A) Acute appendicitis with a thickened, tender oedematous wall. Hyperechoic peri-appendiceal fat is present. (B) Perforation of the inflamed appendix has resulted in the presence of intraperitoneal fluid under the liver. (C) Appendix mucocele, found to be perforated at surgery. (D) Appendicitis with an appendicolith demonstrated.

Inflammatory bowel disease (IBD)

Both barium studies and ultrasound have a useful role to play in the management of patients with IBD. Diagnosis is generally made with conventional barium X-ray studies, whilst ultrasound may be used to monitor disease and identify extraluminal complications of the disease.[30]

Crohn's disease

Is a common cause of inflammation affecting the small bowel and particularly the terminal ileum. It usually presents with pain, diarrhoea and weight loss. The terminal ileum/ileocaecal junction is involved in the majority of cases, and thickened, hypoechoic bowel wall can often be demonstrated in this area.[31] Initial ultrasound assessment may suggest the initial diagnosis and can be used to evaluate the bowel wall and identify other complications of Crohn's disease with sensitivity and specificity comparable to CT.[32] Ultrasound is also used to screen patients at risk, and monitor patients for recurrence of disease following surgery.[33]

Crohn's disease affects the entire thickness of the bowel wall, and one of the common complications is that of intramural abscesses. These can sometimes be seen within the thickened wall as gas-containing, highly echogenic areas. When large, they may perforate resulting in an ill-defined collection of pus, which may be drained percutaneously (Fig. 8.13). Fistulae are another complication of Crohn's and are easier to demonstrate with contrast radiography.

Ulcerative colitis (UC)

Affects the mucosa, rather than the whole wall. On ultrasound it produces a thickened, stratified hypoechoic wall, unlike Crohn's, in which the entire thickness of the wall is affected. A wall thickness greater than 3 mm is considered abnormal. Like Crohn's, small ulcer craters with the wall of the colon in ulcerative colitis may appear as hyperechoic gas-filled foci.

Diverticulitis

Diverticulitis may also be recognized on ultrasound as outpouchings from the bowel wall, most commonly affecting the sigmoid colon (Fig. 8.13C).[19] Acute diverticulitis usually demonstrates hypoechoic and thickened bowel wall, and ultrasound in experienced hands may rival CT in sensitivity and specificity in the diagnosis of acute diverticulitis.[34] Perforation of a diverticulum may give rise to a diverticular abscess, although the presence of air makes ultrasound limited in its evaluation of this condition, and CT is still the method of choice for the complications of diverticulitis.

Doppler in IBD

Inflammatory bowel diseases increase the perfusion of the intestine, decreasing vascular resistance. Hypervascularized bowel wall has been identified in both Crohn's and ulcerative colitis,[35] compared with normal subjects. Doppler of the SMA has revealed an increase in flow velocities (both peak systolic and end diastolic) and a decrease in RI in numerous types of pathological bowel, including Crohn's.[36] However the lack of specificity limits its use in clinical work. Changes in RI have been found to be related to the activity of Crohn's disease,[37] which could prove valuable in monitoring patients with known disease.

Malignant tumours

The most common site for a bowel tumour in the adult is around the caecum. It is useful to target this area in patients with altered bowel habit in whom bowel carcinoma is suspected, although detection with ultrasound is still more usually incidental than deliberate.

The mass tends to be hypoechoic, or of mixed echogenicity, with a small, eccentric, gas-filled lumen and a loss of or disruption of the wall layers. Vigorous Doppler flow can usually be visualized in malignant bowel masses, although it is also present in inflammatory masses (Fig. 8.14). Normal findings of bowel on ultrasound does not, of course, exclude bowel carcinoma.

The finding of a colonic mass would normally prompt a barium enema, to delineate the nature, extent and position of the mass, with subsequent staging by CT if malignancy is confirmed. The advantage of ultrasound over barium enema is that of displaying the tumour itself, rather than just the narrowed lumen.

The role of ultrasound in patients with known bowel carcinoma is to identify and document the presence of distant metastases, particularly in the liver, as metastases from colorectal carcinoma are particularly amenable to curative resection. Bowel tumours should be considered in the list of differential diagnoses when the origin of a mass discovered on ultrasound is unclear.

Endosonography may be used to detect and stage rectal cancers, although it is only able to demonstrate perirectal nodes and cannot evaluate distant disease. Endosonography is ideal however, in the follow-up of rectal cancer, and can detect early recurrence of disease.

Obstruction

Ultrasound has been found to be helpful in the investigation of acute obstruction. It can confirm

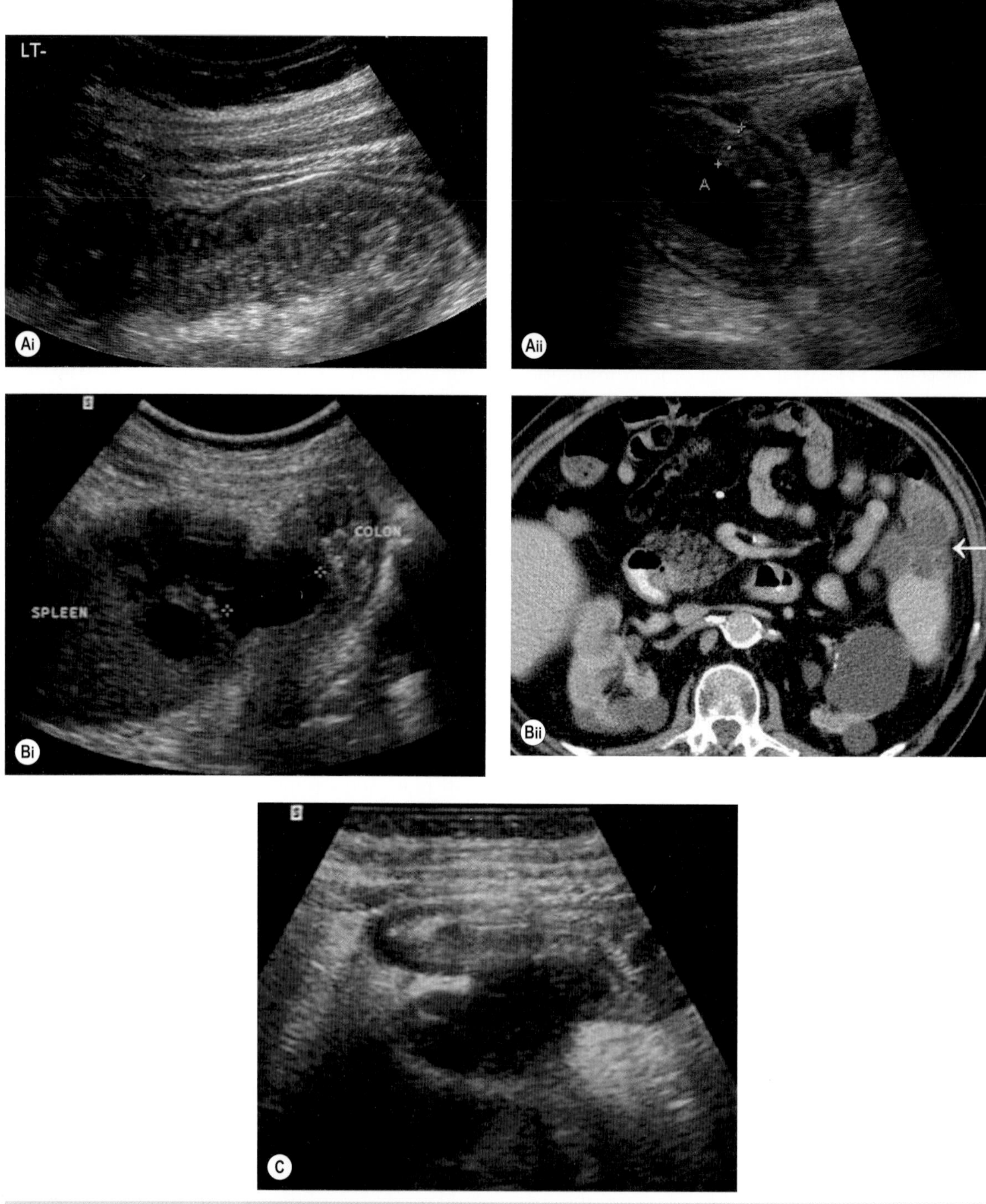

Fig. 8.13 • (Ai) Thickened, bowel wall in active Crohn's disease. (Aii) TS through a loop of thickened inflammatory bowel (9 mm). (Bi) A diverticular abscess arising in the left colon has invaded the spleen. (Bii) Appearances are confirmed at CT. (C) Diverticular abscess arising from the descending colon.

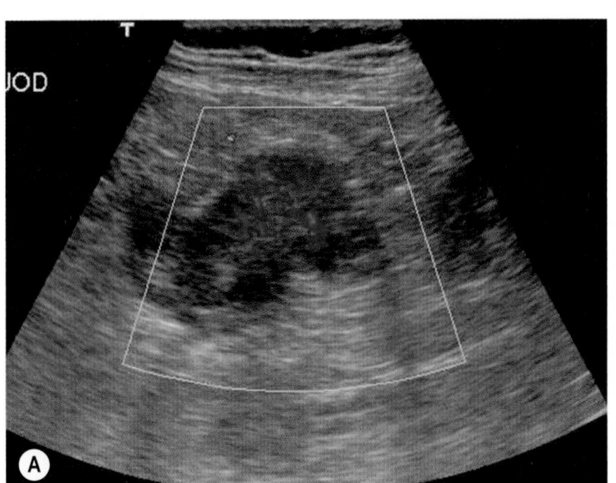

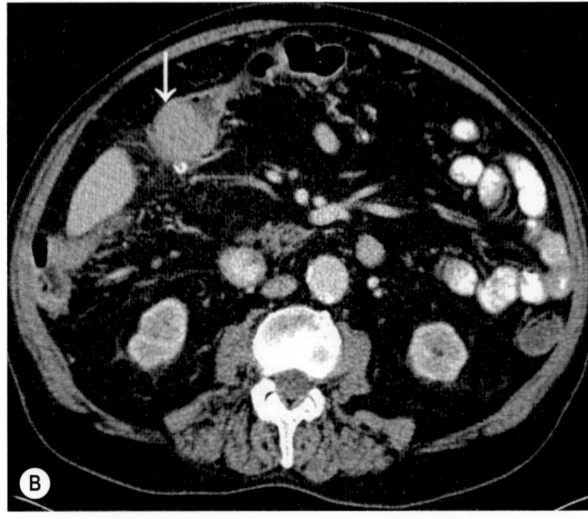

Fig. 8.14 • (A) A suspected bowel carcinoma found in a patient presenting with RUQ pain. (B) CT confirms the carcinoma in the transverse colon (arrow).

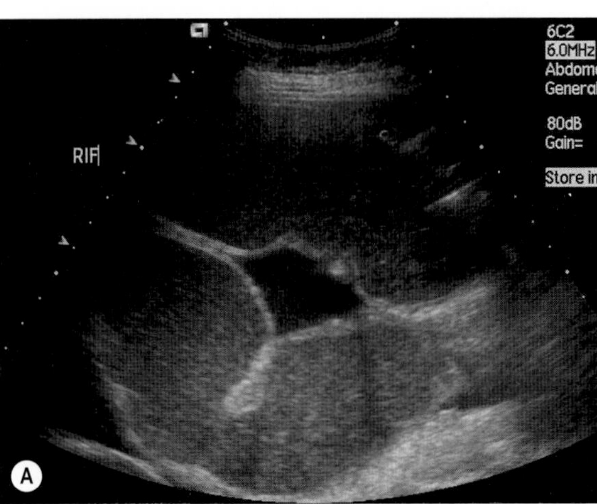

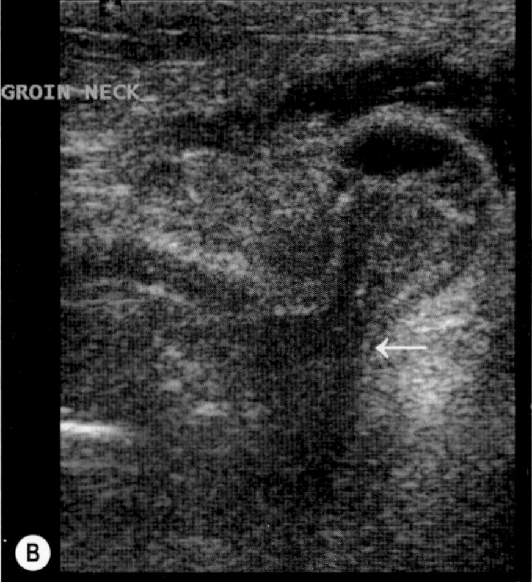

Fig. 8.15 • (A) Dilated, fluid-filled loops of bowel as a result of an obstructing caecal carcinoma. Ascites is also present. (B) A loop of bowel is demonstrated herniating through into the right groin. The neck of the hernia is indicated by the arrow.

obstruction by demonstrating dilated, fluid-filled bowel loops with ineffective peristalsis (Fig. 8.15). These fluid-filled loops of bowel are highly amenable to ultrasound scanning, which has the advantage of being able to directly visualize peristalsis, unlike a plain X-ray. It is possible to trace the dilated bowel to the site of obstruction, distal to which are normal loops of collapsed bowel.[38]

Ultrasound has a sensitivity of 89% in the diagnosis of small bowel obstruction[39] and 88% in establishing the level and cause of obstruction in the colon.[40] This potentially reduces radiation dose and is able to assist in the planning of surgery in such patients. However, identifying the actual site and cause of obstruction is time-consuming and frequently unsuccessful. Patients with suspected bowel obstruction, therefore, usually proceed straight to CT. Ultrasound is also useful in demonstrating herniation of bowel (Fig. 8.15B) especially in acute cases associated with obstruction.

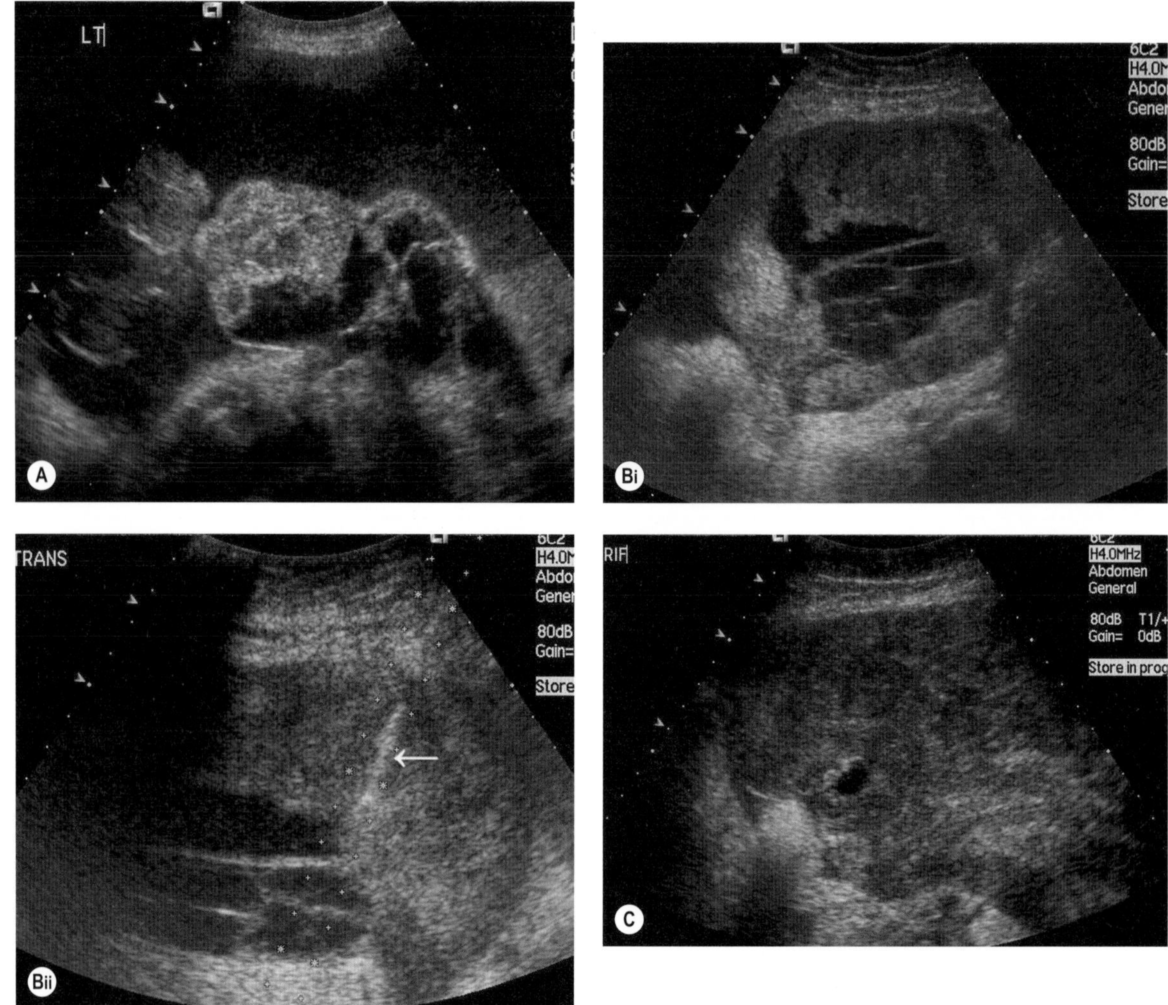

Fig. 8.16 • (A) Late-stage ovarian carcinoma demonstrates abdominal ascites with hyperechoic omental deposits. (Bi) Carcinoma of the peritoneum. An ultrasound-guided biopsy was performed prior to treatment; (Bii) the needle is seen (arrow) entering the solid peripheral area of the mass for histological diagnosis. (C) A large solid peritoneal tumour.

Other retroperitoneal abnormalities

Ultrasound is useful for identifying retroperitoneal masses, but CT and MRI are more effective in establishing the extent and nature of many of these masses, particularly those partly obscured by gas-filled bowel.

The majority of malignant retroperitoneal tumours are renal or adrenal in origin. Other primary tumours, apart from lymphomas, are rare, and include liposarcoma and leiomyosarcoma. These tend to be large when they present, and of variable/complex ultrasound appearance. Encasement of major vessels by tumour is a further characteristic of the retroperitoneal origin of the mass, together with anterior displacement of structures such as the pancreas, kidneys, aorta and IVC.

Ultrasound is also able to identify peritoneal and omental deposits in patients with late-stage carcinoma. These are particularly amenable to diagnosis when surrounded by ascites (Fig. 8.16) and usually arise from gynaecological or urological tumours. Other retroperitoneal masses identifiable on ultrasound include haematomas, psoas abscesses, lymphadenopathy (Fig. 8.17) and pancreatic pseudocysts.

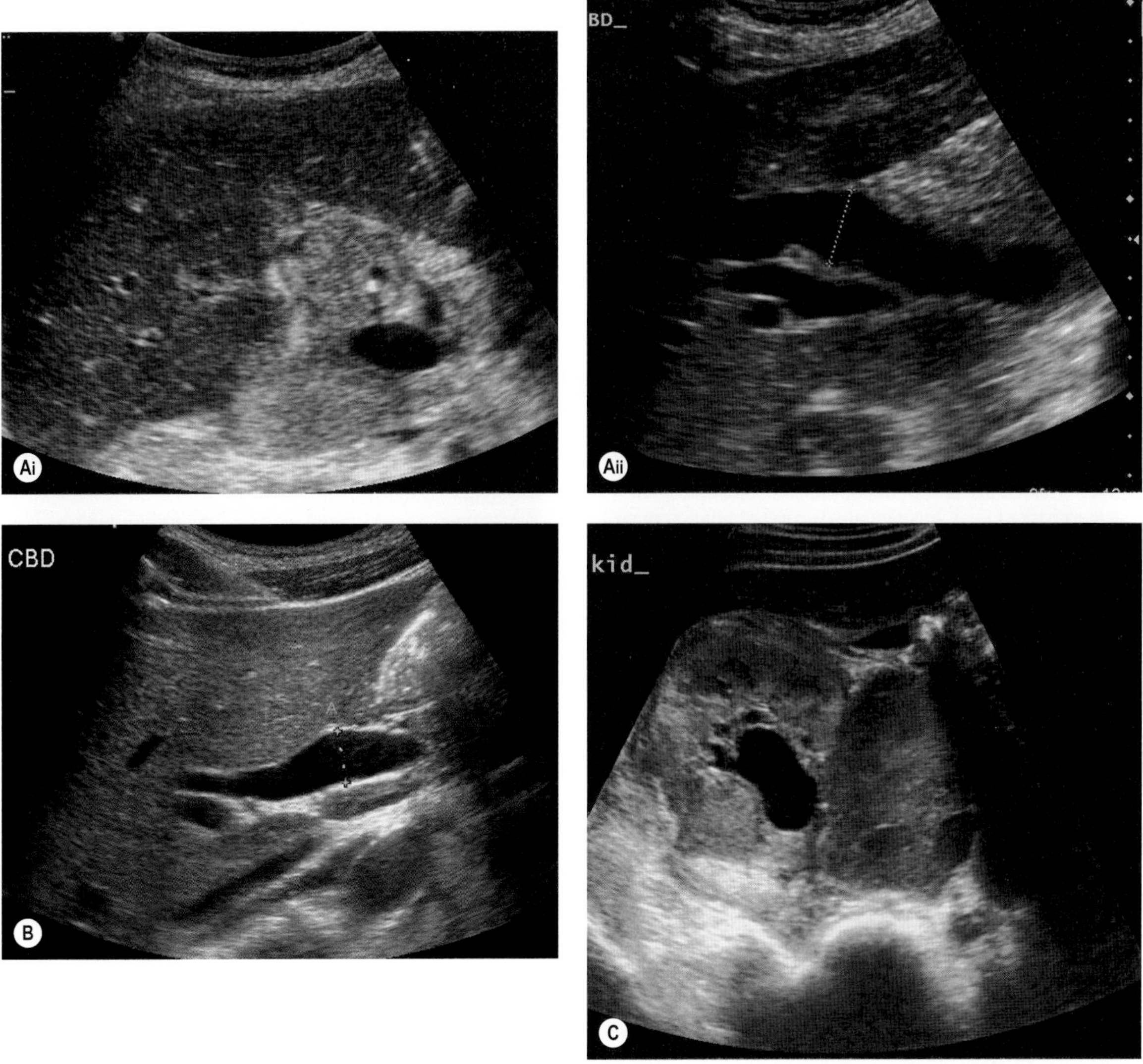

Fig. 8.17 • (Ai) A hyperechoic mass of enlarged lymph node around the porta hepatis is causing obstructive jaundice, with dilatation of the CBD (Aii). (B) Lymphadenopathy may be the cause of obstructive jaundice. Small lymph nodes are present around the porta, dilating the CBD (calipers). (C) Large retroperitoneal lymph node mass causing right renal obstruction.

References

1. Russel JGB. Is screening for abdominal aortic aneurysms worthwhile? Clin Radiol 1990; 41: 182–184
2. Cosford PA, Leng GC. Screening for abdominal aortic aneurysm. Cochrane Database Syst Rev 2007; 18: CD002945
3. Fleming C, Whitlock EP, Beil TL, Lederle FA. Screening for abdominal aortic aneurysm: a best-evidence systematic review for the U.S. Preventive Services Task Force. Ann Intern Med 2005; 142: 203–211
4. Ouriel K. The PIVOTAL study: a randomized comparison of endovascular repair versus surveillance in patients with smaller abdominal aortic aneurysms. J Vasc Surg 2009; 49: 266–269
5. Iezzi R, Basilico R, Giancristofaro D et al. Contrast-enhanced ultrasound versus color duplex ultrasound imaging in the follow-up of patients after endovascular abdominal aortic aneurysm repair. J Vasc Surg 2009; 49: 552–560
6. Clevert DA, Minaifar N, Weckbach S et al. Color duplex ultrasound and contrast-enhanced ultrasound in comparison to MS-CT in the detection of endoleak

following endovascular aneurysm repair. Clin Hemorheol Microcirc 2008; 39: 121–132

7. Mingoli A, Cavallaro A, Sapienza P et al. International registry of inferior Vena Cava leiomyosarcoma: analysis of a world series on 218 patients. Anticancer Res 1996; 16: 3201–3205
8. Singh-Panghaal S, Karcnik TJ, Wachsberg RH, Baker SR. Inferior vena caval leiomyosarcoma: diagnosis and biopsy with colour Doppler sonography. J Clin Ultrasound 1997; 25: 275–278
9. Marchal G, Gelin J, Verbeken E et al. High-resolution real-time sonography of the adrenal glands. J Ultrasound Med 1986; 5: 65–68
10. Bates JA, Irving HC. Adrenal sonography. Electro Medica 1989; 2: 70–75
11. Ilias I, Sahdev A, Reznek RH et al. The optimal imaging of adrenal tumours: a comparison of different methods. Endocr Relat Cancer 2007; 14: 587–599
12. Kasperlik-Zaluska AA, Rosslonowska E, Slowinska-Srzednicka J et al. Incidentally discovered adrenal mass (incidentaloma): investigation and management of 208 patients. Clin Endocrinol 1997; 46: 29–37
13. Fassnacht M, Kenn W, Allolio B. Adrenal tumors: how to establish malignancy? J Endocrinol Invest 2004; 27: 387–399
14. Friedrich-Rust M, Schneider G, Bohle RM et al. Contrast-enhanced sonography of adrenal masses: differentiation of adenomas and nonadenomatous lesions. AJR Am J Roentgenol 2008; 191: 1852–1860
15. Havekes B, Lai EW, Corssmit EP et al. Detection and treatment of pheochromocytomas and paragangliomas: current standing of MIBG scintigraphy and future role of PET imaging. Q J Nucl Med Mol Imaging 2008; 52: 419–429
16. Ng L, Libertino JM. Adrenocortical carcinoma: diagnosis, evaluation and treatment. J Urol 2003; 169: 5–11
17. Wood BJ, Abraham J, Hvizda JL et al. Radiofrequency ablation of adrenal tumours and adrenocortical carcinoma metastases. Cancer 2003; 1: 554–560
18. Kuzmich S, Howlett DC, Andi A et al. Transabdominal sonography in assessment of the bowel in adults. AJR Am J Roentgenol 2009; 192: 197–212
19. O'Malley M, Wilson S. Ultrasound of gastrointestinal tract abnormalities with CT correlation. Radiographics 2003; 23: 59–72
20. Tous F, Busto M. Assessment of abdominal sonography in the diagnosis of tumours of the gastroduodenal tract. J Clin Ultrasound 1997; 25: 243–247
21. Dye CE, Waxman I. Endoscopic ultrasound. Gastroenterol Clin North Am 2002; 31: 863–879
22. Yong AA, Roberts SA. Interventional endoscopic ultrasound. Clin Radiol 2003; 58: 32–43
23. Lennon AM, Penman ID. Endoscopic ultrasound in cancer staging. Br Med Bull 2007; 84: 81–98
24. Deehan DJ, Heys SD, Brittenden J, Eremin O. Mesenteric ischaemia: prognosic factors and influence of delay upon outcome. J R Coll Surg Edinb 1995; 40: 112–115
25. Hoogenburg K, Van-Essen LH, Van Den Dungen JJAM et al. Chronic mesenteric ischaemia: diagnostic challenges and treatment options. J Intern Med 1995; 237: 293–299
26. Danse EM, Van Beers BE, Goffette P et al. Acute intestinal ischaemia due to occlusion of the superior mesenteric artery: detection with Doppler sonography. J Ultrasound Med 1996; 15: 323–326
27. Roobottom CA, Dubbins PA. Significant disease of the celiac and superior mesenteric arteries in asymptomatic patients: predictive value of Doppler sonography. AJR Am J Roentgenol 1993; 161: 985–988
28. Nichols S, Windeler H. Duplex scanning in diagnosis of mesenteric insuficiency. J Diagn Med Sonog 1995; 11: 120–127
29. Zeidan BS, Wasser T, Nicholas GG. Ultrasonography in the diagnosis of acute appendicitis. J R Coll Surg Edinb 1997; 42: 24–26
30. Carucci LR, Levine MS. Radiographic imaging of inflammatory bowel disease. Gastroenterol Clinics North Am 2002; 31: 93–117
31. McLoughlin RF, Downey DR, Rizkalla KS. Sonography of intestinal abnormality in the right iliac fossa. AJR Am J Roentgenol 1996; 167: 1473–1476
32. Horsthius K, Bipat S, Bennink RJ, Stoker J. Inflammatory bowel disease diagnosed with US, MR, scintigraphy and CT: meta-analysis of prospective studies. Radiology 2008; 247: 64–79
33. Andreoli A, Cerro P, Flasco G. Role of ultrasonography in the diagnosis of postsurgical recurrence of Crohn's disease. Am J Gastroenterol 1998; 93: 1117–1121
34. Ripolles T, Agramunt M, Martinez MJ et al. The role of ultrasound in the diagnosis, management and evolutive prognosis of acute left-sided colonic diverticulitis; a review of 208 patients. Eur Radiol 2003; 13: 2587–2595
35. Heyne R, Rickes S, Bock P et al. Non-invasive evaluation of activity in inflammatory bowel disease by Doppler sonography. Zeitschrife fur Gastroenterologie 2002; 40: 171–175
36. Erden A, Cumhur T, Olcer T. Superior mesenteric artery Doppler waveform changes in response to inflammation of the ileocecal region. Abdom Imaging 1997; 22: 483–486
37. Van Oostayen JA, Wasser MNJM, Van Hogezand RA et al. Doppler sonography evaluation of superior mesenteric artery flow to assess Crohn's disease activity: correlation with clinical evaluation, Crohn's disease activity index and alpha-1-antitrypsin clearance in feces. AJR Am J Roentgenol 1997; 168: 429–433
38. Ogata M, Mateer JR, Condon RE. Prospective evaluation of abdominal sonography for the diagnosis of bowel obstruction. Ann Surg 1996; 223: 237–241
39. Schmutz GR, Benko A, Fournier L. Small bowel obstruction: role and contribution of sonography. Eur Radiol 1997; 7: 1054–1058
40. Lim JH, Ko YT, Dee DH et al. Determining the site and causes of colonic obstruction with sonography. AJR Am J Roentgenol 1994; 163: 1113–1117

Ultrasound of the paediatric abdomen

9

Co-written with Terry M. Humphrey

CHAPTER CONTENTS

INTRODUCTION

Ultrasound of the paediatric abdomen requires different techniques and skills from those used in the adult. Although there are a few situations in which knowledge of adult pathology can be applied to the paediatric patient, the child cannot simply be considered a mini version of an adult. The presenting symptoms and pathological processes in the child are generally quite different from those in adults and the operator must be fully aware of the special considerations of the paediatric patient in terms of both diagnosis and technique. This chapter addresses only the most common paediatric situations likely to be encountered in a general department, and further specialist paediatric reading is recommended at the end of the chapter.

Techniques

The operator can minimize any distress to the child, and make the examination considerably easier and quicker, in numerous ways.

(a) The ultrasound environment should be as friendly as possible, with appropriate decorations and toys, and should always be kept warm, (nothing is more likely to make your patient uncooperative than cold gel). Minimize the time the child spends in the scanning room by having everything ready first.

(b) Most children find it reassuring to be accompanied by their carer during the examination.

(c) Separate facilities, such as a dedicated children's waiting area are preferable and more reassuring for the child.

(d) The equipment should incorporate a range of high frequency (5–15 MHz) transducers with small as well as conventional footprints. A small curvilinear transducer is useful for most abdominal work and a high frequency linear probe is essential for bowel sonography and assessment of the acute abdomen. Transducers with a dynamic frequency facility are an excellent choice, as it is easy to switch to the highest possible frequency without having to change the transducer. The use of more than one transducer, i.e. both curvilinear and linear, may be necessary particularly in the assessment of the acute abdomen.

(e) A cine facility on the ultrasound machine is invaluable, and cuts down scanning time. Colour Doppler is essential in the assessment of hepato-biliary problems and the examination of the acute abdomen.

(f) Generally speaking it is necessary to employ a fast frame rate. (The smaller field of view needed for children allows the line density to remain high, maintaining adequate resolution.)

HEPATO-BILIARY PATHOLOGY

Cystic fibrosis

Cystic fibrosis is a common, autosomal recessive multisystem disease. The main organs affected are the lungs, liver and pancreas. Accumulation of mucus in the bronchi rapidly leads to respiratory problems including infections, with a predisposition to abscess formation with destruction of the terminal bronchioles developing into bronchiectasis.

Pancreatic insufficiency, requiring enzyme supplements, is a feature of cystic fibrosis, with gradual fatty replacement and subsequent fibrosis of pancreatic tissue, resulting in increased echogenicity of the pancreatic parenchyma. The pancreas is generally reduced in size. Cysts, calcification and ductal dilatation may also be found.[1] Advances in the management of pulmonary problems associated with cystic fibrosis have led to longer survival and a subsequent increase in the prevalence of chronic liver disease. Annual ultrasound examination is recommended as sonographic changes may be identified in the absence of abnormality on biochemical assessment.[2] The liver may be hyperechoic and the texture becomes coarse and nodular as fibrosis develops (Fig. 9.1). Increased periportal echogenicity may be demonstrated. Eventually cirrhosis develops, causing portal hypertension. Assessment of the portal venous system with colour and spectral Doppler is useful, providing a baseline with which to compare progression of the disease.

The gallbladder is small in up to one third of patients[1,3] (Fig. 9.1D). This microgallbladder meas-

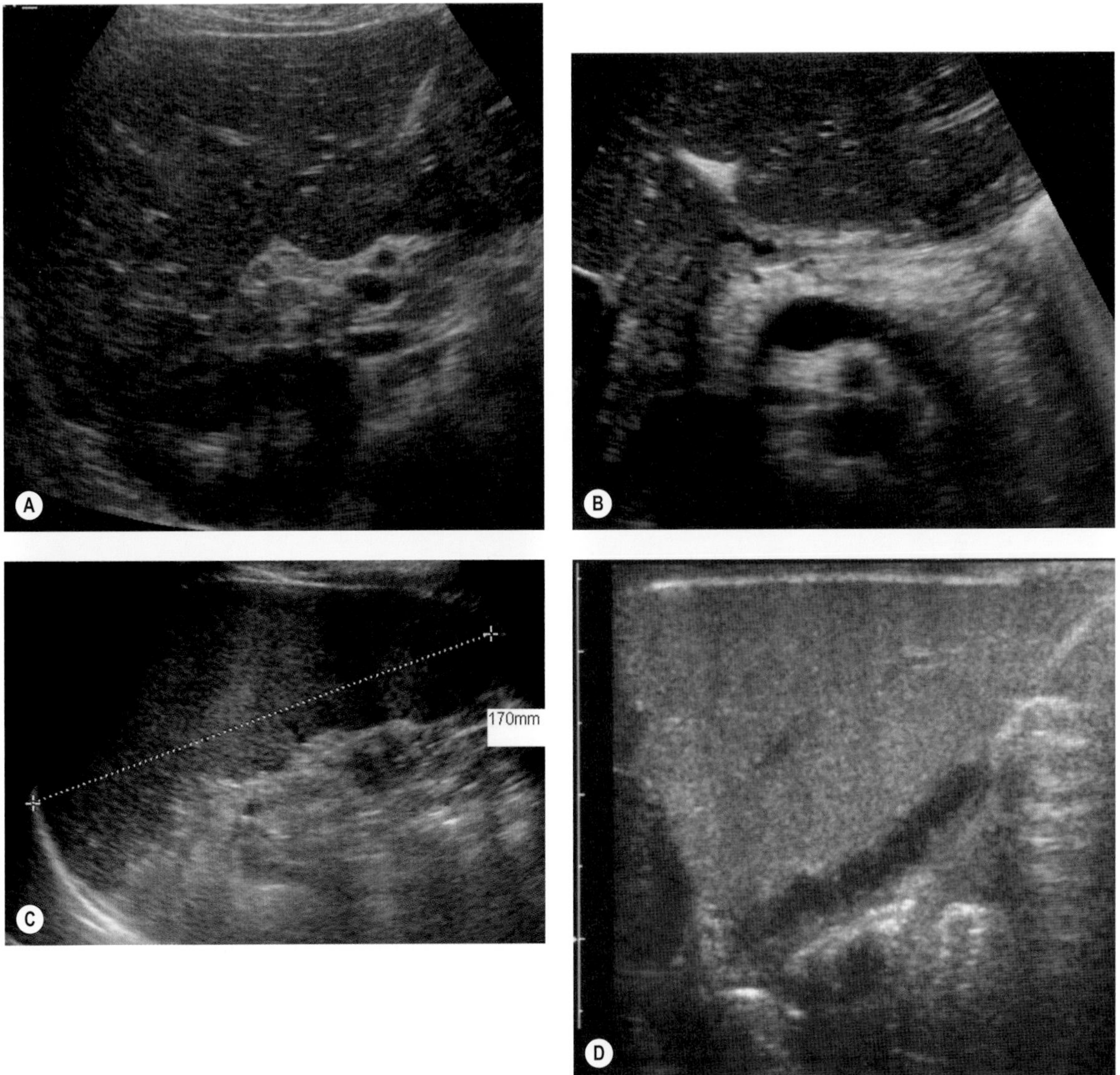

Fig. 9.1 • Cystic fibrosis (CF). (A) Coarse nodular liver. (B) Hyperechoic, coarse pancreas, typical of CF. (C) Enlarged spleen caused by portal hypertension in CF. (D) Microgallbladder. The gallbladder is thick walled and small, despite fasting.

ures less than 3 × 1 × 1 cm after fasting and is filled with mucus. Up to 10% of patients with cystic fibrosis may have gallstones; cholecystitis and biliary strictures may occur.

Neonatal cholestasis and biliary atresia

Babies who have persistent jaundice beyond 2 weeks of age and any neonate with conjugated jaundice should be investigated to exclude biliary atresia.[4] Biliary atresia and neonatal hepatitis are the most common causes of neonatal cholestasis, typically presenting at 1–2 months of age with jaundice, dark urine and pale stools. Early diagnosis of biliary atresia and differentiation from hepatitis and other causes of neonatal cholestasis are crucial to successful treatment. The aetiology of biliary atresia remains unclear but progressive inflammation, destruction and fibrosis of the biliary tree occurs resulting in obliteration of all or part of the bile ducts and gallbladder with the subsequent development biliary cirrhosis.[5]

The presence or absence of a gallbladder is not a reliable sign of biliary atresia, though detailed ultrasound examination in expert hands has revealed that there are ultrasound features that can help make the diagnosis (Fig. 9.2).[6] These include an abnormal gallbladder which may have an irregular wall, abnormal shape or be small. An area of increased echogenicity may be seen anterior to the bifurcation of the portal vein. This is known as the triangular cord sign and represents the fibrotic remnant of the extrahepatic biliary tree. There may be absence of the common bile duct and the intra and extrahepatic biliary tree is not dilated although a cyst is sometimes seen at the porta hepatis. The developing cirrhosis leads rapidly to portal hypertension so there may be hepatosplenomegaly. The

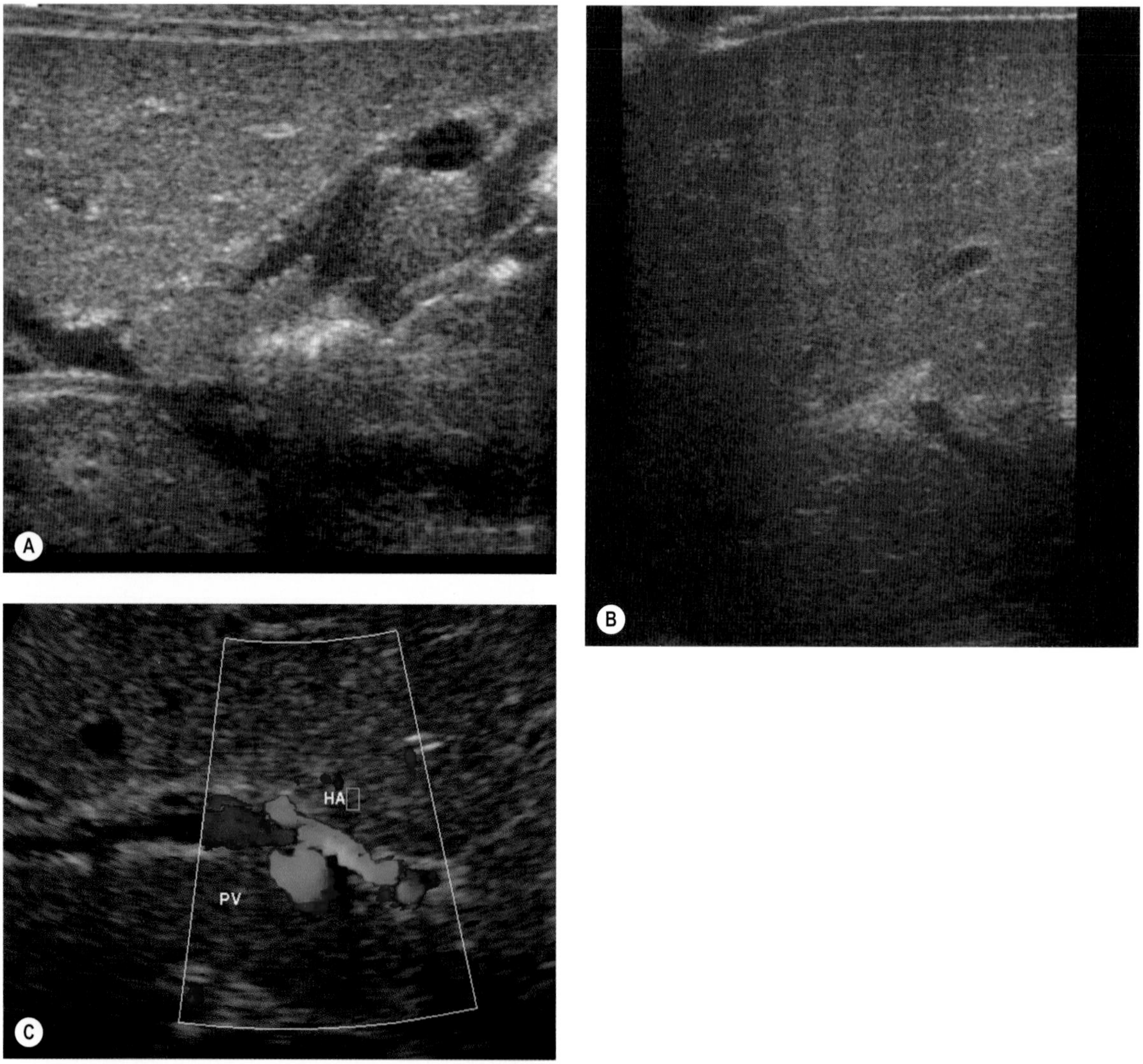

Fig. 9.2 • Biliary atresia (BA). (A) Abnormal irregular walled gallbladder in BA. (B) Triangular cord sign, increased echogenicity seen anterior to the bifurcation of the portal vein in a 5-week-old infant with BA. (C) Hypertrophy of the hepatic artery in BA.

hepatic artery can become hypertrophied and appear dominant.

Approximately 10–20% of infants with biliary atresia have associated congenital abnormalities including situs inversus, polysplenia, preduodenal portal vein and interruption of the IVC with azygous continuation, all of which may be detected on sonography. Sonography can also exclude other less frequent causes of neonatal cholestasis such as a congenital choledochal cyst and obstruction to the common bile duct due to bile inspissation where biliary tract dilatation will be noted. The diameter of the normal CBD should not be greater than 2 mm in the infant up to 1-year-old (or 4 mm in children up to 10 years of age).[7]

Liver biopsy and radioisotope studies are also used to try to differentiate biliary atresia from neonatal hepatitis. Excretion of radionuclide from the liver into the duodenum excludes biliary atresia although a lack of excretion into the duodenum may be seen in both atresia and severe neonatal hepatitis. In some centres MR cholangiography and/or ERCP are used to investigate neonatal jaundice, however, the small duct size and motion sensitivity related to rapid respiratory and heart rate make these investigations challenging.[8] In cases where biliary atresia has not been excluded, laparotomy with intraoperative cholangiogram will be necessary to reach a final diagnosis.

Biliary atresia is usually treatable by early surgery, provided the diagnosis is made before the age of eight weeks at which time irreversible biliary cirrhosis may have developed. Liver transplant may eventually be required, particularly in those presenting late with established biliary cirrhosis.

Choledochal cyst

Choledochal cysts are congenital dilations of the biliary tree that may present at any age, and can be diagnosed in the fetus during routine obstetric scanning. In the neonate the main presenting feature will be cholestatic jaundice but the classical triad of pain, jaundice and a palpable mass is more likely to be seen in the young adult. Choledochal cysts can be classified into five anatomical types as described by Todani et al.[9] The most common form is type 1 which occurs in up to 90% of cases and consists of varying degrees of CBD dilatation over a variable length. In many cases there is an anomalous insertion of the bile duct into the pancreatic duct of Wirsung.

On sonography a well-defined cyst will be identified close to the porta hepatis in continuity with the biliary tree (Fig. 9.3). There may be dilatation of the proximal bile ducts and sludge or calculi may be seen within the cyst. Small choledochal cysts may be seen in association with biliary atresia

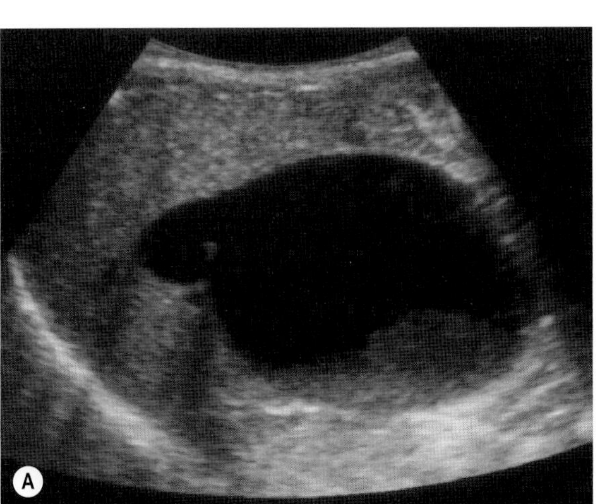

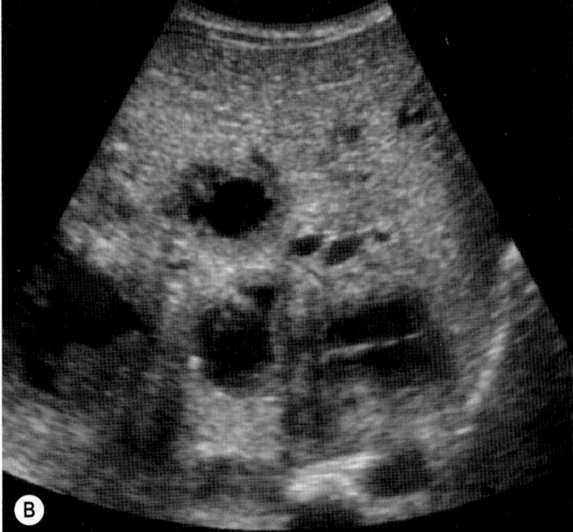

Fig. 9.3 • (A) Large choledochal cyst containing debris seen at the porta hepatis. (B) Liver abscesses seen in a 10-year-old girl with a choledochal cyst.

but in these cases there will be no associated biliary tract dilatation. Further complications of choledochal cysts include: cholangitis, pancreatitis, liver abscess (Fig. 9.3B) and cyst rupture. Definitive diagnosis is made by MR cholangiography although scintigraphy and ERCP may be useful in difficult cases.[10]

Other causes of cholestasis in children and neonates include bile duct stones (more common in girls), sclerosing cholangitis, cystic fibrosis, infections and Alagille's syndrome (a congenital paucity of the bile ducts). Acute cholestasis may also be caused by viral hepatitis, drugs, toxins, metabolic diseases or hypoxaemia.

Hepatoblastoma and hepatocellular carcinoma

Primary, malignant tumours of the liver are comparatively rare in children and frequently present as a large abdominal mass. Large hepatic tumours may present acutely as a result of haemorrhage. Hepatoblastoma is the commonest primary liver malignancy in childhood, generally occurring in children under 3 years of age and may be associated with predisposing conditions such as Beckwith–Wiedemann syndrome and children infected with HIV (Fig. 9.4).[11] Metastatic spread is most frequent to the lungs, brain and local lymph nodes. HCC is more usually associated with chronic liver disease and tends to develop during the later stage of disease with peak incidences of 4–5 years and 12–14 years. Both tumours are associated with increased levels of serum alpha-fetoprotein.

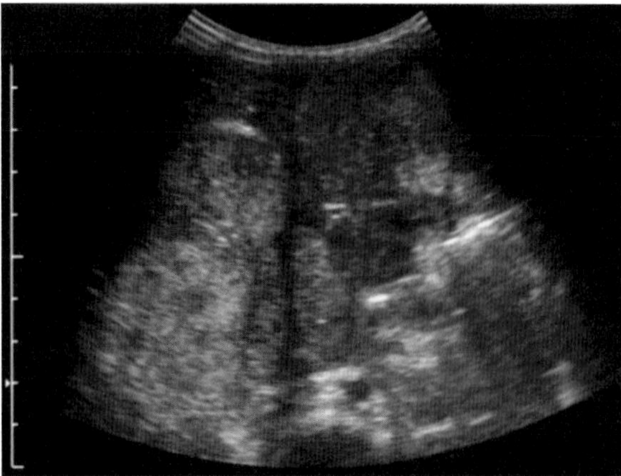

Fig. 9.4 • Large complex mass occupying most of the right lobe of the liver is a hepatoblastoma in this 2-year-old girl.

On ultrasound, these tumours appear solid, heterogeneous and are often large and poorly demarcated from the adjacent liver parenchyma. Areas of necrosis or haemorrhage may be identified in the mass. Occasionally they may be multifocal. Although the two types of tumour are not distinguishable on ultrasound, the clinical history may give a clue and ultrasound guided biopsy can be used to obtain a histological diagnosis. Ultrasound is useful in identifying the extent of the tumour, and when combined with colour flow Doppler imaging, adjacent vascular invasion can be evaluated. CT or MRI complement the ultrasound findings and are essential for staging and assessment of suitability for resection or transplantation.[12] Chemotherapy may be used to shrink the tumour prior to surgery.

Rhabdomyosarcoma is a rare tumour which may originate in the biliary ducts. Children present with painless obstructive jaundice and solid material within dilated intra- and extrahepatic bile ducts can be seen on ultrasound. Rhabdomyosarcoma originates from muscle cells and is the commonest type of soft tissue sarcoma seen in childhood, with a peak incidence before 5 years of age. It occurs in various sites throughout the body.

Other causes of focal liver lesions

Liver metastases may occur from most paediatric malignancies particularly, neuroblastoma, rhabdomyosarcoma and Wilms' tumour (Fig. 9.13C). Leukaemia and lymphoma may also cause focal defects in the liver. Liver involvement may be manifested by hepatomegaly with normal liver texture, a non-specific sign, or by diffuse coarsened liver texture with or without hepatomegaly.

Haemangioendothelioma and haemangiomas

Vascular tumours account for most benign liver tumours in childhood. Haemangioendotheliomas and haemangiomas are benign tumours whose clinical course, prognosis and treatment are similar. The radiological appearances of these lesions overlap and although there is a histological distinction between them, hepatic tissue is not commonly obtained and either term may be used in clinical practice.[13] Infants may be asymptomatic but generally present before the age of 6 months with an abdominal mass, respiratory distress, anaemia and cardiac failure, caused by the shunting of blood from the aorta through the tumour. In rare cases large tumours may bleed spontaneously, resulting in haemoperitoneum. They may present with jaundice and increased transaminase levels and 50% of children also have cutaneous haemangiomas.[14]

These tumours can be solitary or multiple, of varying echogenicity and may have a complex echotexture due to thrombus, calcifications and internal septations (Fig. 9.5). The vascular nature of these lesions is demonstrated by a large coeliac

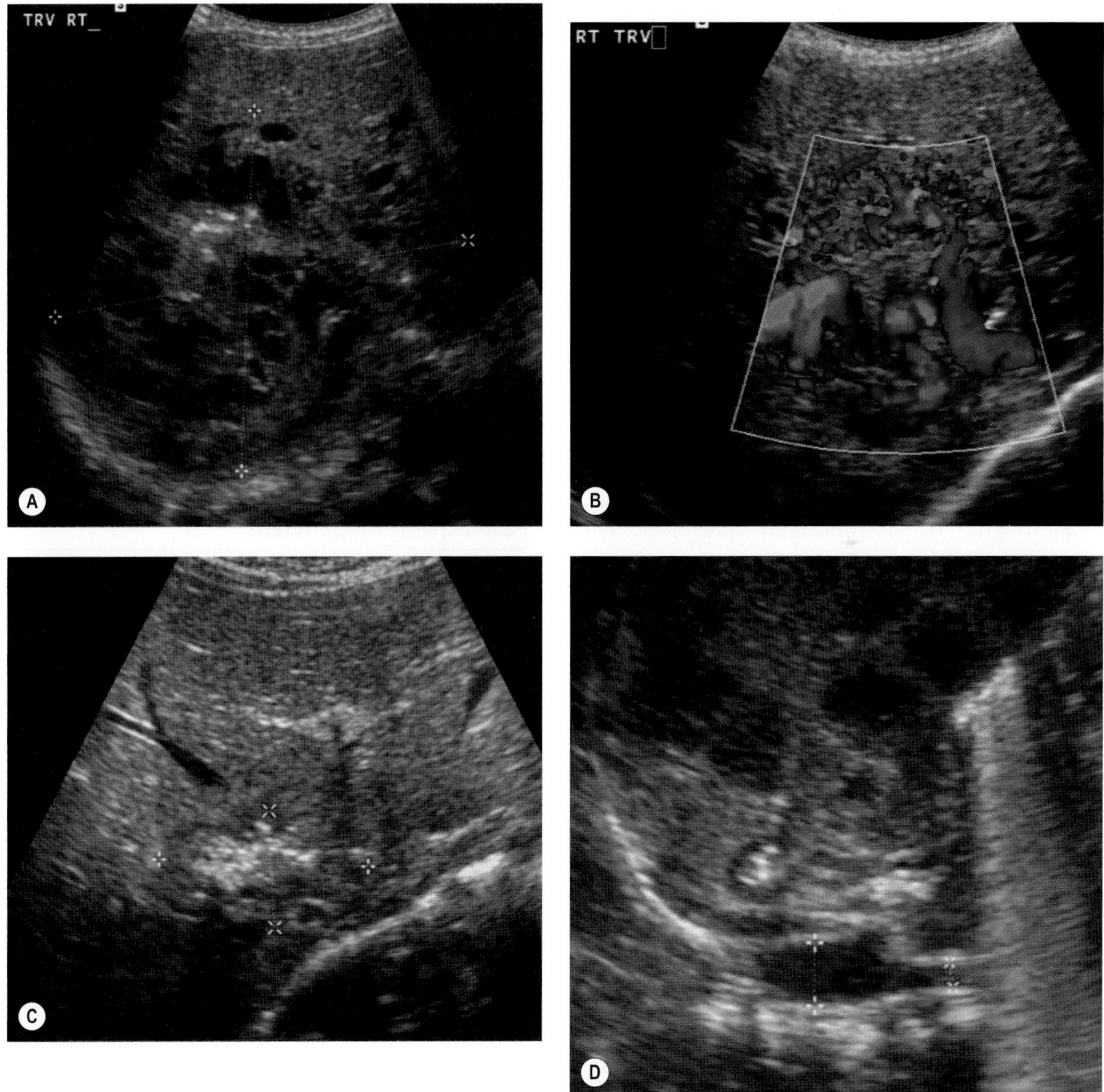

Fig. 9.5 • (A) Large solitary haemangioendothelioma in a 4-week-old girl. (B) Colour Doppler image demonstrates the highly vascular nature of these lesions. (C) After 6 months of steroid treatment, the haemangioendothelioma has shrunk and contains calcification. (D) Aortic tapering is seen due to massive shunting of blood to multiple haemangiomas in the liver of an 8-week-old girl.

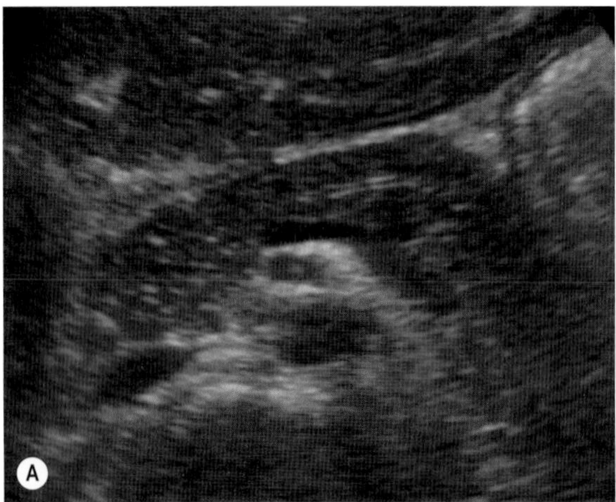

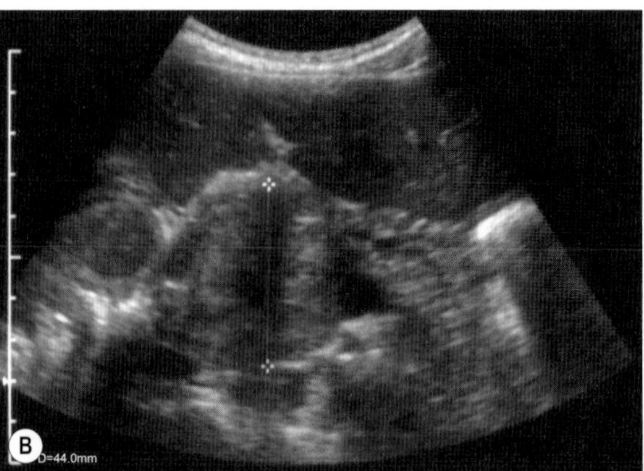

Fig. 9.6 • (A) Normal pancreas in a 5-year-old boy – relatively hypoechoic and bulky in comparison with the adult gland. (B) A complex mass in the head of the pancreas and a dilated pancreatic duct in a 7-year-old boy. Ultrasound-guided biopsy revealed a complex malignant vascular tumour and he underwent a Whipple's procedure.

axis and marked decrease in the size of the aorta below the origin of the coeliac axis (Fig. 9.5D). The main differential diagnosis of multiple haemangioendotheliomas is from metastatic liver disease particularly from disseminated neuroblastoma.

Although most asymptomatic paediatric haemangioendotheliomas regress spontaneously, those complicated by cardiac failure require active treatment. Steroids may be administered and serial ultrasound scans may be used to monitor the gradual resolution of the lesion. Angiographic embolization of the major feeding vessels may be necessary in severe cases that fail to respond to steroid therapy.

PANCREAS

Normal appearances

The acoustic characteristics of the pancreas vary with age. Pancreatic echogenicity is quite variable and is occasionally hypoechoic in neonates compared with the adult gland. In older children echogenicity is equal to or slightly greater than that of the liver. The pancreas is relatively larger in young children than in adults gradually increasing with age, reaching adult size in late teens.[15] The pancreatic duct should not be greater than 2 mm in diameter. The relative hypoechogenicity and relatively larger size of the normal pancreas in childhood should not be misinterpreted as a sign of probable pancreatitis when scanning a child with abdominal pain (Fig. 9.6A).

Pathology of the pancreas

Pancreatic abnormalities are relatively uncommon in childhood. Most ultrasound abnormalities are the result of infiltrative processes associated with other syndromes or diseases (Table 9.1). Focal pancreatic lesions are rare but as with adult practice, the presence of biliary and pancreatic duct dilatation should be treated with suspicion (Fig. 9.6B).

Ultrasound is an ideal investigation for evaluating the paediatric pancreas, as a high frequency probe demonstrates excellent detail. A water-based drink may be given to provide an acoustic window. In cases of blunt injury to the abdomen with suspected pancreatic damage, CT is the imaging modality of choice in the acute situation although sonography should be used during follow-up to detect the presence of a pseudocyst.

URINARY TRACT

Ultrasound is the first line of investigation in both antenatally detected abnormalities and in symptomatic children.

INCREASED ECHOGENICITY	
Cystic fibrosis	Fatty replacement of the pancreas, calcifications, ectatic pancreatic duct, coarse texture, cysts
Pancreatitis	Hereditary Trauma (physical abuse, road traffic accident) Congenital anomaly, e.g. choledochal cyst Drug toxicity Viral and parasitic infection
Haemochromatosis	Pancreatic fibrosis, iron deposition in liver and pancreas
FOCAL LESIONS	
Cysts	Isolated congenital cyst Autosomal dominant polycystic disease Von Hippel–Lindau disease Meckel–Gruber syndrome
Solid lesions	Primary pancreatic neoplasms are very rare in children

Table 9.1 Paediatric pancreatic abnormalities

(a) The bladder should be scanned first, as voiding may often occur during the examination.
(b) Measurements of both kidneys – either length or renal volume – should be taken to highlight any difference in size and to provide a baseline for further growth comparison.
(c) A variety of planes can be used to view the kidneys in children – often a posterior approach is best for obtaining an accurate bipolar length.
(d) Ensure that renal pelvic dilatation is not physiological, by rescanning post-micturition.
(e) Measure the AP diameter of any renal pelvic dilatation in transverse section through the renal hilum.
(f) Always scan the bladder immediately after micturition, paying attention to the ureteric orifices and looking for any ureteric or renal dilatation which may suggest reflux. Measure any residual volume.
(g) Colour Doppler may be helpful in identifying the ureteric orifices, by locating the jets of urine entering the bladder.

Normal appearances

After birth the renal cortex is relatively hyperechoic compared to the adult kidney, in strong contrast to the hypoechoic medullary pyramids. The outline of the kidney is often lobulated due to persistent fetal lobulation. The renal pelvis is relatively hypoechoic, as the fat deposition seen in the adult is not yet present (Fig. 9.7A).

Gradually the cortex becomes less hyperechoic with age, the corticomedullary differentiation lessens and fat deposition in the renal sinus becomes more evident. The outline becomes smooth, although fetal lobulations do persist in some adult kidneys.

Normal postnatal growth of the kidneys, in terms of length and volume, is closely related to the height, weight and age of the child. Charts giving normal age and weight related values should routinely be referred to.[16] Errors do occur in measurements of renal length with a potential error in the order of one year's growth.[17] Thus follow-up measurements for renal growth should not be undertaken at intervals of less than 1 year.

Anatomical variants and pathology

The duplex system

The duplex system is one of the more common congenital anomalies, occurring in up to 9% of referrals.[18] It stems from aberrant budding of the Wolffian duct in utero, and can take a variety of forms, from complete duplication with two kidneys, each with a separate ureter, to a partial duplication involving the kidney only. Complete duplication predisposes to reflux, particularly into the lower moiety and subsequently to infection.

The upper pole moiety of a duplex kidney is more prone to obstruction either secondary to a

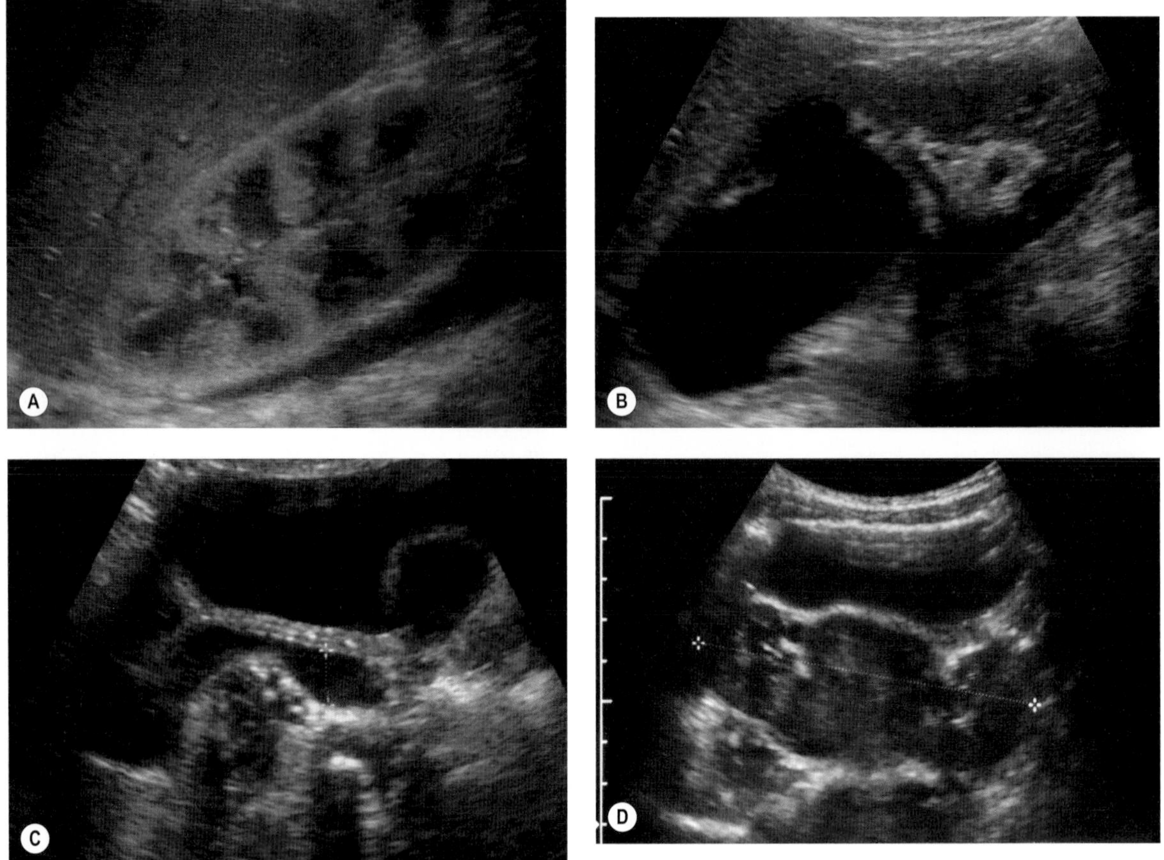

Fig. 9.7 • (A) Normal neonatal kidney, showing hyperechoic cortex, increased corticomedullary differentiation and reduced renal sinus echoes. (B) Duplex kidney. The upper moiety is dilated with a thin cortex, the lower moiety is normal. (C) Dilated ureter (calipers) of the upper moiety of a duplex kidney terminating in a ureterocele seen in the base of the bladder. (D) Renal fusion forming a 'cake' shaped solitary kidney in the pelvis.

ureterocele or less commonly with an obstructed ectopic ureter. In the former case the obstructed upper moiety may be associated with a dilated ureter which can be followed to the bladder where a ureterocele, i.e. a cystic dilatation of the distal ureter, may be seen within the bladder at the ipsilateral vesico ureteric junction (Fig. 9.7B, C). The ureterocele may extend into the urethra causing bladder outlet obstruction which if severe may result in bilateral hydronephrosis.

In the absence of any dilatation, it may be difficult to demonstrate the duplex kidney on ultrasound. Generally, the kidney is longer than normal and two discrete hyperechoic sinus echoes can be seen. Ectopic insertion of the upper pole ureter in a duplex system is a cause of urinary incontinence in girls. It may not be possible to follow an ectopic ureter to its distal end, even when dilated, but one may be able to demonstrate that the ureter is passing distally to the bladder. When there is a strong clinical suspicion of an ectopic ureter an IVU or MR urogram will be required to identify a duplex kidney and site of ureteric insertion.

Renal fusion and ectopia

The horseshoe kidney is the most common form of renal fusion, in which the lower poles of the kidneys are fused with a central isthmus or 'bridge' across the front of the spine. The isthmus frequently lies behind gas-filled bowel and can be difficult to detect. The sonographer should be suspicious of a horseshoe kidney when the lower poles of the kidneys cannot be clearly outlined particularly when both kidneys look a little smaller than expected for age. Always ensure you see the outline of the lower poles clearly by turning the child prone or by scanning coronally through the side if necessary.

A DMSA scan may demonstrate the isthmus or bridge of renal tissue (when the ultrasound scan is equivocal) but only if it is functioning. In some cases the bridge is composed of non-functioning, fibrous tissue. Fusion can take other forms, including an 'L' shape, where one kidney lies horizontally across the midline; crossed fused ectopia where both kidneys lie on the same side; 'H' shaped fusion of the hilar regions; and complete fusion to form a 'cake' shaped solitary kidney (Fig. 9.7D).

Ectopic kidneys occur most frequently in the pelvis. In rare cases the kidney may be situated in the thorax. Ectopic and horseshoe kidneys are often associated with a degree of malrotation of the kidney. This can be associated with a degree of obstruction at the pelviureteric junction, and predisposes to the development of renal calculi.

Renal agenesis

The kidneys form from the ureteric bud, which arises from the pelvic area during the fifth to sixth week of gestation. The bud undergoes numerous divisions, forming the ureters, renal pelvis, calyces and renal tubules. Any interruption of this process may cause renal agenesis or ectopia.

Bilateral renal agenesis is lethal and is usually diagnosed prenatally. The incidence of unilateral renal agenesis is about 1:450 live births and is usually prenatally detected. Ultrasound is useful in confirming the prenatal diagnosis and excluding the presence of an ectopic kidney. A DMSA scan confirms the diagnosis. Renal agenesis is associated with VATER syndrome (Vertebral, Anal, Trachea, oEsophagus and Radius anomalies) and with ipsilateral gynaecological anomalies in girls.

Multicystic dysplastic kidney

The MCDK is generally the result of complete, early ureteric obstruction in utero before 10 weeks, and is frequently diagnosed antenatally. The resulting kidney is non-functioning and contains cysts of varying sizes, separated by hyperechoic 'dysplastic' renal parenchyma (Fig. 9.8A). In general the cysts do not communicate but occasionally some communication can be seen, making differentiation from a severe hydronephrosis difficult.

MCDK is usually unilateral and is considered a benign condition although there is a slight risk of malignancy and hypertension in later life. The kidney gradually involutes and often completely disappears. Surgical removal is unnecessary unless symptomatic due to its large size or is associated with repeated episodes of infection. Provided the contralateral kidney is normal, with good function, the prognosis is good. There is, however, an increased risk of associated urinary tract anomalies, such as ureterocele, vesicoureteric reflux or contralateral pelviureteric junction obstruction, which may predispose to infection. These can be demonstrated with ultrasound and MCUG.

A DMSA scan differentiates MCDK, which is completely non-functioning, from a grossly hydronephrotic kidney – a distinction which may sometimes be difficult to make on ultrasound. Follow-up ultrasound scanning is generally advised in view of the slight increased risk of Wilms' tumour and to monitor the growth of the contralateral kidney.[19]

Polycystic disease of the kidneys

Autosomal recessive polycystic disease of the kidney (ARPCDK; 'infantile') may be diagnosed prenatally. Both kidneys are abnormal being large and hyperechoic, with loss of corticomedullary differentiation (Fig. 9.8B). There is a spectrum of severity of disease and in some cases it may present later in childhood with the milder, juvenile form of the disease. Prenatally the less severe forms appear normal on ultrasound. ARPCDK is associated with hepatic fibrosis and portal hypertension.

Autosomal dominant polycystic disease of the kidney (ADPCDK; 'adult') also has a wide spectrum of severity. Although it tends to present later in life, the more severe forms can present in childhood and can occasionally be diagnosed prenatally. Frank cysts can usually be demonstrated on ultrasound, but may not be detected until the

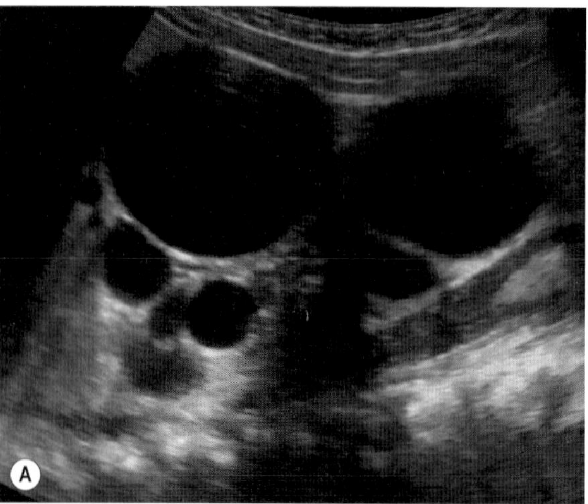

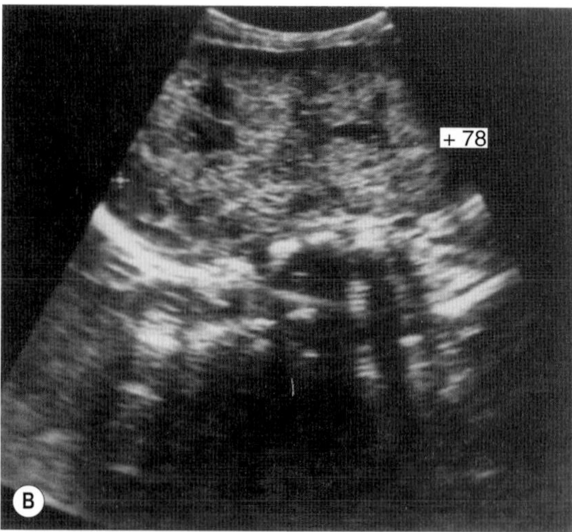

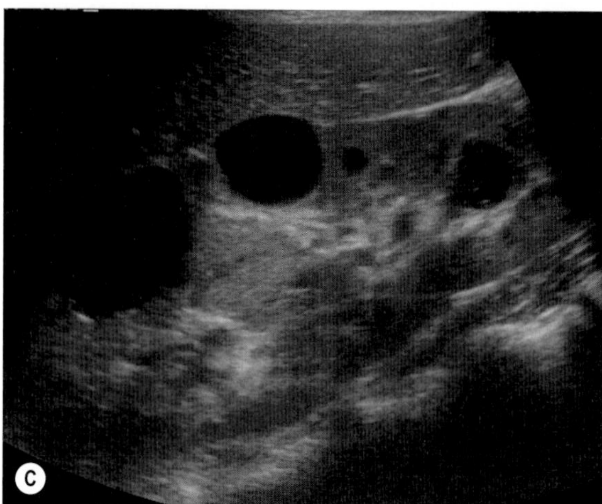

Fig. 9.8 • (A) MCDK. (B) Large hyperechoic kidneys in a neonate with ARPCDK. (C) Frank cysts seen in the kidneys of a 10-year-old girl with ADPCDK.

second or third decade of life (Fig. 9.8C). The disease is also associated with cysts in the liver and pancreas, and with intracranial berry aneurysms.

Renal dilatation

Hydronephrosis is frequently detected antenatally, although the cause may be difficult to demonstrate. Dilatation is due either to obstructive uropathy – e.g. vesico- or pelviureteric junction obstruction, posterior urethral valves, or obstructed upper moiety of a duplex kidney, or it may be non-obstructive, e.g. due to reflux.

Postnatal ultrasound scans should be performed when the infant is more than 4 days old, because there is commonly a period of dehydration immediately after birth. This may cause an obstructed or otherwise dilated kidney to appear normal for the first few days of life. The timing of the first postnatal scan is much debated and varies with local guidelines,[20] however even if normal, a follow-up scan is generally recommended at about the age of 6 weeks.

The presence of any calyceal dilatation or ureteric dilatation, as opposed to dilatation confined to the renal pelvis, is an important factor to note, indicating a greater degree of severity. A measurement of the AP diameter of the dilated intrarenal pelvis is a useful baseline from which to compare subsequent follow-up scans. It should be noted that slight separation of the renal pelvis is a normal finding in the newborn with an AP renal pelvis of 5 mm being the upper limit of normal.

The presence of a baggy, extrarenal pelvis, less than 10 mm, without pelvicalyceal dilatation is usually managed conservatively using ultrasound monitoring to demonstrate any increasing dilatation. Pelvicalyceal system dilatation with a renal pelvic diameter of between 10 mm and 20 mm is more serious and likely to require an assessment of renal function with a MAG3 renogram. Conservative treatment is possible, but surgery may be required for very poor function.

The dilated renal tract is predisposed to infection due to ascending infection in reflux or haematogenous infection in an obstructed system, where a pyonephrosis requiring percutaneous nephrostomy may develop (Fig. 9.9A, B). As a consequence

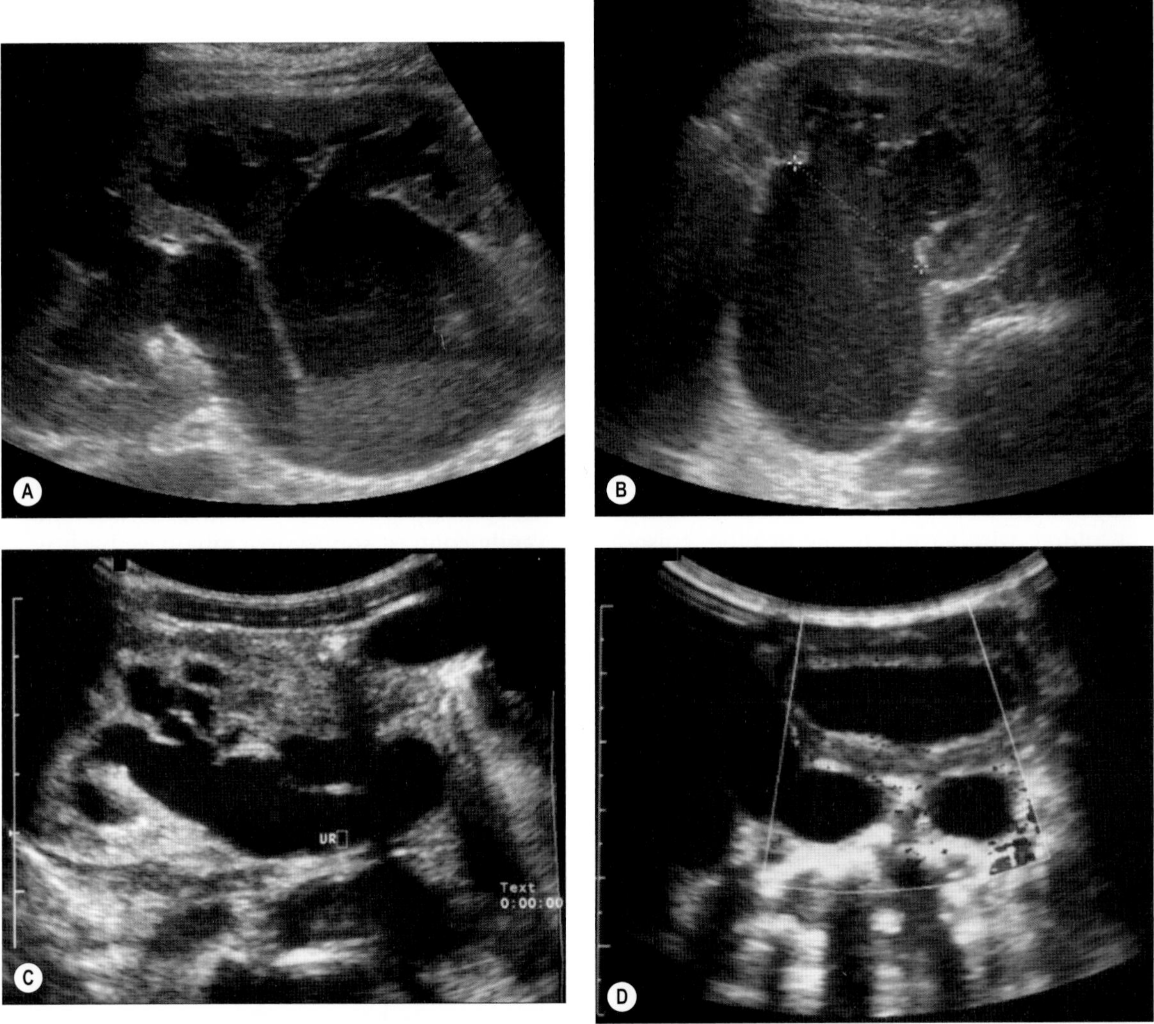

Fig. 9.9 • (A) Longitudinal view and (B) Transverse view of echoes within the dilated pelvicalyceal system of a child with pyonephrosis. (C) Dilated kidney and proximal ureter in a boy with posterior urethral valves. (D) Same patient as in (C). Dilated distal ureters are seen posterior to the thick walled bladder.

antibiotic prophylaxis is frequently advised in the neonate with significant renal tract dilatation.

Bilateral renal tract dilatation in boys may be due to posterior urethral valves with secondary dilatation of the upper tracts due to the urethral obstruction. The diagnosis is confirmed by fluoroscopic micturating cystography. This diagnosis may be suspected sonographically by the association of bilateral hydronephrosis in association with a distended and thick-walled bladder (Fig. 9.9C, D).

Vesicoureteric reflux

Vesicoureteric reflux – the retrograde passage of urine from the bladder up the ureter and into the kidney – predisposes the child to urinary tract infection and the development of reflux nephropathy. In the first year of life only, reflux is more common in boys than in girls and is usually more severe.[21] Conversely after the first year of life reflux is more likely to present in girls and is often less severe. Vesicoureteric reflux is a common cause of hydronephrosis antenatally, accounting for up to 38% of all prenatal urinary tract dilatation, requiring ultrasound follow-up and antibiotic prophylaxis.[22,23] Reflux may either be due to a developmental anomaly at the vesicoureteric junction, or can be the result of a neurogenic bladder, partial outlet obstruction or foreign bodies such as calculi (Fig. 9.10) and the presence of a catheter.

Children who have had one or more episodes of UTI should be investigated to search for an underlying cause and to identify evidence of reflux nephropathy (Box 9.1) and (Table 9.2). Approximately 2% of boys and 8% of girls will develop at least one urinary tract infection, by 10 years of age, requiring investigation and in most centres will account for a substantial proportion of the paediatric sonography performed.

Reflux itself is not reliably diagnosed by ultrasound as it is possible to have intermittent reflux in the presence of a normal ultrasound scan, with a non-dilated urinary tract.[23,24] There may be evidence of thickening of the uro-epithelium of the renal pelvis due to intermittent renal pelvis distension. Uni- or bilateral dilatation may be present to a mild or severe degree and may involve the kidney and/or ureter. It is important to scan the renal pelves and ureteric orifices immediately after micturition, when intermittent dilatation due to reflux may be demonstrated on an otherwise normal scan.

BOX 9.1 Conditions associated with urinary tract infection

(a) Vesicoureteric reflux
(b) Obstruction
- Pelviureteric junction
- Vesicoureteric junction
- Posterior urethral valves
- Duplex kidney with obstructed moiety/ectopic ureter
- Ureterocele

(c) Other structural anomalies
- Duplex and/or ectopic renal anatomy
- MCDK
- Prune belly syndrome

(d) Calculi
(e) Neurogenic bladder

When dilatation *is* seen, the exact cause may be uncertain unless reflux is actually visualized, which is rare and micturating cystography is required. Although most commonly performed conventionally by fluoroscopy using iodinated contrast medium, radionuclide cystography and more recently contrast sonocystography have been used as an alternative, particularly in the older child.[24]

The most common complication of reflux is infection and most children present with at least one episode of UTI. This can cause renal scarring. It is important to make the diagnosis of vesicoureteric reflux and renal scarring early in order to prescribe prophylactic antibiotics in an attempt to avoid the damaging complications caused by reflux of infected urine. The ultrasound appearances of scarring include a focal reduction in cortical thickness, irregular outline, interruption of or loss of the renal capsule echo or a disruption in the renal architecture. Colour flow and power Doppler, may show wedge shaped areas of decreased or absent blood flow (and occasionally increased flow) and can improve the detection rate of focal scarring on sonography.[25] These signs can be difficult to demonstrate in young children's kidneys, particularly

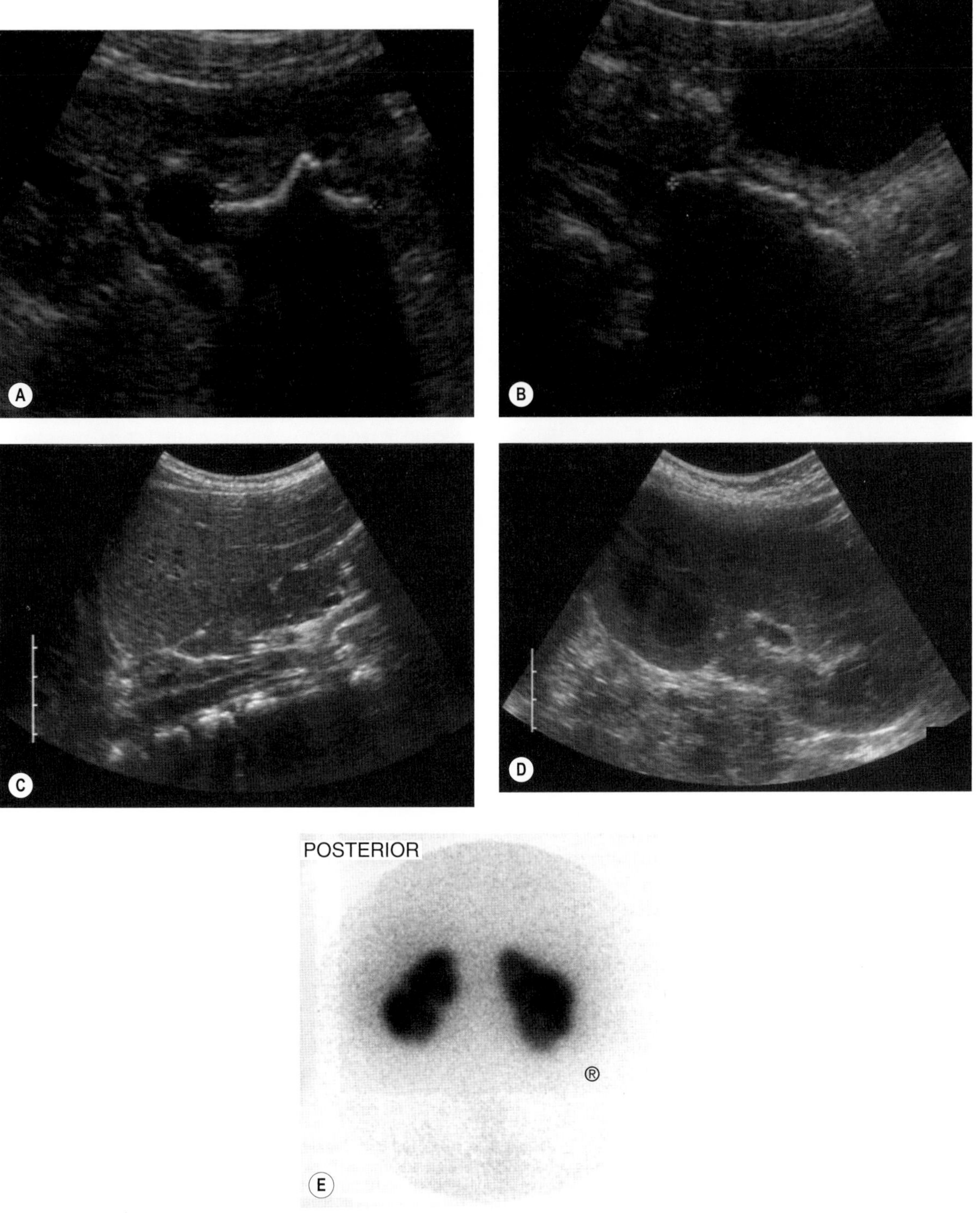

Fig. 9.10 • (A) Partial staghorn calculus seen in the lower pole of a mildly dilated kidney in a 3-year-old boy who presented with fever and urinary tract infection. (B) Same patient as (A). Large calculus is seen in the distal ureter, posterior to the bladder. (C) Small scarred right kidney due to reflux. (D) Hypertrophy of the contralateral kidney. (E) DMSA scan showing bilateral renal scarring due to reflux. Note in particular two wedge-shaped scars in the RK.

Ultrasound	First-line investigation in all cases. Excellent structural detail Limited sensitivity for duplex kidneys, reflux, ureteral pathology and small scars Monitoring of disease progression Monitoring of treatment
Contrast sonocystography	Alternative to X-ray or radionuclide cystography. Poor structural detail, unsuitable for the demonstration of urethral anomalies
Diuretic renogram (dynamic) – Tc^{99M} MAG3	Outlines the pelvicalyceal system. Diagnosis of obstruction and relative renal function by analysis of excretion curves
Radionuclide cystography (Dynamic)	Diagnosis of reflux
Direct (via catheter or suprapubic injection of isotope into the bladder) or indirect (following diuretic renogram.)	
Cortical scintigraphy (static) – Tc^{99M} DMSA	Demonstrates uptake in the renal cortex Superior detection of renal scarring in vesicoureteric reflux and acute pyelonephritis Demonstration of congenital anomalies, e.g. ectopic or solitary kidney Analysis of *differential* renal function
Intravenous urography	Limited use in children Assessment of level of ureteric obstruction Assessment of congenital anomalies, e.g. ectopic ureters and duplex kidney Post-operative evaluation
Micturating cystourethrogram	Accurate diagnosis of reflux, polyps, diverticulae, strictures and urethral anomalies, but involving a significant radiation dose
Plain X-ray	Some calculi – mainly those in the ureter Of limited value in paediatric renal work-up May show gross spinal anomalies
CT	Reserved mainly for confirmation and staging of malignant tumours, due to significant radiation dose Renal trauma Increasingly used for ureteric calculus detection
MRI	Assessment of difficult congenital anomalies and focal masses. Staging of malignancy

Table 9.2 Imaging the paediatric renal tract

when highly lobulated and the most reliable method of scar detection is a DMSA scan (Fig. 9.10E).

Chronic reflux nephropathy leads to failure of renal growth, resulting in a shrivelled, poorly-functioning kidney (Fig. 9.10C). Measurements of the maximum length of the kidneys should be routinely performed, and can be related to age, height and weight.[16] A difference in renal length of more than 10% between the two kidneys should prompt further investigation into renal function with a DMSA scan.

Fungal infection

Candidiasis is a fungal infection which is most commonly seen in infants who are acutely ill or immunocompromised or in sick ventilated

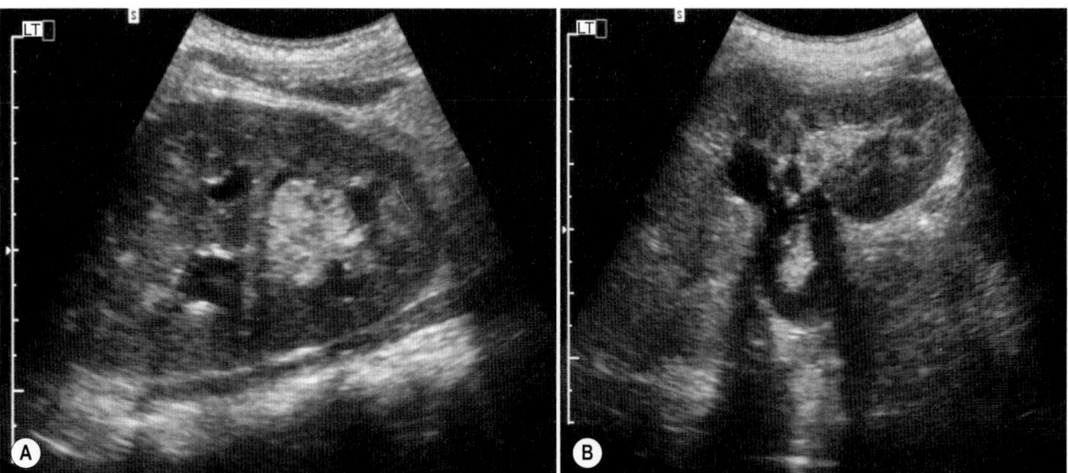

Fig. 9.11 • (A) The dilated collecting system of this kidney is filled with a large, rounded fungal ball of candidiasis infection. (B) The fungus ball is seen to disintegrate, emptying into the renal pelvis.

neonates. Fungal balls dilate and may obstruct the collecting system of the kidney (Fig. 9.11). Ultrasound is particularly useful in making the diagnosis by demonstrating the hyperechoic fungal balls within the dilated collecting system. Fungal infection may also undergo haematogenous spread to the spleen and liver, where it can result in multifocal abscess formation.

Wilms' tumour

The most common paediatric renal malignancy, Wilms' tumours usually present before the age of 3 years. Although the lesion generally occurs in previously fit individuals, there are several known predisposing conditions including hemihypertrophy, Beckwith–Wiedemann syndrome and sporadic aniridia, with a 30–40% incidence in the latter. The tumours are large at presentation, presenting with a palpable abdominal mass, and, less frequently, pain, haematuria and fever. The prognosis when unilateral is generally good.

The ultrasound appearances are of a relatively well-defined heterogeneous mass – predominantly solid but frequently with some necrotic or haemorrhagic areas – often almost completely replacing the kidney (Fig. 9.12). Small focal areas of calcification are seen occasionally. A search should be made for tumour invasion of the renal vein and IVC which occurs in up to 10% of cases. Tumour invasion may extend into the right atrium. Occasionally a large, right-sided Wilms' tumour may compress the IVC but not invade it; colour or power Doppler may be useful in the difficult distinction between compression and invasion on ultrasound. Ultrasound also identifies associated lymphadenopathy, particularly in the para-aortic and paracaval regions, and metastatic liver disease.

In a small percentage of cases, tumour may also be found in the contralateral kidney. This is usually much smaller than the mass on the presenting side and may be acoustically subtle. Up to 7% of contralateral tumours are missed on preoperative imaging due to their small size and the operator must be alert to the possibility of bilateral disease.[26] Occasionally a Wilms' tumour may be found to be predominantly cystic, having the appearances of a large, multiloculated cystic mass. The main differential diagnosis would be of a mesonephric blastoma occurring during the first year of life and histology is required to establish the diagnosis.

In most cases, an ultrasound and chest radiograph are sufficient to correctly diagnose Wilms' tumour but CT of the chest and abdomen is generally used for staging, and to exclude metastatic disease in the chest and liver.[27] Percutaneous biopsy for confirmation of histological type is generally performed. CT or MRI are more sensitive than ultrasound scanning in demonstrating small tumours in the contralateral kidney.

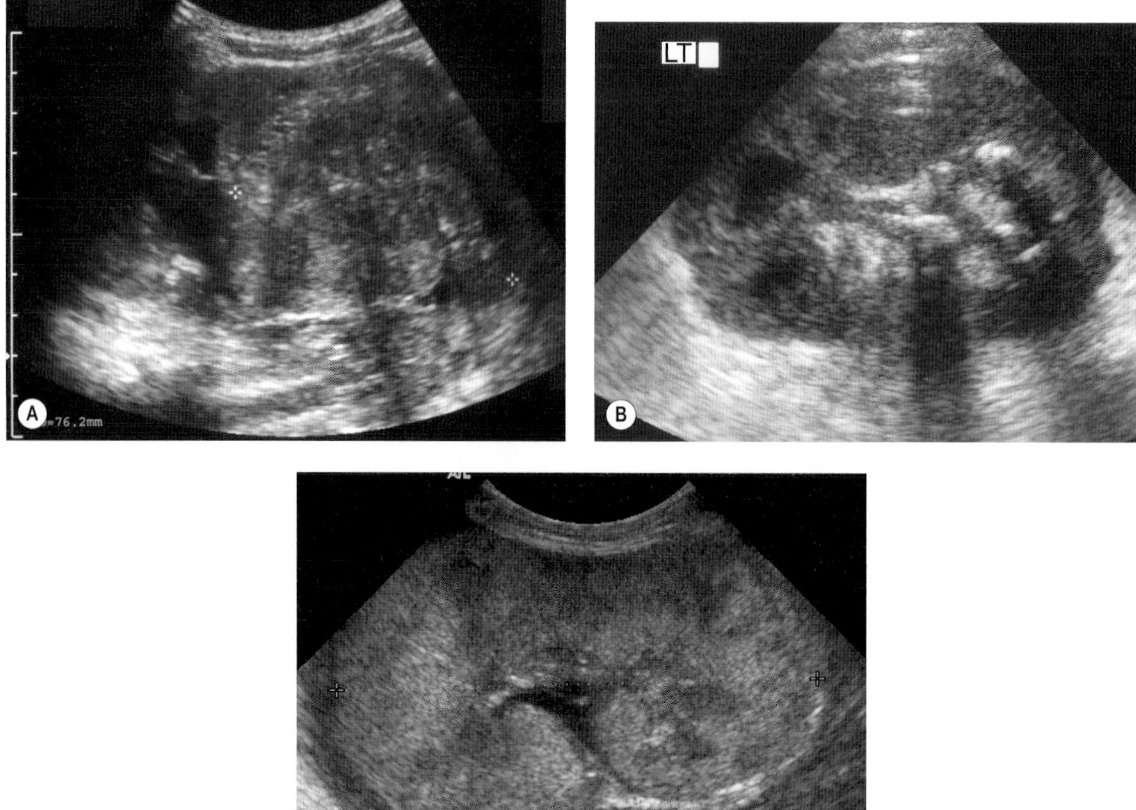

Fig. 9.12 • (A) Wilms' tumour in the left kidney. There is dilatation of the upper pole calyces due to compression by the tumour. (B) Xanthogranulomatous pyelonephritis was the cause of the renal mass in this 8-year-old boy presenting with anaemia and a flank mass. (C) Renal vein thrombosis in a dehydrated neonate, showing an enlarged 'globular' kidney with loss of the normal corticomedullary differentiation.

Xanthogranulomatous pyelonephritis

Xanthogranulomatous pyelonephritis, results from chronic infection in an obstructed kidney and children present with a history of general malaise, low grade fever, flank pain, and may be found to be anaemic. The finding of a palpable abdominal mass on examination often leads to an early diagnosis of a possible Wilms' tumour. On sonography the kidney is diffusely enlarged, with loss of the normal corticomedullary differentiation. The presence of calyceal dilatation with debris and calculi in the collecting system, confirmation of urinary infection in addition to the generalized involvement of the kidney helps to differentiate this condition from Wilms' tumour (Fig. 9.12B). Occasionally CT scanning may also be helpful. The kidney will usually be found to be non-functioning on a DMSA scan and nephrectomy is required.

Renal vein thrombosis

RVT primarily occurs in the neonatal period but may occur in the older child particularly in association with renal malignancy and amyloidosis. Classically the sick neonate is noted to develop gross haematuria in association with a palpable abdominal mass. RVT is usually unilateral but may be bilateral and is associated with acute adrenal haemorrhage when left sided. Sonographically the affected kidney is enlarged and globular and develops an inhomogeneous echogenicity of the renal parenchyma with areas of increased echogenicity due to haemorrhage (Fig 9.12C). Thrombus may be detected in the ipsilateral renal vein and IVC and Doppler sonography shows reduced or absent blood flow in the renal vein and increased resistance in the renal arteries.[28] On follow-up, the kidney may completely recover due to the development of collateral blood flow or early recanalization of the renal vein, but in severe cases the kidney may atrophy and calcify.

ADRENAL GLANDS

Normal appearances

In utero and postnatally, the adrenal glands are large – about a third the size of the kidney – and composed mainly of the bulky, hypoechoic fetal cortex which makes up about 80% of the gland. The neonatal adrenal glands are easily demonstrated on ultrasound. The bulky fetal cortex is sonographically apparent as a thick hypoechoic layer surrounding the thinner, hyperechoic adrenal medulla (Fig. 9.13A). The fetal cortex surrounds

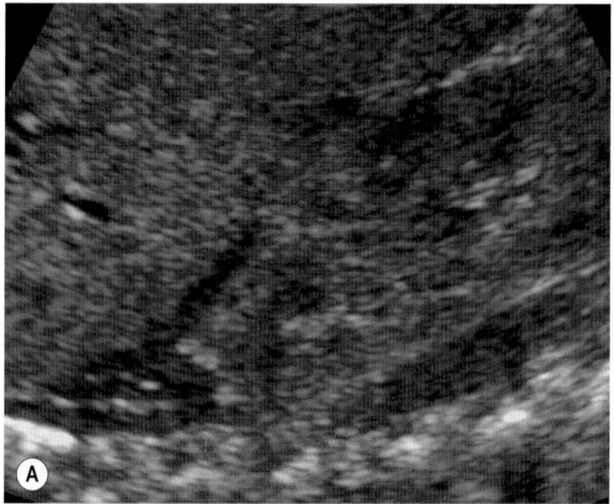

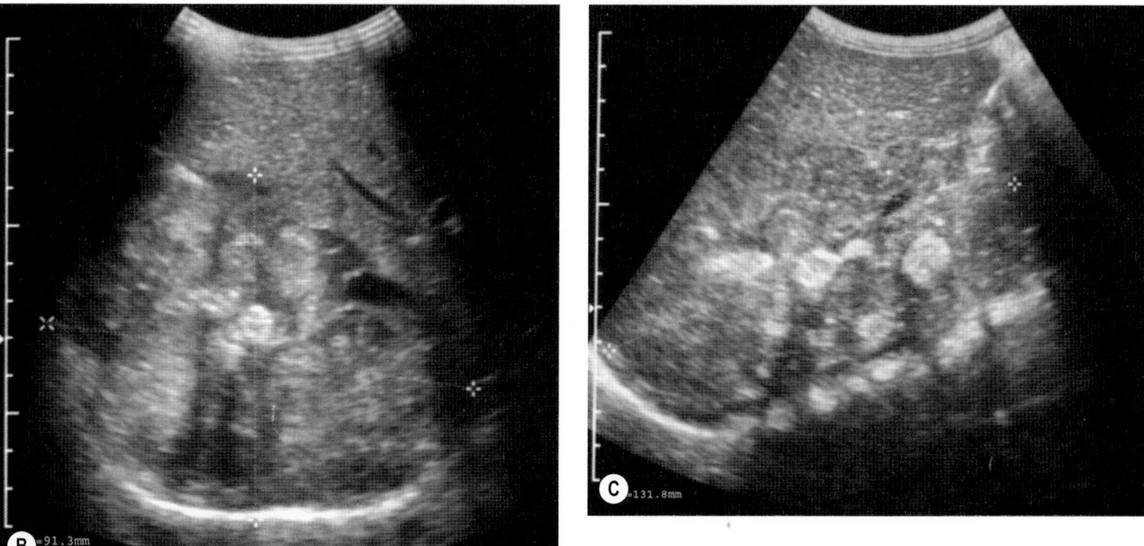

Fig. 9.13 • (A) Normal adrenal gland in a neonate. Note the bulky hypoechoic fetal cortex surrounding the thinner hyperechoic medulla. (B & C) Right adrenal neuroblastoma. Calcification can be seen within the tumour.

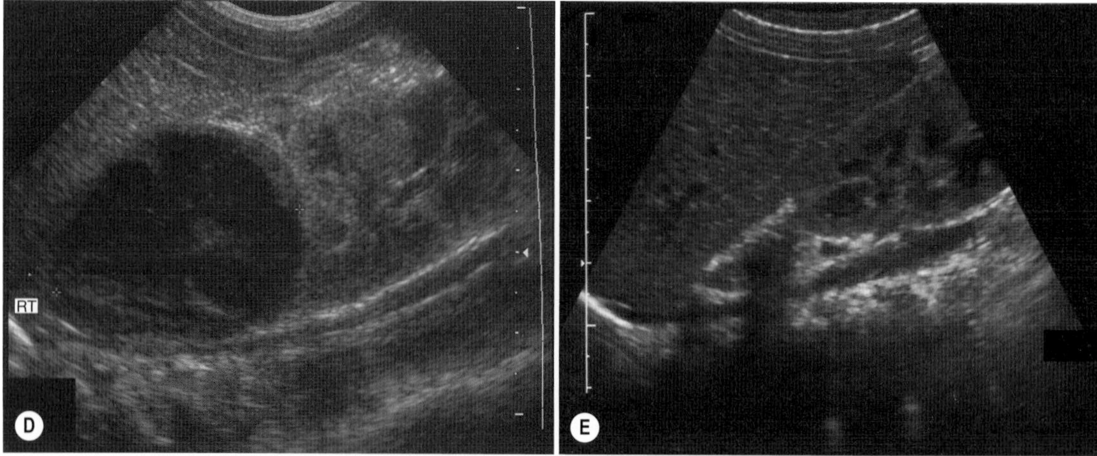

Fig. 9.13, cont'd • (D) Adrenal haemorrhage in a neonate. (E) Same patient as in (D); 3 months later the haemorrhage has resolved and there is calcification in the involuted adrenal gland.

the smaller, permanent cortex and gradually starts to involute after birth. By the age of 2–4 months, the adrenal glands have attained their normal 'adult' configuration of the thin, hypoechoic cortex with a tiny layer of hyperechoic adrenal medulla within.

Neuroblastoma

The neuroblastoma is a malignant tumour arising in the sympathetic chain, most commonly the adrenal medulla. The majority of neuroblastomas present before the age of 4 years with a palpable abdominal mass, and many already have metastases at the time of presentation – to the liver, bone marrow, skin or lymph nodes. Box 9.2 lists the most frequent abdominal tumours occurring in childhood.

The tumour is usually large on presentation, displacing the kidney downwards and laterally. In some cases it may invade the adjacent kidney, becoming difficult to distinguish from a Wilms' tumour. Neuroblastoma is predominantly solid on ultrasound, having a heterogeneous texture and frequently containing calcification. There may be anechoic areas within the lesion due to necrosis or haemorrhage. The tumour margins are ill-defined and infiltrate the surrounding organs and tissues, crossing the midline and encasing vascular structures which may be difficult to differentiate from lymphadenopathy (Fig. 9.13B, C). Nodes tend to surround and elevate the aorta and IVC.

MRI and CT are used for staging, particularly in assessing retroperitoneal spread; bone scintigraphy and MIBG scans are also useful in demonstrating metastases.[29]

BOX 9.2 Paediatric abdominal malignancies

(a) Neuroblastoma
(b) Wilms' tumour
(c) Hepatoblastoma
(d) Hepatocellular carcinoma
(e) Rhabdomyosarcoma
(f) Leukaemia
(g) Lymphoma

Adrenal haemorrhage

After birth, the bulky fetal cortex normally involutes. Adrenal haemorrhage occurs in the neonate as a result of trauma to the vulnerable fetal cortex during delivery or in association with perinatal asphyxia. Haemorrhage may occur in up to 2% of births.[30] This may be uni- or bilateral and may cause a palpable mass and abdominal pain. Ultrasound can be used to follow the resolution of the haemorrhage over a period of weeks; in the initial stages of haemorrhage the adrenal mass is hyperechoic, gradually liquefying into a well-defined mass of mixed echo pattern and becoming cystic (Fig. 9.13D, E). This may completely resolve over a period of some weeks leaving a normal adrenal gland or the gland may become atrophic and calcify. In rare cases an adrenal haemorrhage may progress to an abscess.[31]

Adrenal calcification

Calcification of the gland in babies and infants is usually the result of previous infection or haemorrhage. Adrenal abscess cavities may calcify after successful treatment. Gross calcification in bilateral adrenal glands in association with hepatosplenomegaly in the infant indicates the likely diagnosis of Wolman's disease, an inborn error of lipid metabolism that is invariably fatal.

GASTROINTESTINAL TRACT

Bowel ultrasound in paediatrics is an established and readily accepted investigation, replacing contrast radiology in many cases. Most gastrointestinal tract scanning in paediatrics is best performed with a high frequency (15–7.5 MHz) linear or small footprint curvilinear probe.

Hypertrophic pyloric stenosis

Hypertrophic pyloric stenosis (HPS) is a condition occurring in newborn infants commonly about 6 weeks of age when the pyloric muscle becomes hypertrophied and elongated, restricting the passage of gastric contents, causing projectile vomiting. Prolonged vomiting leads to hypochloraemic alkalosis and when seen in association with a palpable epigastric mass the size of an olive on test feeding, the diagnosis is clear without the need for ultrasonic imaging. However, ultrasound is very successful in demonstrating HPS and is often used to make the diagnosis before protracted vomiting is allowed to occur.[32]

The baby should be positioned comfortably right side down and the stomach and pylorus identified usually just to the right of the midline in the low epigastric region. If the stomach is empty a glucose solution or water (preferable to milk as it does not contain echoes which may obscure vital detail) can be given orally or through a nasogastric tube to aid visualization of the gastric antrum. A small, high frequency linear or curvilinear transducer is best.

	NORMAL PYLORUS	HYPERTROPHIC PYLORIC STENOSIS
Pyloric length	<15 mm	≥16 mm
Pyloric width	<11 mm	≥11 mm
Muscle thickness	<2.5 mm	≥3 mm

Table 9.3 Pyloric muscle dimensions

The pylorus projects into gastric lumen and is outlined by the fluid. Hypertrophic pyloric stenosis can be confirmed by the demonstration of:

(a) Thickened and elongated pyloric muscle
(b) Increased but ineffective peristalsis
(c) Failure of the pylorus to relax and open
(d) Various figures have been quoted for muscle thickness in hypertrophic pyloric stenosis ranging from 2.5 mm to 5 mm but 3 mm is most commonly accepted (Table 9.3).[33]

It must be stressed that the examination is dynamic and measurements of muscle thickness must be interpreted in conjunction with the observations of gastric peristalsis and failure of the pylorus to relax normally. Sensitivity and specificity of 97% and 99% for the diagnosis of HPS have been reported in expert hands (Fig. 9.14). If clinical suspicion persists after a negative ultrasound, a repeat examination after one or two days may be performed to exclude an evolving pyloric stenosis.

Intussusception

Intussusception is the invagination of a segment of bowel into the lumen of the adjacent bowel. It is a common paediatric emergency, especially in younger children aged 3 months to 3 years, and tends to affect the ileocaecal region. The child presents with abdominal pain, sometimes with a

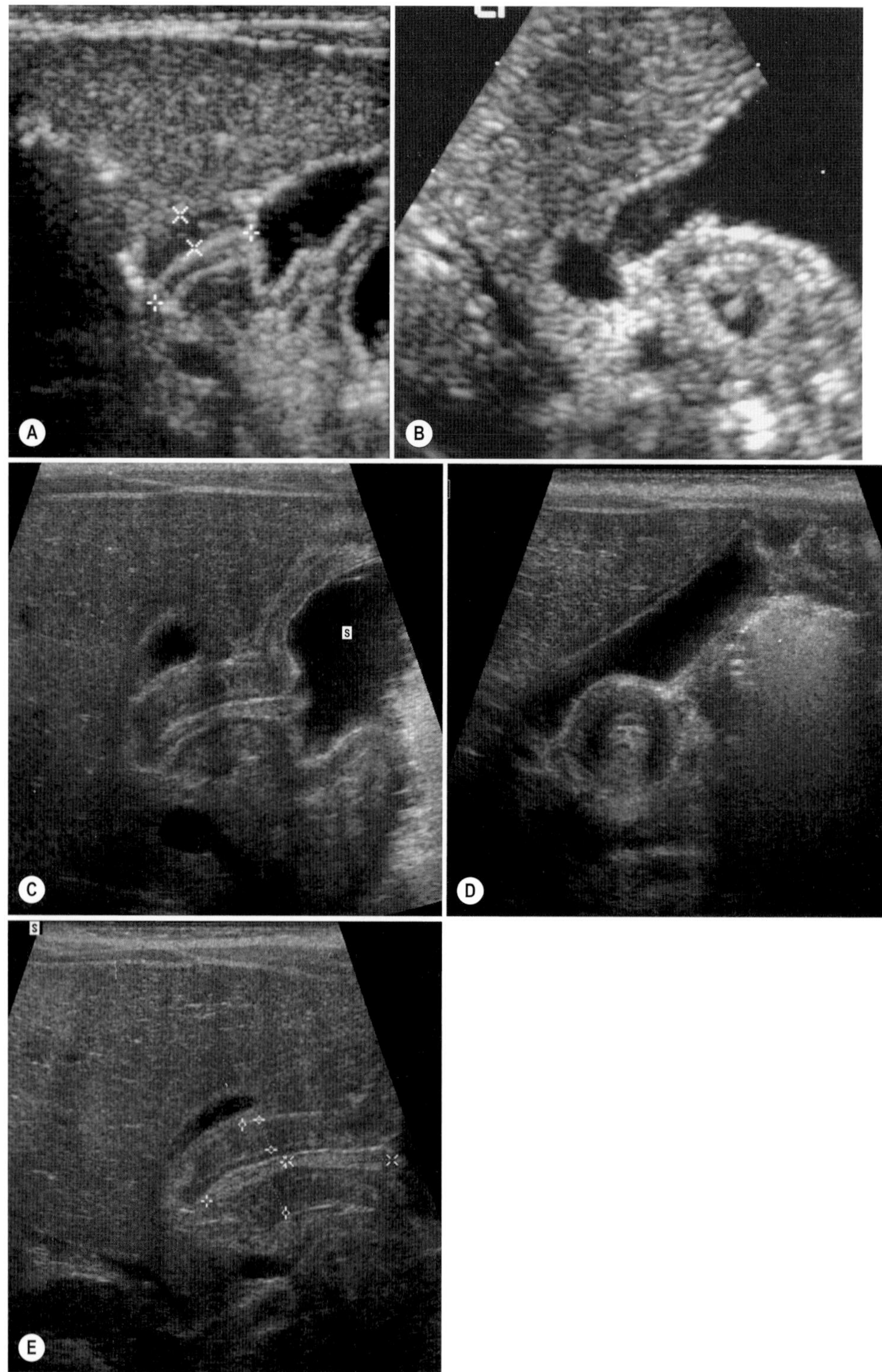

Fig. 9.14 • Hypertrophic pyloric stenosis. (A) Normal pylorus demonstrating measurement of length of pyloric canal and thickness of the muscle. (B) A few minutes later the pylorus relaxed and opened widely, excluding the diagnosis of hypertrophic pyloric stenosis. (C) Thickened and elongated pylorus of hypertrophic pyloric stenosis seen in longitudinal section. S represents a fluid-filled stomach. (D) TS view of the thickened pylorus. (E) Demonstrates the measurements of pyloric length, muscle thickness and pyloric width.

palpable mass, vomiting or rectal bleeding. Intussusception can result in bowel necrosis, and subsequently perforation requiring surgery.

The ultrasound appearances of bowel within bowel are characteristic. In cross section, the bowel assumes a 'doughnut' configuration, with concentric rings of bowel wall (Fig. 9.15). Dilated loops of fluid-filled, obstructed bowel may be demonstrated proximal to the intussusception. The use of ultrasound to diagnose this condition is highly reliable, reducing or eliminating the need for diagnostic enema.[34]

An air enema is most commonly used to reduce the intussusception using inflation pressures of up to 120 mm Hg. Hydrostatic reduction (i.e. with water/saline) under fluoroscopic or ultrasound control is also an accepted treatment.[35]

The main contraindications to attempting a non-surgical reduction are peritonitis and free intraperitoneal air. A number of sonographic features have been reported to be associated with a decreased success rate of non-surgical reduction including a hypoechoic rim greater than 10 mm, absent blood flow on colour flow Doppler sonography, or a large amount of fluid trapped within the intussusception, but these findings are not contraindications to a careful attempt at non-surgical reduction.[32] Approximately 10% of cases recur whether the initial intussusception was treated surgically or non-surgically.[36]

Midgut volvulus

Malrotation of the midgut occurs as a result of failure of normal rotation of the small bowel during intrauterine development, resulting in a shortened mesenteric fixation of the small bowel to the posterior abdominal wall. This predisposes the small bowel to twisting (volving) around the mesenteric vascular axis resulting in bowel obstruction and vascular compromise with a risk of infarction of most of the small bowel if the volvulus is not treated quickly.

Following volvulus the child presents with acute pain, and bile-stained vomiting. The bowel may intermittently twist and untwist resulting in temporary alleviation of symptoms which may make diagnosis more difficult.The definitive diagnosis is usually made fluoroscopically during an upper gastrointestinal contrast study. In malrotation the duodenal jejunal flexure is generally found to be lower and in a more medial position than is normal and if a volvulus has occurred a corkscrew appearance of the volved small bowel may be seen (Fig. 9.16). The proximal duodenum will be dilated secondary to the duodenal obstruction.

Malrotation without volvulus may be suspected during a sonographic examination performed for intermittent abdominal pain, due to the associated malposition of the mesenteric vessels best seen on colour Doppler sonography. The normal relationship of the SMV to the SMA is reversed, with the SMV lying anteriorly and/or to the left of the SMA. Although vessel inversion suggests malrotation, a normal relationship between the SMA and SMV does not exclude it. Occasionally anatomical variations in the position of the mesenteric vessels can be seen in normal individuals and therefore a contrast study is required for confirmation.[37]

When volvulus has occurred the vessels may be noted to be spiralling around a bowel mass i.e. the 'whirlpool sign' (Fig. 9.16).[38] Other ultrasound appearances include a dilated, fluid-filled obstructed duodenum although the obstructed duodenum may be gas-filled, obscuring visualization. This sign is not invariable, however, and contrast fluoroscopy may still be needed to confirm or exclude the diagnosis of a midgut volvulus. Surgery is performed to untwist the bowel, which is then laid carefully in the correct position; attachment is usually unnecessary, as abdominal adhesions tend to stabilize the bowel.

Gastro-oesophageal reflux

Reflux through the gastro-oesophageal hiatus is a common problem associated with neonatal vomiting, leading to oesophagitis. The diagnosis is usually made with a contrast meal, pH probe and isotope milk scan. Reflux can be observed on ultrasound as the retrograde flow of stomach contents through the hiatus and up the oesophagus.

The normal intra-abdominal segment of the oesophagus can be demonstrated through the left lobe of the liver, is usually between 2 cm and 3 cm long, and makes an acute angle with the gastric wall. When episodes of reflux are seen over three times in 10 minutes, this is said to pathological.

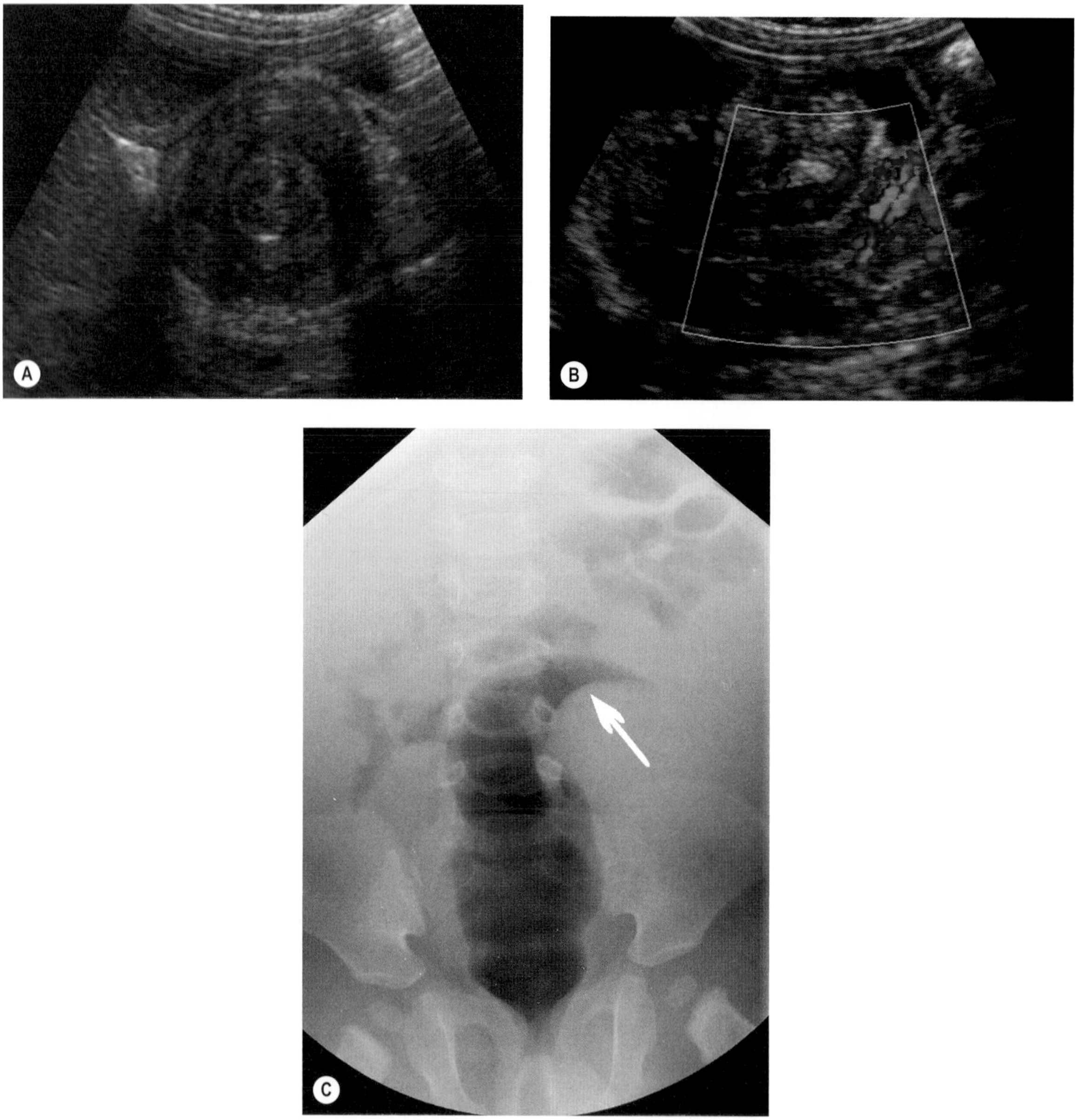

Fig. 9.15 • Intussusception. (A) The characteristic 'doughnut' appearance of bowel within bowel due to an intussusception. (B) Colour Doppler demonstrates blood flow within the intussuscepted bowel and dilated fluid-filled loops of obstructed bowel are seen proximal to it. (C) Air enema; the intussusception is seen indenting into the lumen of the air-filled sigmoid colon during a successful air enema reduction (arrow).

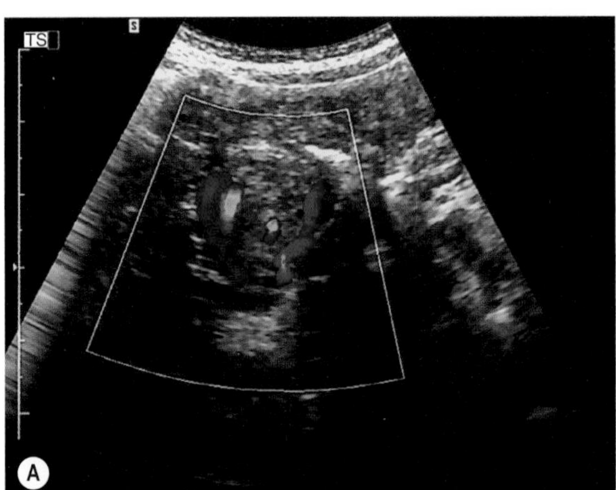

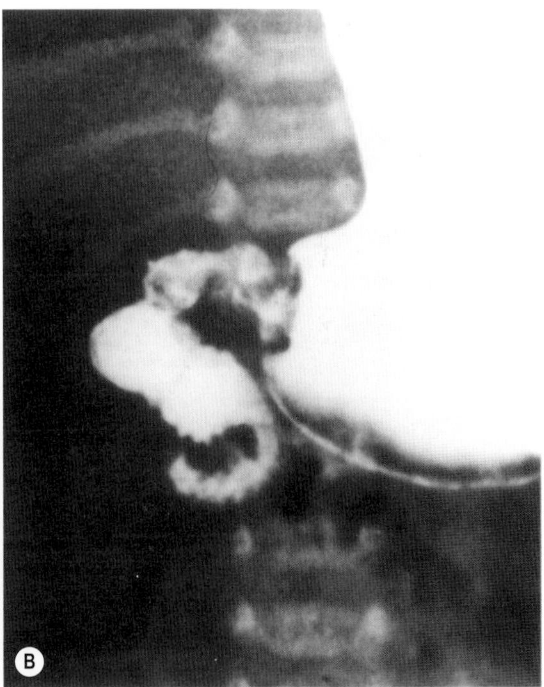

Fig. 9.16 • Volvulus. (A) Mesentery and superior mesenteric vein are twisted around the superior mesenteric artery, which is seen in cross-section at the centre of the film. (B) Barium meal shows corkscrewing of the duodenum away from the midline, consistent with a malrotation and volvulus. (By kind permission of Dr Delia Martinez, Leeds.)

Appendicitis

Ultrasound is the first line of investigation for the child presenting with acute abdominal pain, where the diagnosis is uncertain following clinical assessment. The position of the appendix in small children may vary – pointing upwards, downwards or to the patient's left making the clinical diagnosis difficult, as the pain is not always confined to the right lower quadrant. Ultrasound is particularly useful in establishing the diagnosis of acute appendicitis and in diagnosing other possible causes of acute abdominal pain, such as gynaecological disorders.[39] It is always good practice to perform a full abdominal survey when the clinical presentation is indeterminate.

Ultrasound demonstrates a hypoechoic, thickened appendix, >6 mm thick, with a blind end (Fig. 9.17). Occasionally an appendicolith, with strong acoustic shadowing, is present. The inflamed appendix is not compressible on gentle, graded compression with the transducer. This should be done *very* carefully, and released very slowly to avoid rebound tenderness. Ultrasound cannot reliably exclude appendicitis, especially if the appendix is retrocaecal.

Perforation may not be easy to see with ultrasound, as fluid may disperse through the abdomen with decompression of the appendix itself. However, a frank, peri-appendiceal fluid collection or abscess is easily demonstrable in a proportion of children and may, in some cases, be treated conservatively with antibiotics or drained percutaneously prior to surgery. The presence of free fluid in the abdomen, particularly if clear, is a non-specific finding and is not a reliable indicator of an acute abdomen. If echogenic fluid is seen this is suggestive of intraperitoneal infection in the child with acute abdominal pain, but may be seen in other conditions, e.g. rupture of a haemorrhagic ovarian cyst. If ultrasound is equivocal, the clinicians may decide to observe the child but further imaging with CT scanning can be helpful in a few selective cases. Alternatively a laparoscopic examination may be performed where there is significant clinical concern.

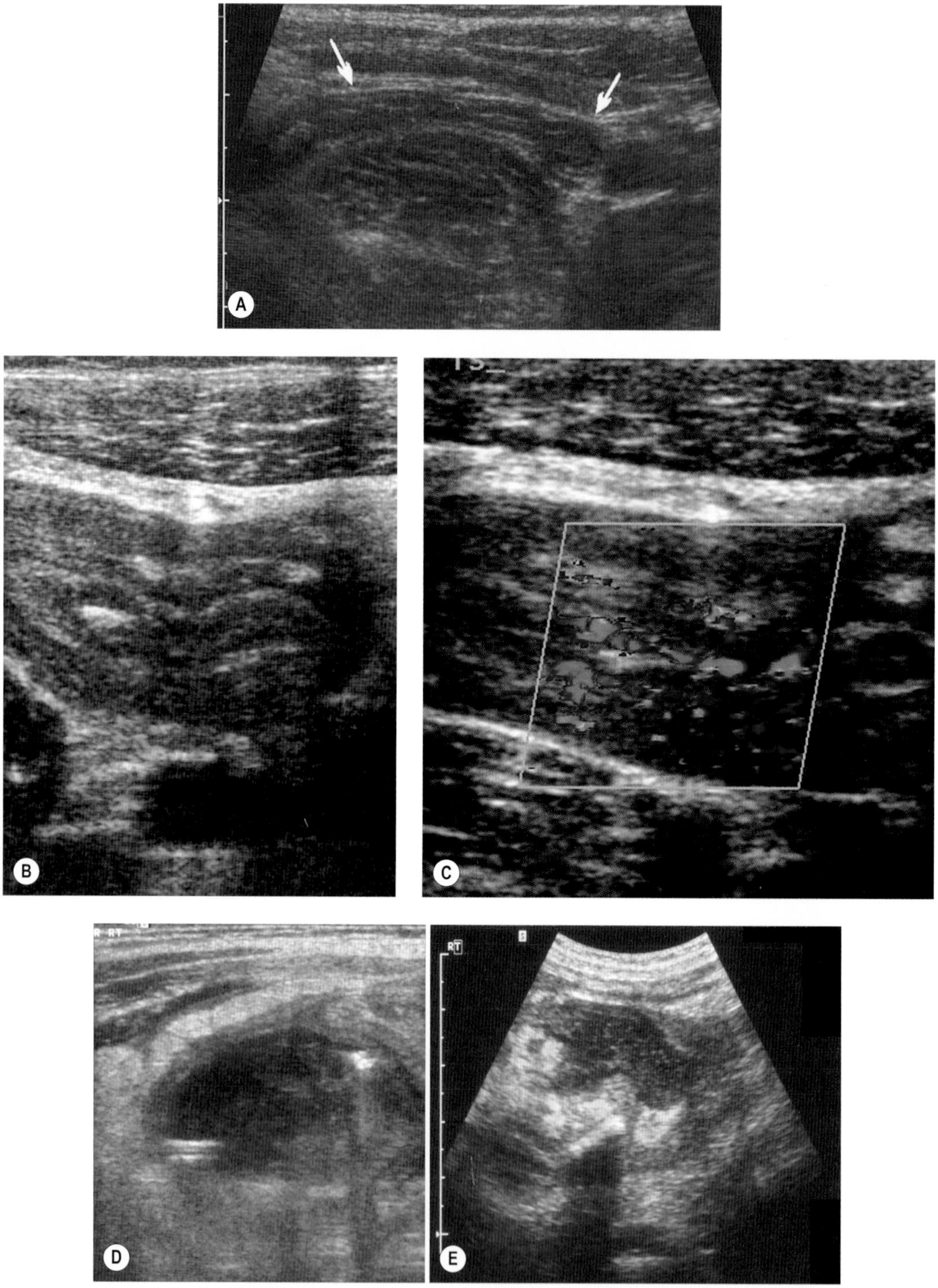

Fig. 9.17 • Appendicitis. (A) The normal appendix (arrows) lying transversely across the psoas muscle. (B) Longitudinal scan through a dilated inflamed appendix containing an appendicolith. (C) Increased vascularity of inflamed appendix seen on colour flow Doppler imaging. (D) Walled off appendix abscess containing fluid and gas. (E) Complex inflammatory mass containing an appendicolith.

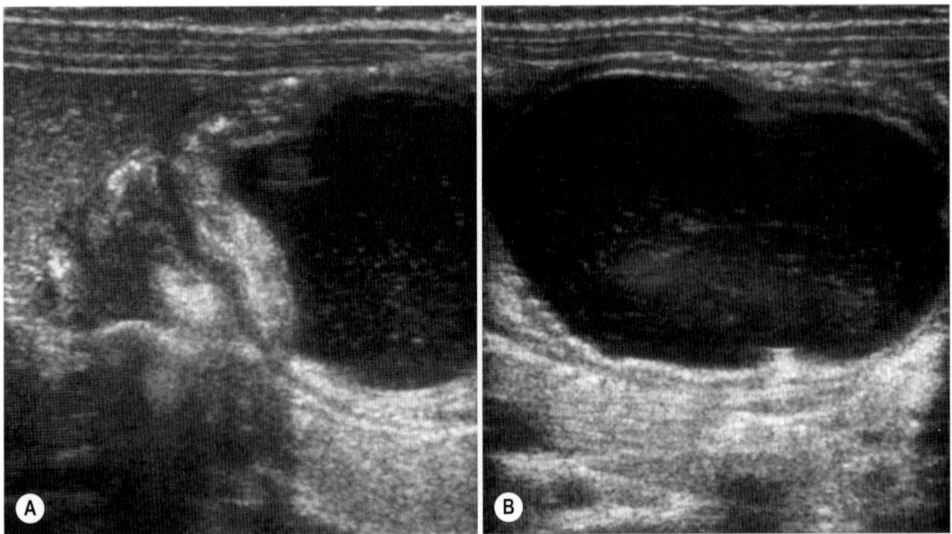

Fig. 9.18 • (A) Duplication cyst with thickened wall adjacent to bowel. (B) Typical 'double' wall seen in enteric duplication cysts.

Enteric duplication cysts

These comparatively rare lesions present in infancy or early childhood with nausea, gastrointestinal bleeding, intestinal obstruction and, occasionally, a palpable mass. Most are intra-abdominal but oesophageal duplication cysts cause a thoracic lesion with respiratory symptoms. Multiple cysts may be present.

The fluid-filled lesion may demonstrate a spectrum of ultrasonic appearances, from anechoic to hyperechoic, sometimes with gravity dependent debris or blood.[34]

The wall is well-defined and a hyperechoic inner rim of mucosa may be identified in some cases of intestinal duplication (Fig. 9.18). The cyst is closely related to the adjacent bowel and this can be appreciated on real time scanning as the bowel peristalses. CT and MRI rarely add anything to the ultrasound information. Contrast radiography may show an extrinsic defect but communication with the cyst is rare.

There are many causes of intra-abdominal cystic masses in children (Box 9.3). The main differential diagnosis in the infant girl is from an ovarian cyst as the ovary is generally an intra-abdominal organ at this age. Useful indicators of an ovarian origin can be detected on careful sonography, by detecting some residual ovarian tissue in the cyst wall, and the finding of a clearly seen multifollicular ovary on one side with absent visualization of a definite ovary on the other side.

BOX 9.3 Abdominal fluid-filled masses in paediatrics – differential diagnoses

(a) Choledochal cyst
(b) Mesenteric cyst
(c) Duplication cyst
(d) Hepatic cyst
(e) Pancreatic pseudocyst
(f) Epidermoid cyst of the spleen
(g) Lymphangioma
(h) Ovarian cyst
(i) Encysted fluid associated with ventriculoperitoneal shunt tubing
(j) Renal cyst or renal dilatation
(k) Cystic renal tumour

References

1. Haber HP. Cystic fibrosis in children and young adults: findings on routine abdominal sonography. AJR Am J Roentgenol 2007; 189: 89–99
2. Williams SM, Goodman R, Thompson A et al. Ultrasound evaluation of liver disease in cystic fibrosis as part of an

annual assessment clinic: a 9-year review. Clin Radiol 2002; 57: 365–370

3. Wilson-Sharpe RC, Irving HC, Brown RC et al. Ultrasonography of the pancreas, liver and biliary system in cystic fibrosis. Arch Dis Child 1984; 59: 923–926
4. Perlmutter DH, Shepherd RW. Extrahepatic biliary atresia: A disease or a phenotype? Hepatology 2002; 35: 1297–1304
5. McEvoy CF, Suchy FJ. Biliary tract disease in children. Pediatr Gastroenterol 1996; 43: 75–98
6. Humphrey TM, Sringer MD. Biliary atresia: US diagnosis. Radiology 2007; 244: 845–851
7. Kim SH, Lim JH, Yoon HK et al. Choledochal cyst: comparison of MR and conventional cholangiography. Clin Radiol 2000; 55: 378–383
8. Lowe LH. Imaging hepatobiliary disease in children. Semin Roentgenol 2008; 43: 39–49
9. Todani T, Watanabe Y, Narusue M et al. Congenital bile duct cysts: classification, operative procedures, and review of thirty-seven cases including cancer arising from choledochal cyst. Am J Surg 1977; 134: 263–269
10. Siegel MJ. Gallbladder and biliary tract. In: Siegel M, ed. Pediatric sonography. Lippincott Williams & Wilkins, Philadelphia, 2002, pp 275–304
11. Takano H, Smith WL. Gastrointestinal tumors of childhood. Radiol Clin North Am 1997; 35: 1367–1389
12. Buetow PC, Rao P, Marshall WH. Imaging of paediatric liver tumours. Magn Reson Imaging Clin North Am 1997; 5: 397–413
13. Davenport M. 2002 Haemangiomas and other vascular anomalies. In: Howard E, ed. Surgery of the liver, bile ducts and pancreas in children. Arnold, London, 2002, pp 219–237
14. Boon LM, Burrows PE, Patiel HJ et al. Hepatic vascular anomalies in infancy: a twenty-seven year experience. J Pediatr 1996; 129: 3346–3354
15. Siegel MJ, Martin KW, Worthington JL. Normal and abnormal pancreas in children: US studies. Radiology 1987; 165: 15–18
16. Han BK, Babcock DS. Sonographic measurements and appearances of normal kidneys in children. AJR Am J Roentgenol 1985; 145: 611–616
17. Ferrer FA, McKenna PH, Bauer B, Miller SF. Accuracy of renal ultrasound measurements for predicting actual kidney size. J Urol 1997; 157: 2278–2281
18. Bisset GS, Strife JL. The duplex collecting system in girls with urinary tract infection prevalence and significance. AJR Am J Roentgenol 1987; 148: 497–500
19. Haines DS, Bates CM, Ingraham S et al. Management and etiology of the unilateral multicystic dysplastic kidney: a review. Pediatr Nephrol 2009; 24: 233–241
20. Refai Z, El-Rifai R. National audit of the management of antenatal renal pelvis dilatation. Arch Dis Child 2008; 93: 546
21. Assael BM, Guez S, Marra G et al. Congenital reflux nephropathy; a follow-up of 108 cases diagnosed perinatally. Br J Urol 1998; 82: 252–257
22. Tibballs JM, De Bruyn. Primary vesicoureteric reflux – how useful is postnatal ultrasound? Arch Dis Child 1996; 75: 444–478
23. Zerin JM, Ritchey ML, Chang CCH. Incidental vesicoureteral reflux in neonates with antenatally detected hydronephrosis and other renal abnormalities. Radiology 1993; 187: 157–160
24. Mackenzie S. Radiological investigation of paediatric UTI. Imaging 2001; 13: 285–294
25. Dacher JN, Pfister C, Monroe M et al. Power Doppler sonographic pattern of acute pyelonephritis in children: comparison with CT. AJR Am J Roentgenol 1996; 166: 1451–1455
26. Ritchey ML, Shamberger RC, Hamilton T et al. Fate of bilateral renal lesions missed on preoperative imaging: A report from the National Wilms Tumor Study Group. J Urol 2005; 174: 1519–1521
27. Scott DJ, Wallace WHB, Hendry GMA. With advances in medical imaging can the radiologist reliably diagnose Wilms' tumours? Clin Radiol 1999; 54: 321–327
28. Lau KK, Stoffman JM, Williams S et al. Neonatal renal vein thrombosis: Review of the English language literature between 1992 and 2006. Pediatrics 2007; 120: 1270–1284
29. Kaste SC, McCarville MB. Imaging pediatric abdominal tumors. Semin Roentgenol 2008; 43: 50–59
30. Felc Z. Ultrasound in screening for neonatal adrenal haemorrhage. Am J Perinatol 1995; 12: 363-366
31. Steffens J, Zaubitzer T, Kirsch W, Humke U. Neonatal adrenal abscesses. Eur Urol 1997; 31: 347-349
32. Pauravi V. Ultrasound evaluation of acute abdominal emergencies in infants and children. Radiol Clin North Am 2004; 42: 445–456
33. Hernanz-Schulman M. Infantile hypertrophic pyloric stenosis. Radiology 2003; 227: 319–331
34. Strouse PJ. Sonographic evaluation of the child with lower abdominal or pelvic pain. Radiol Clin North Am 2006; 44: 911–923
35. Chan KL, Saing H, Peh WCG et al. Childhood intussusception: ultrasound-guided Hartmann's solution hydrostatic reduction or Barium enema reduction? J Pediatr Surg 1997; 32: 3–6
36. Applegate KE. Intussusception in children: imaging choices. Semin Roentgenol 2008; 43: 15–21
37. Lampl B, Levin TL, Berdon WE et al. Malrotation and midgut volvulus: a historical review and current controversies in diagnosis and management. Pediatr Radiol 2009; 39: 359–366
38. Pracros P, Sann L, Genin G et al. Ultrasound diagnosis of midgut volvulus: the 'whirlpool' sign. Pediatr Radiol 1992; 22: 18–20
39. Puig S, Staudenherz A, Felder-Puig R Imaging of appendicitis in children and adolescents: useful or useless? A comparison of imaging techniques and a

critical review of the current literature. Semin Roentgenol 2008; 43: 22–28

General reading

Applegate KE. Seminars in roentgenology. 2008; 43: 1–82

Carty H, Brunelle F, Stringer DA, Kao SCS. Imaging children, 2nd edn. Churchill Livingston, Edinburgh, 2005

Siegel MJ. Pediatric sonography, 3rd edn. Lippincott Williams & Wilkins, Philadelphia, 2002

Stringer DA, Babyn PS. Pediatric gastrointestinal imaging and intervention. BC Decker, Ontario, 2000

Ultrasound of the acute abdomen

10

CHAPTER CONTENTS

INTRODUCTION

Ultrasound continues to play a vital role in the initial evaluation of the acute abdomen. Ultrasound may be used as a first line investigation in order to make a definitive diagnosis (such as in acute cholecystitis in RUQ pain) or can be used as a triage tool to direct subsequent patient management appropriately. As with all ultrasound techniques, the value of the test is in the high sensitivity and specificity provided by a trained, experienced operator.

The introduction of smaller, portable and hand-held ultrasound machines has greatly increased the accessibility of ultrasound which is potentially useful in emergency situations. However, this is only the case if the scanning technique is adequate, as untrained operators may potentially seriously misdirect or delay appropriate management. Small hand-held machines are usually of suitable quality to perform a limited examination – for example looking for hydronephrosis, free fluid or guiding drainage – but the image quality is inferior to that of the more expensive, larger machines and the operator must take care to understand and recognize the limitations of the image in order to avoid misinterpretation.

CT has become increasingly accessible in most trauma centres, and has the advantage of demonstrating structures not demonstrable on ultrasound. This means that trauma victims with multiple injuries are often best served by immediate and comprehensive CT. However, the risk to the patient from the radiation dose must be carefully balanced by the potential benefit of the diagnostic process.[1] Women with probable gynaecological pain, some paediatrics and the acutely ill, unstable patients are likely to benefit from a comprehensive ultrasound examination by a trained practitioner with good-quality equipment.

The accuracy of the ultrasound scan is directly attributable to the skill and experience of the operator.[2] For instance, a detailed knowledge of the anatomy, and therefore potential communications, of the peritoneal and retroperitoneal fascial spaces is essential in order to understand the significance and likely origin of an abdominal fluid collection. A left iliac fluid collection may simply be due to local causes such as a diverticular abscess, but could be the result of fluid tracking from a leaking aortic aneurysm or an acutely inflamed or ruptured pancreas.

A further significant advantage of ultrasound is that it is usually an 'interactive' process. Asking the patient to locate the pain directs the operator to the underlying pathology, for example in acute bowel inflammation or acute cholecystitis. Clinical signs, such as *erythema ab igne* which results from pain relief by the patient applying a hot water bottle to the symptomatic area, may also help to focus the examination. The operator should be alert to potential clues and be prepared to step outside standard scanning protocols, adapting to the many possible presentations of trauma or other acute abdominal conditions. Many of the following conditions are dealt with in other relevant chapters, but there are issues that are specific to the patient who presents acutely.

TRAUMA

Blunt or penetrating trauma to the torso, frequently due to a road traffic accident (RTA) or other forms of accident or violence, is a frequent cause of referral to most emergency departments. Internal organ injury as a result of trauma is extremely difficult to assess clinically, especially as many patients are admitted unconscious or in a highly unstable condition. Such trauma patients may require emergency laparotomy and ultrasound has been shown to be an invaluable tool in the triage process.[3,4] CT has the advantage of being able to recognize other injuries which may be present, such as bony, spinal or retroperitoneal trauma which may not be accessible to ultrasound investigation, and is often the first choice for imaging in multiple injury trauma patients.

FAST

FAST (focused assessment with sonography for trauma) has become widely adopted in many trauma centres. This system uses a limited scan by emergency physicians to identify the presence of free fluid on ultrasound. Results are highly dependent on proper training, and a number of standardized training and accreditation programmes have been devised, notably by the American College of Emergency Physicians.[5] FAST scanning involves a minimum four-view examination, principally to detect the presence of fluid which may result from the rupture of internal organs. The four-view scan should include the right and left flanks (for hepatorenal space, perisplenic regions and spaces above and below the diaphragm), the subcostal region (to include the pericardial space) and the pelvis (retrovesical and retrouterine spaces).[6]

Free fluid is associated with numerous types of injury including rupture of the liver, spleen, kidney, pancreas or bowel (Fig. 10.1). Free fluid in the pelvis may be difficult to detect (due to overlying bowel and underfilled bladder) unless the patient is put into the Trendelenburg position, allowing it to collect in the pelvis under the influence of gravity. Ultrasound is more successful in detecting free fluid than in detecting organ injury directly.[7,8] One study reported a 98% sensitivity for detection of fluid, but only 41% of organ injuries could be demonstrated.[9] FAST has so far failed to demonstrate any population benefit[10] and its use is difficult to support on evidence-based grounds. However, there may be evidence for a reduction in the interval between admission and surgery for some patients, with potential resource benefits.[11]

The published studies have concentrated only on the presence or absence of free fluid, rather than a comprehensive assessment of the abdomen by suitably qualified sonographers. There is a clear case for the latter, especially if the patient is unstable and cannot be moved, as ultrasound is able to offer valuable information about the viscera which can direct management quickly and appropriately.

Visceral rupture

Direct visualization of organ rupture is difficult unless a haematoma or other collection is seen. Laceration or contusion may be demonstrated in the liver, kidneys or spleen, but less easily in the pancreas and very infrequently in the bowel. A subtle change in texture may be observed by the experienced operator, or a fine, high reflectivity linear band representing an organ tear (Fig. 10.1B–D). The use of CEUS is particularly helpful in assessing liver and spleen damage, especially in the absence of haematoma or before a haemoperitoneum is established.[12,13]

Small visceral lacerations not visible on ultrasound may become apparent when imaged with CT. In particular, pancreatic damage (often due to the sudden pressure of a seat belt across the abdomen during road accidents) may not be obvious immediately post-trauma on either ultrasound or CT.[14] Damage to the pancreatic duct (Fig. 10.1E) causes leakage of pancreatic fluid into the abdominal cavity, resulting in pancreatitis and

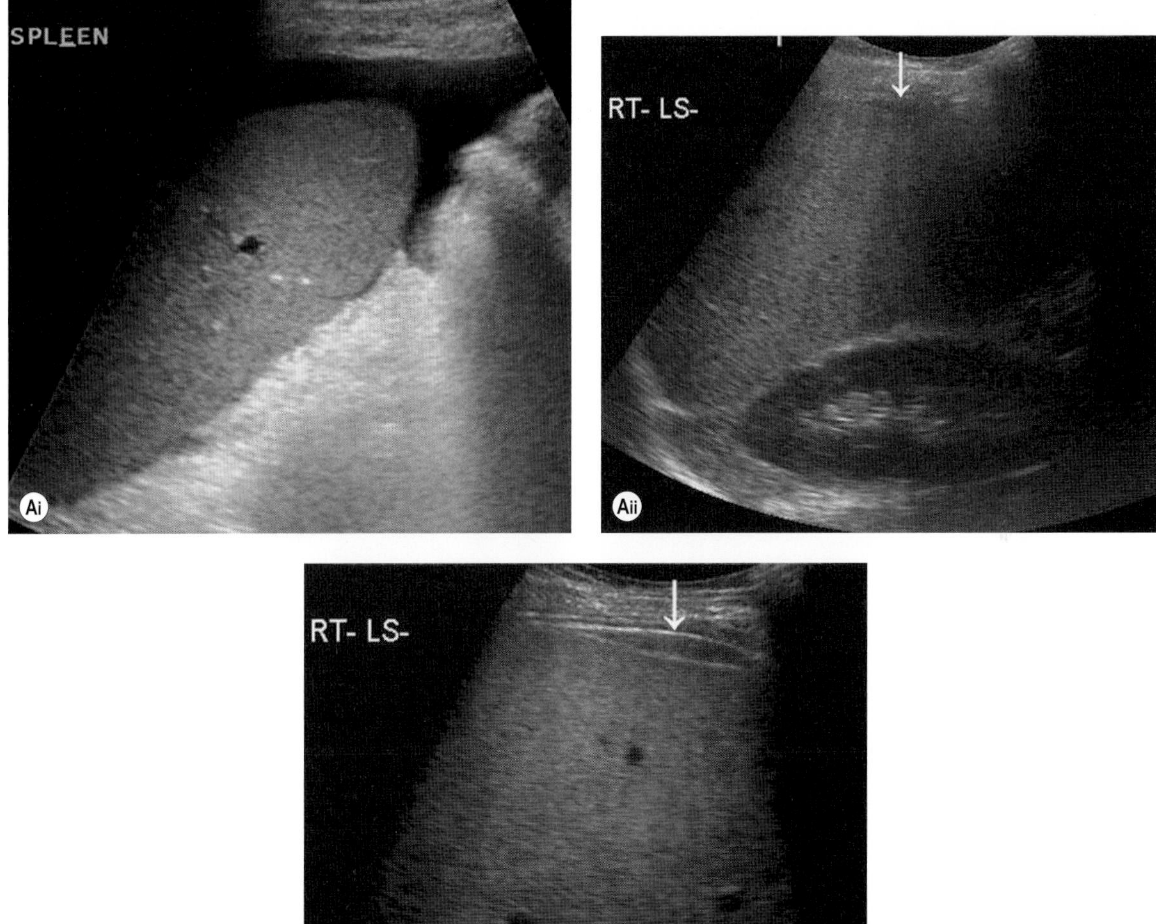

Fig. 10.1 • (Ai) The presence of free fluid in a trauma patient infers organ injury. (Aii) Free fluid may be difficult to detect immediately following trauma. This patient has a trace of free fluid following blunt trauma (arrow) which is more clearly demonstrated. (Aiii) When the focal zone is placed in the near field.

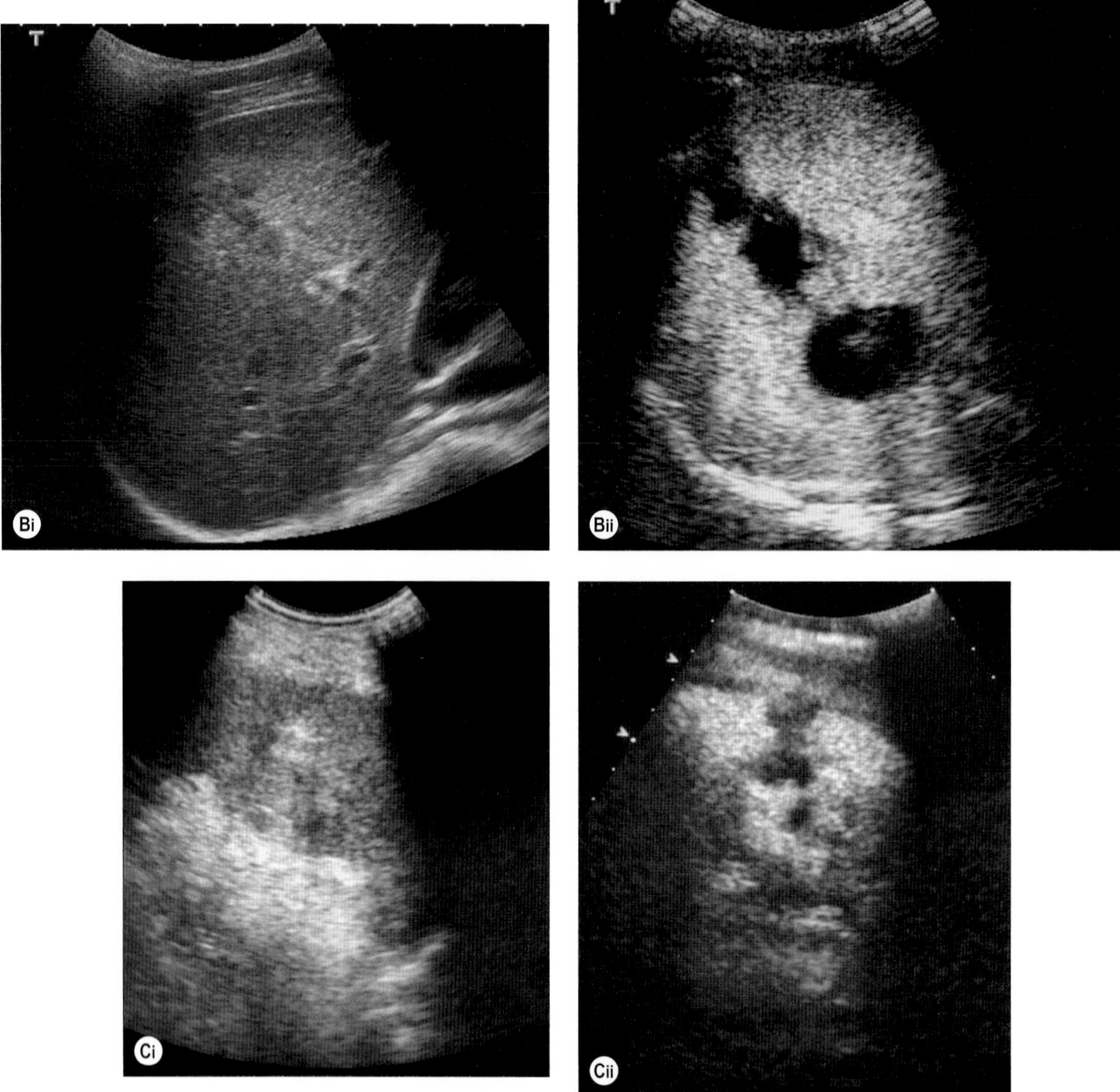

Fig. 10.1, cont'd • (Bi) A patient with a RUQ injury following trauma has altered echotexture in the liver, but no frank haemoperitoneum at this stage. (Bii) CEUS clearly demonstrates the extent of the injury in the sinusoidal phase, as a non-vascular rupture. (Ci) Laceration of the spleen immediately following a road traffic accident demonstrates hardly any free fluid. (Cii) CEUS confirms a splenic laceration which was managed conservatively.

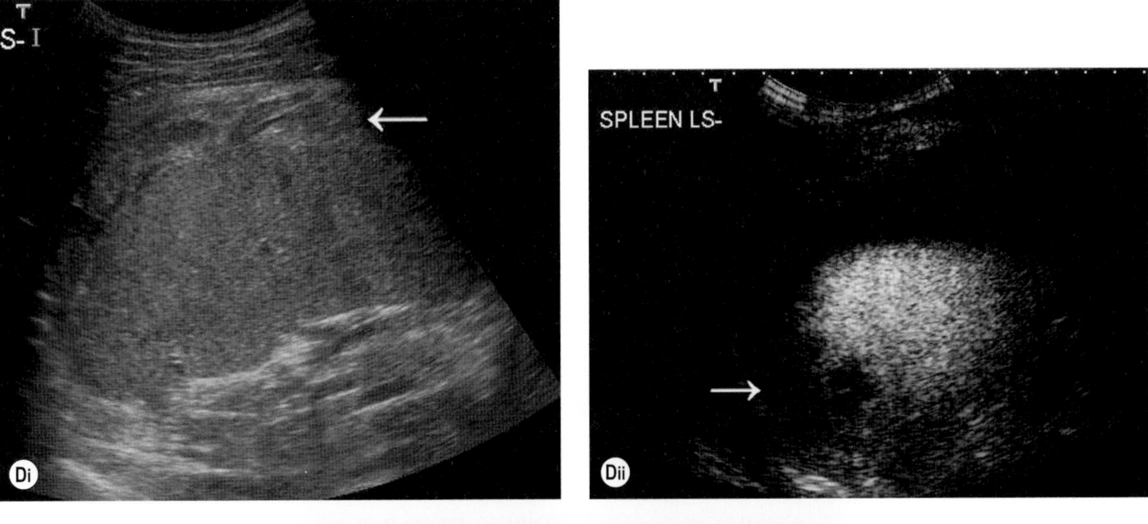

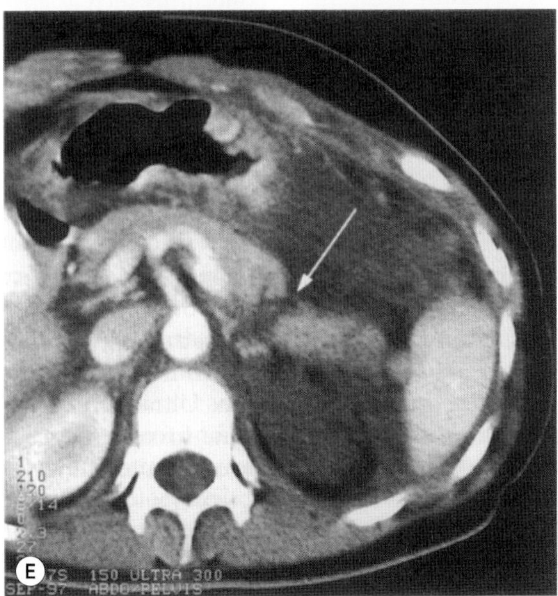

Fig. 10.1, cont'd • (Di) 48 hours after injury a solidifying haematoma (arrow) is seen around the spleen with no free abdominal fluid. (Dii) CEUS demonstrates the injury at the dome of the spleen (arrow). (E) CT demonstrating pancreatic fracture (arrow) in the tail of pancreas following a road traffic accident. Ultrasound was not able to demonstrate the fracture but did demonstrate free fluid following the accident and also diagnosed devascularisation of the left kidney (no Doppler flow within the kidney) following a severed left renal artery, also confirmed on CT.

possible pseudocyst formation or peritonitis. Free fluid may be present as the result of vessel, rather than organ, rupture. A reduction or loss of blood flow to all or part of the relevant organ, for example the kidney, may be demonstrated using colour and power Doppler ultrasound or CEUS.

The finding of free fluid in women should prompt a detailed scan of the pelvis where possible. Gynaecological masses may rupture or haemorrhage, presenting acutely, and in women of childbearing age ectopic pregnancy should be included in the list of differential diagnoses.

When visceral trauma is treated conservatively, follow-up ultrasound may be used to monitor the resolution of any fluid collections or haematoma.

GASTROINTESTINAL TRACT

Most acute presentations of gastrointestinal tract pathology are due to obstruction or inflammation (see Chapter 8). Appendicitis, and its possible complications, is one of the most common reasons for referral (see also Chapter 8) (Fig. 10.2). Ultrasound has a high sensitivity for acute appendicitis, particularly in children. Although the detailed assessment of the primary gastrointestinal pathology usually requires evaluation by an experienced operator with a high-frequency linear probe, many useful indicators can be found with the basic curvilinear abdominal probe.

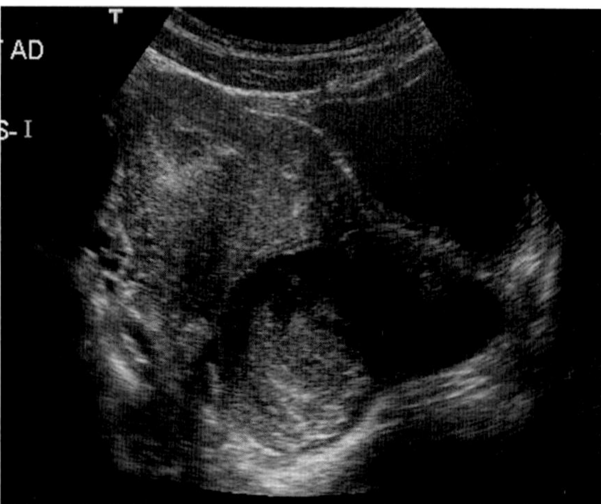

Fig. 10.2 • An appendiceal abscess in a patient with acute abdominal pain.

Dilated loops of fluid-filled bowel, which may also show 'overactive' peristalsis, should alert the operator to the possibility of acute intestinal obstruction. Such segments frequently lie proximal to the obstructing lesion, and so the point at which they appear to end should be the subject of detailed examination. Ultrasound is highly accurate in demonstrating obstruction. However, it is less successful in finding its cause and contrast CT or other bowel studies are usually undertaken when obstruction is diagnosed.

With both intestinal obstruction and focal pain it may be necessary to examine the hernial orifices. A small but symptomatic epigastric hernia often goes unnoticed unless a detailed, high frequency scan of the abdominal wall is performed. Fluid collections such as abscesses may also point to the diseased segment, for example in Crohn's disease or acute diverticulitis. Such inflammatory bowel conditions may well present with an established history, which helps the operator to focus the ultrasound examination accordingly.

Perforation of an abdominal viscus can produce small amounts of ascites. This is usually 'mucky', i.e. containing particulate or gas bubble echoes, and may be localized close to the perforation site, around the duodenum or within the lesser sac. Although gas is usually regarded as an obstacle to ultrasound diagnosis, recent studies have shown that specific patterns of gas echoes can make ultrasound more sensitive than plain radiography in the diagnosis of pneumoperitoneum.[15]

HEPATO-BILIARY EMERGENCIES

Ultrasound scanning is invariably the first-line investigation for suspected biliary tract emergencies. These include inflammatory conditions causing RUQ and epigastric pain, mostly acute cholecystitis or gallstone pancreatitis, and the various causes of obstructive jaundice (Fig. 10.3). If possible, interventional treatment should be delayed until a detailed imaging assessment of the cause of biliary obstruction has been made, since the presence of a biliary stent can compromise subsequent imaging by CT, MRI or EUS. Similarly, biliary stents frequently cause bile duct wall thickening and may introduce gas into the biliary tree. These will prevent the diagnosis of cholangitis or ductal calculi with ultrasound, and may impede

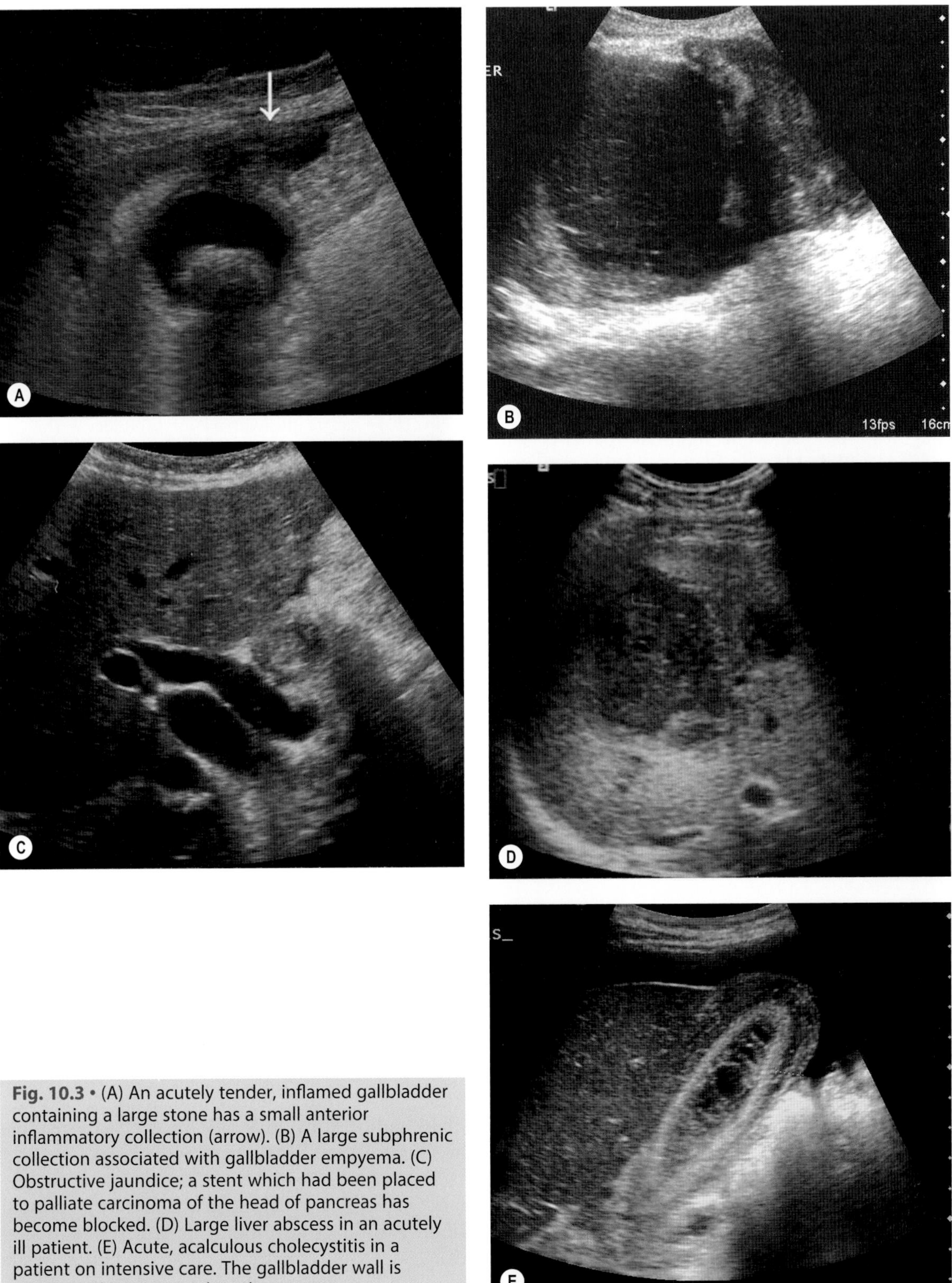

Fig. 10.3 • (A) An acutely tender, inflamed gallbladder containing a large stone has a small anterior inflammatory collection (arrow). (B) A large subphrenic collection associated with gallbladder empyema. (C) Obstructive jaundice; a stent which had been placed to palliate carcinoma of the head of pancreas has become blocked. (D) Large liver abscess in an acutely ill patient. (E) Acute, acalculous cholecystitis in a patient on intensive care. The gallbladder wall is grossly oedematous and tender.

detailed Doppler investigation of, for example, the portal vein.

There is an increasing trend towards less invasive diagnostic and therapeutic procedures, which has improved the mortality rate from biliary emergencies. The use of MRCP and EUS can avoid a diagnostic ERCP.[16] If urgent biliary drainage is required, particularly when the bile is infected, this can quickly be effected by endoscopic stent placement or sphincterotomy.[17] Endoscopic sphincterotomy and stone extraction have been found to be preferable to surgery, particularly in cases of severe gallstone pancreatitis where patients may be poor operative risks[18] and in cases of stone-related cholangitis.

Ultrasound-guided bedside cholecystostomy may also be useful in high-risk patients with infected gallbladders and is an effective treatment for acalculous cholecystitis brought on by prolonged post-operative fasting.[19]

The liver itself may be acutely tender in systemic venous congestion due to cardiac failure, acute hepatitis, or the presence of an intrahepatic abscess. The management of liver abscesses is determined by their size, number and cause. Ultrasound is used to guide diagnostic aspiration and drainage procedures, and most types of hepatic abscess can be treated successfully using these techniques combined with appropriate antibiotics therapy.

THE ACUTE PANCREAS (see also Chapter 5)

Most cases of acute pancreatitis are suspected clinically, with raised amylase levels and often a history of recurrent epigastric pain pointing to the diagnosis of acute pancreatitis (Fig. 10.4). Although pancreatitis may be due to abdominal trauma, it is more frequently due to gallstone obstruction or alcohol abuse. The pancreas often appears normal even when acutely inflamed, so ultrasound examination should focus on the possible causes (such as gallstones, biliary dilatation or evidence of alcoholic liver disease) and complications (pseudocysts, portal or splenic vein thrombosis). MRCP and EUS offer an accurate and less invasive diagnosis than ERCP, which is reserved for therapeutic stone removal or stent placements.[20]

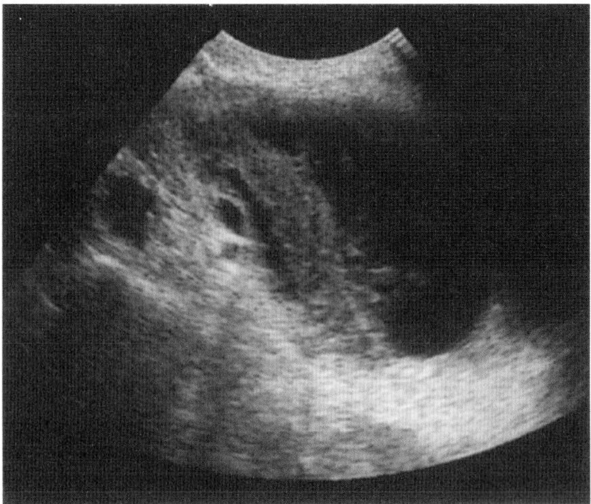

Fig. 10.4 • Pancreatitis with a large pseudocyst. The patient was acutely tender and the cyst was drained under ultrasound guidance.

Many pancreatic pseudocysts are now managed successfully by endoscopic ultrasound-guided transgastric drainage.[21]

RENAL TRACT EMERGENCIES (see also Chapter 7)

Ultrasound is the first-line investigation in the assessment of acute loin pain, which in the absence of trauma is commonly due to acute urinary tract obstruction and/or renal infection (Fig. 10.5). Less common acute presentations include renal vein thrombosis or spontaneous haemorrhage – usually from a renal tumour or cyst.

Ultrasound is also useful in assessing patients with acute renal colic due to suspected ureteric calculus, and readily detects stones, obstruction and other causes of pain (Fig. 10.5E). Low-dose unenhanced multislice CT is increasingly the method of choice for locating ureteric calculi,[22,23] but even with this technique diagnostic pitfalls exist.[24] Abdominal ultrasound with or without plain radiography may still provide comparable accuracy where CT resources are limited.[25,26]

The main limitation of ultrasound in acute ureteric obstruction is that obstruction may be present in the early stages without collecting system dilatation. But the minimally dilated renal pelvis, which would normally be dismissed as unremarkable in

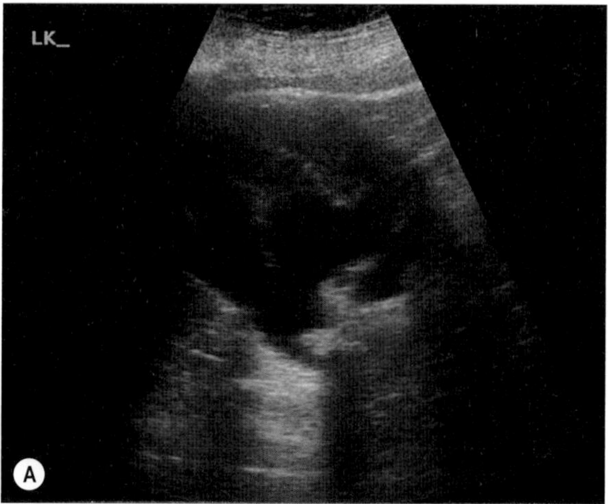

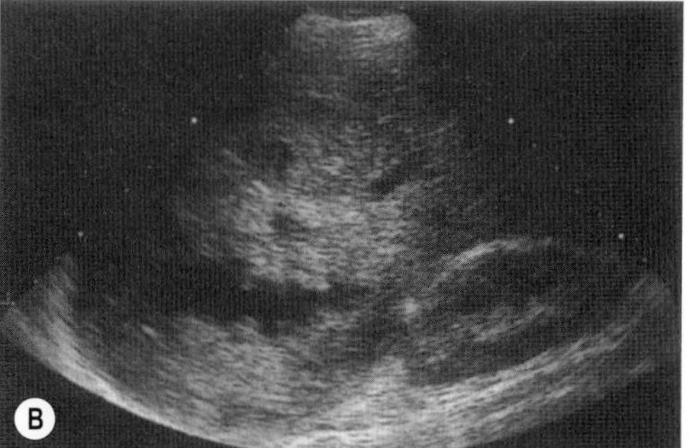

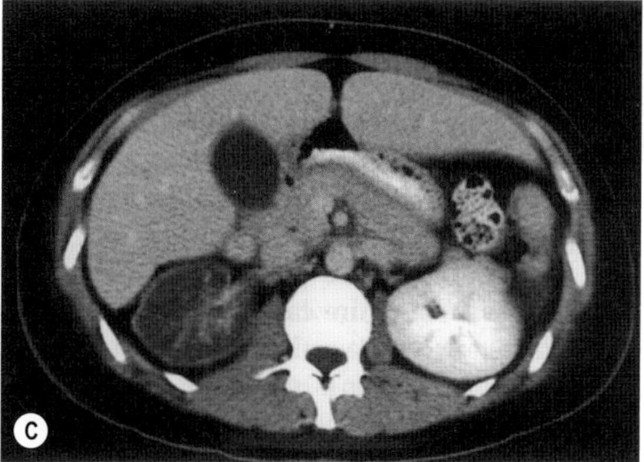

Fig. 10.5 • (A) Obstructed kidney with pelvicalyceal system dilatation and a stone at the pelviureteric junction. (B) Severe laceration to the liver following a road traffic accident. (C) The same patient's CT scan confirms the liver injury and demonstrates an avascular right kidney (compared with the normal LK) due to laceration of the renal vessels.

a patient with a full bladder, should raise the operator's suspicion in the patient with acute loin pain. Doppler ultrasound of the kidneys shows a higher resistance index in the obstructed kidney than in the normal side.[27] Upper tract obstruction can be relieved via cystoscopy-guided ureteric stent placement. Ultrasound-guided percutaneous nephrostomy may be required if this is not practicable, or if there is evidence of infection.

Renal infection with parenchymal involvement (acute pyelonephritis) may be the cause of severe acute loin pain with fever, but ultrasound examination mostly shows no abnormality. Occasionally the skilled operator using high-specification equipment may be able to identify segmental areas of high reflectivity, showing *decreased* blood flow with power Doppler. The diagnosis of this condition is usually based on clinical criteria, but these segments can be demonstrated with CT if necessary.

OTHER RETROPERITONEAL EMERGENCIES (see also Chapter 8)

Ultrasound has an established role in identifying the presence of an abdominal aortic aneurysm, but should not be used to assess subacute leakage or rupture. However where rupture is suspected, and no previous imaging results are available, ultrasound can be a timesaving triage tool to exclude an aneurysm from the differential diagnosis of abdominal pain. Suitable trained emergency department clinical staff can perform this quickly and successfully.[28] Rupture of an aortic aneurysm is a catastrophic event, and although an urgent contrast-enhanced CT can be helpful, emergency surgery based on clinical findings should not be delayed by imaging investigations.

Ultrasound is also the first investigation of choice for demonstrating suspected psoas abscess or haematoma (Fig. 10.6).[29]

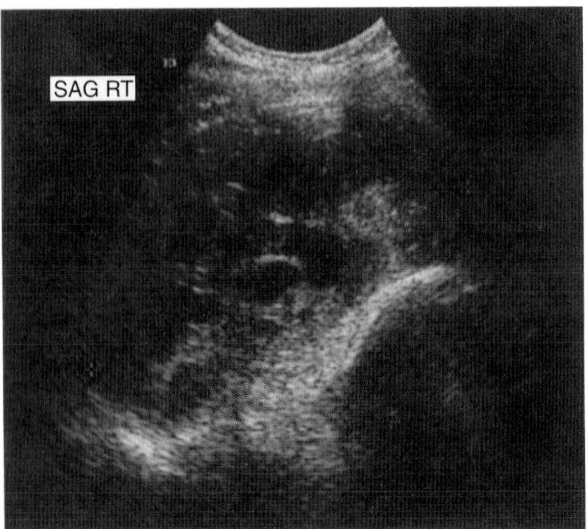

Fig. 10.6 • A large, right-sided psoas haematoma.

References

1. Sodickson A, Baeyens PF, Andriole KP et al. Recurrent CT, cumulative radiation exposure, and associated radiation-induced cancer risks from CT of adults. Radiology 2009; 251: 175–184
2. Forster R, Pillasch J, Zielke A. Ultrasonography in blunt abdominal trauma: influence of the investigator's experience. J Trauma 1993; 34: 264–269
3. Porter RS, Nester BA, Dalsey WC et al. Use of ultrasound to determine the need for laparotomy in trauma patients. Ann Emerg Med 1997; 29: 323–330
4. McGahan JP, Rose J, Coates TL et al. Use of ultrasonography in the patient with acute abdominal trauma. J Ultrasound Med 1997; 16: 653–662
5. American College of Emergency Physicians. Use of ultrasound imaging by emergency physicians [policy statement]. Ann Emerg Med 1997; 30: 364–365
6. Scalea TM, Rodriguez A, Chiu WC et al. Focused assessment with sonography for trauma (FAST): results from an international consensus conference. J Trauma 1999; 46: 466–472
7. Bode PJ, Neizen RA, Van Vugt AB. Abdominal ultrasound as a reliable indicator for conclusive laparotomy in blunt abdominal trauma. J Trauma 1993; 34: 27–31
8. Lentz KA, McKenney MG, Nunez DB et al. Evaluating blunt abdominal trauma. J Ultrasound Med 1996; 15: 447–451
9. Rothlin MA, Naf R, Amgwerd M. Ultrasound in blunt abdominal and thoracic trauma. J Trauma 1993; 34: 488–495
10. Stengel D, Bauwens K, Sehouli J et al. Emergency ultrasound-based algorithms for diagnosing blunt abdominal trauma. Cochrane Database Syst Rev 2005; 2: CD004446
11. Melniker LA, Leibner E, McKenney MG et al. Randomized controlled clinical trial of point-of-care, limited ultrasonography for trauma in the emergency department: the first sonography outcomes assessment program trial. Ann Emerg Med 2006; 48: 227–235
12. Thorelius L. Emergency real-time contrast-enhanced ultrasonography for detection of solid organ injuries. Eur Radiol 2007; 17 Suppl 6: F107–F111
13. Valentino M, Serra C, Pavlica P, Barozzi L. Contrast-enhanced ultrasound for blunt abdominal trauma. Semin Ultrasound CT MR 2007; 28: 130–140
14. Gupta A, Stuhlfaut JW, Fleming KW et al. Blunt trauma of the pancreas and biliary tract: a multimodality imaging approach to diagnosis. Radiographics 2004; 24: 1381–1395
15. Chen SC, Wang HP, Chen WJ et al. Selective use of ultrasonography for the detection of pneumoperitoneum. Acad Emerg Med 2002; 9: 643–645
16. Lee YT, Chan FK, Leung WK et al. Comparison of EUS and ERCP in the investigation with suspected biliary obstruction caused by choledocholithiasis: a randomized study. Gastrointest Endosc 2008; 67: 660–668
17. Lameris JS, Van-Overhagen H. Imaging and intervention in patients with acute right upper quadrant disease. Baillieres Clin Gastroenterol 1995; 9: 21–36
18. Cohen SA, Siegel JH. Biliary tract emergencies: endoscopic and medical management. Crit Care Clin 1995; 11: 273–294
19. Ginat D, Saad WE. Cholecystostomy and transcholecystic biliary access. Tech Vasc Interv Radiol 2008; 11: 2–13
20. Baillie J. Endoscopic therapy in acute recurrent pancreatitis. World J Gastroenterol 2008; 14: 1034–1037
21. Norton ID, Clain JE, Wiersema MJ et al. Utility of endoscopic ultrasonography in endoscopic drainage of pancreatic pseudocysts in selected patients. Mayo Clin Proc 2001; 76: 794–798
22. Tack D, Sourtzis S, Delpierre I et al. Low-dose unenhanced multidetector CT of patients with suspected renal colic. AJR Am J Roentgenol 2003; 180: 305–311
23. Tamm EP, Silverman PM, Shuman WP. Evaluation of the patient with flank pain and possible ureteral calculus. Radiology 2003; 228: 319–329
24. Colistro R, Torreggiani WC, Lyburn ID et al. Unenhanced helical CT in the investigation of acute flank pain. Clin Radiol 2002; 57: 435–441
25. Catalano O, Nunziata A, Altei F, Siani A. Suspected ureteral colic: primary helical CT versus selective helical CT after unenhanced radiography and sonography. AJR Am J Roentgenol 2002; 178: 379–387
26. Patlas M, Farkas A, Fisher D et al. Ultrasound vs CT for the detection of ureteric stones in patients with renal colic. Br J Radiol 2001; 74: 901–904
27. Rodgers PM, Bates JA, Irving HC. Intrarenal Doppler ultrasound studies in normal and acutely obstructed kidneys. Br J Radiol 1992; 65: 207–212
28. Kuhn M, Bonnin RL, Davey MJ et al. Emergency department ultrasound scanning for abdominal aortic aneurysm: accessible, accurate, and advantageous. Ann Emerg Med 2000; 36: 219–223
29. Monnier-Cholley L, Arrive L, Taboury J et al. Non-vascular retroperitoneal emergencies. Ann Radiol (Paris) 1996; 39: 72–77

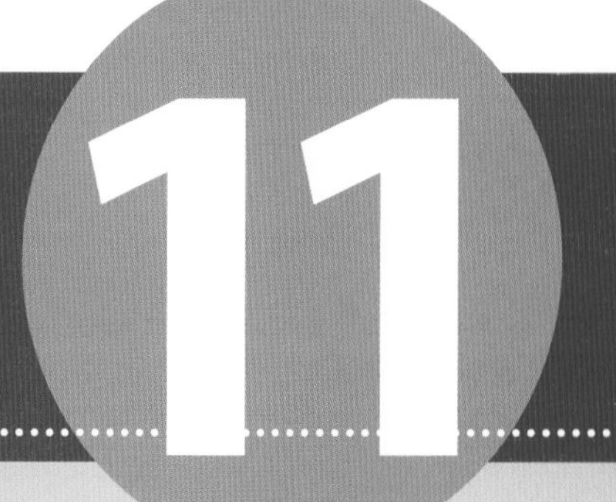

Interventional techniques

Co-written with Grant Baxter

CHAPTER CONTENTS

INTRODUCTION

The use of ultrasound-guided minimally invasive procedures, including diagnostic biopsy, therapeutic drainage and treatment techniques, is accepted and essential practice in the management of many conditions. These minimally invasive methods are responsible for improvements in patient mortality and morbidity, when compared to more invasive options, together with increased patient acceptability and cost effectiveness.

The relative speed and ease with which these procedures can be carried out has resulted in a reduction of the diagnostic laparotomy and more prompt and appropriate patient treatment. While both ultrasound and CT may be used for many of these procedures, in general, ultrasound is often the first-line method as it is effective in the vast majority, generally more accessible, and does not carry a radiation risk. In addition, ultrasound has the advantage of 'real-time' placement, avoiding structures which could otherwise be damaged and effecting accurate and safe placement of the needle or drain.

ULTRASOUND-GUIDED BIOPSY: GENERAL CONSIDERATIONS

Percutaneous biopsy of organs, masses or focal visceral lesions is an integral part of the diagnostic process for many patients. Although changes on ultrasound may confirm the suspected clinical suspicion, i.e. a hyperechoic liver may indicate fatty change, a nodular liver, cirrhosis, or enlarged hyperechoic kidneys or glomerulonephritis, imaging alone is insufficient and frequently non-specific and a definitive histological diagnosis is required. The advantages of using ultrasound to guide such procedures are numerous:

- The needle tip is directed, in real time, along the biopsy path and visualized within the lesion.
- Greater precision is obtained; needle guidance is essential for all small lesions and lesions at depth.
- Fewer needle passes are required to obtain the desired result and so post procedure complications are minimized.
- The best route can be utilized and vital structures, such as blood vessels, avoided.
- Confidence in the biopsy result - particularly a negative one - is increased due to direct visualization of the needle tip in the lesion.
- All the advantages of ultrasound over other imaging methods apply (quick, direct vision, no radiation hazard, low cost). The limitations due to bone and air-filled structures also apply.
- The capability to perform bedside procedures for critically ill patients and to use in conjunction with other imaging techniques, for example fluoroscopy, is advantageous.

With ultrasound the biopsy procedure is quick, safe, accurate and usually acceptable to the patient. There are several accepted methods of performing a guided biopsy, but certain generic rules are common to the procedure, regardless of the organ under investigation.

- A written request form from a medical practitioner with the results of any previous investigations should be available. The reason for biopsy should be appropriate.
- Assessment of blood clotting status – normally the prothrombin time should be within 3 seconds of the control, platelet count >75 000 /mL and INR (international normalized ratio < 1.2).
- Identification of possible contraindications to biopsy. Contraindications are relative and include the biopsy pathway, an uncooperative patient and uncorrectable coagulation, and should be assessed on an individual basis.
- Careful explanation of the procedure to the patient, including risks and benefits.
- Informed consent for the procedure.
- Procedure should be performed in a quiet and clean environment. Infection control measures should be observed, and steps taken to preserve pre-, peri- and post-procedure sterility.
- A pre-biopsy scan is performed to identify a suitable biopsy route avoiding vital structures.
- Satisfactory care of the patient both during and after the biopsy procedure with relevant observations of vital signs. A pulse oximeter and appropriate nurse cover are recommended.
- Appropriate preparation of the specimen.

Analgesia

For the vast majority of biopsy procedures a local anaesthetic is administered following localization of the biopsy site with ultrasound. Lidocaine (1% or 2%) is commonly used; the volume will depend on patient build, depth of lesion, patient anxiety, etc. It is also useful to inject the anaesthesia under ultrasound guidance, so that lidocaine can be targeted exactly to the biopsy route, enabling effective pain relief throughout. Usually a short period of time, commonly 3–4 minutes, is allowed to pass so that the anaesthetic can work, after which, a small scalpel incision is made in the skin to facilitate the biopsy needle's introduction, with little or no discomfort to the patient. In cases of simple aspiration with a 22G needle or smaller, local anaesthetic is usually unnecessary.

Patients who are particularly apprehensive may require pre-procedure medication with a sedative such as diazepam or similar anxiolytic agent, however, this is uncommon. Very occasionally intravenous analgesia and/or sedation may be required during the procedure; it is often a good idea to have an intravenous cannula in situ prior to biopsy.

The use of general anaesthesia for children is common practice to enable the procedure to be carried out quickly and accurately while the child remains still.

Methods of ultrasound guidance

There are various ways of performing ultrasound-guided procedures i.e. guided, freehand or 'blind'. The choice of method depends on the procedure in question, equipment and the experience and skill of the operator.

Blind biopsy

With this method ultrasound may be used to localize a position on the skin surface overlying the organ to be biopsied. This may be acceptable when performing 'blind' biopsies of the liver when only a reflective sample of liver tissue is required. Nevertheless, it is good practice even in these situations, to visualize the needle during the procedure.

Biopsy guidance

Most manufacturers provide a biopsy guide which fits snugly onto the transducer head and provides a rigid pathway for the needle (Fig. 11.1) These are now common and a widely accepted method of biopsy. The fixed biopsy guide contains a groove for a series of plastic inserts ranging from 14G to 22G size, depending upon the size of the biopsy needle. It is usual to use one size greater than the needle (i.e. a 16G insert for an 18G needle) as the needle tends to move more freely. The guide is sterilized and fitted onto the transducer over a sterile sheath.

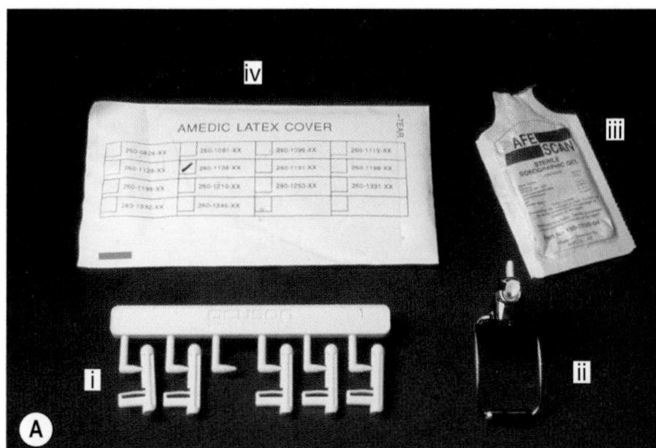

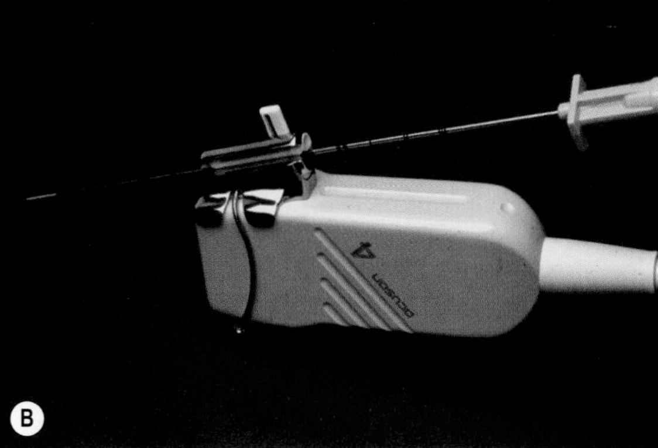

Fig. 11.1 • (A) Necessary component parts to perform an ultrasound-guided biopsy procedure. A series of plastic inserts (Ai) range in size from 14G to 22G. The appropriate insert is inserted into a fixed biopsy guide (Aii). The procedure is performed with sterile jelly (Aiii) and a sterile probe cover (Aiv) if required.
(B) The assembled biopsy guide.

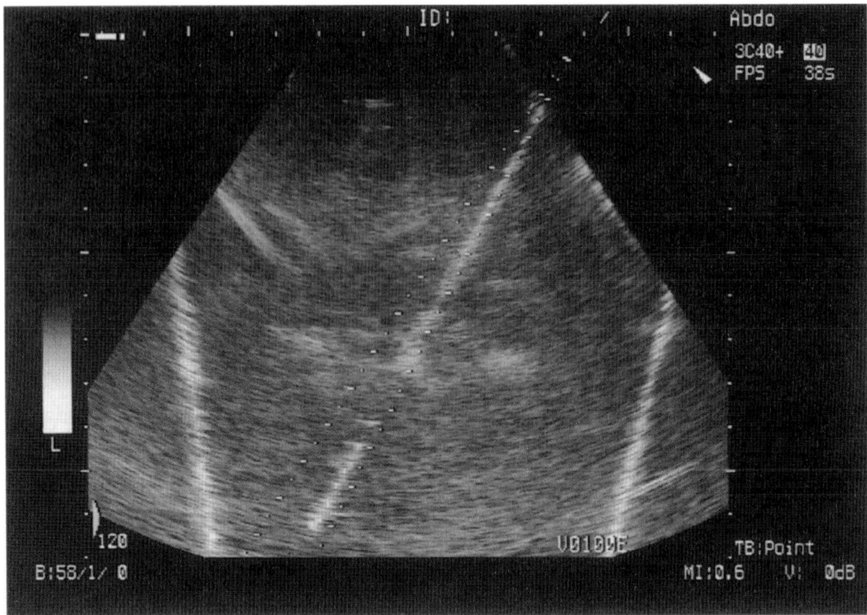

Fig. 11.2 • Testing the alignment of the biopsy guide. The electronic pathway is activated on the image and the needle is scanned as it is passed into a jug of water.

The needle pathway is displayed on the ultrasound monitor electronically – as a line or narrow sector – through which the needle passes. The operator then scans in order to align the electronic pathway along the chosen route, the needle inserted, and the biopsy taken. These attachments should be tested regularly to ensure the needle follows the correct path (Fig. 11.2).

Freehand

A freehand approach, in which the operator scans with one hand and introduces the needle near to the transducer with the other, may be used for larger or more superficial lesions. This technique is commonly used for breast biopsy and biopsy in the head and neck. The needle is inserted from one end of the probe. Generally speaking the angle utilized is shallow in comparison with the fixed guide systems for deeper structures. This technique is also used for drainages.

Equipment and needles

The core of tissue for histological analysis is obtained with a specially designed needle consisting of an inner needle with a chamber or recess for the tissue sample and an outer, cutting needle which moves over it i.e. the Tru-cut needle. The biopsy is obtained in two stages – first the inner needle is advanced into the tissue, then the outer cutting sheath is advanced over it and the needle withdrawn containing the required tissue core (Fig. 11.3). The use of a spring-loaded 'gun' to operate these needles is now commonplace (Fig. 11.4). It is designed to enable operation of the needle with one hand, (whilst being able to hold the probe

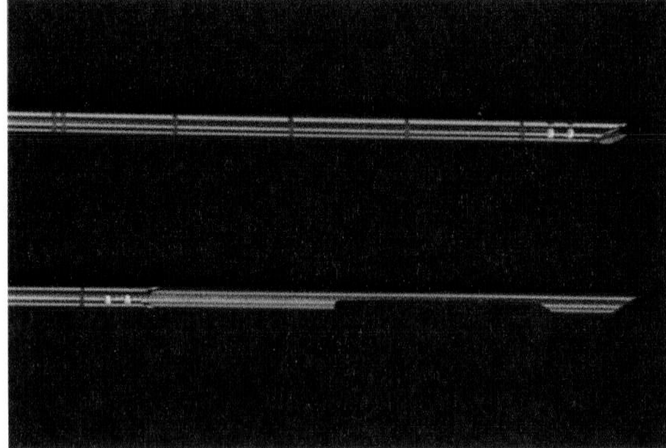

Fig. 11.3 • Biopsy needle closed (top) and open (bottom).

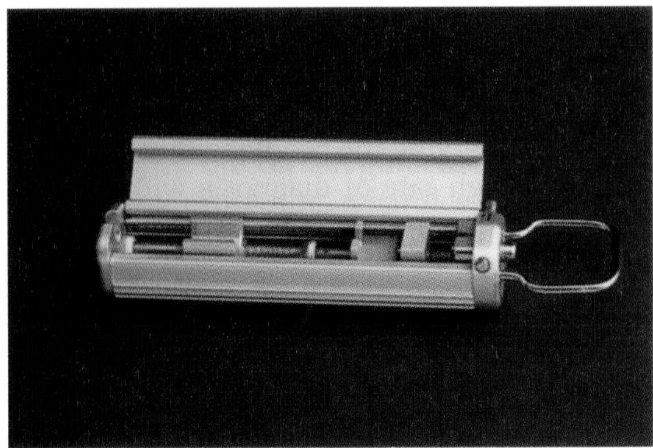

Fig. 11.4 • Non-disposable spring-loaded gun designed to operate the cutting needle.

with the other) and has the advantage of being sterile and disposable.

The whole needle is advanced into the tissue, just in front of the area to be biopsied. By pressing the spring-loaded control, the inner part is quickly advanced into the lesion, followed rapidly by the cutting sheath over it. Needles can be obtained in a variety of sizes, generally 14, 16, 18 or 20G. Most focal lesions are biopsied with a standard 18G needle. As a general principle, as the needle advances approximately 1.5–2.0 cm during biopsy, it is advisable to position the needle tip on the edge of a lesion to obtain a good histological sample as most lesion necrosis tends to be centrally located. Because the gun enables the operator to scan with one hand and biopsy with the other, the needle can be observed within the lesion, yielding a high rate of diagnosis with a single pass technique,[1] and minimizing post-biopsy complications.

Fine needle histology, involving the use of needles of 21G or less, reduces even further the possibility of post-procedure complications. These are generally not used as only small amounts of tissue are obtained for analysis and as thin needles they are apt to bend more easily, and are therefore more difficult to see and retain within the plane of the scan. Biopsy of deep lesions is therefore more difficult if not impossible.

Fine needle aspiration cytology

Cytology is the analysis of cells rather than a core of tissue obtained for histology. This is generally more difficult to interpret pathologically, as the characteristic architecture and intercellular relationships seen in a histological sample are absent. It has the advantage, however, of allowing a finer needle to be used which can be passed through structures, e.g. the stomach, blood vessels, on route to the site of interest, with no adverse effects.

Fine needles for cytology are of size 21G or smaller. They are of a simple design with a bevelled, hollow core and no cutting mechanism. The needle is introduced under ultrasound guidance to the required position. Fragments of tissue are removed into the needle by applying negative (sucking) pressure with a syringe to the needle, while moving the needle to and fro to loosen the tissue. These can then be expelled onto a microscope slide and smeared. The main disadvantage of this technique is that it requires a highly trained and specialized pathologist to interpret the samples (whereas all trained pathologists can view histological specimens). In addition for many conditions histological diagnosis is required, although cytology remains a useful tool in the breast and thyroid.

ULTRASOUND-GUIDED BIOPSY PROCEDURES

Liver biopsy

The most common reason for ultrasound-guided biopsy is for metastatic disease. The liver is one of the most common sites for metastases and histology may be required to confirm the diagnosis, or, more usually, to identify the origin of an unknown primary lesion (Figs 11.5–11.7). Biopsy of suspected HCCs is generally avoided, as it is associated with a poorer treatment outcome and there is a small risk of tumour seeding. CEUS and/or MRI can now characterize many lesions, avoiding the need for biopsy in an increasing number of cases. Focal lesion biopsy is generally safely and accurately performed with an 18G needle which yields reliable tissue for histological analysis. In general, an accuracy of 96% should be achievable.[2]

In addition to focal lesion biopsy another common reason for liver biopsy is to assess the presence/absence of parenchymal liver disease, severity of disease and where appropriate, the aetiology of the disease process. This is often performed in patients with abnormal liver function tests with no evidence of biliary obstruction. The

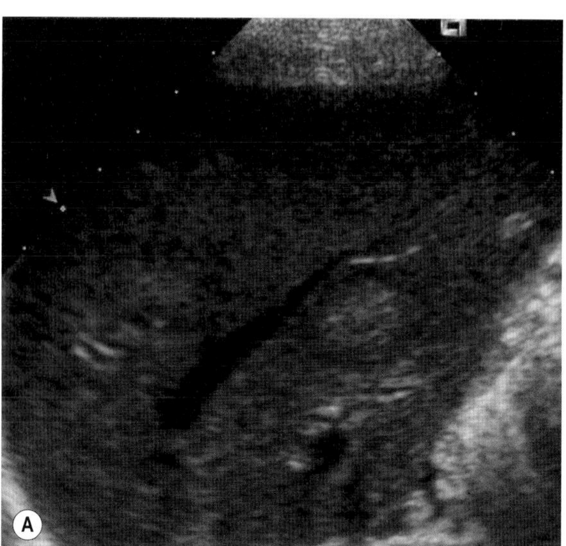

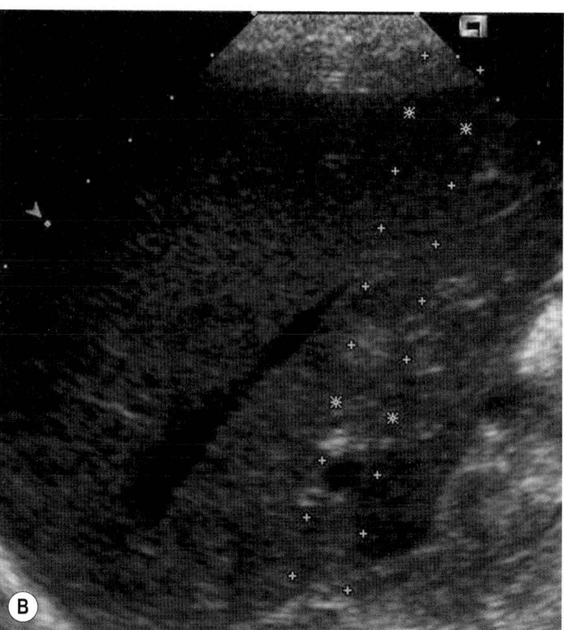

Fig. 11.5 • (A) A liver lesion is identified in the right lobe prior to biopsy. (B) A route is chosen avoiding the adjacent hepatic vein.

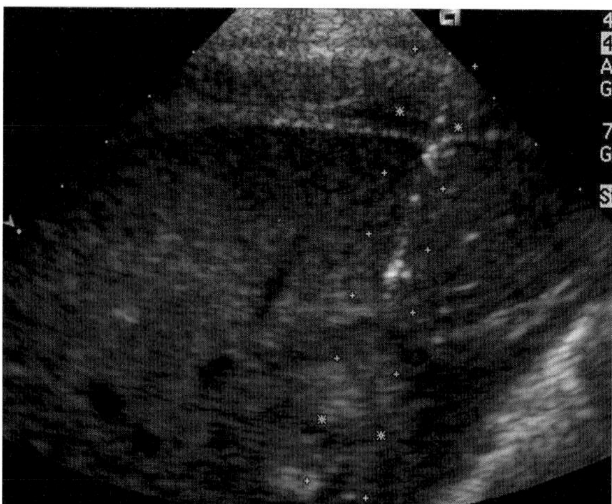

Fig. 11.6 • The needle is introduced into the liver, just in front of the lesion under ultrasound guidance.

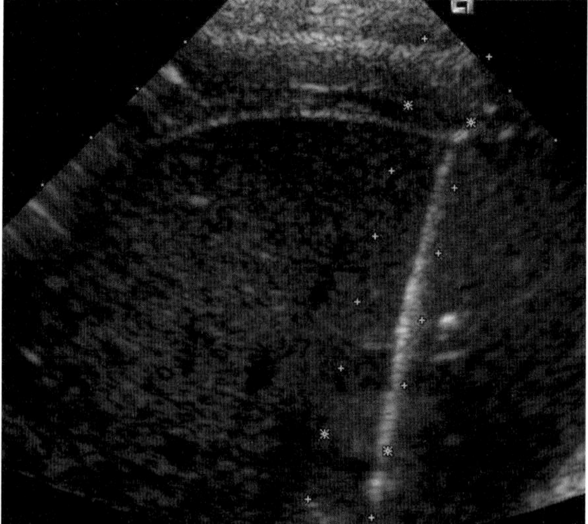

Fig. 11.7 • The gun is fired, propelling the needle tip into the lesion . This visually confirms the biopsy has been taken from the correct area.

clinical history and serological analysis can be helpful in determining aetiology however biopsy is often required. This is usually performed with a 14G or 16G Tru-cut needle. Often the liver is simply identified with ultrasound and a suitable mark made on the skin, often in the mid axillary line and the biopsy performed through the right lobe. Although this is acceptable for this type of biopsy, ultrasound guidance during the procedure is still preferable to the 'blind' technique in order to avoid large vessels and reduce the subsequent risk of haematoma. Biopsy may also be performed

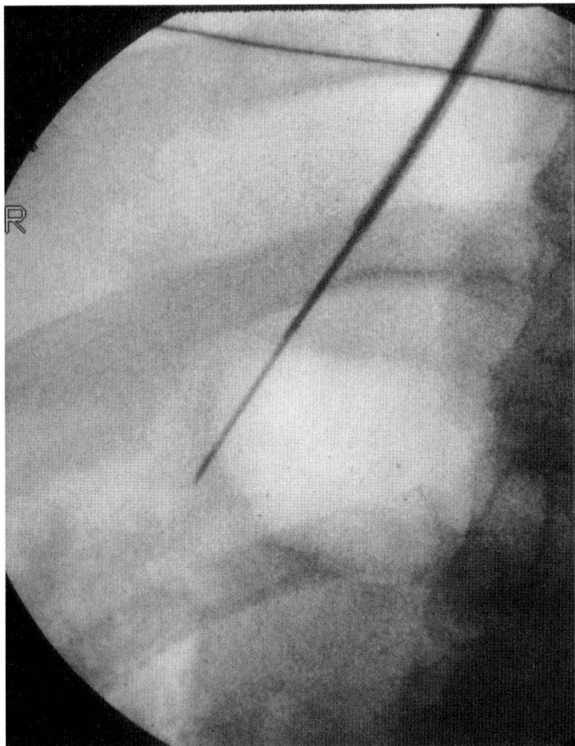

Fig. 11.8 • Transjugular biopsy of the liver. Access is via the right internal jugular vein, through the right atrium and into the IVC and hepatic veins. Once the catheter is wedged in the hepatic vein the cutting needle is released and a biopsy is taken.

for patients with suspected rejection following hepatic transplantation.

Where coagulation profiles are not correctable (and most generally are) liver biopsy can be performed using a 'plugged' technique or, more commonly, by the transjugular route (Fig. 11.8).

Pancreatic biopsy

The commonest reason for biopsy of the pancreas is in patients presenting with obstructive jaundice due to a mass in the head of the gland. A fine needle technique enables the mass to be accessed through the stomach and left lobe of liver without complications, however, an 18G needle biopsy is advisable to try to reduce false-negative results due to the well-known situation of a carcinoma being associated with an element of peripheral inflammation. Pancreatic biopsies are often better performed under CT control (Fig. 11.9) particularly when lesions are small, patients big and/or the lesion is difficult to identify with ultrasound. In those patients with negative biopsies very often interval CT scans are performed to see if the lesion is static or progressive.

Native kidney biopsy

Histology is frequently required in order to direct further management of diffuse renal disease. Biopsy of solid, renal masses are rarely performed as the diagnosis of renal cell or transitional cell carcinoma is usually clear from imaging. Biopsies are still performed, however, in those patients who are not having surgery to confirm the diagnosis, as this is often required prior to chemotherapy or new therapeutic regimens.

Biopsy of the native kidney is performed in the majority of centres under ultrasound guidance. Contraindications to biopsy include hydronephrosis, which may be more appropriately treated with catheterization or nephrostomy, or small kidneys, i.e. <8 cm longitudinal axis, these appearances being indicative of chronic renal impairment. Kidneys >9 cm can potentially be biopsied, however, other factors including cortical thickness, age, clinical history and the requirement for definitive diagnosis will all have a bearing on whether biopsy is performed or not. Hydronephrosis and kidney size are easily assessable with a pre-biopsy scan.

In most cases the biopsy is performed with the patient prone over a small bolster to maximize access to the kidney. The shortest route, avoiding adjacent structures, is selected – subcostally, traversing the cortex of the lower pole and avoiding the collecting system and major vessels is recommended. With ultrasound guidance, either kidney may be chosen and accessibility will vary between patients. The depth of penetration and angle of approach are carefully assessed. Biopsy is normally with a 16G needle.

The patient's cooperation is required in suspending respiration at the crucial moment. This avoids undue damage to the kidney as the needle is introduced through the capsule. The needle should be positioned just within the capsule prior to biopsy so that the maximum amount of cortical tissue is obtained for analysis as the throw of the needle may be up to 2 cm (Fig. 11.10).

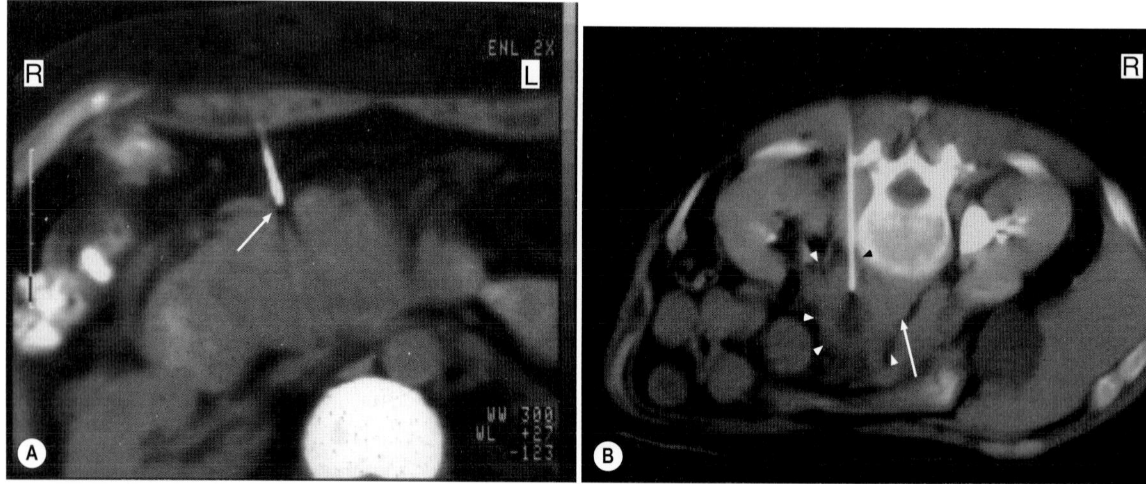

Fig. 11.9 • (A) CT-guided biopsy of a pancreatic head mass. The tip of the biopsy needle (arrow) is positioned in the periphery of the lesion so that when the biopsy is taken a good core of tissue is obtained. Note the artefact from the needle tip. (B) CT-guided biopsy of a retroperitoneal lymph node mass (arrowheads). The mass lies adjacent to the aorta (arrow) however this is protected from the needle by the angle of approach and its relationship to the vertebral body. CT is the preferred biopsy method of choice for deep structures within the retroperitoneum.

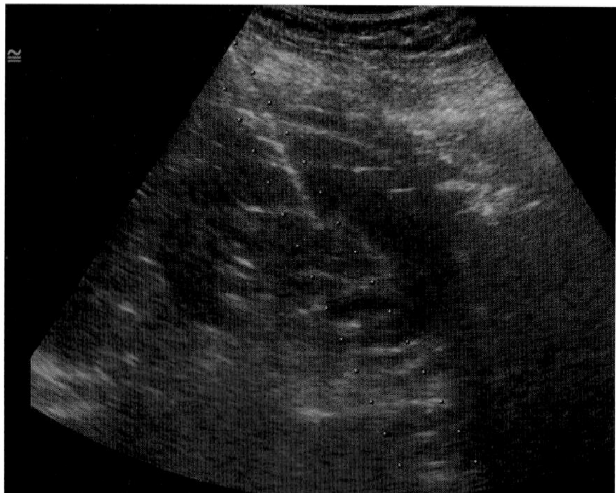

Fig. 11.10 • Ultrasound-guided biopsy of the native left kidney. The tip of the needle was positioned on the outer aspect of the kidney. With a 2 cm jump of the needle on firing, a good core of renal parenchyma is obtained.

Renal transplant biopsy

Biopsy is a valuable tool in the post-operative management of a transplant recipient (Chapter 7), enabling the cause of graft dysfunction to be identified, in particular differentiating acute tubular necrosis from acute rejection. Ultrasound guidance is essential in order to reduce complications such as haematoma, vascular damage (which may result in an AV fistula or pseudoaneurysm formation) and laceration of the renal collecting system.

A single pass technique, using the spring-loaded biopsy gun with an 18G needle is usually sufficient for histological purposes, however two passes may be required so that electron microscopy and immunofluorescence can also be performed. The procedure is well tolerated by the patient and the complication rate low at less than 5%.[3]

A full scan of the kidney is first performed to highlight potential problems (e.g. perirenal fluid collections) and to establish the safest and most effective route. The transplanted kidney lies in an extraperitoneal position and the chosen route should avoid puncturing the peritoneum, to minimize the risk of infection. Unlike the native kidney, the upper pole of the transplanted kidney is usually chosen to avoid major blood vessels and the ureter, which pass close to the lower pole.

The biopsy aims to harvest glomeruli, and the chosen route should therefore target the renal cortex. An angle is chosen to include the maximum thickness of cortex and where possible, avoid the renal hilum (Fig. 11.11).

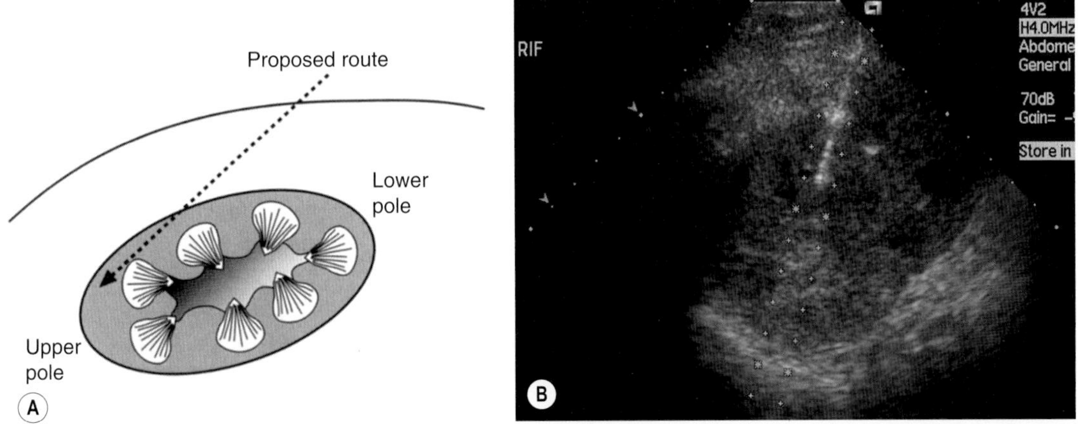

Fig. 11.11 • (A) The transplanted kidney lies in the iliac fossa and is biopsied with the patient supine. (B) The needle is seen entering the cortex of a transplanted kidney.

AUTHOR	YEAR	NUMBER OF BIOPSIES	MORTALITY RATE	MAJOR COMPLICATION
Fornari et al.[4]	1989	10 800	1:5400	1:530
Nolse et al.[6]	1990	8000	1:2700	1:540
Smith[7]	1991	164 000	1:3300	–

Table 11.1 Complications of ultrasound-guided biopsy

COMPLICATIONS OF ULTRASOUND-GUIDED BIOPSY

Post-procedure complications such as haematoma requiring blood transfusion and trauma to adjacent viscera occur very infrequently when ultrasound guidance is used. As expected, the risk of complications is less in fine needle biopsy than with larger needles,[4] however, there is no significant difference in complication rate between a standard 18G Tru-cut needle and a 22G Chiba needle.[5] The mortality and major complication rates vary but using a standard 18G needle these are approximately 0.018–0.038% and 0.18–0.187%, respectively, mortality being due to haemorrhage in 70%. As a working figure this means the mortality is approximately 1 in 3300–5400 and morbidity 1 in 530 biopsies (Table 11.1).[4,6,7] The risk of haemorrhage is increased in patients with coexistent cirrhosis and is more likely to occur with malignant than benign lesions.[8,9] As with any procedure of this nature, there is a very small risk of infection, which can be minimized by using an aseptic technique.

Tumour seeding of the biopsy tract is an uncommon complication of biopsy and reports of tumour seeding are associated with repeated passes into the mass using large needles. Although much talked about, tumour track seeding is in fact rare occurring in approximately 1 in 20 000 biopsies.[7,10] The best known tumours for this are mesothelioma and hepatoma. Complications following abdominal biopsy are increased with multiple passes and are at least in part related to the skill and experience of the operator.

If the biopsy result is negative or unexpected then a number of scenarios should be considered and include sampling error, poor histological specimen, sonographic or pathological misinterpretation or indeed a true negative finding. A repeat biopsy is sometimes justified.

ULTRASOUND-GUIDED DRAINAGE

Many fluid collections are the result of surgical intervention and often cannot be differentiated apart on ultrasound alone. Diagnostic aspiration is used to establish their exact nature which may include haematoma, lymphocoele, urinoma, biloma, pseudocysts and others.

Post-operative haematomas are usually treated conservatively and tend to resolve spontaneously. Insertion of a drain into such a collection is at high risk of converting the collection into an abscess.

Paracentesis

Drainage of abdominal ascites is most often carried out in terminally ill patients, in whom accumulation of fluid has become uncomfortable, often affecting breathing and mobility, or preceding chemotherapy. Patients with refractory and/or infected ascites also benefit from paracentesis. Ultrasound guidance has the advantage of being able to assess the volume of fluid, selecting a suitable site and a route avoiding bowel and omental deposits (Fig. 11.12A).

Abscess drainage

Ultrasound-guided drainage of abscesses is now the preferred treatment when the collection can be visualized on ultrasound and a safe route chosen. Abscesses may result from post-operative infection, inflammatory bowel conditions, such as Crohn's disease or appendicitis, or other sources of infection, particularly in immunosuppressed patients. Drains come in different sizes and generally the thicker the pus the larger the bore of drain that is required. Whilst aspiration is initially performed to confirm the nature of the collection, very often a drain is left in situ which together with appropriate antibiotic therapy is usually effective. At the very least it normally leads to an improvement in the overall clinical condition to allow treatment and can in itself be a definitive cure.

Ultrasound is particularly useful in cases of hepatic abscesses and in draining the subphrenic, pericolic and subhepatic areas (Fig. 11.12). Superficial collections, usually associated with wound sites, are also readily accessible to ultrasound. Collections obscured by bowel gas are best drained under CT guidance (Fig. 11.13).

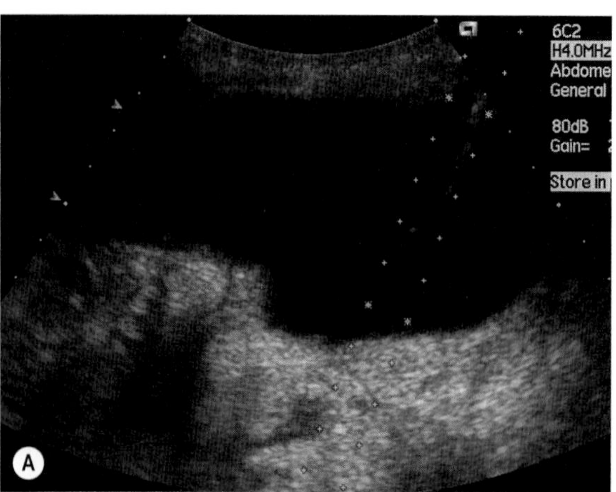

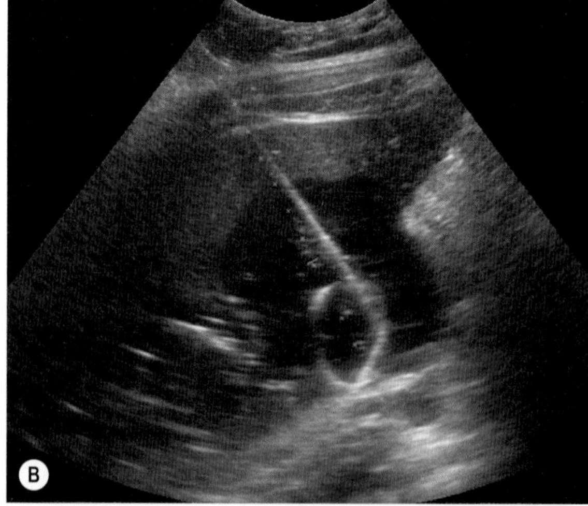

Fig. 11.12 • Ultrasound-guided drainage. (A) Paracentesis under ultrasound guidance. Such procedures are often repeated regularly in the terminally ill and ultrasound guidance facilitates an acceptable, pain-free procedure, focussing the area of local anaesthetic injection and avoiding omental deposits. (B) Post-operative subhepatic collection. This has been accessed with an 18G needle and guidewire inserted.

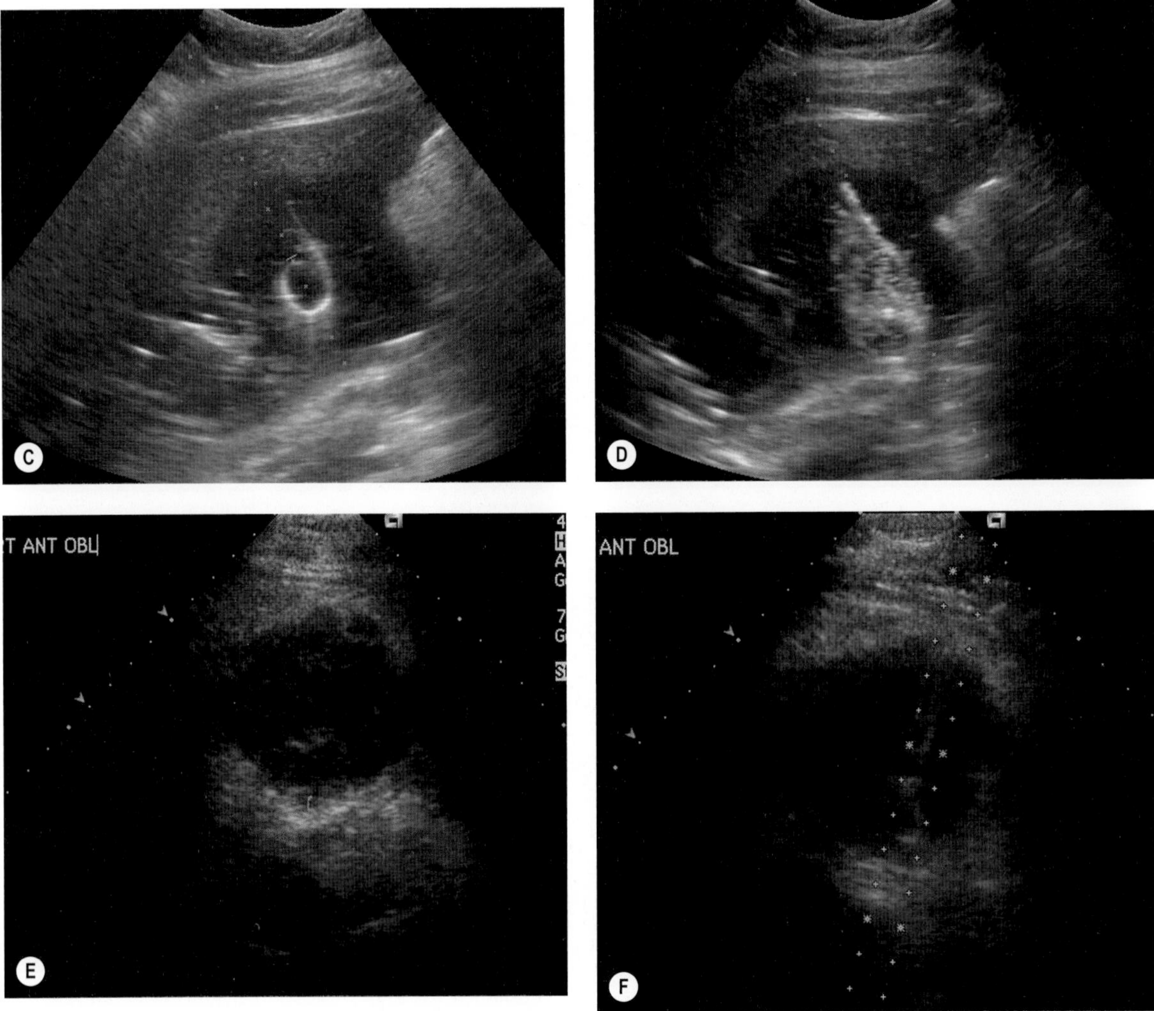

Fig. 11.12, cont'd • (C) Guidewire has been withdrawn and an 8Fr pigtail catheter is seen within the collection. (D) A small amount of saline is injected via the catheter to confirm position within the collection. A renal abscess (E) undergoing ultrasound-guided drainage (F).

Gallbladder drainage

Gallbladder drainage under ultrasound control is a temporary, palliative procedure which tends to be reserved for particularly ill patients with septicaemia, as a method of stabilizing their condition prior to surgery. Drainage of, for example, a gallbladder empyema, buys useful time – reducing the risk of perforation and subsequent peritonitis and improving clinical status prior to surgical removal. Although the portable nature of ultrasound allows a bedside procedure to be performed, particularly useful in patients under intensive therapy who cannot be moved, these procedures carry a high risk to the patient and full anaesthesia, nursing and medical support is required (see Chapter 3, Fig. 3.31).

Nephrostomy

Renal obstruction in which the pelvicalyceal system is dilated may be alleviated by the percutaneous introduction of a nephrostomy tube under ultrasound guidance. This procedure relieves pressure in the renal collecting system and avoids potential,

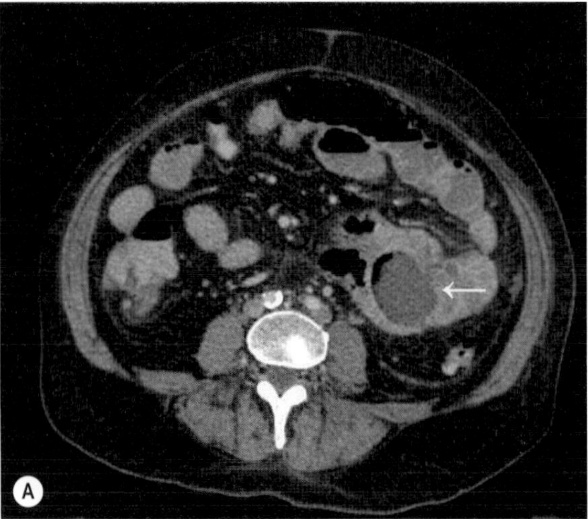

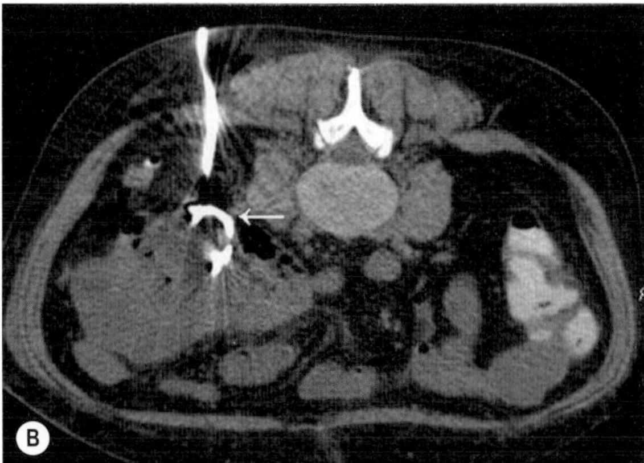

Fig. 11.13 • (A) CT scan through the lower abdomen and upper pelvis. This shows an abscess cavity (arrows) which has tracked superiorly almost certainly from a perforated diverticulum more inferiorly.
(B) This would almost certainly not be drainable with ultrasound. The surrounding small bowel loops means that a posterior approach is required and so CT is the modality of choice. The abscess cavity was accessed with an 18G needle and an 8Fr drain (arrow) left in situ.

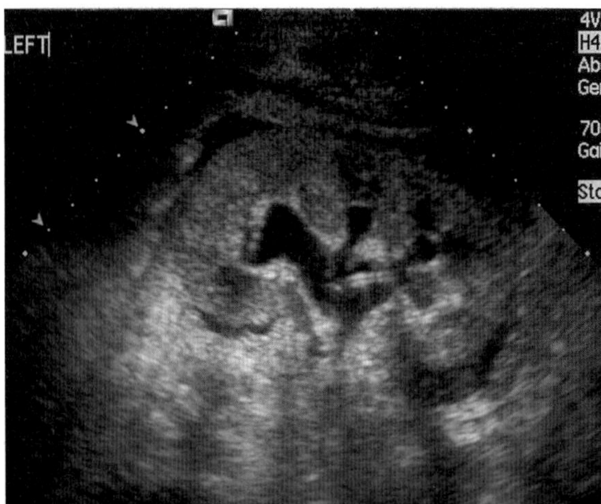

Fig. 11.14 • Longitudinal ultrasound scan of the left kidney immediately following nephrostomy. A small rim of fluid, probably urinoma, surrounds the previously obstructed kidney.

irreversible damage to the renal parenchyma (Fig. 11.14). Although the procedure may be carried out completely under ultrasound control it is more normal for the procedure to be performed in a screening room where both a combination of ultrasound and X-ray screening can be used to maximal effect.

Cyst drainage

The percutaneous treatment of renal and hepatic cysts, by simple aspiration may afford only temporary relief as they frequently recur, but a more permanent result may be achieved by injecting a sclerosant, for example, absolute alcohol, tetracycline, into the cyst. In addition, percutaneous treatment of hydatid liver disease, (traditionally avoided because of the risk of spreading parasites along the needle track and causing further infection) has been successfully performed by the injection of a scolicidal agent,[11] avoiding the need for surgical removal.

Other applications include the drainage of pancreatic pseudocysts with the insertion of a cystogastrostomy tube with combined fluoroscopy and ultrasound guidance, through which the cyst is allowed to drain into the stomach. This is usually performed endoscopically.[12]

INDIRECT ULTRASOUND GUIDANCE

Not infrequently drainage of fluid, for example from the pleural cavity, may be performed away from the ultrasound department in the ward or clinic. Ideally this is done under guidance with a portable scanner, to minimize complications.

Iatrogenic splenic trauma has been known due to the 'blind' insertion of a drain in the case of left pleural effusion. Guidance from the British Thoracic Society[13] and the National Patient Safety Agency[14] to perform such procedures under ultrasound guidance, following proper training, has reduced such incidents.

INTRAOPERATIVE ULTRASOUND

IOUS is a vital component of many surgical procedures, providing an immediate, real-time impact on surgical procedures and the diagnosis and treatment of lesions. Its applications are varied and its dynamic nature, mobility and high resolution make it ideal for surgical work.

Hepatic IOUS

A frequent application in the abdomen is in the diagnosis of liver metastases prior to surgical resection. Resection of metastases, particularly from colorectal carcinoma, is a potential cure. However results are unsuccessful if small lesions, undetected pre-operatively, are not removed at operation. Despite improvements in pre-operative imaging, IOUS can still provide additional useful information in up to 47% of patients undergoing resection for metastatic disease.[15]

The direct contact of the IOUS probe with the liver surface, avoiding attenuative subcutaneous tissue, enables a high frequency (7.5–10 MHz) probe to be used, and various probe designs are available to suit the different clinical scenarios.[16] IOUS can demonstrate lesions too small to be detected on pre-operative imaging, and as a result can change operative management[17,18] in terms of altering the resection line to include more tissue, remove additional hepatic segments or to abandon the operative procedure altogether in unsuspected widespread disease.

A combination of surgical palpation, which detects small surface lesions, and IOUS, which detects small, deep lesions, has the highest diagnostic accuracy. IOUS is quick to perform in the hands of an experienced operator and its contribution to the success of surgery is invaluable (Fig. 11.15).[19]

IOUS is particularly useful when there has been a delay between pre-operative imaging (usually MRI) and surgery, as progression of disease may have occurred during this interval, or when pre-operative imaging is equivocal, (for example differentiating tiny cystic from solid lesions). IOUS is often able to offer a definitive diagnosis and when doubt still exists guided biopsy under ultrasound control may be performed. In addition to lesion detection it is able to demonstrate vascular invasion by tumour and to clearly demonstrate, in real time, the relationship of the tumour to adjacent vascular structures – essential for planning a resection line. The greater the margin of normal tissue around the resected tumour, the better the long-term prognosis.

IOUS is also used to locate deep lesions for ultrasound-guided biopsy or ablation, and in hepatic transplantation when confirmation of vessel patency may be required (Fig. 11.15E).

Other applications of IOUS

IOUS is used in many surgical procedures, including urological, vascular and gastrointestinal tract scanning. Ultrasound evaluation of the common duct for calculi following cholecystectomy can identify small fragments which may not be easily palpable through the duct wall. Using this technique the duct is less susceptible to injury which may be associated with direct examination or the introduction of X-ray contrast agents. Pancreatic scanning is particularly useful in identifying small tumours of the body and tail of pancreas for curative resection[20] and in differentiating small pancreatic retention cysts from solid nodules.[21]

The treatment of tumours by percutaneous ultrasound-guided techniques, rather than surgical resection, is becoming more common. However, it may not always be possible to achieve success percutaneously and techniques have been developed to ablate tumours during open surgery. Radiofrequency, microwave ablation and cryotherapy are techniques that have had considerable success in the treatment of liver lesions including both metastases and HCC (Fig. 11.16).[22–24]

The success of such techniques depends to a large extent on patient selection. Those with very large and/or multiple lesions tend to have a poor prognosis compared with patients with smaller, well-confined disease. However, these techniques continue to develop and are likely to offer hope to

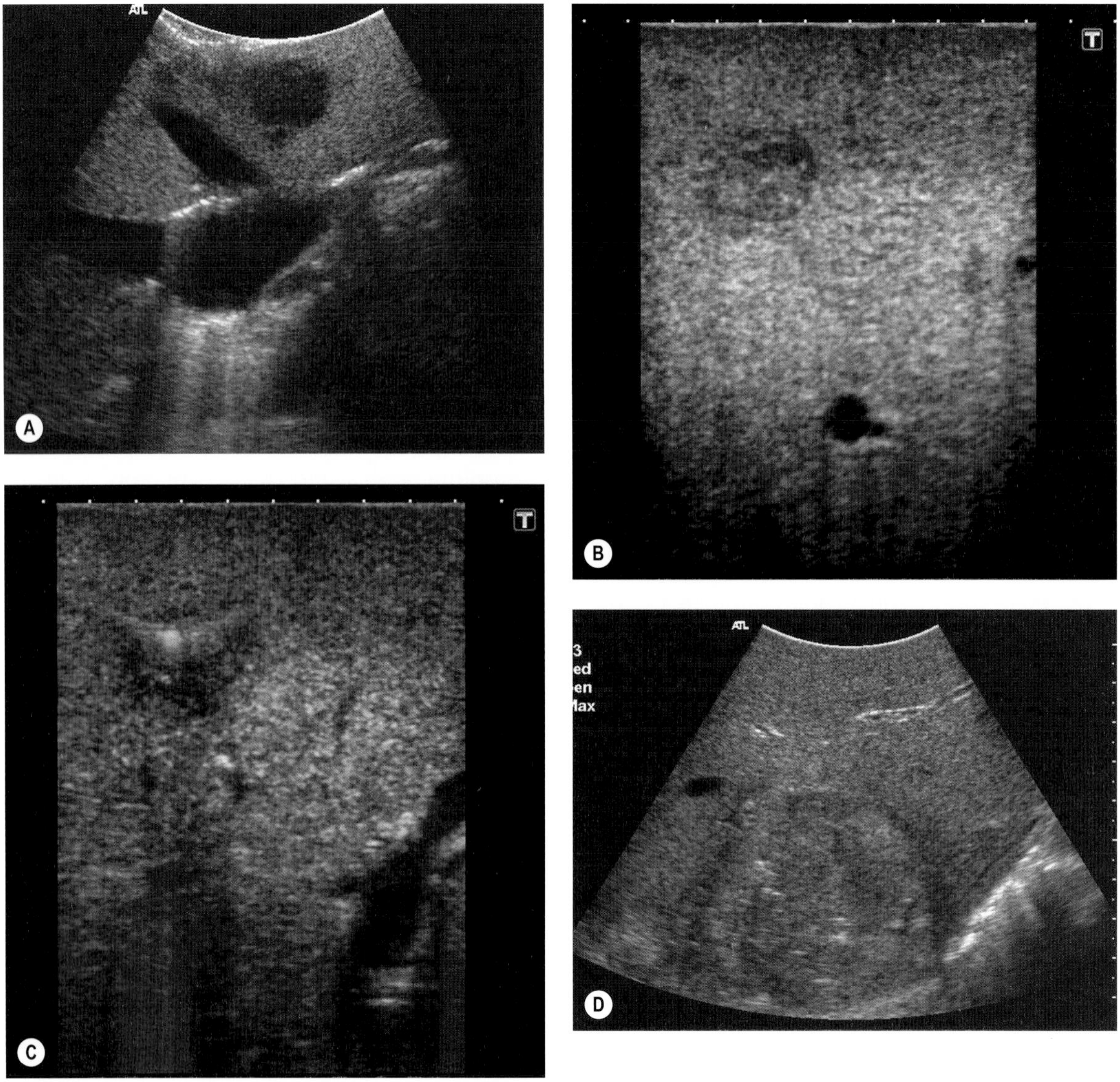

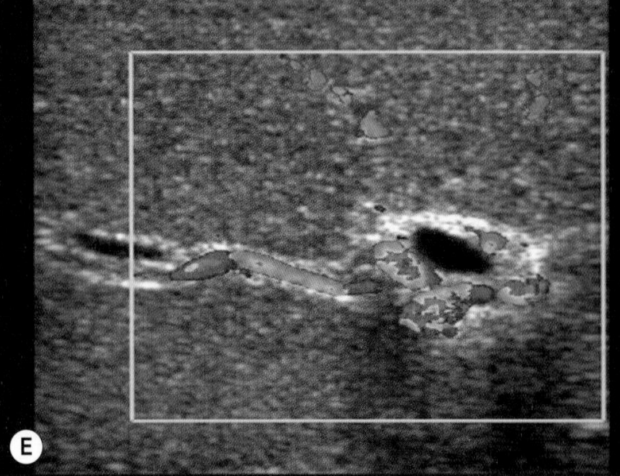

Fig. 11.15 • Intraoperative ultrasound. (A) A metastasis lies close to the hepatic vein, leaving a small but sufficient margin prior to resection. (B) A small extra metastasis, not seen pre-operatively, is located during liver resection. (C) This metastasis is ablated intraoperatively under ultrasound guidance. The tip of the probe can be seen in the lesion. (D) A large metastasis is demonstrated prior to resection. (E) Doppler is useful in confirming vessel patency in a transplant prior to skin closure.

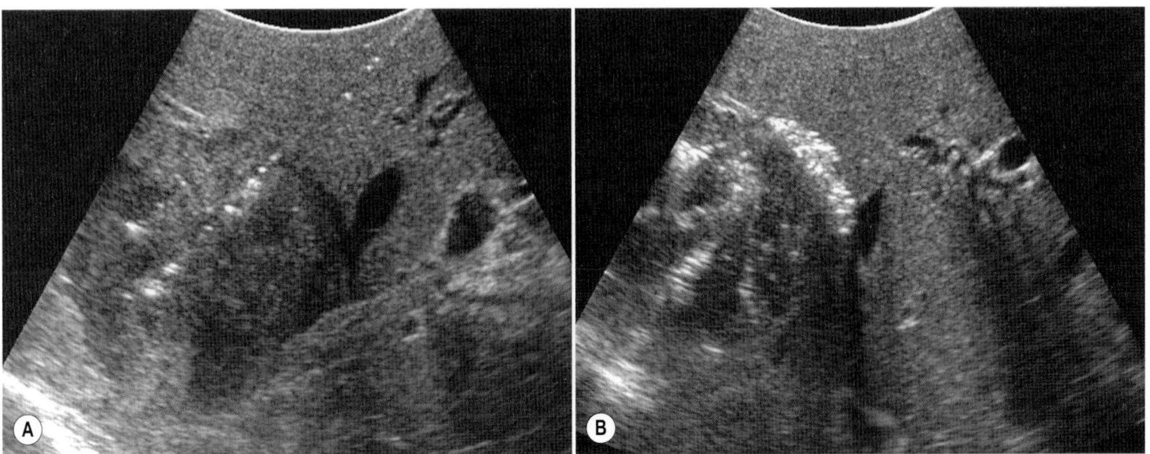

Fig. 11.16 • Radiofrequency ablation. (A) The RF probe is introduced into the metastasis under IOUS guidance. (B) The lesion is gradually ablated: the area of ablated tissue gives off tiny bubbles, enhancing the acoustic reflection.

many patients currently untreatable with conventional methods.

LAPAROSCOPIC ULTRASOUND

A laparoscopic approach, in contrast to open surgery, reduces patient morbidity, with reduced blood loss and lower complication rates.[25] The disadvantage for the surgeon of reduced field of view, and of not being able to palpate the organ, can be mitigated to a large extent by the use of laparoscopic ultrasound. Dedicated laparoscopic ultrasound probes may be passed through the laparoscopic port during surgical procedures to investigate the liver, biliary tree, pancreas and other viscera without the need for open surgery (Fig. 11.17).

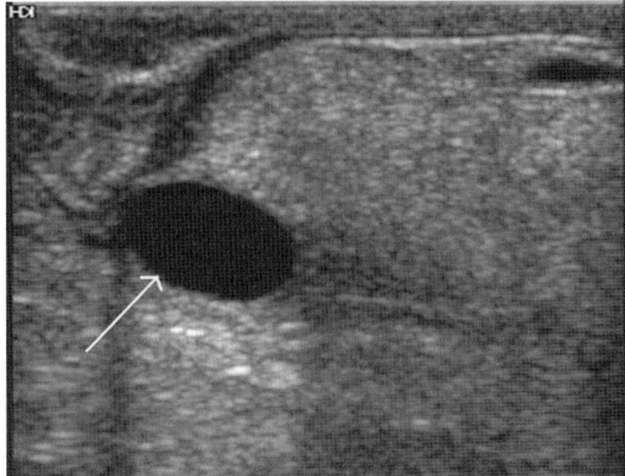

Fig. 11.17 • Laparoscopic ultrasound demonstrating the normal CBD (arrow) in the head of pancreas.

The trend towards laparoscopic, rather than open cholecystectomy has increased the need for accurate laparoscopic exploration of the biliary ductal system to confirm the presence or absence of stones. Laparoscopic ultrasound is better at demonstrating stones in the duct and anatomical ductal variations than conventional intraoperative cholangiography,[26] has the added advantage of lack of radiation and also reduces the rate of injury to the duct when compared with conventional techniques.[27]

Laparoscopic ultrasound has also proven advantageous in staging patients with hepatic tumours for liver resection,[28] demonstrating deep tumours not visible on surgical laparoscopy, or by pre-operative imaging methods, and so avoiding the need to proceed to open hepatic resection in some patients. Patients with pancreatic head and ampullary carcinomas are potentially resectable in only a minority of cases. Pre-operative imaging is known to underestimate the extent of the disease, and so many patients traditionally undergo a staging laparotomy before resection is attempted. However, over a third of patients previously considered resectable will demonstrate occult metastases –

often in the peritoneum. Staging laparoscopy does not demonstrate intrahepatic metastases, and the use of laparoscopic ultrasound at this stage greatly increases the accuracy of staging and influences the surgical decision.[29]

Laparoscopic ultrasound is also useful in staging patients with gastric cancer[30] and colorectal cancer.[31] Curative resection of bowel cancer can be performed either with open surgery or laparoscopic resection. Laparoscopic ultrasound can be used to examine the liver to confirm the absence of metastases – particularly useful in a laparoscopic resection as the surgeon is unable to palpate the liver under these circumstances.

The treatment of primary and secondary hepatic tumours by percutaneous methods

In patients with colorectal carcinoma the presence of liver metastasis is the most accurate predictor of survival. Resection of liver metastases is known to increase the lifespan of patients, with good quality of life and an overall 5-year survival of 20–45%, and up to 60% in unifocal disease. Without surgery the 5-year survival in this patient group is effectively zero. However, not all patients with liver metastases are deemed suitable for resection, being poor surgical risks or having lesions which are either too large or affect too many hepatic segments. Percutaneous ablation of liver tumours is a viable option for control of liver metastases, prolonging survival time after initial diagnosis and, in some cases, shrinking tumours to enable future curative resection. Various methods have been investigated, using ultrasound guidance.

Alcohol injection has proved effective for HCC,[32,33] shrinking tumours over a period of time and causing necrosis within them, but can be painful and requires repeat attendances. (It is not effective for metastatic liver disease. This is thought to reflect the fact that HCC is a 'soft' tumour and so the alcohol can be instilled effectively into the tumour whereas metastasis are 'hard' lesions and often the alcohol seeps out of the lesion.)

Radiofrequency (RF) thermal ablation, microwave coagulation and laser ablation are minimally invasive percutaneous therapeutic techniques. Ablation of liver metastases using RF is a method of ultrasound-guided therapy for liver metastases and hepatocellular carcinoma in which RF, applied to monopolar electrodes either individually or with multiprobe arrays, is guided into the lesion to be treated. RF tissue ablation through an 18G needle uses fewer probes than laser. It is an outpatient procedure consisting of one to four sessions and has been reported to achieve complete necrosis of liver metastases in 67% of lesions.[34] It is a simple, safe and potentially effective treatment for liver metastases, associated with a low rate of complications (in one study only one small area of haemorrhage was observed in 75 sessions)[35] together with a significant rate of shrinking or stabilization of the metastases.

Such minimally invasive treatments are not regarded as curative, but can successfully debulk the burden of tumour in the liver, extending survival time and impeding the progress of disease until further treatment can be given. In some cirrhotic patients with HCC, the only viable curative option is transplantation, for which the patient may be too ill. Ablation of existing tumours effectively maintains their position on the transplant waiting list, ensuring a more favourable prognosis when surgery finally takes place.

Ablation is also used in patients with renal tumours, in particular those with multiple lesions in whom nephrectomy is not an option.

HIGH INTENSITY FOCUSED ULTRASOUND

High intensity focused ultrasound uses high intensity sound, directed accurately at a lesion, to destroy the tissue. The focussed beam produces heat which causes coagulation necrosis. Currently there are several ongoing trials for various types of cancer, including hepatic, renal and pancreatic, but its efficacy is yet to be firmly established and it is not yet in general use. This percutaneous technique is able to focus very accurately on a lesion without needle puncture. Its sphere of effective tissue destruction can be carefully controlled, and results are promising, particularly for tumours which are difficult to treat by other means.[36]

ENDOSCOPIC ULTRASOUND

Some of the limitations of conventional ultrasonography in biliary and pancreatic imaging can be overcome by the use of endoscopic probes and miniprobes.

Endoscopic probes are either radial or linear arrays which are incorporated into the end of an endoscope. They have a frequency of 7.5–12 MHz and are used to image the pancreas, biliary tract, portal vein and adjacent structures within 5–6 cm of the probe. Radial probes may be used in the pre-operative staging of a number of diseases including oesophageal, gastric, pancreatic and lung cancer, while linear array probes are used for interventional procedures, commonly fine needle aspiration analysis of mediastinal lymph nodes, solid organ assessment, for example pancreas, occasionally liver, adrenals, pseudocyst drainage and coeliac plexus neurolysis.

Endoscopic ultrasound is more sensitive and specific than spiral CT, MRI or transabdominal ultrasound in the detection of small pancreatic masses, and its diagnostic ability can be further enhanced by the use of endoscopic ultrasonically guided fine needle aspiration cytology[37] and biopsy. It may also detect early changes of pancreatitis that are not visible on ERCP, and one of its main uses is in staging pancreatic tumours – predicting their respectability, identifying small lymph node metastases and assessing vascular invasion.[38] It is particularly accurate in identifying small pancreatic insulinomas,[39] often difficult or impossible to identify on conventional cross-sectional imaging despite a documented biochemical abnormality, and thus guiding subsequent surgical procedures. Endoscopic ultrasound is also used in the detection of biliary calculi – particularly in the normal-calibre CBD – with a much higher accuracy than other imaging techniques, and without the potential additional risks of ERCP.[40] Other less-established uses of endoscopic ultrasound include gastrointestinal examinations, in which invasion of gastric lesions into and through the wall of the stomach can be assessed,[41] anal ultrasound, which is used to visualize the sphincter muscles in cases of sphincter dysfunction, the staging of colorectal carcinomas and the demonstration of bowel wall changes in inflammatory bowel conditions.[42]

The miniprobe has a higher frequency – 20–30 MHz – and may be passed down a conventional endoscope. It therefore has the advantage of a one-stage gastrointestinal tract endoscopy/ ERCP, rather than requiring a separate procedure. It may be inserted into the common duct of the biliary tree to assess local tumour invasion and to clarify the extent and/or nature of small lesions already identified by other imaging methods. It shows remarkable accuracy in the detection of CBD tumours and other biliary tract disease when compared with other imaging modalities.[43] It may be used in the staging of oesophageal and gastric cancer, and is especially useful when a tight oesophageal stricture prevents the passage of the endoscope itself.[42] The layers of the oesophageal or gastric wall, and the extent of tumour invasion, can be accurately assessed.

The miniprobe is also used in patients with suspected pancreatic carcinoma, e.g. in patients with a negative CT but who have irregularity of the pancreatic duct on contrast examination. The probe can be passed into the pancreatic duct during ERCP to detect small lesions, assess the extent of the tumour and predict resectibility.[44] It is superior to conventional endoscopic ultrasound in the detection of the smaller, branch tumour nodules, and can also detect local retroperitoneal or vascular invasion in areas adjacent to the probe.

The use of endoscopic ultrasound is limited to specialist centres. A steep learning curve together with the expense of the equipment, is likely to restrict its widespread use, however, as its applications expand and its value becomes proven, it is likely to become a more routine investigation at many centres.[42]

ULTRASOUND CONTRAST AGENTS IN THE ABDOMEN

CEUS cannot be considered an 'invasive' procedure, but a general overview is included here for convenience. See the relevant chapters for specific CEUS applications and appearances.

History

Ultrasound contrast media have been well-established for cardiac imaging since the 1980s. The first clinical use of such an agent was in 1968 and involved the injection of saline to identify echoes from the mitral valve.[45] These early contrast agents were composed of relatively large (by today's standards) microbubbles of air in solution. They were unstable, short-lived and the bubbles were too large to pass through the capillary beds – hence their use exclusively for cardiac ultrasound.

Since those early years there have been a number of developments in the field of contrast ultrasound. Agents such as Albunex (Molecular Biosystems, San Diego, USA) consisting of albumin-coated microbubbles, were small enough to pass through the pulmonary capillaries and enter the left side of the heart, however, they were too weak to withstand systolic pressure and could not therefore enter the blood pool in any appreciable quantity. A more stable suspension was then produced consisting of small microbubbles – in the order of 2–5 µm – which passed through the pulmonary capillary bed after intravenous injection, and acted as a true blood pool agent. This was called Levovist (Schering, Berlin, Germany) and is a galactose-based agent (99.9%) containing palmitic acid (0.1%) for stability, which traps air which is subsequently released when the bubbles burst. As the first stable blood pool agent it could be used for examining the abdominal viscera and vasculature.

By coincidence, microbubbles of this size, can pass through the pulmonary capillaries and resonate at frequencies used in clinical diagnostic ultrasound (1–20 MHz). This resonance causes a much greater capacity for scattering the beam than that from a non-resonating particle and thus a stronger signal is produced of up to 25 dB on both grey-scale and Doppler. The Doppler signal from a 'contrast enhanced' blood vessel is greatly increased, and early agents were actually designed to identify blood flow in vessels where the Doppler signal was difficult to detect – the so-called 'Doppler Rescue'. Nowadays, Doppler equipment is much more sensitive, and this particular role for contrast is reserved for a minority of difficult cases (Fig. 11.18).

Vessels too small to be identified on normal grey-scale or non-enhanced Doppler scans can be identified when using a microbubble agent (Fig. 11.18) and harmonic software aids and improves visualization of microvasculature. When insonated with ultrasound of a certain frequency, microbubbles emit a secondary harmonic frequency twice

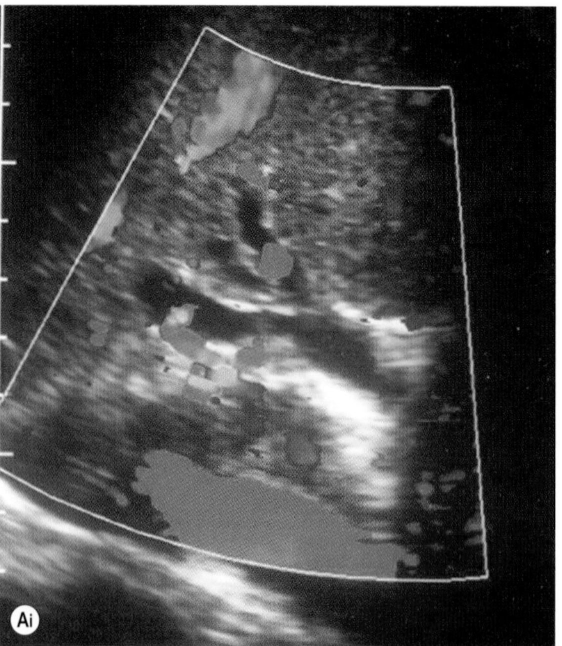

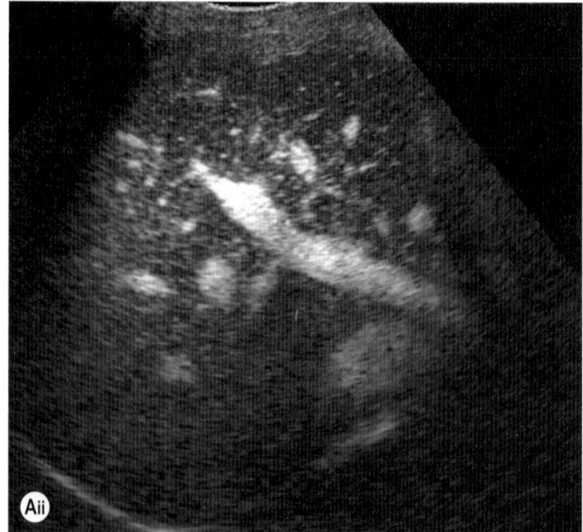

Fig. 11.18 • CEUS for vascular patency: (Ai) Pre-injection of contrast, no flow could be demonstrated in the PV. (Technical limitations prevented the vessel being imaged at a more suitable angle to the probe). (Aii) Post-injection, contrast is seen, confirming vessel patency.

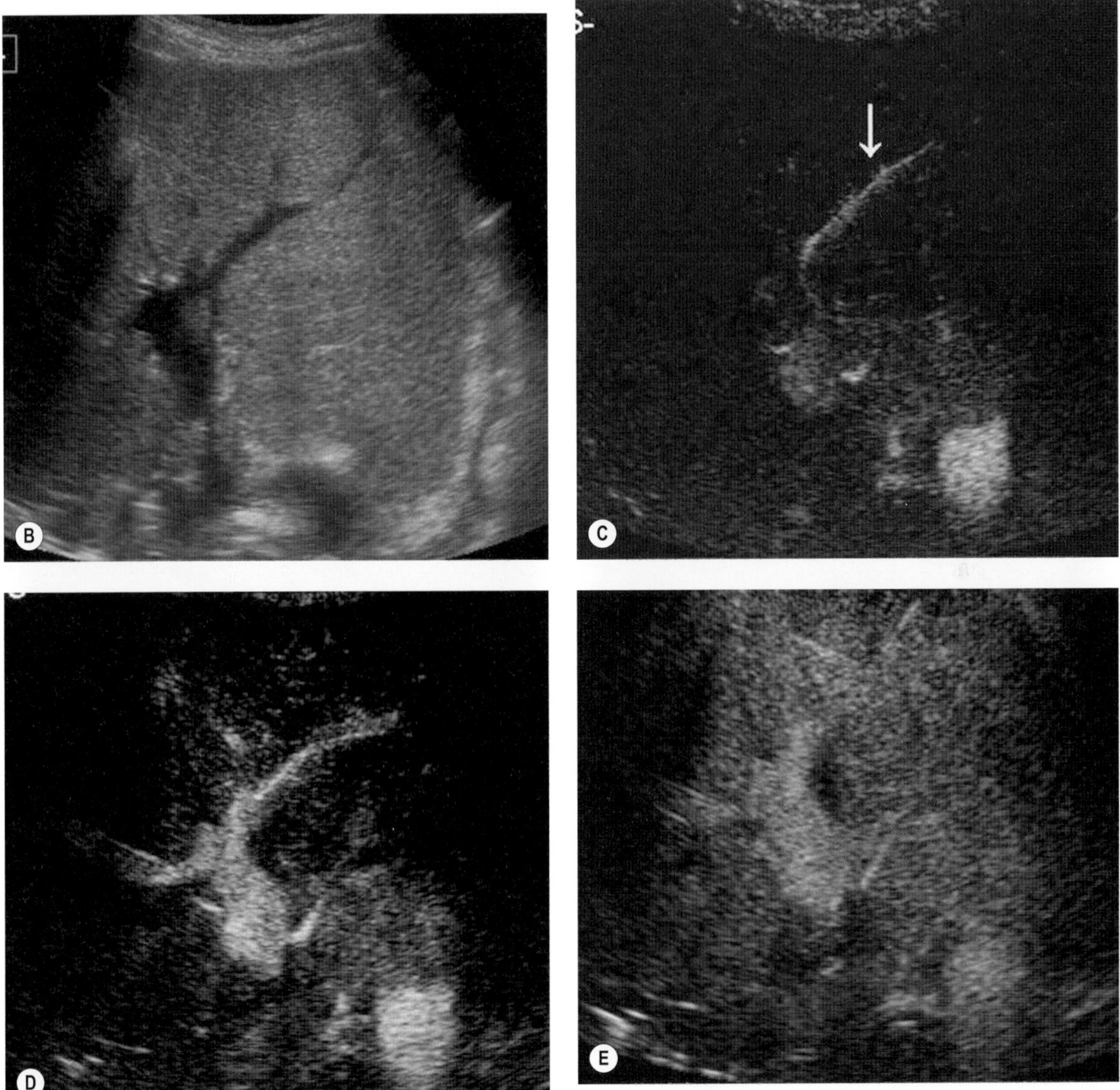

Fig. 11.18, cont'd • (B) No arterial flow could be demonstrated with Doppler in this split graft liver transplant. (C) Contrast demonstrates a narrow but patent artery (arrow). (D) The portal vein starts to enhance a few seconds later, and (E) The liver take up of contrast in the sinusoidal phase is normal, obviating the need for angiography.

that of the incident wave, in addition to the primary harmonic. As the second peak is a purer signal this increases the sensitivity, enabling smaller vessels with slow flow to be successfully detected and distinguished from surrounding tissues. Many harmonic based pulse methods are used with contrast agents and some of the more popular ones include pulse and phase inversion, e.g. pulse inversion is a dual pulse technique, 180° out of phase, resulting in summation of signal from non-linear scatterers, i.e. microbubbles, and cancellation of signal from linear scatterers, i.e. tissue.

Technique

The beauty of CEUS is that it can be done at the time of scanning, to augment the diagnostic information. Administration is by IV cannula – usually not smaller than 20G, otherwise the pressure of injection triggers some bubble burst and reduces the effectiveness of the examination.

A machine with pulsed inversion harmonics software is necessary to evaluate the microvasculature throughout the vascular phases. Some machines have the ability to use a side-by-side display of the fundamental and contrast images. This is particularly useful when the lesion is tiny and easy to 'lose' during scanning. A cine facility is advisable, so that the cycle of contrast take up can be comprehensively recorded and evaluated later. A low MI must be used to avoid bubble burst.

Each agent has recommendations for administration, and contraindications, which should be observed. Sonovue (Bracco, Italy), the most frequently used abdominal agent in the UK, has a

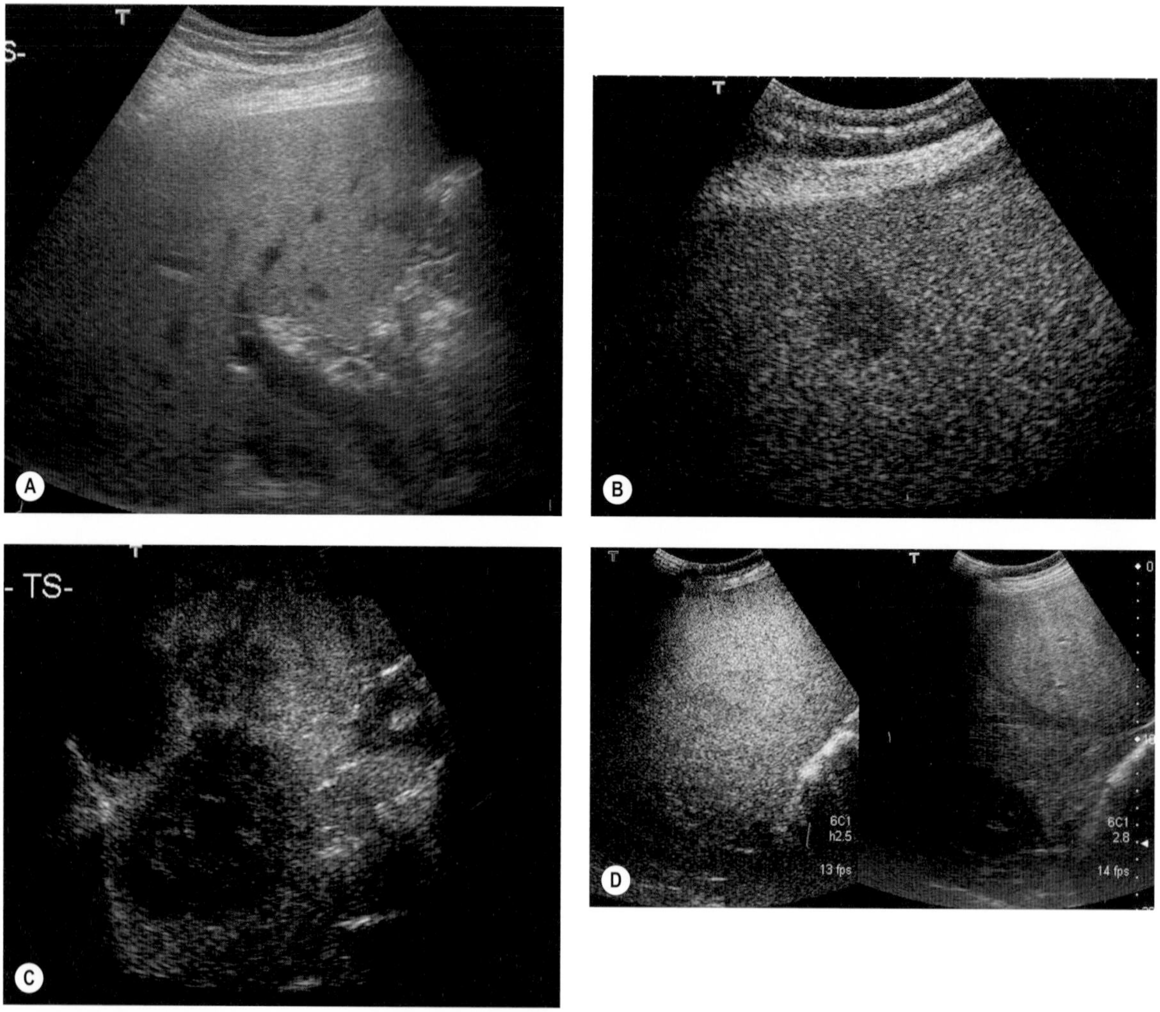

Fig. 11.19 • CEUS for metastases: (A) Conventional ultrasound of the liver showing no abnormality. (B) The same case as (A), demonstrates a metastasis as a hypoenhancing lesion in the sinusoidal phase. (C) Multiple metastases are seen as 'defects' in the sinusoidal phase of contrast take up. (D) A patient with a history of previous carcinoma and abnormal LFTs has normal contrast take up in the sinusoidal phase (left-hand image) confirming no metastases.

relatively good safety profile and patient acceptance level, and is non-nephrotoxic, giving it an advantage over some other radiological contrast agents.

The range of potential applications for CEUS is considerable, and its benefits for the patient are now well established.[46,47]

CLINICAL APPLICATIONS OF CEUS

Vascular patency

In cases where Doppler information is sub-optimal, CEUS enhances the signal from the blood pool and increases diagnostic confidence. This may obviate the need for other, more invasive angiographic investigations.[48] It can be useful in patients with chronic liver disease for the investigation of venous thrombosis[49] and in confirming the vascular patency and perfusion of transplanted organs, such as the hepatic artery.

Lesion characterization

The characterization of hepatic masses is also improved with contrast agents as these agents are preferentially taken up by the hepatosplenic parenchyma enabling evaluation of the characteristic vasculature of lesions through the arterial, portal and sinusoidal phases (see Chapter 4). There is growing evidence to support the differentiation of lesions within the liver, not previously possible with conventional ultrasound[50,51] and certainly microbubble agents are helpful in the diagnosis of capillary haemangiomas, hepatomas and FNH.

Lesion detection

While the usual limitations to ultrasound lesion detection apply (for example poor acoustic access due to body habitus or bowel gas), there is good evidence to support the use of CEUS in the detection of focal liver disease.[52] Ultrasound contrast remains in the intravascular space (unlike CT and MRI agents, which clear from the blood pool into the extracellular space). In the liver, the bubbles resonate during the late (or sinusoidal phase) to produce a greatly enhanced, 'bright' signal. This produces a greatly increased contrast resolution between normal liver and the 'filling defects' of the metastases, which do not take up the contrast in the sinusoidal phase, enabling the operator to demonstrate small, often subcentimetre lesions with confidence (Fig. 11.19).

CEUS is proven to be useful in many clinical scenarios,[46] including characterization of liver lesions, detection of metastases, vascular patency, leaking aortic grafts, blunt trauma, characterization and follow-up of renal lesions, follow-up of oncology patients, guidance for percutaneous ablation and the follow-up of ablated lesions to detect tumour recurrence. This will assume elevated importance in patient management as the medical community recognizes and strives to reduce the adverse effects of cumulative diagnostic radiation.[53]

References

1. Ishii C, Yamada T, Irie T et al. Clinical evaluation of renal biopsy using automated biopsy gun under ultrasonography. J Clin Radiol 1996; 41: 233–236
2. Reading CC, Charboneau JW, James EM, Hurt MR. Sonographically guided percutaneous biopsy of small (3 cm or less) masses. AJR Am J Roentgenol 1988; 151: 189–192
3. Wilczek HE. Percutaneous needle biopsy of the renal allograft. Transplant 1990; 50: 790–797
4. Fornari F, Civardi G, Cavanna L et al. Complications of ultrasonically guided fine needle abdominal biopsy: results of a multi center Italian study and review of the literature. Scand J Gastroenterol 1989; 24: 949–955
5. Martino CR, Haaga JR, Bryan PJ et al. CT guided liver biopsies: eight years experience. Work in progress. Radiology 1984; 152: 755–757
6. Nolsoe C, Nielsen L, Torp-Pedersen S et al. Major complications and deaths due to interventional ultrasonography: a review of 8000 cases. J Clin Ultrasound 1990; 18: 179–184
7. Smith EH. Complications of percutaneous abdominal fine needle biopsy. Radiology 1991; 178: 253–258
8. Di Stasi M, Buscarini L, Bolondi L et al. Ultrasound-guided fine-needle liver biopsy: a multi-centre survey of pre-procedure evaluation practices and complication rates. J Intervent Radiol 1995; 10: 43–48
9. Livraghi T, Lazzaroni S, Civelli L et al. Risk conditions and mortality rate of abdominal fine needle biopsy. J Intervent Radiol 1997; 12: 57–64
10. Ryd W, Hagmar B, Eriksson O. Local tumour cell seeding by fine needle aspiration biopsy. Acta Pathol Microbiol Immunol Scand 1983; 91: 17–21
11. Salama H, Abdel-Wahab MF, Strickland GT. Diagnosis and treatment of hepatic Hydatid cysts with the aid of echo-gioded percutaneous cyst puncture. Clin Infect Dis 1995; 21: 1372–1376
12. Yong AA, Roberts SA. Interventional endoscopic ultrasound. Clin Radiol 2003; 58: 32–43

13. Laws D, Neville E, Duffy J. BTS guidelines for the insertion of a chest drain. British Thoracic Society. Thorax 2003; 58 Suppl ii: 53–59
14. National Patient Safety Agency. Rapid Response Report NPSA/2008/RRR003. Risks of chest drain insertion. National Patient Safety Agency, London, 2008.
15. Conlon R, Jacobs M, Dasgupta D, Lodge JPA. The value of intraoperative ultrasound during hepatic resection compared with improved preoperative magnetic resonance imaging. Eur J Ultrasound 2003; 16: 211–216
16. Kennish S, Smith J. Intraoperative ultrasound. In: Meire H, Cosgrove D, Dewbury K, Farrant P, eds. Clinical ultrasound, 3rd edn. Churchill Livingstone, Edinburgh, in press
17. Solomon MJ, Stephen MS, Gallinger S, White GH. Does intraoperative ultrasonography change surgical decision making during liver resection? Am J Surg 1994; 168: 307–310
18. Fortunato L, Claor M, Hoffman J et al. Is CT portography (CTAP) really useful in patients with liver tumours who undergo intraoperative ultrasonography (IOUS)? Am Surg 1995; 61: 560–565
19. Bates JA, Conlon RM. Intraoperative ultrasound in hepatic resection. In: Paterson A, Price R, eds. Current topics in radiography. Saunders, Edinburgh, 1995
20. Correnti S, Liverani A, Antoni G et al. Intraoperative ultrasonography for pancreatic insulinomas. Hepato-Gastroenterol 1996; 43: 207–211
21. Kubota K, Noie T, Sano K et al. Impact of intraoperative ultrasonography on surgery for cystic lesions of the pancreas. World J of Surg 1997; 21: 2–77
22. Morris DL, Ross WB. Australian experience of cryoablation of liver tumours: metastases. Surg Oncol Clin North Am 1996; 5: 391–397
23. Sato M, Watanabe Y, Ueda S et al. Microwave coagulation therapy for hepatocellular carcinoma. Gastroenterology 1996; 110: 1507–1514
24. Ogawa M, Shibata T, Takami M et al. Long-term survival in two cases of multiple liver metastases successfully treated with intraoperative ultrasound-guided microwave tumour coagulation (MTC.) Jpn J Cancer Chemother 1995; 22: 1679–1683
25. Buell JF, Thomas MT, Rudich S et al. Experience with more than 500 minimally invasive hepatic procedures. Ann Surg 2008; 248: 475–486
26. Rothlin MA, Schob O, Schlumpf R, Largiader F. Laparoscopic ultrasonography during cholecystectomy. Br J Surg 1996; 83: 1512–1516
27. Machi J, Johnson JO, Deziel DJ et al. The routine use of laparoscopic ultrasound decreases bile duct injury: a multicenter study. Surg Endosc 2009; 23: 384–388
28. John TG, Greig JD, Crosbie JL et al. Superior staging of liver tumours with laparoscopy and laparoscopic ultrasound. Ann Surg 1995; 220: 711–719
29. John TG, Greig JD, Carter DC, Garden OJ. Carcinoma of the pancreatic head and periampullary region: tumour staging with laparoscopy and laparoscopic ultrasonography. Ann Surg 1995; 221: 156–164
30. Conlon KC, Karpeh Jr MS. Laparoscopy and laparoscopic ultrasound in the staging of gastric cancer. Semin Oncol 1996; 23: 347–351
31. Marchesa P, Milsom JW, Hale JC et al. Intraoperative laparoscopic liver ultrasonography for staging of colorectal cancer: an initial experience. Dis Colon Rectum 1996; 39 Suppl: S73–S78
32. Livraghi T, Giorgio A, Marin G et al. Hepatocellular carcinoma and cirrhosis in 746 patients: long-term results of percutaneous ethanol injection. Radiology 1995; 197: 101–108
33. Ohnishi K, Ohyama N, Ito S, Fujiwara K. Small hepatocellular carcinoma: treatment with US-guided intratumoral injection of acetic acid. Radiology 1994; 193: 747–752
34. Rossi S, Di Stasi M, Buscarini E et al. Percutaneous RF interstitial thermal ablation in the treatment of hepatic cancer. AJR Am J Roentgenol 1996; 167: 673–759
35. Solbiati L, Ierace T, Goldberg SN et al. Percutaneous US-guided radio-frequency tissue ablation of liver metastases. Treatment and follow-up in 16 patients. Radiology 1997; 202: 195–203
36. Dubinsky TJ, Cuevas C, Dighe MK et al. High-intensity focused ultrasound: current potential and oncologic applications. AJR Am J Roentgenol 2008; 190: 191–199
37. Cahn M, Chang K, Nguyen P. Impact of endoscopic ultrasound with fine needle aspiration on the surgical management of pancreatic cancer. Am J Surg 1996: 172: 470–472
38. Tio TL, Sie LH, Kallimanis G et al. Staging of ampullary and pancreatic carcinoma: comparison between endosonography and surgery. Gastrointest Endosc 1996; 44: 706–713
39. Pitre J, Soubrane O, Palazzo L, Chapuis Y. Endoscopic ultrasonography for the preoperative localisation of insulinoma. Pancreas 1996; 13: 55–60
40. Amouyal P, Amouyal G, Levy P et al. Diagnosis of choledocholithiasis by endoscopic ultrasonography. Gastroenterology 1994; 106: 1062–1067
41. Wojtowycz AR, Spirt BA, Kaplan DS, Roy AK. Endoscopic ultrasonography of the gastrointestinal tract. Ultrasound Q 1995; 13: 139–152
42. McLean A, Fairclough P. Review: endoscopic ultrasound – current applications. Clin Radiol 1996; 51: 83–98
43. Gillams AR, Lees WR. Recent developments in biliary tract imaging. Gastrointest Endosc Clin North Am 1996; 6: 1–15
44. Taki T, Goto H, Naitoh Y et al. Diagnosis of mucin-producing tumour of the pancreas with an intraductal sonographic system. J Ultrasound Med 1997; 16: 1–6
45. Gramiak R, Shah PM. Echocardiography of the aortic root. Invest Radiol 1968; 3: 356–366
46. Claudon M, Cosgrove D, Albrecht T et al. Guidelines and good clinical practice recommendations for contrast

enhanced ultrasound (CEUS) — update 2008. Ultraschall Med 2008; 29: 28–44

47. Sidhu P. The EFSUMB guidelines for contrast-enhanced ultrasound are comprehensive and informative for good clinical practice: will radiologists take the lead? Br J Radiol 2008; 81: 524–525
48. Schlief R. Developments in echo-enhancing contrast agents. Clin Radiol 1996; 51 Suppl 1: 5–7
49. Braunschweig R, Stern W, Dabidian A et al. Contrast enhanced colour Doppler studies of liver vessels. Abstract. Echocardiography 1993; 10: 674
50. Cosgrove D. Ultrasound contrast enhancement of tumours. Clin Radiol 1996; 51 Suppl 1: 44–49
51. Leen E, Mcardle CA. Ultrasound contrast agents in liver imaging. Clin Radiol 1996; 51 Suppl 1: 35–39
52. Harvey CJ, Pilcher JM, Eckersley RJ et al. Advances in ultrasound. Clin Radiol 2002; 57: 157–177
53. Sodickson A, Baeyens PF, Andriole KP et al. Recurrent CT, cumulative radiation exposure, and associated radiation-induced cancer risks from CT of adults. Radiology 2009; 251: 175–184

Bibliography, resources and further reading

Allan P, Dubbins P, Pozniak M, McDicken N. Clinical Doppler ultrasound. Churchill Livingstone, Edinburgh, 2000

Bisset RAL, Khan AN. Differential diagnosis in abdominal ultrasound. Ballière Tindall, London, 2002

The British Medical Ultrasound Society (BMUS). Available at: www.bmus.org.

Brooke JR, Ralls PW. Sonography of the abdomen. Raven Press, New York, 1995

Carty H, Brunelle F, Shaw D, Kendall B. Imaging children. Churchill Livingstone, Edinburgh, 1994

Damjanov I. Pathology for the health-related professions. Saunders, Philadelphia, 1996

Gebel M. Ultrasound in gastroenterology and epatology. Blackwell Science, Berlin, 1999

Lees WR, Lyons EA. Invasive ultrasound. Martin Dunitz, 1996

Meire H, Cosgrove D, Dewburt K, Farrant P. Clinical ultrasound – abdominal and general ultrasound, 2nd edn. Churcill Livingstone, Edinburgh, 2001

Nightingale J, Law R. Gastrointestinal imaging. Churchill Livingstone, Edinburgh, 2010

Radiographics. www.radiographics.rsna.org

Sonoworld. www.sonoworld.com

Williams P. Gray's anatomy. Elsevier, Edinburgh, 1999

Index

Notes

As the subject of this book is ultrasound and its variants, subentries under these terms relate to the theory and techniques of these methods. All other references can be found under specific anatomical features or individual diseases/disorders.

To save space in the index, the following abbreviations have been used:

CEUS – contrast enhanced ultrasound
CT – computed tomography
MRCP – magnetic resonance cholangiopancreatography

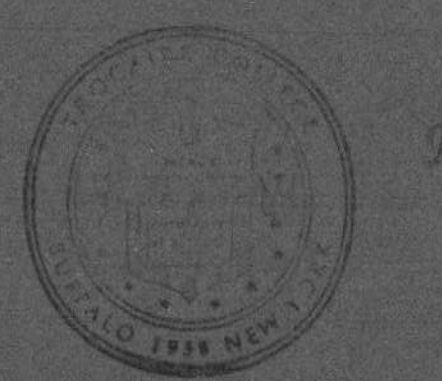